Learning and Teaching in Clinical Contexts

Learning and Teaching in Clinical Contexts

A Practical Guide

Editors

Clare Delany PhD, MHlthMedLaw, MPhysio, BAppSci (Physio)
Associate Professor, Department of Medical Education, The University of Melbourne, and Clinical Ethicist, The Royal Children's Hospital Melbourne

Elizabeth Molloy PhD, BPhysio (Hons), FANZAHPE
Professor of Work Integrated Learning, Department of Medical Education, Melbourne Medical School, The University of Melbourne

ELSEVIER

ELSEVIER

Elsevier Australia. ACN 001 002 357
(a division of Reed International Books Australia Pty Ltd) Tower 1, 475 Victoria Avenue, Chatswood, NSW 2067

International Standard Book Number: 978-0-7295-4272-2

Notice

Practitioners and researchers must always rely on their own experience and knowledge in evaluating and using any information, methods, compounds or experiments described herein. Because of rapid advances in the medical sciences, in particular, independent verification of diagnoses and drug dosages should be made. To the fullest extent of the law, no responsibility is assumed by Elsevier, authors, editors or contributors for any injury and/or damage to persons or property as a matter of products liability, negligence or otherwise, or from any use or operation of any methods, products, instructions, or ideas contained in the material herein.

Cataloging-in-Publication Data

 A catalogue record for this book is available from the National Library of Australia

---

Senior Content Strategist: Melinda McEvoy
Senior Content Development Specialists: Tamsin Curtis & Martina Vascotto
Senior Project Manager: Anitha Rajarathnam
Edited by Kate Stone
Proofread by Forsyth Publishing Services
Cover and Internal Design by Georgette Hall
Index by Innodata Indexing
Typeset by Toppan Best-set Premedia Limited
Printed in China by 1010 Printing International Ltd.

Contents

About the authors

Associate Professor Clare Delany
PhD, MHlthMedLaw, MPhysio, BAppSci (Physio)

Clare Delany is known nationally and internationally for research and practice in health professional ethics, clinical reasoning, critical reflection, resilience for clinical learning and translation of educational theory into health workplace environments. Her work has mostly centred on physiotherapy; however, she reaches beyond that profession to teach and research in health professional education and higher education more broadly. Clare is Chair of the University of Melbourne 'Education, Fine Arts, Music and Business' Human Research Ethics Committee and has served as Vice President of the Physiotherapists' Registration Board in Victoria and Chair of the Australian Physiotherapy National Professional Standards Panel. Clare is author or co-author of more than 90 publications in peer-reviewed journals and has co-edited two books: *Clinical Education in the Health Professions* and most recently *When Doctors and Parents Disagree: Ethics, Paediatrics and the Zone of Parental Discretion*. Clare's research expertise is in the area of qualitative methodology and methods and this is applied across broad subject areas of clinical ethics, clinical education and paediatric bioethics. At the Department of Medical Education, The University of Melbourne, Clare is responsible for coordination of research higher degrees and the masters year of the EXCITE (Excellence in Clinical Teaching) program. Clare is also a clinical ethicist at the Royal Children's Hospital Children's Bioethics Centre in Melbourne. This role involves conducting clinical ethics consultations, education and research in paediatric bioethics.

Professor Elizabeth Molloy
PhD, BPhysio (Hons), FANZAHPE

Elizabeth Molloy is Professor of Work Integrated Learning in the Department of Medical Education, Melbourne Medical School, The University of Melbourne. Prior to this role, she was Director of the Health Professions Education and Educational Research Centre at Monash University. She has published more than 90 peer-reviewed journal articles, book chapters and books, with a focus on workplace learning, feedback, assessment, professional transitions and clinical teacher professional development. Previous edited books include *Clinical Education in the Health Professions* and *Feedback in Higher and Professional Education*. Elizabeth's clinical background is physiotherapy and her PhD (2006) examined the culture of feedback in the health workplace. As well as teacher education (short courses and postgraduate award courses), Elizabeth is involved in designing and researching innovations to improve the preparation of undergraduate and postgraduate students to engage in workplace learning. Elizabeth is currently working on two nationally funded grants examining how feedback can be designed in the university and work-based setting. She is also a Fellow of the Australian and New Zealand Association for Health Professions Education.

Contributors

Rola Ajjawi BAppSc (Hons), PhD
Centre for Research in Assessment and Digital
Learning, Deakin University, Melbourne,
Victoria, Australia

Joanna Bates MDCM
Professor, Family Medicine, University of British
Columbia;
Scientist, Centre for Health Education
Scholarship (CHES), University of British
Columbia, Vancouver, British Columbia, Canada

Margaret Bearman BSc (Hons), PhD
Associate Professor, Centre for Research and
Assessment in Digital Learning, Deakin
University;
Adjunct Associate Professor, Monash Centre
for Scholarship in Health Education, Monash
University, Melbourne, Victoria, Australia

David Beckett BA (Hons), MA, MEd, PhD,
Cert IV, TPTC
Professor, Melbourne Graduate School of
Education, The University of Melbourne,
Melbourne, Victoria, Australia

Stephen Billett BA, DipT Teaching, MEdSt,
PhD, PhD honoris causa
Professor, Education and Professional Studies,
Griffith University, Brisbane; Visiting Research
Professor, Gold Coast Hospital and Health
Service, Southport, Queensland, Australia

David Boud BSc (Hons), PhD
Professor and Director, Centre for Research in
Assessment and Digital Learning, Deakin
University, Geelong, Victoria, Australia;
Emeritus Professor, Faculty of Arts and Social
Science, University of Technology Sydney,
Sydney, New South Wales, Australia;
Research Professor, Institute for Work-Based
Learning, Middlesex University, London, UK

Damian J. Castanelli MBBS, MClinEd, FANZCA
Consultant Anaesthetist, Department of
Anaesthesia and Perioperative Medicine,
Monash Health, Melbourne;
Adjunct Lecturer, Department of Anaesthesia
and Perioperative Medicine, Monash
University, Clayton, Victoria, Australia

Huiju Carrie Chen BA, MD, MSEd, PhD
Associate Dean of Assessment and
Educational Scholarship, Professor, Pediatrics,
Georgetown University, School of Medicine,
Washington, DC, USA

Paul Crampton BSc (Hons), MSc, PhD
Research Fellow, Monash Centre for
Scholarship in Health Education, Monash
University, Melbourne, Victoria, Australia;
Research Department of Medical Education,
University College London, London, UK

James GM Crossley MA, MBBS, MEd, MRCP,
MRCPCH, DM
Professor, The Medical School, University of
Sheffield, Sheffield, South Yorkshire, UK

Phillip Dawson BCompSc (Hons), PhD
Associate Professor, Centre for Research in
Assessment and Digital Learning, Deakin
University, Geelong, Victoria, Australia

Charlotte Denniston BPhysio (Hons)
Assistant Lecturer, Monash Centre for
Scholarship in Health Education, Monash
University, Clayton, Victoria, Australia

Rachel Helen Ellaway BSc, PhD
Professor, Community Health Sciences,
Cumming School of Medicine, University of
Calgary, Calgary, Alberta, Canada

Althea Jane Gamble Blakey BHSc, MHSc (Clin
Ed), PhD (Med Ed)
Otago Medical School, University of Otago,
Dunedin, Otago, New Zealand

Lynn Gillam BA (Hons), MA, PhD
Professor, Melbourne School of Population and
Global Health, University of Melbourne, Melbourne;
Academic Director, Children's Bioethics Centre,
Royal Children's Hospital, Parkville, Victoria,
Australia

Clinton Golding BA, DipProfEthics,
MA (Hons), PhD
Associate Professor, Higher Education
Development Centre, University of Otago,
Dunedin, Otago, New Zealand

Mark Goldszmidt MDCM, MHPE, PhD
Associate Director, Centre for Education
Research & Innovation, University of Western
Ontario, London, Ontario, Canada

Gerard J. Gormley MB BCh BAO, DMH,
DRCOG, MD, PGCMedEd, FHEA, FRCGP
Professor, Centre for Medical Education, Queen's
University Belfast, Belfast, County Antrim, UK

Suzanne Gough BSc (Hons), MA (Ed), PhD,
PGCert AP, PFHEA
Senior Lecturer, Health Professions,
Manchester Metropolitan University,
Manchester, UK

Jennene Greenhill BA, GDipNsg, MSPD, PhD
Professor, Flinders University Rural Health SA,
Flinders University, Renmark, South Australia,
Australia

Nigel Hart BSc (Hons), MB BCh BAO,
MMedSc (Ed), MD, FRCGP
Senior Lecturer, Centre for Medical Education,
Queen's University Belfast, County Antrim;
Associate Director, General Practice
Department, Northern Ireland Medical and
Dental Training Agency, Belfast, Northern
Ireland, UK

Eric S. Holmboe BSc, MD
Senior Vice President, Milestones, ACGME,
Chicago, Illinois;
Professor Adjunct, Medicine, Yale University,
New Haven, Connecticut;
Adjunct Professor, Medicine, Feinberg School
of Medicine Northwestern University, Chicago,
Illinois, USA

Carolyn Johnston LLB, LLM, MA, PhD
School of Medicine, Faculty of Health, Deakin
University, Geelong;
Senior Research Fellow, Melbourne Law
School, Melbourne, Victoria, Australia

Jennifer Johnston BCh, MB, MPhil, PhD,
MRCGP
Clinical Senior Lecturer, Centre for Medical
Education, Queen's University Belfast, Belfast,
Northern Ireland, UK

Anna Jones BA (Hons), MEd, PhD
Senior Teaching Fellow, GKT School of
Medical Education, King's College London,
London, UK

Fiona Kent BPhysio, GCEBP, MHPE, PhD
Senior Lecturer, Faculty Medicine, Nursing and
Health Sciences, Monash University,
Melbourne, Victoria, Australia

Sue Kilminster MPhil, MA, RGN, RSCN
Faculty Lead for Health, Professional Education
Research, University of Leeds, Leeds, UK

Jill Klein BA, PhD
Professorial Fellow, Department of Medical
Education, Melbourne Medical School, The
University of Melbourne;
Professor, Melbourne Business School, Carlton,
Victoria, Australia

Lorelei Lingard BA, MA, PhD
Director, Centre for Education Research and
Innovation; Professor, Department of Medicine,
Schulich School of Medicine and Dentistry;
Professor, Faculty of Education, Western
University, London, Ontario, Canada

Jason M. Lodge BPsych (Hons), MHEd,
MLS&T, PhD
Principal Research Fellow, ARC Science of
Learning Research Centre, Associate Professor
of Educational Psychology, School of
Education, The University of Queensland,
Brisbane, Queensland, Australia

Rosalind McDougall BSc, BA (Hons), BPhil, PhD
Research Fellow in Ethics, Melbourne School
of Population and Global Health, The University
of Melbourne, Melbourne, Victoria, Australia

Judy McKimm BA (Hons), MBA, MA(Ed),
SFHEA
Professor of Medical Education, School of
Medicine, Swansea University, Swansea, West
Glamorgan, UK

Samantha McLeod BSc, Grad ip (Health
Psych), MA (Gifted Ed), PhD (App Sci)
Director, Principal Psychologist, The SAM
Centre, Preston West, Victoria, Australia

Lynn Valerie Monrouxe BSc, PGDip, PhD
Director of Chang Gung Medical Education
Research Centre, CG-MERC, Chang Gung
Memorial Hospital, Linkou, Taiwan

Haavi Morreim JD, PhD
Professor, Internal Medicine, University of
Tennessee College of Medicine; Principal
Center for Conflict Resolution in Healthcare
LLC, Memphis, Tennessee, USA

Debra Nestel PhD, FAcadMEd, FSSH
Professor of Surgical Education, Department of
Surgery, University of Melbourne; Professor of
Simulation Education in Healthcare, Monash
Institute of Health and Clinical Education,
Monash University, Melbourne, Victoria,
Australia

Gillian Nisbet DipNutr, BSc (Hons), MMEd, PhD
Work Integrated Learning, Faculty of Health Sciences, The University of Sydney, Sydney, New South Wales, Australia

Christy Noble BPharm, PGCertClinPharm, MEd, PhD
Principal Medical Education Officer and Principal Allied Health Research Fellow, Medical Education Unit and Allied Health, Gold Coast Health, Southport;
Senior Lecturer (Adjunct), School of Medicine, Griffith University, Southport;
Senior Lecturer (Adjunct), School of Pharmacy, University of Queensland, St Lucia, Queensland, Australia

Gabriel Reedy MEd, PhD, CPsychol, CSci, AFBPsS, FAcadMEd, SFHEA
Senior Lecturer in Clinical Education, Programme Director, Masters in Clinical Education, Faculty of Life Sciences and Medicine, King's College London, London, UK

Charlotte Emma Rees BSc (Hons), MEd, PhD
Professor, Faculty of Medicine, Nursing & Health Sciences, Monash University, Clayton, Victoria, Australia

Christopher Roberts MBChB, MMedSci, PhD
Associate Professor, Sydney Medical School, University of Sydney, Sydney, New South Wales, Australia

Samantha Lee Sevenhuysen BPhys, PhD
Elective Surgery Manager, Surgery Program, Monash Health, Dandenong;
Teaching & Research Associate, Department of Physiotherapy, Monash University, Frankston, Victoria, Australia

Malissa K. Shaw BA, MSc, PhD
Post-Doctoral Fellow, Chang Gung Medical Education Research Centre, Chang Gung Memorial Hospital, Linkou, Taiwan

Linda Sweet BNg, MNgS, GradCert Ed, PhD
Associate Professor, School of Nursing and Midwifery, Flinders University, Bedford Park, South Australia, Australia

Joanna Hong-Meng Tai BMedSc (Hons), MBBS (Hons), PhD
Research Fellow, Centre for Research in Assessment and Digital Learning, Deakin University, Geelong, Victoria, Australia

Olle ten Cate PhD
Professor, Center for Research and Development of Education, University Medical Center Utrecht, Utrecht, The Netherlands

Stephen Trumble MBBS, MD, FRACGP
Head of the Department of Medical Education, Melbourne Medical School, University of Melbourne, Melbourne, Victoria, Australia

J. M. Monica van de Ridder PhD
Assistant Professor, Office of Medical Education Research and Development (OMERAD);
Faculty Affairs and Development (FAD);
Director of the Clinician Educator Mentoring Program (CEMP);
College of Human Medicine, Michigan State University, Grand Rapids, Michigan, USA

Christopher Watling MD, MMEd, PhD
Associate Dean, Postgraduate Medical Education, Schulich School of Medicine and Dentistry, Western University, London, Ontario, Canada

Tim J. Wilkinson MBChB, MClinEd, PhD, MD, FRACP, FRCP
MBChB Program Director, University of Otago, Christchurch, New Zealand

Miriam Zukas BSc (Hons)
Professor, School of Social Science, History and Philosophy, Birkbeck, University of London, London, UK

Reviewers

Julie Ash BSc (Hons), BMBS, PhD
Senior Lecturer in Clinical Teaching & Learning,
College of Medicine and Public Health,
Flinders University, Adelaide, South Australia,
Australia

Jane Conway RN, BHSc, BN (Hons1),
GradCert HRM, GradDip FET, MEd, DEd
Associate Dean, Teaching and Learning,
Faculty of Medicine and Health, The University
of New England, Armidale, New South Wales,
Australia

Lorna Davin PhD
Senior Lecturer Medical Education, Program
Coordinator Health Professional Education,
School of Medicine, University of Notre Dame,
Fremantle, Western Australia, Australia

Sara Geale RN, PhD
Director of Clinical Education, School of
Nursing and Midwifery, The University of
Newcastle (UON), Callaghan, New South
Wales, Australia

Koshila Kumar PhD
Coordinator – Clinical Education Programs,
Prideaux Centre for Research in Health
Professions Education, Flinders University,
Adelaide, South Australia, Australia

Acknowledgments

In this book we set out to weave education theory and education practice with stories about learning in real clinical contexts. This endeavour was only possible because we had contributors who could bring experience, critical understanding of the research and imaginative ideas. We would like to thank all of the contributors to this book for generously sharing their expertise, ideas and scholarship of learning and teaching in clinical workplaces. In particular, we would like to thank Associate Professor Margaret Bearman for her close reading and critical feedback on the opening and closing chapters. The combined efforts of all chapter authors are a wonderful example of a community of scholars offering their rich knowledge and asking further critical questions to enhance our understanding of how we may contribute more effectively to clinical learning and teaching. We are very grateful to them all.

We would also like to thank the many students, teachers and clinicians who have enrolled in postgraduate programs in clinical education and in research higher degree programs examining learning through work. Their stories and their curiosity about how education theories can influence teaching approaches have provided stimulus for this text.

We hope you enjoy and learn from this book as much as we have enjoyed and learned from editing it.

Clare Delany and Elizabeth Molloy

Section 1

Preparing learners for workplace learning

1

Becoming a clinical educator

Clare Delany and Elizabeth Molloy

Introduction

Learning in clinical workplace settings is integral to shaping the professional development and skill sets of future health practitioners. However, clinical workplace environments are complex and dynamic, and the learning and teaching which occurs can similarly be complex, unpredictable and at times chaotic, but also rich and full of possibilities. The purpose of this book is to identify and exploit these rich dimensions of work-based education. Each chapter seeks to inform and encourage clinical educators from a broad range of disciplines and contexts to rethink and redesign clinical teaching practices, and to contribute to the development of a collective professional clinical educator identity which integrates both clinician and educator roles.

The last decade has seen a large growth in 'medical' or 'clinical' education as a legitimate scholarly, stand-alone field. There are now multiple dedicated 'health professions education', 'nursing education' and 'medical education' peer-reviewed journals rising up the impact factor charts, along with education-based studies featuring in clinical journals. This literature covers a spectrum of topics from practical 'how to teach methods' aimed at the on-the-ground clinical educator through to discussions of theoretical paradigms and authoritative pedagogies relevant to learning and teaching in clinical contexts. At the practical teaching methods end, authors have distilled and translated educational theory into practical and concrete tips and strategies to apply in specific teaching situations (Aronson, 2011; Joyner & Young, 2006; Steinert et al., 2016; Vickery & Lake, 2005). At the theoretical end, there is a burgeoning literature on educational theories relevant to both understand and shape workplace learning and teaching processes (Bunniss & Kelly, 2010; Nestel & Bearman, 2015).

The expanding scholarship of clinical education is also influencing expectations of clinicians responsible for educating students and trainees on clinical placements. Previous apprenticeship-style models of learning, where students were assumed to develop adequate competencies based on time spent on clinical placements, are now recognised as being educationally inadequate (Frenk et al., 2010; Higgs, 2009). Clinical education has moved well beyond prescriptive teaching or a reliance on shadowing senior clinicians. It involves purposefully orienting student experiences to encourage self-regulated and reflective learning. It also involves designing incremental learning tasks which build learners' sensitivity to important cues (including input from patients, caregivers, other team members, near and same-level peers, administrators and regulators).

An evidence-based approach to clinical education means that clinicians must also account for their education practice through teaching evaluations, explicit contributions to curricular design and research (Hu et al., 2015; Stalmeijer et al., 2010), and evidence of learning outcomes achieved. Along with learning outcomes related to procedural skill development, clinical educators are expected to actively develop students' capabilities for their future practice, including broad-based competencies enabling participation in 'patient and population-centred health systems as members of locally responsive and globally connected teams' (Frenk et al., 2010, p 1924). This expands the breadth and depth of clinical education beyond discipline-based competencies and includes covering areas of critical thinking (Golding, 2011; Ajjawi & Higgs, 2011; Delany & Golding, 2014), evaluative judgment (Tai et al., 2015), self-regulation of learning (Molloy et al., 2013), professionalism (Rees et al., 2013), emotional regulation for professional practice (Lewis & Rees, 2013; Gillam et al., 2013) and resilience to cope with pressures and challenges (Delany et al., 2015; Klein et al., 2017).

In addition to responding to expanding scholarly expectations, clinical educators must attend to the balance between meeting service delivery demands where individual patients are at the centre of the care process and learner needs for experiential and individualised learning (Frenk et al., 2010). The challenging task of balancing patient care and safety with student learning needs is further compounded by shifting service models where patients have shorter stays in hospital, students have shorter workplace rotations and regulatory requirements for trainees proscribe and seek to specify shorter hours of clinical work. The impact of these changes has led to fragmented learning experiences with reduced opportunities to build continuity in supervisory relationships. The changes in service models have also influenced the types and validity of workplace-based assessments. For example, within a single clinical placement, students may encounter multiple supervisors, and the assigned 'supervisor of training' (responsible for formal feedback sessions and making high-stakes decisions about progress) may have few opportunities to directly observe learners. A lack of direct observation of performance by supervisors (Castanelli et al., 2016) and a reliance on a synthesis of 'second-hand' feedback from multiple sources can, in turn, inhibit the building of trusting and sustained relationships between learners and clinical educators, which are critical for development-based discussions (Watling et al., 2016).

Clinical educators have responded to the visions for, and challenges of, clinical education in two main ways. The first is via the development of professional development programs within health institutions, enabling clinicians to attend seminars or short courses which offer practical tips, teaching strategies and heuristics of clinical supervision which can be incorporated quickly into their practice. A second response is via increasing availability and uptake in accredited and formalised postgraduate coursework and research higher degree programs, designed to build scholarship around workplace learning and teaching (Steinert et al., 2016). Both responses demonstrate a trend by clinicians towards a deeper investment in their role as educators within health workplaces, to empower learners to be the best they can be in their chosen health disciplinary area. This represents the key impetus for this book.

Becoming a clinical educator

Most clinicians don't set out to be a clinical educator but rather the role is thrust upon them as part of their clinical work. Their uptake of pathways towards clinical education expertise is largely influenced by their own professional inclinations, interests or identities relating to education and clinical practice or via the affordances or barriers provided by their specific clinical workplace environment (Bearman et al., 2017; Clement et al., 2016). This means that they do not have the luxury of sustained exposure to and immersion in pedagogy relevant to their 'classroom'. They do not have the opportunity to construct knowledge about relationships between education theory and practice (as do teachers undertaking teacher training as their primary discipline), or the opportunity to regularly trial and learn from teaching experience.

This represents a very different educational career progression when compared with the pathway towards becoming a clinician. For clinicians, career progression is characterised by an interplay of specific experiences and targeted learning, role-modelling through collegial relationships and multiple other workplace opportunities. For example, becoming a nurse, a doctor, a surgeon, a physiotherapist or any other health practitioner means, at a minimum, developing a set of discipline-specific competencies in the form of identifiable skills. It also involves absorbing a particular type of professional identity; learning to think in a critical and reflective way and developing character-based attributes and values which seek to promote the interests of patients. As the field of clinical education expands and is underpinned by both theory and evidence, pathways will similarly emerge enabling clinicians to develop stronger professional identities as clinical educators (Higgs, 2009; Hager & Hodkinson, 2011; Frenk et al., 2010).

Our aim, in bringing an eminent group of authors together to contribute their wisdom, is to provide accessible material to support clinicians along these pathways. The book provides a wealth of strategies and tips for 'how to teach'. However, practical teaching ideas are not confined to how to 'do teaching' in a single encounter in the workplace. Instead the book is designed to demonstrate the integrated nature of three key threads within the field and practice of clinical education: theory, method and context. In each chapter, authors identify and explain the first main *thread underpinning theoretical frameworks* (such as cognitive, psychological, sociocultural, experiential and ethical traditions), which underpin the second *thread of specific learning and teaching strategies* designed to generate more productive and transformative outcomes for learners. Theory and practice are then described via a *third thread, a case example within a particular context*. A key goal of the book is to support clinicians to *become* clinical educators who embrace their professional roles as designers and planners of student learning experiences (Boud & Molloy, 2013).

Engaging with this book

A unique feature of this text is the use of cases to illustrate the emergent nature of learning and teaching in the workplace, influenced by personalities, tasks, contexts, experiences, emotions and relationships (Cruess et al., 2015; Cruess et al., 2016). Each of the contributors situates their discussion of clinical education theory and practice within a case study or story, reflective of typical challenges encountered by both learners and educators in clinical placement settings. A feature of the cases is their discursive nature. Unlike routine 'medical case' presentations (Passi et al., 2013) where the key clinical features are presented with current treatment and responses packaged into a standard bare bones clinical case format, each of the authors has opted to 'tell a story'. The stories are rich in detail. They describe conversations between people; highlight how students, clinicians, educators or patients are feeling; point out helpful and unhelpful relationship patterns; and emphasise aspects of the context that work to influence communication, interpretation, understanding and learning. In this way, the cases exemplify the features of learning and teaching in clinical education. They are complex, chaotic, changeable, and yet rich and full of potential (Strand et al., 2015). Many of the authors use a form of narrative analysis in their cases to highlight the learning possibilities and educationally important moments which may otherwise have been passed over as seemingly insignificant or routine activities and details of the clinical workplace. The cases are listed and the main elements of the story summarised in Table 1.1 at the end of the chapter.

Readers can dip into this book in several ways. They can refer to the cases to identify a learning and teaching topic or detail relevant to their own work; they can identify particular pedagogies and associated teaching practices from the titles of the chapters; or they can select broad phases of clinical learning and teaching from the four overall book sections (preparing learners for workplace learning; education approaches within clinical learning contexts; assessment for learning in the workplace; and leadership and faculty development in health professions education).

The chapters have the following core elements:
- an introduction to the education concept or topic;
- a case study which illuminates key elements relevant to the topic;

- educational theory related to the topic;
- bringing pedagogy to practice via elaboration and resolution of the case study;
- potential directions for evaluation and research;
- practical tips from expert practitioners.

Preparing learners for workplace learning

Chapters 2–6 highlight the transition from university to the clinical setting as a critically intensive learning period with the consequent need for educators to prepare students in particular ways, to take advantage of the rich learning opportunities. The chapters in this section present strategies to foster a capacity to think critically, to develop resilient responses for the inevitable setbacks and learning challenges encountered in clinical workplaces, to recognise and respond to ethical dimensions of learning and clinical practice, and to be prepared for and have skills to address workplace-based conflict.

In Chapter 2, Miriam Zukas and Sue Kilminster, well known for their previous writing about transitions as heightened times for learning, discuss transitional periods within health professional training (including moving from university to clinical placements, moving from one rotation to another and beginning new clinical positions). They refer to these transitions as 'critically intensive learning periods' (CLIPS), and suggest that educators should take advantage of these periods by developing strategies which go beyond preparing standard information about learning expectations. Instead, the focus is on assisting learners to 'attune' to important aspects of transitional periods and 'new' environments.

In Chapter 3, Clinton Golding, Tim Wilkinson and Althea Gamble Blakey discuss the importance of critical thinking as a foundational and fundamental component of health professional practice. They provide concrete examples of critical versus uncritical thinking approaches and suggest that educators need to be aware of and be able to articulate the types of critical thinking they are looking for. Their practical teaching strategies include approaches to making the specific critical thinking required in a given area of clinical practice visible to students and giving students frequent and regular opportunities to use this type of critical thinking.

In Chapter 4, Clare Delany, Jill Klein and Samantha McLeod draw on their combined backgrounds of education and clinical and behavioural psychology to describe dimensions of resilience relevant to learning and practising in clinical workplaces, and grounded in psychological theory. Specific strategies educators can use both to explicitly teach and to more broadly cultivate resilience for clinical learning and future health professional work are also discussed.

In Chapter 5, Clare Delany, Rosalind McDougall, Lynn Gillam and Carolyn Johnston pose the question: What pedagogy and teaching methods can clinician educators use to bridge the gap between formally taught ethical principles and professional ideals, and the everyday ethical challenges students and trainees encounter in their clinical work? The teaching strategies they present to answer this question are distilled from clinical ethics consultation processes (formal processes for considering and resolving ethical challenges and complexities, usually embedded in the hospital work context). This chapter is written for clinical educators who may not have prior training, formal qualifications or specific expertise in teaching ethics.

In Chapter 6, Haavi Morreim pre-empts a key message of this book, that providing health care and education within the workplace are high stakes and complex activities relying on effective communication, teamwork and clinical decision-making. In clinical placement contexts, the potential for conflict arises when people from diverse disciplinary backgrounds bring differing conceptions of what counts as treatment in a patient's best interests, who should be empowered to make treatment decisions and how learners are best supported and included in clinical decision-making and practice. Skills in conflict management are essential to patient safety, learner progress and organisational efficiency and effectiveness. This chapter introduces conflict resolution strategies which can be used in clinical education settings.

Education approaches within clinical learning contexts

A common theme in the 11 chapters which make up the second section of the book is an emphasis on the role of educators to see themselves as designers or curators of educational experiences for students. Each chapter in this main section of the book zooms in on an aspect of the clinical learning environment which can be deliberately used by educators to build formative learning experiences and to empower students to take an active role in their own education.

In Chapter 7, Joanna Bates, Rachel Ellaway and Christopher Watling highlight the important influence that context has on clinical learning and teaching. The chapter helps clinical educators to better understand and make more effective use of their clinical workplace contexts for teaching. Drawing from a case study that describes the experience of a community-based clinical educator and her clinical trainee, the authors draw on aspects of sociocultural learning theory to explore how and what learners take in from the clinical workplace contexts in which they are immersed. The authors then describe pedagogical strategies that clinical educators can use to purposefully direct and enhance their trainees' learning from clinical workplace contexts.

In Chapter 8, Malissa Shaw, Paul Crampton, Charlotte Rees and Lynn Monrouxe explore the theoretical constructs of professionalism, and factors influencing the formation of professional identities. They consider the differences between acting professional and internalising, or embodying, professionalism, and they discuss education approaches to assist learners to not only learn about, but also embody professional identities.

In Chapter 9, Mark Goldszmidt and Lorelei Lingard introduce two theories (sociomateriality and rhetorical genre theory) that they have found to be particularly powerful to scaffold workplace learning and teaching strategies. Sociomateriality allows educators to view clinical placements, including the people and material entanglements that exist within them, as assemblages or material constructs which can be used to support dual missions of clinical education and patient care. Rhetorical genre theory is introduced to help educators consider how they use genre in their disciplinary practice and communication, and how they can use their own repertoires to see which ones best support clinical learners.

In Chapter 10, Stephen Trumble introduces the idea of a clinical educator as a coach, where the role becomes one of providing learners with a trusted, respected and goal-oriented perspective on their performance. The role of the clinical coach is described as neither a 'sour armchair critic' nor an 'enthusiastic cheerleader'. Instead, the chapter sets out how clinical coaches need to find the right mix of challenge and support to drive and support learning and professional transformation.

In Chapter 11, Clare Delany and David Beckett discuss how developing expertise for clinical practice is a rich and highly relational activity. It requires a learner to think and act independently, to self-regulate and monitor the impact of their practice on others, and also to move beyond these individual cognitive-based learning processes into building relationships and collaborating with colleagues from different disciplines. They suggest that a critical pedagogical task for the clinical educator that follows from this idea is one of translation — not via a technical or mechanical explanation, or mere transfer of knowledge about skills and techniques, but rather, translation as a process of creatively opening up spaces for learners to participate in practice-based dialogue and supported exploration of routine practice. At a practical level, this involves simple and sensible conversations such as talking through what needs to be done, why it should be done, what would be better to do and how a different outcome could be achieved (next time).

In Chapter 12, Joanna Tai, Samantha Sevenhuysen and Phillip Dawson focus on peer learning. They highlight that although many peer learning interventions have originated from a need to host more learners on a clinical placement, educators need a sound understanding of educational theory applicable to peer learning. They also point out that collaborative learning approaches are key to ongoing workplace practice. The chapter provides practical teaching strategies and ideas for clinician educators who wish to implement peer learning in their setting.

In Chapter 13, Debra Nestel and Suzanne Gough discuss key educational aims and features of simulation-based education, including its potential for promoting transference of learning in the clinical setting. Two simulation frameworks (Integrated Simulation and Technology Enhanced Learning [ISTEL] and a national training program in Australia [NHET-Sim]) are discussed to assist educators to design simulation programs and activities. The brief and the debrief are privileged aspects of the design in these examples, and the authors suggest that adoption of these mechanisms in clinical education may heighten the capacity for deeper learning.

In Chapter 14, Fiona Kent and Gillian Nisbet discuss how clinical education can be designed to prepare future clinicians for work within interprofessional teams and within complex systems. They distinguish between formal approaches to interprofessional learning (such as pre-designed and scheduled, with set learning outcomes and structured activities for a target group of learners) and informal interprofessional learning (unstructured, experiential learning occurring as part of everyday work practice) and suggest both present valuable educational opportunities for interprofessional learning.

In Chapter 15, Stephen Billett, Christy Noble and Linda Sweet identify how routine healthcare activities such as handovers, ward rounds and team meetings are all examples of pedagogically rich activities. They consider how these activities might be used to promote novices, students or new workplace entrants' learning. They also highlight the importance of these pedagogically rich activities for ongoing development of healthcare practitioners across and within their working lives, including supporting effective interprofessional working and learning.

In Chapter 16, Jennifer Johnston, Nigel Hart and Gerard Gormley discuss primary care as a particular paradigm of health practice. They identify principles of primary care pedagogy, drawn from social theories of learning, highlighting the importance of context and the relationships between people, as valuable educational concepts which can be used in this workplace setting.

In Chapter 17, Margaret Bearman, Damian Castanelli and Charlotte Denniston discuss the notion of underperformance, and argue for the need to go beyond remediation strategies to address gaps in knowledge, skills and attitudes, after learners actually fail. The chapter offers educational strategies, informed by two different but complementary theories, 'communities of practice' and 'self-determination theory', to assist both the learner and the clinical supervisor to make the best out of the situation at hand. The authors challenge us to consider the question: How can learners who underperform be assisted to build their capacities?

Assessment for learning in the workplace

The four chapters in the third section focus more closely on a crucial aspect of clinical learning: workplace-based assessment. Assessment plays a fundamental role in tertiary and post-tertiary qualifications in determining a learner's knowledge and skills. However, as each of the chapters in this section highlights, assessment can and should also play a role in shaping learning.

In Chapter 18, James Crossley refers to a golden rule of assessment as 'choose or design an assessment process that is likely to measure the learning you're interested in, and has measurement characteristics consistent with the purpose of your assessment'. He introduces strategies for applying this golden rule to workplace-based assessments, emphasising that assessment in the workplace requires educators to acknowledge and incorporate unique contextual affordances to the desired learning with the learning outcomes from workplace-based assessment.

In Chapter 19, Rola Ajjawi and David Boud propose sustainable assessment as an approach which focuses on building the capacity of learners to make evaluative judgments or decisions about the quality of their own work and that of others. They suggest that if assessment is focused on the role of the learner as active, engaged and responsible for learning, some of the limitations of fragmented and disconnected learning and assessment can be addressed.

In Chapter 20, Olle ten Cate and Carrie Chen discuss the concept of entrustable professional activities as a framework for linking workplace-based competency domains as they exist in workplace settings. The authors highlight how this framework takes into account future performance with an unknown case and addresses not just learner ability but also deeper and more sustained professional learning concepts including learner integrity, reliability and humility.

In Chapter 21, Elizabeth Molloy and Monica van de Ridder reiterate the potential for feedback to influence clinical learning, but also highlight a range of influences that prevent it from achieving this promised learning potential. They examine an alternative way to view feedback, anchored in constructivism, so that feedback is a process learners can actively engage in and use to their short-term advantage (improved performance on their next task) as well as longer-term benefit (development of self-regulatory skills).

Leadership and faculty development in health professions education

In the final section of the book, five chapters step away from the coalface of teaching and learning and discuss the professional development journey which clinical educators must make as they embrace their role to educate and empower health professional learners. Features of the journey include not only knowing about but also using evidence, embracing innovation and recognising threshold moments which mark progression towards educational professionalism and leadership.

In Chapter 22, Gabrielle Reedy and Anna Jones explore the development of a clinician as educator using two theoretical frameworks: signature pedagogies and threshold concepts. They discuss how these theoretical concepts can support clinicians to more fully understand the ways in which clinicians shape their own career paths. They suggest that clinicians' traditional roles can be reframed so that clinicians/teachers become less 'custodians of knowledge' and more 'facilitators of learning'.

In Chapter 23, Jennene Greenhill and Judy McKimm bring together leadership, followership and change theories to argue for the relevance of adaptive, connected styles of leadership for health and education systems. Drawing from these theoretical constructs, they discuss strategies for transformational and collaborative leadership and highlight the importance of 'soft' power, as a way of encouraging 'followers' to recognise and act on their leadership potential as agents for change through the use of role-modelling within education contexts.

In Chapter 24, Eric Holmboe argues that innovative approaches are urgently needed to enable clinical education to keep pace with changes occurring in medical and healthcare delivery science. He calls for clinical educators to embrace principles and lessons from disruptive innovations and diffusion of innovations. Longitudinal integrated clerkships and work-based assessments are presented as effective examples of these innovation processes in clinical education.

In Chapter 25, Rola Ajjawi, Jason Lodge and Chris Roberts discuss the challenge of translating the increasing body of educational research into the practice of clinical education. They propose an interdisciplinary and collaborative framework for knowledge translation that utilises shared decision-making and design thinking. Shared decision-making facilitates tailoring evidence to specific disciplinary contexts. Design thinking is used to inform how clinical educators can and should make judgments about what is 'educationally desirable' in particular situations in collaboration with educational experts.

In the concluding chapter, Chapter 26, the editors Elizabeth Molloy and Clare Delany pick up the threads of the chapters and discuss how this book challenges current approaches to clinical education. The changing landscape of clinical learning and the ongoing tension between learning and service demands means that educators must become designers of experiences to 'milk' the educational value of clinical placement experiences. The notion of 'becoming' is highlighted as a key theme in the book, both in terms of the ongoing developing expertise and identity of the clinician, but also the emerging identity of the clinical educator. They emphasise the challenge for us all to think differently (with the help of theory), to try things on for size and, most importantly, to evaluate the effect of the approaches in terms of student learning and/or patient outcomes.

Conclusion

The book as a whole aims to capture the rich possibilities for learning and professional growth within clinical workplaces. Each chapter shares a common purpose to encourage clinicians who are also educators to be aware of, but also to move beyond, the 'tips and tricks' of learning and teaching approaches. The book highlights the powerful role of storytelling and how narratives can raise awareness of the shared vulnerability of both the novice and the expert within the context of a complex work environment. The importance of context in learning is articulated across all chapters, and the illustrative case studies and the foregrounding of theory (sociocultural, critical, psychological and education-based) help to advance our understanding of clinical education.

This book was not developed as a prescriptive 'how to' text. Our goal as editors was to showcase a range of educational challenges, concepts and options to encourage the reader to see beyond learning outcomes and to embrace the broader notion of educational design, to better support patient care and student learning.

TABLE 1.1: Case studies

Chapter	Brief description	Page number
2	*Case 2.1 Hectic first day with little support* Val is in her first year after qualification, working in an urban hospital. After a brief handover from a junior doctor she was replacing, Val finds she receives little support from nurses and other colleagues to deal with a complicated patient requiring senior staff to oversee the consent for surgery.	16
	Case 2.2 Poor communication within the team Jaz is a second-year doctor working alongside nurses who are younger but technically more senior. This leads to some tensions in team communication.	16
	Case 2.3 A day where support and planning were visible and helpful Viv (specialist trainee) and Anna (fifth-year medical student) began the day by discussing what Anna wanted to focus on, while Viv made suggestions as to which patients to look at; they each had a copy of a printed bed list upon which they were writing notes.	17
3	*Cases 3.1–3.7 Learning and teaching critical thinking* Educators discuss different types of critical thinking they would like students to use. For example, Angela wants her clinical students to develop as independent, proactive thinkers; Maya wants her students to be independent thinkers or to show initiative, flexibility and adaptability in their judgments; and Akira wants his clinical students to learn to evaluate.	33, 34, 35, 37, 38, 39, 40
4	*Case 4.1 Learning and teaching resilience* Sophie is a senior physiotherapist wanting to include resilience training within her teaching (although she doesn't feel very resilient herself). Win is an international student in her final year of physiotherapy training. She discusses what assists her and what is less helpful in building resilience for learning.	47, 54
5	*Cases 5.1 and 5.2 Teaching ethics* A medical student experiences poor communication with a patient, feeling sorry for the patient but unsure of what to do in response.	59
	A junior doctor is left with responsibility for patient care decisions overnight and feels uncomfortable and unsure of a decision to perform a pregnancy test without consent from the patient.	59
6	*Cases 6.1 and 6.2 Educating for conflict resolution* Carl, age 48, had been admitted earlier in the month for gastrointestinal pain and then discharged home, feeling better but with no clear diagnosis (although several important potential diagnoses had been ruled out). A few days later he returned and was readmitted. Several days later, when Carl pegged his abdominal pain at most as a 3 on a scale of 10, the team informed him he would be discharged that afternoon. Carl objected, insisting that he should feel completely fine and well before going home. The doctors see a conflict brewing.	73
	Alice is a 14-month-old toddler admitted to the neurology floor in a paediatric hospital for what is probably nothing more than a simple febrile seizure. Although frightening to parents, a febrile seizure is usually just a convulsion that accompanies a fever. Over the past two days the nurse manager has increasingly insisted to Alice's mother that the child should be transferred to the paediatric intensive care unit (PICU). The second-year resident has now been called at 3 am. She is convinced the child does not need PICU care, but is not sure what to say to the mother.	74

TABLE 1.1: Case studies — cont'd

Chapter	Brief description	Page number
7	*Case 7.1 The influence of workplace context* Sean (senior medical student) is struggling to make sense of an unfamiliar clinical workplace context-rural setting, and Sandy (family doctor) is struggling to understand Sean's challenges in adapting to his new circumstances.	86
8	*Cases 8.1–8.3 Supporting the development of professional identity* While on a clinical placement, Hui-Wen observes a doctor (her teacher) disregarding the patient's description of her current mental status, and displaying impatience with the patient. Hui-Wen suggests that the doctor appeared to lack empathy but nevertheless interprets the doctor's behaviour as professional, largely because of his seniority.	105
	Daniel, a medical student, narrates two professionalism dilemmas that he encountered during his emergency department placement, acknowledging both incidents as examples of suboptimal care, but also explaining different responses as he develops his own view of professionalism.	109
	The hidden curriculum can be addressed by suggesting strategies for students to reflect on their clinical experiences and professionalism dilemmas.	111
9	*Case 9.1 Scaffolding learning for independence* Carl and Yvonne are newly hired general internists (first-year doctors) who will also be taking on a student supervision role. They discuss their prior learning experiences with three different types of supervisors and discuss the pros and cons of each approach: Dr M gives a lot of responsibility to students and lets the team operate independently; Dr D is highly efficient with patients and has a didactic approach to teaching students; and Dr E is highly efficient in planning for teaching and caring for patients but it is difficult to know how he manages both.	116, 126
10	*Case 10.1 Integrating coaching* Therese has been a general practitioner in a large rural town for many years and she reflects on different models of coaching which may be needed for two students, one of whom is very cautious, while the other appears to be overly confident in her approach.	137, 144
11	*Case 11.1 Supporting and translating practice for junior clinicians* Carl is in his first year of medical practice as an intern, in the emergency department. He discusses the impact of two different supervisory approaches on his capacity to understand and undertake his role. One supervisor takes a sequential teaching approach and limits Carl's involvement. The second supervisor expects him to manage a case load independently.	155
12	*Case 12.1 Peer learning* Ben and Michelle are senior physiotherapists who have been asked by their affiliated university to use peer learning within students' clinical placement. They discuss how they can best set this up to cater for different student learning needs.	165, 168
13	*Cases 13.1 and 13.2 Simulation as a teaching tool* Two simulation cases are described in detail. Scenario about two acutely deteriorating medical in-patients: the example is designed to enhance effective teamwork and explore unconscious bias.	185
	Scenario where a patient presents in severe pain in the emergency department: the example is designed to promote patient-centred communication skills and clinical judgment.	188

Continued

TABLE 1.1: Case studies — cont'd

Chapter	Brief description	Page number
14	*Case 14.1 Interprofessional education through peer learning* Jackie is a physiotherapist in a subacute rehabilitation centre. Her colleagues from medicine, nursing, occupational therapy and social work frequently ask whether their students can spend some time watching her in the gym to increase their students' understanding of what a physiotherapist does. Jackie would like to use concepts about peer learning to make better use of this interprofessional learning opportunity.	195
15	*Cases 15.1–15.3 Recognising and using pedagogically rich workplace activities* Final-year nurses attending a routine handover miss some key learning opportunities which could increase their understanding and awareness of their role in caring for patients both within and outside of the hospital.	208, 216, 217
16	*Cases 16.1 and 16.2 Learning in community-based contexts* Fiona is a 22-year-old medical student at a UK-based medical school. For the first time she will experience a one-to-one learning relationship with a clinical educator in a general practice setting.	225
	Educators use webcams and video-conferencing technology to enable geographically dispersed healthcare professionals to link in from 'spokes' to a central 'hub' for case-based discussions.	228
17	*Cases 17.1 and 17.2 Identifying and working with underperformance* Kate is a supervisor of anaesthetic training and prepares to support Antoine, an anaesthetic registrar who is six years post medical school graduation.	237, 239, 243, 248
	Ethan is a junior occupational therapist and is the primary supervisor of two third-year occupational therapy students. He needs to formulate ways of supporting both students.	238, 240, 243, 248
18	*Case 18.1 Workplace-based assessments* As the assessment lead for a hospital's multi-professional education team, you have been asked to devise and implement workplace-based assessments, but there is resistance to this method from your colleagues.	255, 267
19	*Case 19.1 Assessments which have a positive influence on longer-term learning* Sam is a clinical educator at a medium-sized regional hospital and Frances is a student in the final year of her health professional study. Both Sam and Frances discuss their preparation and responses to a mid-term formative assessment.	282
20	*Case 20.1 Assessment through entrustable professional activities (EPAs)* Caroline is a clinical educator who works in a community clinic that serves as a required ambulatory clinical placement for medical students and paediatric residents from the university. Caroline discusses two first-year paediatric residents working with her in clinic. David performs at a level that is typical for an average first-year resident. He requests support in thinking through clinical cases and frequently asks questions both to ensure he is providing appropriate care and to improve his learning. In contrast, Amy is a resident with an impressive fund of knowledge and clinical skills but a recent experience observing Amy has made Caroline uncomfortable with Amy's performance.	288, 298

TABLE 1.1: Case studies — cont'd

Chapter	Brief description	Page number
21	*Case 21.1 Written and verbal feedback: why, when, how* Pearl is in her final year of medical school and so far has performed well in her studies. This is Pearl's first exposure to a rehabilitation facility and based on advice from peers, Pearl anticipates that the pace will be slower here than in the acute setting, and that need for diagnostic skills will be reduced. Contrary to her expectations, five days in, Pearl feels as if she is at sea.	310, 312, 315
22	*Case 22.1 Faculty development: building the skills of 'clinician as educator'* Maria, an emergency medicine trainee, was an enthusiastic and capable doctor who was comfortably on track for finishing her training and was looking forward to her career as a consultant. However, over time and based on several opportunities in both clinical practice and teaching others, Maria began to realise the synergies between her educator and clinician role. She began to conceptualise that her role as an educator was to provide something much more than her trainees could get in a book, and therefore required much more from her than just knowing content.	328
23	*Case 23.1 Leadership in health professional education* You have been asked to establish a new program to educate the next generation of health professionals in an underserved community. As a leader of this project, you focus on collaborative communication and engagement with the community and local health service managers. Introducing change to health services in small communities requires more than political knowledge, community and university support; it also requires a collaborative and shared leadership approach between all stakeholders.	242
24	*Cases 24.1 and 24.2 Disruptive innovation in health professions education: how might this model guide change?* Medical students are assigned a group of patients and they follow these individuals longitudinally over the course of the year. This affords them 'educational continuity' and represents an example of disruptive innovation.	353
	The rise of new workplace-based assessments is helping to disrupt prior approaches to assessment.	355
25	*Case 25.1 Translating educational research into educational practice* A senior clinical educator, Rosa, who is based in general practice approaches the health professional education unit at her local university for some advice about the re-design of their eight-week primary care placement. Rosa wants to develop her students' clinical reasoning skills. She struggles with balancing her service and educational roles while giving more to her learners.	372

References

Ajjawi, R., & Higgs, J. (2011). Core components of communication of clinical reasoning: A qualitative study with experienced Australian physiotherapists. *Advances in Health Sciences Education*, 1–13.

Aronson, L. (2011). Twelve tips for teaching reflection at all levels of medical education. *Medical Teacher, 33*(3), 200–205.

Bearman, M., Tai, J., Kent, F., et al. (2017). What should we teach the teachers? Identifying the learning priorities of clinical supervisors. *Advances in Health Science Education*, doi:10.1007/s10459-017-9772-3.

Boud, D., & Molloy, E. (2013). *Feedback in higher education*. London: Routledge.

Bunniss, S., & Kelly, D. (2010). Research paradigms in medical education research. *Medical Education, 44*, 358–366.

Castanelli, D., Jowsey, T., Chen, Y., et al. (2016). Perceptions of purpose, value, and process of the mini-Clinical Evaluation Exercise in anesthesia training. *Canadian Journal of Anaesthesia, 63*, 1345–1356.

Clement, T., Brown, J., Morrison, J., et al. (2016). Ad hoc supervision of general practice registrars as a 'community of practice': Analysis, interpretation and re-presentation. *Advances in Health Sciences Education*, *21*, 415–437.

Cruess, R. L., Cruess, S. R., Boudreau, J. D., et al. (2015). A schematic representation of the professional identity formation and socialization of medical students and residents: A guide for medical educators. *Academic Medicine*, *90*(6), 718–725.

Cruess, R. L., Cruess, S. R., & Steinert, Y. (2016). Amending Miller's pyramid to include professional identity formation. *Academic Medicine*, *91*(2), 180–185.

Delany, C., & Golding, C. (2014). Teaching clinical reasoning by making thinking visible: An action research project with allied health clinical educators. *BMC Medical Education*, *14*(1), 20.

Delany, C., Miller, K., El-Ansary, D., et al. (2015). Replacing stressful challenges with positive coping strategies: A resilience program for clinical placement learning. *Advances in Health Sciences Education*, 1–22.

Frenk, J., Chen, L., Bhutta, Z., et al. (2010). Health professionals for a new century: Transforming education to strengthen health systems in an interdependent world. *The Lancet*, *376*(9756), 1923–1958.

Gillam, L., Delany, C., Guillemin, M., et al. (2013). The role of emotions in health professional ethics teaching. *Journal of Medical Ethics*, *40*, 331–335.

Golding, C. (2011). Educating for critical thinking: Thought-encouraging questions in a community of inquiry. *Higher Education Research and Development*, *30*(3), 357–379.

Hager, P., & Hodkinson, P. (2011). Becoming as an appropriate metaphor for understanding professional learning. In L. Scanlon (Ed.), *'Becoming' a professional: an interdisciplinary analysis of professional learning* (pp. 33–56). Dordrecht, Netherlands: Springer.

Higgs, J. (2009). Ways of knowing for clinical practice. In C. Delany & E. Molloy (Eds.), *Clinical education in the health professions* (pp. 25–37). Sydney: Elsevier.

Hu, W. C., Thistlethwaite, J., Weller, J., et al. (2015). 'It was serendipity': A qualitative study of academic careers in medical education. *Medical Education*, *49*(11), 1124–1136.

Joyner, B., & Young, L. (2006). Teaching medical students using role play: Twelve tips for successful role plays. *Medical Teacher*, *28*(3), 225–229.

Klein, J., Delany, C., Fischer, M., et al. (2017). A growth mindset approach to preparing trainees for medical error. *BMJ Quality & Safety*, doi:10.1136/bmjqs-2016-006416.

Lewis, N., & Rees, C. (2013). *Distributed emotional intelligence: a resource to help medical students learn in stressful settings first do no self-harm*. Oxford: Oxford University Press.

Molloy, E., Borello, F., & Epstein, R. (2013). The impact of emotion in feedback. In D. Boud & E. Molloy (Eds.), *Feedback in higher education* (pp. 50–71). London: Routledge.

Nestel, D., & Bearman, M. (2015). Theory and simulation-based education: Definitions, worldviews and applications. *Clinical Simulation in Nursing*, *11*, 349–354.

Passi, V., Johnson, S., Peile, E., et al. (2013). Doctor role modelling in medical education: BEME Guide No. 27. *Medical Teacher*, *35*(9), e1422–e1436.

Rees, C., Monrouxe, L., & McDonald, L. (2013). Narrative, emotion, and action: Analysing 'most memorable' professionalism dilemmas. *Medical Education*, *47*(1), 80–96.

Stalmeijer, R. E., Dolmans, D. H. J. M., Wolfhagen, I. H. A. P., et al. (2010). The Maastricht Clinical Teaching Questionnaire (MCTQ) as a valid and reliable instrument for the evaluation of clinical teachers. *Academic Medicine*, *85*, 1732–1738. doi:10.1097/ACM.0b013e3181f554d6.

Steinert, Y., Mann, K., Anderson, B., et al. (2016). A systematic review of faculty development initiatives designed to enhance teaching effectiveness: A 10-year update—BEME Guide No. 40. *Medical Teacher*, *38*, 769–786. doi:10.1080/0142159X.2016.1181851.

Strand, P., Edgren, G., Borna, P., et al. (2015). Conceptions of how a learning or teaching curriculum, workplace culture and agency of individuals shape medical student learning and supervisory practices in the clinical workplace. *Advances in Health Sciences Education*, *20*(2), 531–557.

Tai, J. H.-M., Canny, B., Haines, T., et al. (2015). The role of peer-assisted learning in building evaluative judgement: Opportunities in clinical medical education. *Advances in Health Science Education*, 1–18.

Vickery, A. W., & Lake, F. R. (2005). Teaching on the run tip 10: Giving feedback. *Medical Journal of Australia*, *183*(5), 267.

Watling, C., LaDonna, K., Lingard, L., et al. (2016). 'Sometimes the work just needs to be done': Socio-cultural influences on direct observation in medical training. *Medical Education*, *50*, 1054–1064.

2

Understanding transitions in health professional learning

Miriam Zukas and Sue Kilminster

Introduction

Students make transitions: from university to clinical practice, from one healthcare setting to another, one level of participation to another. Health professionals also make transitions: from one site of practice to another; one specialist area to another; from providing care to managing others who are providing care; from learner to educator. The career structure and training requirements of each profession determine the frequency and type of transitions within that profession, but they are a particularly noticeable feature of clinical training, compared to other professional groups. The general view within the existing clinical education literature is that pedagogical interventions to facilitate transitions should focus on the development of the individual's knowledge, skills or identities. For example, authors have recommended preparing learners to be resilient or providing them with simulated experiences ahead of the transition (for example, Chambers et al., 2016; Cho et al., 2017; Teunissen & Westerman, 2011a).

We take a different view. We believe that the unfamiliar contexts in which learners and clinicians find themselves are not just backdrops for transitions in which individuals apply the knowledge, skills and personal qualities that have already been developed elsewhere; nor are they communities of practice in which learners and healthcare professionals participate in legitimate peripheral activities and, gradually over time, become expert participants in that community. Instead, we believe that participants have a (very) short period in which to learn 'how we do things around here'. Further, the material and social phenomena which constitute healthcare practice actively configure and organise what is to be done and how it is to be done. These phenomena involve people (patients, other professionals, families), materials (instruments, wards, drugs, for example) and texts (protocols, scripts, research materials, patient records). Such worlds also have histories, micropolitics and cultures, including ways of doing things 'around here'.

What happens in transitions is uncertain, unpredictable and emergent; what needs to be known and learnt is not fixed but contingent, unstable and the effect of the 'webs of relations' constituting the sociomaterial context. Of course, this is not to deny that making a transition — whether early on in one's training or mid-career — is not emotionally challenging for individuals (see, for example, Chapter 4 of this book; Brennan et al., 2010; Bullock et al., 2013). But our purpose here is to propose a different approach for clinical educators preparing learners for transitions. Instead of arming learners with knowledge, competences and personal qualities to ensure that they are able to participate even as peripheral healthcare professionals, one task is to prepare and help learners in transition to attune quickly to the specificity and immediacy of clinical practice; a second is to understand that the transition itself is a crucial time for learning. And a third task is to attend to the sociomaterial relations at work (Cuyvers et al., 2016), as we will show later.

To set the context, we begin with three case studies, drawn from a research project we undertook several years ago, which sought to better understand the links between transitions and medical performance (Kilminster et al., 2010; Kilminster et al., 2011), particularly in relation to learning responsibility in practice. Our cases are based on work-shadowing of, and interviews with, trainee doctors working on elderly patient wards early in their transition into a new position. Although our examples are highly specific in terms of setting, profession and stage of transition, we propose that they echo a variety of experiences of transitions that reflect those of all health professionals, both in their initial entry into work and later in their working lives. We then go on to develop our theoretical argument, before marshalling this theoretical perspective to analyse the three cases from the point of view of the context, the educator and the learner. We finally consider a number of strategies to support transitions.

Case study 2.1

Val is in her first year after initial medical qualification, working in an urban hospital. She had undertaken her first two rotations in the same hospital, and this — her third — was on one of the two elderly medicine wards (each on different floors). On her first day, both of the consultants and the registrars were on leave, and only Val and a locum junior doctor were on duty. She had received a briefing handover the day before from the junior doctor she was replacing.

There was a patient who had been due for discharge, but became sick later in the day. However, the locum junior doctor announced, just as they were 'sorting the patient out' (a colloquial term frequently used by clinicians), that 'I need to go now to get the shuttle bus back', and Val was left on her own. To her relief, the on-call doctor was someone she had worked with on a previous rotation, 'so he kind of just took over and said it was fine and did everything, but I felt that it shouldn't have been his responsibility in that it should have been sorted out by the day team'. When asked whether anyone else could have helped, Val said the nurses were 'quite abrupt and short — I didn't really feel like we were part of the team. It was kind of sometimes — not like me against them, but they weren't always particularly helpful with things, and this was quite a sick patient as well.'

In addition, on her first day, there was a patient who was going to have a percutaneous endoscopic gastrostomy (PEG) tube inserted in a surgical procedure. The patient had learning difficulties and, said Val, couldn't communicate. When the patient was taken down for her operation, 'they said that there wasn't the appropriate consent form in her notes which had to be a registrar or above, and because we didn't have anyone else to do it, we didn't know who to contact'. So the patient was returned to the ward because she didn't have the consent form 'and we couldn't get someone to fill one in'.

Case study 2.2

Jaz, in his second year after qualification, has started work on an elderly ward with Liz, a general practitioner (family medicine) trainee, and Pam, another foundation year doctor. (The foundation year is the first year of work after initial qualification as a doctor.) The team meet first thing in the morning to discuss the patients on the wards and the outliers (seven or eight) — patients in the care of the ward but placed elsewhere in the hospital for one reason or another. They discuss who will do which jobs, and Jaz volunteers to look after the outliers. He leaves the ward. Liz says that she and Pam like Jaz to go and look after outliers, and he likes it as 'it's easier'. Liz says that it is hard to deal with Jaz because he is older than she is. Liz and Pam join Jane, a locum consultant, on the ward and begin to see patients. The work flows easily between Liz, Pam and Jane, with many brief exchanges about patients, usually to give information. There are also jokes and some teasing, as one of them is getting married.

Two hours later, Jaz bleeps to say he needs help with a cannula.

After twenty minutes, another caller bleeps Liz. She refers the caller to Jaz, and tells them to bleep him twice because he does not answer his bleep very often. Liz and Pam have a little joke about this afterwards.

An hour later, Liz goes to the ward where Jaz needs help, gathering the necessary equipment, joking with a couple of nurses, and having a brief chat with Jaz himself. He continues to write up a drug chart while she inserts the cannula.

As they are leaving, Liz checks that Jaz is okay and tells him that they may be going to lunch soon. He does not respond. Afterwards, Liz repeats that she finds it difficult to deal with Jaz, especially as she is younger than him, although technically his senior.

Case study 2.3

The 25-bed medical ward in which Viv (a specialist trainee) and Anna (a fifth-year medical student) were placed was well staffed and pleasant. Anna and Viv began the day by discussing what Anna wanted to focus on, while Viv made suggestions as to which patients to look at; they each had a copy of a printed bed list upon which they were writing notes. Barry, a newly qualified junior doctor, arrived a few minutes later and started reading the case notes. Viv talked with him, and they agreed to see the first patient together so that he understood how things were 'done around here'. As they reviewed Mr H, Viv explained what she usually did. She then wrote a comprehensive note in Mr H's file. Viv kept explaining things to Barry before they looked at Mr H's X-ray together and discussed it. Viv then continued to write notes, saying, 'Dr P likes us to document everything'.

A little later, Anna returned to talk with Viv, who reviewed the patient Anna had just seen and asked Anna lots of questions. She suggested that Anna check something out on the computer as she (Viv) was logged on. A little later, Anna and Viv agreed that Anna would examine a patient with Viv observing. Viv then reviewed the notes Anna had written and asked further questions, before giving Anna a teach-in about anaemia.

The consultant (Dr P) arrived unexpectedly, and they agreed to do the ward round altogether. Dr P gave a comprehensive summary of one patient as a 'teach-in' to Anna and Barry; Viv didn't say anything. Dr P said she was going to examine the patient herself because the patient could be aggressive, and proceeded with the examination, after which everyone returned to the desk. Dr P ran through another patient's notes with Anna, Barry and Viv, before they all went in to see that patient. Anna undertook the examination at Dr P's suggestion. Viv checked something with Dr P about his aspirin prescription, and Dr P confirmed what should happen. Then Dr P suggested that they all watch the patient's breathing, clearly directing comments at Anna and Barry, but Viv watched and learned, too, as she reflected in an interview afterwards.

Viv and Anna then discussed another patient's heart murmur — Viv went to listen because Anna wasn't sure what she had heard. Viv reviewed a patient on her own, before she and Anna reviewed a patient with Parkinson's disease; during the review, Viv explained how to examine for Parkinson's. Anna then practised what she had learnt on the patient, before Viv and Anna wrote up notes and discussed the case.

Learning and transitions

What makes for a good transition? Happily, in our research and in our own experiences, as case study 2.3 shows, we have seen 'good' clinical learning environments. They were very different, but all were able to support effective transitions for health professional students and staff. But this is incommensurate with the research literature, which has tended to focus on the problems and difficulties associated with transitions. Teunissen and Westerman (2011b) suggest that transitions are experienced as problems because of a shift in purpose: the 'learning orientation' of university-based education clashes with the 'performance orientation' of workplace-based medical education. In the former, medical students are taught what they need to know in practice, and learning is the primary focus. In the latter, patients' needs are primary, and learning is of secondary importance, occurring as an outcome of patient-centred activities. They suggest that junior doctors (and healthcare professionals more broadly) are caught between the learning orientation of clinical training schools and the performance orientation of clinical workplaces. Learners' responses to this clash depend, say Teunissen and Westerman, on coping strategies, including what they term 'metacognitive' skills, which will help learners develop the ability to learn in new contexts, and on the ways in which workplaces provide guidance and legitimacy such that new healthcare professionals are able to combine work and learning.

While we see why students, novice healthcare professionals and their supervisors might characterise the transition as a clash of purpose, we believe that a theoretical reorientation towards practice-based and sociomaterial accounts of learning will not only expand our understanding of what is happening, but also help establish that performance (practice) is learning, too. We believe this has significant implications for clinical educators as well. In order to establish why we think this, we begin by summarising briefly 'families' of learning theory, and show how they have been implicitly or explicitly drawn on in the literature to think about transitions. Hager et al. (2012) identify three main families of learning theory and their relationship to practice.

Cognitive psychology-based theories

The first, the family of cognitive psychology-based theories was, until relatively recently, the dominant view of learning in clinical education. In summary, in the formal education system, the individual learner undergoes change through rational and cognitive processing of knowledge. In the transition to practice, they apply their newly acquired knowledge more or less successfully to caring for patients. They might reflect on what happens, and change that knowledge or their practice as a result. Learning is thus regarded as a 'thing' that is taken in by the individual ('acquired'), and then carried from location to location in order to reapply it ('transferred'). It is held inside the body (in the mind, usually), but the body itself is not implicated in the learning process. The social, cultural, organisational and material world in which the learner is embedded is understood to be the background for the learner and their learning, but it is seen as a separate matter, the primary focus being the individual.

This underlying theoretical assumption about learning gives rise to the concept of preparedness for practice — 'something possessed by the individual and his/her knowledge and skills rather than having a contextual dimension' (Monrouxe et al., 2014, p 11). However, a satirical contribution by Rosenstock and Sparks (2016) to a special edition of *Medical Education* is a wonderful example of the issues facing those working in what they call 'the real world of medicine'. Tongues firmly in their cheeks, Rosenstock and Sparks propose a new curriculum of administration-based learning in which students learn what apps to use to diagnose a rash and how best to select the right form for the right patient — in other words, they propose a curriculum constituted by 'how we do things around here'. In the same edition, Evans et al. (2016) suggest a FARCICAL approach (Fostering A Relevant Curriculum that Is Closer to Actual Life), in which core competencies include doctor as negotiator, storyteller and treasure-hunter.

More serious research with healthcare professionals also suggests that it seems impossible to acquire that kind of knowledge in their preparation for practice. For example, Kellett et al. (2015) asked foundation doctors (F1s) and their supervisors about the transition to practice. It was instructive that many F1s were surprised by the amount of administration they were required to undertake (for example, ordering blood tests, chasing up results, clerking), and did not know where to go for help or how to get hold of the relevant paperwork. Many F1s found prioritisation and managing multiple demands very challenging, particularly when they were on-call, and they, as well as the supervisors, noted that these skills developed over time. Both F1s and supervisors identified the areas in which F1s had the least 'real' prior responsibility as those in which F1s struggled: for example, although F1s felt confident about history-taking and record-keeping, they found that diagnosis and treatment were very different as an F1 from their experience as student where decisions had seemed much clearer. Supervisors thought that F1s found it challenging to deal with acutely ill patients with complex and multiple problems.

The question for us is whether or not these areas of struggle might be mitigated through preparing students in some way. Is the concept of preparedness (e.g. Alexander et al., 2014; Wiener-Ogilvie et al., 2014) useful here? Kellett et al., for example, recommend that 'practice in how to appropriately manage time including how to prioritise tasks' (p 953) is provided to students. They also suggest that students and F1s are provided with life skills training to enable them to cope in the transition to working as an F1. Life skills training lies well beyond the conventional understandings of what healthcare professionals need, but, as with the majority of responses to the issue of transitions in health professional learning, they still centre on acquiring 'skills' and personal attributes as some kind of preparation for what is to come.

The basis for these approaches is an implicit assumption that actual clinical practice — what is to come — is predictable and manageable, orderly and 'knowable'. However, what is apparent from Kellett et al.'s work, our vignettes, junior doctors' memoirs and personal accounts is that clinical work is usually none of these things: it is often disorderly, hectic, non-sequential. Our argument is therefore that, while anything that assists students to anticipate working life and clinical practice is helpful, the notion of 'preparedness' is misguided for several reasons: first, and most importantly, we do not think the underlying assumptions about learning hold in relation to 'preparedness'.

Take, for example, the recommendation that students are given practice in how to appropriately manage time, including how to prioritise tasks. This suggests that managing time and prioritisation are skills which students can acquire and transport from one place to another. While we believe that managing time and prioritising tasks are very challenging for those making the transition to health professional roles, we do not think they can be abstracted from the work that students undertake and the workplace contexts, because they are relational: managing one's time in a well-supported, multi-professional team with moderately sick patients is quite different from managing one's time when there are no other health professionals around and more than one patient is critically ill. Second, if work is uncertain, unstable and multiple, and working life and relationships are so variable, then what, precisely, constitutes 'preparedness'? Third, if we accept that workplaces and learners vary considerably, isn't 'preparedness' a function of the relationship between the work, the workplace and the learner themselves (as well as the patients, supervisors, other clinical professionals)?

Sociocultural theories

More recently, many clinical educators have become interested in sociocultural theories of learning (Mann, 2011; see also Chapter 7 of this volume). One important distinction between sociocultural and cognitive-psychology theories is their conceptualisation of context. Although cognitive psychology theories as employed in clinical education treat contexts as variable and specific, sociocultural theories link learning to context quite explicitly. Such theories are premised on the understanding that learning occurs through participation and active engagement in the authentic activities of the community. Novice learners undertake authentic but peripheral work (legitimate peripheral participation) as they enter communities of practice, and through that work their learning is shaped by social, organisational, cultural and other contextual factors. Learning is therefore recognised as being both embodied and embedded in the specific context and practices of the community of practice — a process sometimes conceptualised as *situated learning*. Learning is thus no longer a product or 'thing', but instead is understood to be integrated with performance through the notion of 'participation'. Learning is viewed as 'becoming', in which knowledge, values and skills are not separate from practice. Thus, Teunissen and Westerman's (2011b) distinction between learning and performance orientations falls away, because these are not distinct but integral — learning does not exist without performance, and vice versa.

These concepts have been deployed in relation to placement learning and to transitions (e.g. Morley, 2016; Morris, 2012; Noble & Billett, 2017; Thrysoe et al., 2010), and they have been useful because they disrupt the ideas of knowing and learning as pre-empting and preceding practice. If knowing and learning emerge in practice, we can no longer regard practice as something that can be tackled only once learners are ready. Nor can we ignore the specificity of context. However, such theories have also been challenged because they frequently fail to analyse power relations in work (Roberts, 2006), an issue to which we return in our case study analysis. Often they do not address the question of the conservatism of communities, and how communities of practice might (or might not) change. They also say little about the detailed place of context, particularly aspects of context which are non-human, such as materials — for example, prescriptions, protocols, equipment (Fenwick, 2013).

More specifically in relation to transitions, there is frequently a disjuncture between one level of clinical responsibility and another. For example, as Kellett et al. (2015) identify, even the most junior doctors have to deal with patients with complex and multiple problems. The tasks that learners undertake are likely to vary considerably, depending on the issues presented by different patients, which other healthcare workers are present, whether it is day or night, and where the patients might be (e.g., in the case of outliers, as in case study 2.2 above).

Further, clinical teams are not stable communities of practice, as characterised by Lave and Wenger (1991), but shifting and transient as a result of shift-working and frequent changes in staffing (as in case study 2.1 above). And the clinical workplace is often populated by intersecting — even competing — populations, such as the nurses in case study 2.1. Finally, the practices themselves are not stable — they change because of alterations to policies and regulations, technological transformations, protocols, etc.

Post-Cartesian theorisations

The third family of theories — what Hager et al. (2012) call 'post-Cartesian' theorisations — challenge modernist views about subjectivity and representation, and question received notions of identity and knowledge. They include, for example, theories which employ Foucault's critique of the rational, unified self, and his emphasis on how power/knowledge influence the way clinical learning is understood (e.g., Bleakley et al., 2011; Hodges et al., 2014). They also include a loose collection of theories, often termed *sociomaterial* (Fenwick et al., 2011), which do not distinguish clearly between social phenomena and materiality. Instead, they propose that dynamic and entangled social and material forces assemble and reassemble to constitute everyday practice (Fenwick, 2015; see also Chapter 9 of this volume). They encompass a diverse range of ideas, including complexity theory, cultural historical activity theory and actor–network theory (ANT), each with quite different premises, yet they share certain commitments.

All build on the idea that learning 'is not fully decidable in advance; rather it emerges from contexts and practices in unanticipated and unpredictable ways' (Hager et al., 2012, p 6). Contexts are dynamic, practices are unstable and emergent — that is, they are not fully specifiable in advance, but are changing and evolving all the time. Learning transpires in and through practice, rather than preceding practice. So, too, does knowing, which can never be disentangled from specific activities and interests (Nicolini, 2011). In the language of complexity theory, learning is 'emergent'.

A second common commitment is to the focus on 'materials as dynamic and enmeshed with human activity' (Fenwick & Dahlgren, 2015, p 361). The theoretical challenge is to the fundamental distinction between human and non-human. Theorists argue that not only is practice inseparable from learning (and knowing), but so too are materials, or what Fenwick (2013) calls 'things that matter'. Materials are more than 'assistants' to practice and knowing: they actively shape those practices (see, for example, Goldszmidt, 2017; Zukas & Kilminster, 2014). The material is everywhere — 'both organic and inorganic, technological and natural: flesh and blood; forms and checklists; diagnostic machines and databases; furniture and passcodes; snowstorms and dead cell zones and so forth' (Fenwick, 2013, p 47). So, too, is the social — the 'symbols and meanings, desires and fears, and cultural discourses'. Thus practices are more than human — they are 'continuously changing *gatherings* [sic] of human and non-human elements that act on one another in unpredictable ways' (Fenwick & Dahlgren, 2015, p 361). To understand learning in transition, we have to go beyond human meanings and human agency. Instead of learning being the result of the acquisition of knowledge, skills and personal attributes, or being able to participate in a community of practice, learning is embedded in material action and interaction, and emerges in practice — that is, learning is enacted.

A third understanding is the focus on the relationships between humans, things, technologies and so on, and what these relationships produce, rather than on the individuals themselves. Taking an example of a doctor, we usually think of doctors as individuals with certain attributes (knowledge, skill, particular attitudes) who are able to move freely among patients in their care, 'applying' their knowledge and skills. But when we look carefully, doctors depend on security passes, passwords, other doctors' notes, signatures, medicines, nurses, patients, beds in order to practise — to doctor. In other words, from a sociomaterial point of view, being a doctor is not a given status conferred by passing one's exams (as so many junior doctors know): the doctor is an effect of a network of immense complexity: patients, passes, notes, nurses, other doctors, instruments, drugs, hospital wards, and much more. The sociomaterial way to speak of this is as an 'assemblage': 'a process of bundling, of assembling … in which the elements put together are not fixed in shape, do not belong to a larger pre-given list but are constructed at least in part as they are entangled together' (Law, 2004, p 42). Thus, passes and nurses, in the example above, are part of the assemblage of the doctor in transition; but assemblages or networks — webs of relations — are fluid, ever-changing, interdependent and co-existing — with actors (nurses, passes, doctors) associated with many different networks. Thus, we can say that the enactment or assemblage of a doctor is fluid, unstable, entangled and messy. Learning is an effect of the assemblage, rather than an acquisitive or sociocultural process.

These 'sociomaterial' (Fenwick, 2013) theories, ranging from complexity theory to actor–network theory, have recently been attracting interest in clinical education — specifically in medical education. While much of the attention to date has been theoretical (Ajjawi & Bearman, 2012; Bleakley, 2012; Fenwick, 2013; Fenwick & Dahlgren, 2015; Goldszmidt & Faden, 2016; Goldszmidt, 2017; McMurtry et al., 2016), a somewhat limited number of empirical studies, focused, on the whole, on simulation (e.g., Dahlgren et al., 2016; Hopwood et al., 2016) is emerging from the clinical education literature. (Also see Chapter 9 of this volume.)

But that is not to say that there haven't been empirical sociomaterial studies in clinical settings: sociomaterial researchers who are interested in understanding how medicine, science and technology shape the world have undertaken a number of important and provocative case studies of clinical practice — for example, on lower-limb artherosclerosis (Mol, 2002), diabetes (Mol, 2008), caring in a nursing home (Gherardi & Rodeschini, 2016), and even medical records (Berg, 1996).

Mol's ethnographic study of lower-limb artherosclerosis has been particularly influential in showing how the GP, the radiographer, the ultrasound specialist and the surgeons are working with four different versions of artherosclerosis, which may connect but are not the same. The ultrasound specialists looked for Doppler differences, which reflect changes in the speed of blood flow. The surgeons open blood vessels and scrape out arterial plaque. The standard assumption is that there is a disease out there, with different perspectives on it from the surgeon or the ultrasound specialist. Mol's counter-argument is that different clinical practices *enact* different artherosclerosis — these are not the same thing from different perspectives. Mol calls this *ontological multiplicity*, while others tend to use the phrase *multiple ontologies*. Bleakley (2012), for example, has explored how an appreciation of multiple ontologies might be employed in medical education research to problematise what might be thought of as 'evidence'. And, of course, such an appreciation could inform and problematise understandings of, and teaching about, interprofessional education and multidisciplinary team work.

We think the notion of multiple ontologies is helpful, too, for thinking about transitions to practice. Practice is multiple and not singular. Networks of relations between things, people and texts give rise to practice, rather than practice determining what is to be done. Although practices appear settled, they are not: they are 'stabilised' in particular sets of relations, but can be interrupted or discarded. If we understand, therefore, that practices are also multiple, then, in preparing individuals for practice — whether at the start of or later on in their careers — we have some challenges that cannot be resolved through preparedness as it is usually understood — that is, through, for example, simulation-based education (Cleland et al., 2016). To some extent, we regard this notion of 'preparedness' in the same way that Whitehead and Kuper (2017) have written about competence-based education. Whitehead and Kuper illuminated how ideas circulate and become 'matters of faith' ('stabilised' in the language of sociomateriality) in a process that they call *faith-based medical education (FBME)*. Once such FBME is established, they argue, to challenge it is heretical. So, too, with the concept of 'preparedness'.

An immediate riposte to our proposal is to suggest that we are disregarding the importance of scientific and clinical knowledge, skills and other attributes. We are not, but we are sceptical about received ideas regarding knowledge, learning and practice, such as those that are implicitly derived from cognitive theories. We are arguing that a reformulation of our understanding of the relationship between learning and practice is essential, in line with both sociocultural and sociomaterial theories. One consequence of such a reformulation is a focus on the transition itself as a 'learning period', rather than relying on the idea of 'preparedness' (Kilminster et al., 2011). To crystallise this idea, we have coined the concept of transitions as *critically intensive learning periods (CILPS)* (Kilminster et al., 2010; 2011). We use the term 'critical' in the sense of 'critical period', a term derived from developmental psychology that refers to a limited time in which some event can occur, usually resulting in some kind of transformation; by 'intense' we mean the immediacy invoked by the immediate requirement to deliver patient care. In the transition, therefore, 'learning shifts from its sole emphasis on preparing for this world by acquiring knowledge representations to a process of participating wisely in situ' (Fenwick, 2013, p 50).

The implications for clinical educators, clinical contexts and learners themselves — who might be established professionals in transition between one career stage or setting and another, as well as those earlier in their career — will be developed throughout the rest of the chapter. In summary, we need to move away from the idea that there is an education–service dichotomy (or learning–performance orientations as discussed earlier) with respect to transitions, where education prepares learners with knowledge, skills and personal attributes that will see them through the transition, and the transition is focused on service, with additional education when necessary. (See also Chapter 9 of this volume.) Any transition is a CILP, although the trajectory depends on many issues — moving roles within a familiar setting may require a less intense transition than taking up an unfamiliar role within a strange context (see, e.g., Chapters 7 and 9 of this volume). Transitions in which educational activity is required at least enables the recognition and legitimation of learning; transitions later in careers are still CILPS, even if learning is not explicitly acknowledged (see, e.g., Harris and Delany, 2013). Thus, the concept is informed by sociomateriality because expertise is understood to reside in sociomaterial relations.

If we regard transitions as CILPs, then the task for educators is somewhat different from that which many clinical educators, at least initially, adopt — the pedagogical activity is not confined to bedside or classroom. Indeed, what we mean by 'education' needs to be expanded to include the working context, other professionals, patients, and healthcare itself. As with knowing and learning, caring is ongoing and emergent. Caring is, as Mol (2008) and others have demonstrated, a 'sociomaterial process that cannot be prescribed or embedded in tasks, routines or coordination mechanisms; rather, it is performed while people and technology work together' (Gherardi and Rodeschini, 2016, p 281). Thus, healthcare, patient care and clinical education are inextricable from one another. It is extremely difficult to conceive of situations in which patient care is poor yet clinical education is good. Work, caring, knowing and learning are not separate activities; they are all implicated in the transition, and in preparing for transitions.

Analysing the case studies

In the following section we unite our sociomaterial perspective with the case studies described above, and analyse the issues of transition from three points of view: from the perspective of the 'context' (ward, culture, community) in which the transition is happening; from the perspective of the clinical educator seeking to manage the transition; and from the point of view of the learner making the transition. If the analytical separation of perspectives appears to be antithetical to the argument we have been making above about the entanglement of people, contexts and things, it might be more useful to deploy the language of multiple ontologies of learning and practice.

Contextual issues

Case study 2.3 demonstrates how daily practices as well as deliberate pedagogical moments effect learning: how work, caring, knowing and learning are inseparable. Medical student Anna was working; she was seeing patients and discussing them with the senior trainee, Viv. Throughout the morning we observed, both social and material actors were enrolled in bringing about Anna's learning: for example, both Anna and Viv had copies of bed lists on which they made notes about future actions, using the lists to agree on the next steps to be taken in patient care. The practices of reading and writing notes were simultaneously clinical and pedagogical, as were the notes themselves. When a new junior doctor, Barry, began work on the ward that morning, within a short time he was not only made aware of 'how we do things around here' through explicit instruction from Viv, but also engaged in site-specific practices of note-taking, because Dr P, the consultant, 'likes us to document everything'. Later, Dr P, the detailed notes, an appropriate patient and the team of three all worked together to assemble Anna as someone capable of examining a patient.

The material and social relations are entangled throughout, with respect to learning. When Anna checked something out on the computer, the computer was more than a knowledge-carrying device that transmitted information to Anna; instead, the learning engendered by the computer was enmeshed with the specific patient's issues, the patient's notes, the case discussions with Viv, and so on. And that learning might or might not predict what Anna would do in future with a similar patient case. These caring practices — reading notes, preparing for patients' specific issues, including how to handle them, discussing patients, seeking further information on the computer about the patient, deciding on a care plan — are all sites of knowing (Nicolini, 2011). Learning is not determined in advance, but is emergent in specific activities and practices.

This was a typical working day, probably very recognisable to our readers: the work was not 'slowed down' by teaching and learning; rather, work and learning were inseparable, with explicit teaching moments contributing to patient care. In discussing 'how we do things around here', Viv was attuning Barry explicitly to the specificities of this ward, this consultant, this hospital. In turn, Viv was noticing both Anna and Barry's actions and effects; she was also being attuned, for example, to refinements in noticing when Dr P drew attention to a patient's breathing, Those initial relationships and activities are acutely significant parts of the CILP.

On her first day, Val was physically isolated (by a floor) from the only other doctor on duty. When a patient who was due to undergo a surgical procedure was returned to the ward because consent had not been obtained by the right level of doctor, neither Val nor her colleague knew how they could find an appropriate person to sign the form. (The regulations determined that, because the patient could not communicate, consent had to be obtained from a registrar or a health professional of a more senior level.) There were others who knew how to get things done around here — the nurses on the ward. But Val felt that they were 'quite abrupt and short', and that they were not part of the same team, so she did not ask and they did not tell her how to resolve the problem by finding someone qualified to obtain consent. In sociomaterial terms, the assemblage of the patient having a surgical procedure failed as the web of relations — the forces and interactions that get things done through networks acting upon one another — broke down. But such assemblages are unstable and precarious: as others have noted (Groopman, 2007; Mol, 2008), daily care is often about 'just making it up', not only because of the limitations of clinical knowledge, but also because of the messiness of procedures, disorderly materials, bodies, technologies and so on. Caring and learning both rely on asssemblages succeeding, or — in the language of actor–network theory — being translated and mobilised. Val's brief initiation into the ward suggested that the connections needed to translate her into an efficient junior doctor were far from local practice.

These two cases illuminate not only the cultures of learning in these two hospital wards, but also what is needed to ensure effective transitions for those early in their careers. Readers will recognise that the same issues arise even when clinicians are much further along the career path: the processes by which humans and non-humans make stable and durable connections in webs of relations require minute negotiations to succeed, and there is often little time to assemble those networks. By adopting a sociomaterial perspective and recognising that the transition or placement is itself 'pedagogical', the clinical setting, patients, administrative procedures, site-specific practices and so on become much more than a backdrop or context for learning: they are all enrolled in the web of relations that effect learning.

Educator perspectives

What might our three case studies tell us as educators? First, transitions are predictably unpredictable: while we hope that our learners will find themselves in contexts like Anna and Viv's, we also recognise that the circumstances giving rise to Val's horrible first day are not that uncommon. Senior colleagues go on holiday or become ill; forms do not get completed; final buses leave; patients become sick when no one else is around. Second, transitions are enacted sociomaterially: technologies, hospital layouts, relations between professional groups, micropolitics and patients' notes all constitute the webs of relations that enact and re-enact practice. And third, in the best circumstances, these practices effect learning as well as caring. Val now knows who to seek out for questions of consent. Viv watches the patient's breathing even though she is not the target for Dr P's intervention. However, Jaz seems likely to need help with cannulation in the future, because he attends to a drug chart while Liz cares for the patient. In the two latter cases, attuning to what is happening in practice could be — is — learning. That is what we mean when we say that transitions themselves are critically intense learning periods.

And yet this is not reflected in much of the discussion about the preparation of learners for transitions, or the transitions themselves. The work of clinical educators is determined, to a large extent, by the professional, regulatory and academic bodies of their health profession. These bodies have requirements about clinical learning and experience. Their proscriptions and prescriptions vary in detail and specifics, but are all essentially concerned with ensuring safe and effective professional practice by newly qualified health professionals. Many of the assumptions inherent in these regulatory requirements derive from an implicit theoretical stance very similar to the one outlined as our first 'family' above (i.e. cognitive psychological theories). In short, learning is understood as an individual, acquisitive process. Such assumptions shape what is expected from health professional educators — both those based in universities and higher education institutions and those based in clinical practice (e.g. Chambers et al., 2016). We see this when regulations include stipulations of the number of 'training hours' or 'formal learning', as well as the requirements for practice.

As we have argued, these assumptions about learning and practice in health professionals' education are not theoretically sustainable. The fundamental assumption — 'that all of the learning needed for successful performance in an occupation can be specified in advance and imparted in a formal course' (Hager, 2011, p 17) — is unjustifiable from the evidence before us. And yet, much of the work directed towards 'preparing' students for clinical experience (and all of the monitoring of that experience) actively perpetuates the notion that learning and education, work and service are separate both in time and practice.

Further issues arise from a belief that what is to be known in transitions can be derived from standardised curricula that specify learning outcomes, and pedagogical events such as simulation-based education (Cleland et al., 2016). Again, underlying assumptions about knowledge and skill — that they are cognitive processes that need to be rehearsed until they reside in long-term memory — enable the discourse about the drive for reliability, and assurances that everyone gets the same experiences. Such standardisation is justified not only as smoothing the transition, but also in terms of fairness and equality. Again, we believe this is misguided. While the educator's desire to ensure that everyone is treated equally and is not oppressed and discriminated against is laudable, we know that working life is contingent, relational, uncertain. It is not that we propose that, in preparing learners for work, we treat them inequitably or unfairly; rather, we suggest that the clinical experiences they participate in will not and cannot be uniform, nor do they replicate what is not possible to replicate. It is therefore much more important to understand the nature of the learning and practice, and help our learners to do the same.

So, returning to our cases. Bearing in mind her clinical education role, Liz (case study 2.2) might have asked Jaz to help her with inserting the cannula; the cannula (and patient) might have been part of the web of relations translating Jaz into someone who has learned cannulation, even with difficult cases. She might even have made explicit that an invitation to lunch was much more than simply the chance to eat, but was an educational opportunity for Jaz. She might also have sought to attune Jaz to managing his bleep more effectively. Meanwhile, Val (case study 2.1) might have been alerted by her clinical educator to the importance of establishing good relations with the nursing staff even before starting work on the ward. Given the theoretical assumption that learning emerges in the complex relations between the human actors and the materiality of the workplace, we believe that educators are charged not with preparedness and ensuring all learners get the same experiences and so on, but with a rather different set of pedagogical tasks that reflect that the transition itself is a CILP. As a consequence, learners could be supported in their clinical placements to attune to what is new, what is troubling, what is different, what is challenging; to notice not only doctors and bodies, but nurses, other professions, paperwork, ward layout — in short, to attend carefully to 'how things are done around here', and to see this as essential in their future transitions.

Learner perspectives

Case study 2.3 shows a pedagogically rich workplace, saturated with what seemed to us to be exemplary care for patients, and contrasts radically with case study 2.2 at Hospital B. Jaz was sent to look after the outliers while Liz, a GP trainee, and Pam, a junior doctor, worked together on the wards with Jane, a locum consultant. Jaz was working on his own at some physical distance away from the easy relationships between the other three. When he called for help with a cannula and Liz arrived after some time, she inserted the cannula without engaging Jaz; he continued to write up a drug chart while Liz got on with the work. So, while we have argued that learning is emergent in daily practices, it is not inevitably the case. Here, the web of relations between cannulas, patients and their veins, doctors, knowledge and so on does not bring about Jaz's learning, because, for whatever reason, he does not attune to what Liz is doing when she inserts the cannula. We can only speculate that Liz does not call Jaz over because, as she says on two occasions, she finds it hard to work with him because he is older than her. Perhaps Jaz finds it hard, too, to observe Liz for the same reason. Nevertheless, these social, generational and spatial (with Jaz away from the ward) relations do not promote caring and learning. There is no doubt that Jaz's absence from shared work and informal time together at lunch at best delays his transition and his participation in the everyday practices through which learning is enacted.

Current assessment practices teach students that their priority in any placement is to get 'signed off' on certain activities or observations or experiences. One result is that they learn to understand work and learning as separate activities; learning only happens if it is labelled as such, and results in some sort of certification in their logbook. It is common for students on placement to be taken away from, or out of, clinical settings for 'clinical teaching'. While the content of such teaching clearly has an important place in health professionals' education, this practice reinforces the notion that the activity of learning has to be labelled. In our view, teaching students something about professional learning and practice would help them to understand the processes in clinical settings.

In our research, the people who made the most effective transitions were those who understood that the transitional process itself was important. Some made contact with previous post-holders, as Val (case study 2.1) had done, or visited the workplace before they started. Some individuals paid careful attention to establishing relationships quickly with others, because they understood that such relationships were essential in helping them make successful transitions. One participant, for example, brought chocolate biscuits each time she moved sites, so that she would have a reason for interacting with other professions informally, and therefore be able to ask for help or information when she needed it. Thus, in relation to 'preparing' learners for transitions, we believe it would be helpful for them to understand those transitions as critical intensive learning periods — CILPS. In other words, they are learning to take part in clinical activity but do not arrive in it fully formed. This is the case regardless of stage of career or the nature of the transition: how we 'do things around here' always requires learning.

Perhaps one of the most important aspects of those transitions is to notice in practice, actual practice, rather than focus on getting 'signed off'. This might, as Dr P advised when she asked her team to watch a patient's breathing, be focused on the patients themselves. We believe that such patient noticing is highly likely to be learnt and developed, but we believe the material world might be ignored. Non-clinical matters, such as ward layouts, notices, paperwork, finding passwords, lunch-break conventions, might be seen as trivial. However, we believe that they are highly significant in effecting learning. For example, a new member of the medical team who fails to notice Dr P's enthusiasm for documenting everything is likely to find their transition more challenging than one who attunes to local practice.

And how we 'do things around here' is always open to tinkering or interruption. Val needed to learn the workarounds (which would have been practised in the hospital) for ensuring that appropriate consent was given, even if there was no registrar on the ward. She might even have interrupted the 'black box of practice', in which doctors were not 'part of the team' with nurses, by asking them what to do.

In summary, we suggest that learners', educators' and healthcare professionals' views of learning and performance as clashing orientations need to be challenged and alternative understandings of the entwining of learning and practice offered.

Strategies to support transitions

We have shown, above, how practice and learning are integral, and outlined some consequent implications for the context, educators and learners. This analysis has illustrated various strategies for supporting transitions from these three points of view: context, educator and learner. We will now summarise them briefly, bearing in mind that patient care needs to be sustained during any transition.

Context

In order to support transitions effectively, the clinical placement/clinical setting needs to accommodate the learners and recognise that transitions are crtical intensive learning periods. For example, Viv (from case study 2.3) explained in a follow-up interview that the medical team on the ward had previously undertaken work to try to ensure that the transitions of trainee doctors were more effective. Viv described how, on their first day at the hospital, the trainees attended a lunchtime induction meeting where they were given information about 'kind of what goes on and it was all written information about what the ward does — what it covers; how do you get X-rays; and I thought that document was probably the most useful thing. ... [I] t was very up to date — they sort of handed it out and went through it. We read all the pages, or pretty much all of them, and they sort of read out and just clarified what things meant and asked questions and things… I've never had one before so I thought it was brilliant really.' This might seem to contradict the fundamental premise that we cannot fully capture and formalise the implicit and unpredictable clinical workplace, but nevertheless many local practices are systematic, and any attempt to explain and/or organise those local practices for trainees would be welcome. Such specific actions follow from the strategic understanding that the transition or placement is itself 'pedagogical', the clinical setting, patients, administrative procedures, site-specific practices and so on effect learning. This understanding is essential for all health professionals, regardless of whether or not they are explicitly involved in supporting learners' transitions.

Educators

Educators are charged with working with learners to understand that the transition itself is a critical intensive learning period. As a consequence, learners could be supported in their clinical placements to attune to what is new, what is troubling, what is different, what is challenging; to notice not only doctors and bodies, but nurses, other professions, paperwork, ward layout — in short, to attend carefully to 'how things are done around here', and to see this as essential in their future transitions.

A good example of this occurred during a follow-up study after our original research on transitions. The emergency clinical team in one UK hospital tried to use some of these understandings about practice and learning and CILPs. First, they discussed our research findings, and considered how they might be applied in the hospital's emergency department. The focus was the importance of involvement in clinical activity — trying to include medical students in the clinical team, enabling them to take part in clinical activities; that is, working while ensuring that patient care was not compromised. Previously, medical students had observed in aspects of clinical activity in a relatively unstructured and unsupervised way; they had also received some clinical teaching away from the immediate clinical areas when time permitted. Instead, during this study, the medical students were included as part of the clinical team. This inclusion was materialised, and therefore visible to everyone, because the students began to wear uniforms and had name badges. It was also authentic and practical, because students saw patients, carrying out tasks alone where appropriate or with supervision when not, and cases were 'talked through'. The students were also expected to do some 'out of hours' work at evenings and weekends. Everyone involved — students and clinicians — was positive about the outcomes. The students' 'supernumerary' or superfluous status disappeared, and they believed they were treated (nearly) as junior doctors; their involvement did not noticeably delay or slow clinical work, and it helped demonstrate how learning is integral to practice. Additionally, learning as practice became more overt. This unusual example therefore outlines a number of strategies that might be taken by health professional educators.

Learners

Currently the emphasis is on the individual learner: that individuals need to be prepared for transitions, and that they will arrive in a new setting as a fully formed participant. This proposition is generally accepted by everyone, including the learners, who believe that work and learning are separate. In our view, teaching students something about professional learning and practice would help them to understand the processes in clinical settings. Instead of 'preparing' for transitions, it would be helpful to understand those transitions as critical intensive learning periods (CILPS). This would enable learners, and educators, to explicitly recognise the complicated, messy nature of clinical practice, as distinct from the specific prescriptions of learning outcomes, logbooks and current workplace assessments.

Perhaps one of the most important aspects of those transitions is to notice practice; certainly with a focus on patients, but also on such matters as ward layouts, notices, paperwork, finding passwords, lunch-break conventions. The analysis of the learner perspectives in case study 2.3 shows how it is essential to attune to what is happening in that setting. As Fenwick (2013) suggests, learners might give attention to 'minor, even mundane, fluctuations and uncanny slips' (p 51) so that they learn how to 'participate wisely in situ'.

PRACTICAL TIPS

- When learners and clinicians find themselves in unfamiliar contexts, they have a (very) short period in which to learn 'how we do things around here'.
- Instead of arming learners with knowledge, competences and personal qualities to ensure that they are able to participate even as peripheral healthcare professionals, one task is to prepare and help learners in transition to attune quickly to the specificity and immediacy of clinical practice; a second is to understand that the transition itself is a crucial time for learning.
- A theoretical reorientation towards practice-based and sociomaterial accounts of learning will not only expand our understanding of what is happening, but also help establish that performance (practice) is learning, too.
- Learners', educators' and healthcare professionals' views of learning and performance as clashing orientations (the education/service dichotomy) need to be challenged, and alternative understandings of the entwining of learning and practice offered.
- Specific actions follow from the strategic understanding that the transition or placement is itself 'pedagogical', that the clinical setting, patients, administrative procedures, site-specific practices and so on effect learning. This understanding is essential for all health professionals, regardless of whether or not they are explicitly involved in supporting learners' transitions.

Conclusion

In this chapter we have considered sociomateriality and its relevance to clinical practice, and explained why we believe this is important in understanding transitions. We have also argued that much of the learning associated with transitions needs to happen quickly (as it is a 'critically intensive learning period'), and therefore requires clinical educators and learners to be oriented towards learning in and through work, rather than through preparation; we have outlined some consequences of this reorientation to transitions in clinical settings. Consequently, we have argued that the emphasis moves from the learner having to accommodate to the setting, towards the setting accommodating to the learner.

References

Ajjawi, R., & Bearman, M. (2012). Sociomateriality matters to family practitioners as supervisors. *Medical Education*, 46, 1141–1151.

Alexander, C., Millar, J., Szmidt, N., et al. (2014). Can doctors be prepared for practice? A review. *The Clinical Teacher*, 11, 188–192.

Berg, M. (1996). Practices of reading and writing: The constitutive role of the patient record in medical work. *Sociology of Health and Illness*, 18(4), 499–524.

Bleakley, A. (2012). The proof is in the pudding: Putting actor–network theory to work in medical education. *Medical Teacher*, 34(6), 462–467.

Bleakley, A., Bligh, J., & Browne, J. (2011). *Medical education for the future: Identity, power and location*. London: Springer.

Brennan, N., Corrigan, O., Allard, J., et al. (2010). The transition from medical student to junior doctor: Today's experiences of tomorrow's doctors. *Medical Education*, 44, 449–458.

Bullock, A., Fox, F., Barnes, R., et al. (2013). Transitions in medicine: Trainee doctor stress and support mechanisms. *Journal of Workplace Learning*, 25(6), 368–382.

Chambers, M., Hickey, G., Borghini, G., et al. (2016). *Preparation for practice: The role of the HCPC's standards of education and training in ensuring that newly qualified professionals are fit to practise*. http://www.hcpc-uk.co.uk/publications/research/index.asp?id=1144.

Cho, K. K., Marjadi, M., Langendyk, V., et al. (2017). Medical student changes in self-regulated learning during the transition to the clinical environment. *BMC Medical Education*, doi:10.1186/s12909-017-0902-7.

Cleland, J., Patey, R., Thomas, I., et al. (2016). Supporting transitions in medical career pathways: The role of simulation-based education. *Advances in Simulation*, 1(14), doi:.org/10.1186/s41077-016-0015-0.

Cuyvers, K., Donche, V., & Van den Bossche, P. (2016). Learning beyond graduation: Exploring newly qualified specialists' entrance into daily practice from a learning perspective. *Advances in Health Sciences Education*, 21(2), 439–453.

Dahlgren, M. A., Fenwick, T., & Hopwood, N. (2016). Theorising simulation in higher education: Difficulty for learners as an emergent phenomenon. *Teaching in Higher Education*, 21(06), 613–627.

Evans, N. R., Warne, B., & Wood, D. F. (2016). Developing a pragmatic medical curriculum for the 21st century. *Medical Education*, 50, 1192–1194.

Fenwick, T. (2013). Sociomateriality in medical practice and learning: Attuning to what matters. *Medical Education*, 48, 44–52.

Fenwick, T. (2015). Sociomateriality and learning: A critical approach. In D. Scott & E. Hargreaves (Eds.), *The Sage handbook of learning* (pp. 83–93). London: Sage.

Fenwick, T., & Dahlgren, M. A. (2015). Towards socio-material approaches in simulation-based education: Lessons from complexity theory. *Medical Education*, 49, 359–367.

Fenwick, T., Edwards, R., & Sawchuk, P. (2011). *Emerging approaches to educational research: Tracing the sociomaterial*. Abingdon: Routledge.

Gherardi, S., & Rodeschini, G. (2016). Caring as a collecting knowledgeable doing: About concern and being concerned. *Management Learning*, 47(3), 266–284.

Goldszmidt, M. (2017). When I say … sociomateriality. *Medical Education*, 51(5), 465–466.

Goldszmidt, M., & Faden, L. (2016). Is medical education ready to embrace the socio-material? *Medical Education*, 50, 162–164.

Groopman, J. (2007). *How doctors think*. Boston, MA: Houghton-Mifflin.

Hager, P. (2011). Theories of workplace learning. In M. Malloch, L. Cairns, K. Evans, et al. (Eds.), *The Sage handbook of workplace learning* (pp. 17–31). London: Sage.

Hager, P., Lee, A., & Reich, A. (2012). Problematising practice, reconceptualising learning and imagining change. In P. Hager, A. Lee, & A. Reich (Eds.), *Practice, learning and change* (pp. 1–11). London: Springer.

Harris, A., & Delany, C. (2013). International medical graduates in transition. *The Clinical Teacher*, 10(5), 328–332. doi:10.1111/tct.12021.

Hodges, B. D., Martimimakis, M. A., McNaughton, N., et al. (2014). Medical education … meet Michel Foucault. *Medical Education*, 48, 563–571.

Hopwood, N., Rooney, D., Boud, D., et al. (2016). Simulation in higher education: A sociomaterial view. *Educational Philosophy and Theory*, 48(2), 165–178.

Kellett, J., Papageorgious, A., Cavenagh, P., et al. (2015). The preparedness of newly qualified doctors — views of foundation doctors and supervisors. *Medical Teacher*, 37(1), 949–954.

Kilminster, S., Zukas, M., Roberts, T., et al. (2010). Learning practice? Exploring the links between transitions and medical performance. *Journal of Health Organization and Management*, 24(06), 556–570.

Kilminster, S., Zukas, M., Roberts, T., et al. (2011). Preparedness is not enough: Understanding transitions as critically intensive learning periods. *Medical Education*, 45, 1006–1015.

Lave, J., & Wenger, E. (1991). *Situated learning: Legitimate peripheral participation*. Cambridge: Cambridge University Press.

Law, J. (2004). *After method: Mess in social science research*. Abingdon: Routledge.

McMurtry, A., Rohse, S., & Kilgour, K. N. (2016). Socio-material perspectives on interprofessional and collaborative learning. *Medical Education, 50*, 169–180.

Mann, K. V. (2011). Theoretical perspectives in medical education: Past experience and future possibilities. *Medical Education, 45*, 60–68.

Mol, A. (2002). *The body multiple: Ontology in medical practice*. London: Duke University Press.

Mol, A. (2008). *The logic of care: Health and the problem of patient choice*. Abingdon: Routledge.

Monrouxe, L., Bullock, A., Cole, J., et al. (2014). *UK medical graduates preparedness for practice: Final report to the GMC*. http://www.gmc-uk.org/How_Prepared_are_ UK_Medical_Graduates_for_Practice_SUBMITTED_ Revised_140614.pdf_58034815.pdf. (Accessed 14 April 2017).

Morley, D. (2016). Applying Wenger's communities of practice theory to placement learning. *Nurse Education Today, 39*, 161–162.

Morris, C. (2012). Reimagining 'the firm': Clinical placements as time spent in communities of practice. In V. Cook, C. Daly, C., et al. (Eds.), *Work-based learning in clinical settings* (pp. 11–25). London: Radcliffe Publishing.

Nicolini, D. (2011). Practice as the site of knowing: Insights from the field of telemedicine. *Organization Science, 22*(3), 602–620.

Noble, C., & Billett, S. (2017). Learning to prescribe through co-working: Junior doctors, pharmacists and consulting. *Medical Education, 51*, 442–451.

Roberts, J. (2006). Limits to communities of practice. *Journal of Management Studies, 43*(3), 623–639.

Rosenstock, J., & Sparks, G. M. (2016). Training physicians for the real world of medicine: Administration-based learning. *Medical Education, 50*, 1189–1191.

Teunissen, P. W., & Westerman, M. (2011a). Opportunity or threat: The ambiguity of the consequences of transitions in medical education. *Medical Education, 45*(1), 51–59. doi:10.1111/j.1365-2923.2010.03755.x.

Teunissen, P. W., & Westerman, M. (2011b). Junior doctors caught in the clash: The transition from learning to working explained. *Medical Education, 45*, 966–972.

Thrysoe, L., Hounsgaard, L., Bonderup Dohn, N., et al. (2010). Participating in a community of practice as a prerequisite for becoming a nurse—trajectories as final year nursing students. *Nurse Education in Practice, 10*(6), 361–366.

Whitehead, C. R., & Kuper, A. (2017). Faith-based medical education. *Advances in Health Sciences Education, 22*, 1–3.

Wiener-Ogilvie, S., Bennison, J., & Smith, V. (2014). General practice training environment and its impact on preparedness. *Education for Primary Care, 25*(1), 8–17.

Zukas, M., & Kilminster, S. (2014). The doctor and the blue form: A sociomaterial account of professional learning. In T. Fenwick & M. Nerland (Eds.), *Reconceptualising professional learning: Changing knowledges, practices, and responsibilities* (pp. 38–51). London: Routledge.

3

Cultivating critical thinkers

Clinton Golding, Tim Wilkinson and
Althea Gamble Blakey

Introduction

We want our clinical students to be critical thinkers. This seems obvious, even self-evident. Critical thinking is vital for a health professional (Alfaro-LeFevre, 2015; Cooke et al., 2010; Huang et al., 2014; Maudsley & Strivens, 2000; Norman, 2005), and is particularly important for dealing with the uncertainty, unpredictability and ambiguity of clinical settings (Brookfield, 2008; Facione & Facione, 1996; Fonteyn & Ritter, 2008; Gordon et al., 1994). It is essential for making professional judgments and decisions, for independent practice, and for personal growth.

But despite the positive regard we have for critical thinking, what exactly do we mean by this? 'Critical thinking' seems a vague and nebulous term (Davies, 2015; Moore, 2013), and its meaning seems to change in different disciplinary and professional contexts (Jones, 2007, 2009; McPeck, 1981). Even though we want to foster critical thinking, we tend to be unclear about exactly what we mean by this, unclear about what this would involve in our particular clinical setting, and so we are unclear about what we want from our clinical students, and how to teach them critical thinking.

The aim of this chapter is to enable clinical educators to respond to this general lack of clarity about critical thinking. In order to cultivate critical thinking in your clinical students, you must first clarify what you mean by this nebulous term, in your particular context, and then you can articulate what you want from your students, and understand how you might cultivate their critical thinking (Blakey, 2016; Delany et al., 2013; Delany & Golding, 2014; Golding, 2011). So, we will first enable you to understand what kind of critical thinking you want to cultivate in your clinical students, and then offer suggestions for how you might enable your clinical students to be critical thinkers in this way.

First, we will discuss in more detail what we mean by critical thinking and being a critical thinker in clinical education. Then we will discuss four theoretically informed perspectives about how to cultivate critical thinking and critical thinkers:

1. be explicit about what you want;
2. cultivate critical thinking by making it visible;
3. give your students regular and frequent opportunities to practise critical thinking;
4. provide an educative environment that supports the development of critical thinking.

For each of the four perspectives, we also discuss practical strategies for cultivating critical thinking in clinical settings, and we include frequent examples. As our theoretical frame for these four perspectives, we employ a kind of theoretical eclecticism, or pragmatist bricolage (Brandon, 2004; Levi-Strauss, 1966), where we use bits and pieces of theories that we have found to be useful.

We finish this introduction with two caveats about the chapter. First, we will not identify everything relevant to cultivating critical thinking, but will instead focus on some important foundations. Second, while we give examples of critical thinking (and uncritical thinking) in a clinical context, these are not prescriptive. You might articulate this in a different way, because in your context you are interested in a different aspect of critical thinking.

Being a critical or an uncritical thinker

To introduce what we mean by a 'critical thinker', in Table 3.1 we illustrate the difference between an uncritical thinker and a critical thinker in a clinical context (while acknowledging that there is a continuum between the two). We hope the examples illustrate that critical thinking is essential for being an independent health professional. The sentences in italics in the table below indicate examples of what a clinical student might say or do.

There are various reasons why a clinical student may not demonstrate clinical thinking, and these reasons overlap with the concerns from other chapters in this book. For example, a clinical student might not yet demonstrate critical thinking in the clinical setting because they are still becoming accustomed to the differences between class learning and clinical learning. Alternatively, they might lack a fully developed professional identity (Chapter 8), and are still learning to be an independent practitioner rather than a more passive classroom learner (Chapter 9), so the increased cognitive load from their new learning may make it more difficult to learn critical thinking as well. Also, if they are unfamiliar with the new contexts in which they are working, they may find critical thinking more difficult because they do not yet have the experience or the language needed for critical thinking in the new clinical contexts.

Because of the overlap between the development of critical thinking and the concerns from other chapters, the process of learning to be a critical thinker parallels the clinical learning discussed in other chapters. For example, learning to be a critical thinker is similar to learning to be an independent clinician (Chapter 9), and similar to developing a professional identity (Chapter 8). It is important to see this chapter as one lens on clinical learning, which will be enhanced by considering the other lenses.

Our clinical students can, and often do, graduate as critical thinkers, without any deliberate attempt to cultivate critical thinking. They might have 'absorbed' it by 'osmosis' from what they see and hear from their educators and the clinical professionals they observe, and some might independently develop as critical thinkers even without the guidance of teachers. However, this leaves the cultivation of critical thinking mostly to chance, and we are more likely to be successful if we deliberately cultivate this thinking in our students. We can start by developing critical thinking in the pre-clinical aspects of their course, but students still need to learn critical thinking in the clinical environment. The next four sections explain four different theoretically informed strategies for cultivating critical thinking in a clinical environment. For each section we focus on one practical implication of various educational theories.

Be explicit about what you want

The examples in the right-hand column of Table 3.1 illustrate what we mean by being a critical thinker, but it is still a vague and ambiguous account, which is likely to need modification in different health professional contexts. Because of this, and to avoid confusion when cultivating critical thinking, the first theoretically informed strategy is for clinical educators to be explicit and precise about what they mean by

TABLE 3.1: What a clinical student in nursing, physiotherapy, medicine or other allied health practice would do if they were a critical thinker, or if they were not, with examples in italics

Uncritical thinkers would ...	Critical thinkers would ...
Check everything with their supervisor before doing anything. *Is this right? Which dressing shall I use?*	Show initiative and make independent judgments, which they justify. But they also evaluate their judgment and seek further information if required. *This is the usual dressing to use in this situation because of hospital policy and best health benefits, so we should probably use this one. But I have also read that this other dressing has these advantages. What do you [my clinical supervisor] think?*
Mechanically use the tools and strategies they have learned, without making independent judgments for themselves. *After learning how to greet a patient they might inflexibly stick to the script: First, they greet the patient 'Hello', then, even if the patient is crying and obviously upset, they next ask 'How are you feeling today?' because this was the script they had learned.*	Flexibly use the tools and strategies they have learned. They deliberate in response to complex and uncertain environments, and choose to deviate from or modify how they use the strategies when this is useful for the situation. *Although they have learned a script for greeting a patient, they use this flexibly: First, they greet the patient 'Hello', then, if the patient is crying and obviously upset, they deviate from the script and acknowledge the patient's feelings: 'Gosh, you seem upset. Is there something we should talk about first?'*
Disregard some of what they have learned because they do not apply their abstract knowledge in a clinical setting, even when it seems obviously relevant. *When asked 'What is the cause of this child's breathlessness?', they might list all of the causes of breathlessness, and include diagnoses that could not apply in this situation: 'It might be smoking-related emphysema.'*	Use their knowledge and apply this to their current situation. They can 'join the dots' themselves. *When asked 'What is the cause of this child's breathlessness?', they would first rule out impossible diagnoses, and would instead consider the most likely diagnoses: 'Given the risk factors and prevalence in the community, it is probably ..., but I would also need to exclude ...'*
Jump to conclusions. They would not reflect on their thinking, nor examine the potential pros and cons of their deliberations or their judgments. So, they also make assumptions that they never check, and they are prone to various biases. They seem completely unaware of their own thinking processes. *It's x!*	Evaluate their limitations, and their judgment process. So, they notice when they are outside their expertise, and then they seek further information and guidance to help make a better judgment. They uncover and notice their assumptions and then challenge them, and they are aware of their own thinking processes and can evaluate and improve what they are doing. *I think it might be x, but I've never seen x before, only read about it, and I'm not sure about prevalence. I need some more information ...*

critical thinking. The implication is that you should stop talking about critical thinking and instead talk about the specific kinds of thinking you are interested in (Blakey, 2016; Hilsdon & Bitzer, 2007).

Diversity and confusion about critical thinking

Each clinical teacher and each clinical student is likely to have a different, more or less vague conception of critical thinking. For example, even if everyone agrees that critical thinking is about making independent judgments, one student might think this means never asking for help, while another student thinks this means always challenging and disagreeing with those in authority, while one clinical teacher might think it means weighing up options before making a tentative conclusion, and another clinical teacher thinks it means knowing when to ask for help.

To add to this confusion, as well as variations in our personal understandings of critical thinking, there are also diverse understandings in the literature. Critical thinking has been an important concept throughout the literature (Barnett, 1997; Facione, 1990; Paul, 1993), but it has also become a nebulous term, defined in multiple ways by different authors. As Davies summarises:

> 'Critical thinking in higher education' is a phrase that means different things to many people … Does it mean a propensity for finding fault? Does it refer to an analytical method? Does it mean an ethical attitude or a disposition? … Critical thinking in higher education can encompass debates about critical pedagogy, political critiques of the role and function of education in society, critical feminist approaches to curriculum, the development of critical citizenship, or any other education-related topic that uses the appellation 'critical.' Equally, it can be concerned to develop general skills in reasoning — skills that all graduates might possess. (Davies, 2015, p 41)

Some authors isolate critical thinking as a specific 'kind' of thinking, or a specific cognitive 'move'. For example, Paul (1993, p 25) defines critical thinking as 'reason and logic', and in a similar way Ennis (1987) defines critical thinking as 'reasonable rational thinking concerned about what to do or believe' (1987, p 10). A more complex definition of critical thinking can be found in Facione (1990), which summarises the consensus of several expert views on critical thinking:

> Critical thinking is purposeful, self-regulatory judgment which results in interpretation, analysis, evaluation and inference, as well as explanation of the evidential, conceptual, methodological, criteriological or contextual considerations upon which that judgment is based. (Facione, 1990, p 10)

Other authors disagree with giving a universal definition of critical thinking, and argue that critical thinking is not a general kind of thinking, but is different in every context. For example, McPeck (1981) argues that critical thinking about one subject matter is different from critical thinking about other subject matter, and Moore (2004) argues that critical thinking in English is completely different from critical thinking in physics.

To add further confusion, critical thinking also seems to overlap with other kinds of thinking. Critical thinking is often thought to include elements of reflective thinking, which is sometimes called critical reflection (Brookfield, 1987), and clinical reasoning and ethical reasoning are both thought to involve critical thinking. Research often acknowledges this messy overlap between critical thinking and other kinds of thinking, such as clinical reasoning, reflection and metacognition (Brookfield, 2008; Christensen et al., 2008; Forneris, 2004). For more on reflective thinking for clinical practice, see Mann (2008), Aronson (2011), and Fook and Gardner (2012). For more on clinical reasoning, see Norman (2005) and Eva (2005), and for more on ethical thinking see Chapter 5 of this book.

The literature on critical thinking shows how difficult it is to pin down, and this is one of the reasons why it is such a challenging concept to work with in practice. Given the diversity of definitions about critical thinking (and we have only scratched the surface), 'critical thinking' is a good example of a concept that Sartori (1970) describes as having been 'conceptually stretched' because of its multiple, conflicting meanings, so it is now a 'blunted' conceptual tool.

Stop talking about critical thinking and be specific about the thinking you want

While 'critical thinking' is important, the term itself is problematic, so it may be easier to cultivate critical thinking if we refrain from using this confusing term and say what we really mean.

When clinical educators use the term 'critical thinking' this is likely to lead to misunderstanding, or the pursuit of incompatible goals by teacher and students (Blakey, 2016). A clinical teacher might want their students to be critical in the sense of being proactive or showing initiative, but if they merely ask for 'critical thinking' their students are likely to misunderstand. Instead of being proactive, they may think they should argue with the clinical educator, and challenge what they say. Then both the clinical teacher and the student will be frustrated: the teacher will be frustrated that their student doesn't understand being an independent practitioner, and instead seems to be belligerent, and the student will be frustrated because they thought they were doing what they were asked to do. The problems can escalate if the teacher starts to think the student is lazy because they are not being independent, and then the student might react by demanding more guidance, which, ironically, is the opposite of what the teacher wanted. Such frustrations can create disharmony between teacher and student, and potentially for the whole student group (Biggs & Tang, 2011; Blakey, 2016).

Instead of talking about critical thinking in general, it is better to be specific about the particular kind of thinking you are interested in, and why you want your students to develop this thinking.

Case study 3.1

Angela specifically states that she wants her clinical students to develop as independent, proactive thinkers, and then she explains that this means:

- making your own judgments on the basis of evidence and reasons;
- being aware of different sources of information and evidence upon which you can base your judgments;
- noticing where you do not have enough information or evidence to make an informed judgment;
- gathering further evidence when required — for example, by talking with patients and other health professionals, or by reading around the topic on your own.

Then, Angela explains why this thinking is important: 'You need to master independent thinking so you can be a professional, working on your own. You cannot rely on others to do your thinking work for you, so you have to be able to make your own judgments, and justify these. You also need to recognise where you need more information before you can make an informed judgment, or when you need to ask for assistance.'

If you are explicit about the thinking you want, you can also evaluate whether, and to what extent, your students are developing as critical thinkers (Delany & Golding, 2014; Golding, 2011). Your explicit description provides criteria for judging whether or not your students are critical thinkers. For example, you can evaluate their critical thinking based on whether your students make judgments based on evidence and reasons. These criteria will not be explicit if you use the term 'critical thinking' without explanation.

So, if you want your students to be critical thinkers, first decide what specific kinds of thinking you want. The illustration of a critical thinker that we gave in Table 3.1 might be helpful.

Case study 3.2

This is Maya's description of the critical thinking she wants: 'I want my students to be independent thinkers or to show initiative, flexibility and adaptability in their judgments; I want them to deliberate in response to complex and uncertain environments where they apply their knowledge, check assumptions, and evaluate the pros and cons before making careful judgments; and I want them to be critically reflective where they identify their own assumptions and potential biases, and where they reflect on what they are doing well and how to improve.'

The specific kind of thinking you want likely involves a process of thinking, or a series of steps or stages. To cultivate critical thinking you need to be explicit about the whole process and all its steps or stages, so students can understand it from start to finish (Billett, 2016). For example, making an independent judgment involves the following thinking process:

1. You first consider the situation and what you know so you can make an initial judgment (for instance, a judgment about what you will do or say).
2. One of the pitfalls of making an independent judgment is jumping to a conclusion or premature closure without considering alternatives, so next you consider alternative judgments. You might ask: 'If my initial judgment turned out wrong, what might be correct instead?'
3. Then you evaluate whether the alternatives are plausible and consistent with the evidence, or whether you have evidence to discount the alternatives.
4. Finally, if you can't discount the plausible alternatives, you gather further information until you can rule out all but one alternative, which is your independent judgment.

Case study 3.3

Akira wants his clinical students to learn to evaluate. In his clinical context, evaluation involves the following thinking steps:

1. You first articulate the claim, conclusion or judgment you want to evaluate.
2. Then you identify all the pros, and then all the cons (like two lawyers on opposing sides of a case).
3. Finally, you weigh up the relative weight of the pros and cons, and make a final considered judgment (like a judge).

When you articulate the thinking you want, you should make your description consistent with the descriptions used by other clinical educators who also work with your students. When one clinical educator asks their students to evaluate, they should mean the same thing as the other educators who also ask for evaluation. If different clinical educators use the same terms to refer to different kinds of thinking, their students will be confused, and it will be harder for them to learn to be critical thinkers. For example, it will be difficult for students if one clinical teacher uses the term 'reflection' to mean 'figuring out how to improve next time', while another teacher uses it to mean 'uncovering your assumptions' — they are using the same term to talk about two different kinds of thinking.

Even if all of the clinical teachers who work together have one common description of the thinking they want, they can still be asking for different things because they want more or less sophisticated versions of that thinking. For example, if evaluating is described as giving reasons, one clinical teacher might ask for a simple form of evaluation that involves just giving a reason, whereas another teacher asks for a more sophisticated form of evaluation that involves giving reasons for *and* against, before weighing up which side is stronger.

You might also work on developing a shared description of the kinds of critical thinking wanted across a whole course, department or program. This is like building a common language of thinking. To do this you may need to have department- or program-wide discussions about what is meant by critical thinking, evaluation and analysis, for example, and how everyone is going to use these terms so that teaching will be consistent for the students. Note that this is not a discussion about the correct use of these terms, because they have multiple legitimate meanings. This is a conversation about how the terms will be used across a program.

Nonetheless, it is inevitable that there will be some variation about how thinking is labelled and described by different clinicians. Our clinical students will likely be working with practitioners from multiple contexts who may be using the same terms in more or less vague, ambiguous and inconsistent ways. Because of this, we need to assist students to discover what their clinical educators really mean. One useful strategy is to encourage them to say something like the following to their clinical educators: 'I've noticed that different clinicians use the term "reflection" in different ways. What do *you* mean by "reflection"?'

In summary, the term 'critical thinking' is too vague for educative purposes, and we need more precise terms, descriptions and processes which are used consistently by different teachers, and across the different levels of education. When students learn evaluative thinking with one teacher in their first year, they should have a clear description of what this thinking involves. And, ideally it should be the same kind of thinking as the evaluative thinking wanted by a different teacher in the same year, and the same kind of thinking the student will need when they reach their second and third year (although it will be a more sophisticated version of this thinking).

Make critical thinking visible

To cultivate critical thinking, it is essential to be specific about the particular kinds of thinking you are interested in, but this is not enough. Even if thinking is given a specific label, the process of thinking tends to be invisible and mysterious for students. They can see a clinician talking with a patient or a client and then magically making a judgment, but calling this reflection or evaluation doesn't illuminate the apparent magic trick. The student only sees the judgment the clinician makes, not the thinking process that led to this judgment. So, the second theoretically informed strategy is to cultivate critical thinking by making it visible for students (Hattie, 2009; Ritchhart & Perkins, 2008).

Give a concrete description of the thinking

Making thinking visible starts with a concrete description. It is not enough to name the specific type of thinking you want to cultivate, nor to give an abstract description. Whatever abstract name and description you give will be prone to the same sort of misunderstanding we described about the general term 'critical thinking'. For example, a clinical teacher and their students can all have different ideas about what counts as 'evaluating whether the alternatives are plausible and consistent with the evidence'. It is important to also give a *concrete* description of what someone does who engages in this kind of thinking, and in the clinical context you are in (Delany & Golding, 2014).

Case study 3.3 (continued)

Akira describes what a clinician does when they are evaluating a judgment they have made; for instance, about the success of a treatment. They might ask: What are the reasons for thinking it successful? What are the reasons for thinking it unsuccessful?

One way to develop a concrete description is to 'reverse-engineer' your own thinking (Golding, 2011), and articulate short phrases or questions, the thinking behaviours, that identify what a thinker does at each stage in the thinking process (Delany et al., 2013; Delany & Golding, 2014). In other words, you reflect on how you think critically, and then articulate what you do, as a professional, as you critically think through the problems and tasks you face in your clinical practice. For example, when we, the authors of this chapter, reverse-engineered our own critical thinking, we realised that when we were thinking critically we would watch for when we lacked full knowledge, and then we would seek further information. We would say: 'I need to know more about … before I can make an informed judgement.' Before we reverse-engineered our critical thinking, we did not realise that this was an essential component of critical thinking, so our previous students would not have known to do this. See Table 3.2 for more examples.

TABLE 3.2: Some aspects of critical thinking with an explicit description, including the behaviours of critical thinkers

Critical thinking task or thinking move	Description of the thinking	Pitfalls	Behaviours such as questions and sentence starters
Justifying	Giving reasons to back up or support conclusions, decisions and judgments	Fast thinking, and merely reciting what you have been taught, or accepting your first though	Slow down and justify: *Why?* *I think what I should …, because …*
Justifying (more sophisticated)	Comparing evidence and reasons for and against before making a considered judgment	Fast thinking	*What are the reasons for? What are the reasons against? On balance, which is the strongest position?*
Considering alternatives	Suspending judgment until a range of alternatives has been considered. This might also be called open-mindedness or flexible thinking	Being blinkered in your thinking. Sticking with the first thing you think of. Premature closure (Croskerry, 2002; Croskerry et al., 2013a, 2013b)	*What are other possibilities? What else could it be? Another possibility might be …*
Evaluating alternatives	Justifying why you accept one alternative, and why you reject the alternatives	Confirmation bias where you only consider evidence that confirms your initial thought (Croskerry, 2002; Croskerry et al., 2013a, 2013b)	Slow down further, and justify why you rejected the alternatives: *Why might someone else accept a different alternative? Why do I reject the alternatives? I can rule this out, because …*

Continued

TABLE 3.2: Some aspects of critical thinking with an explicit description, including the behaviours of critical thinkers — cont'd

Critical thinking task or thinking move	Description of the thinking	Pitfalls	Behaviours such as questions and sentence starters
Dealing with complex and uncertain situations	Noticing when you do not have full knowledge, being comfortable with uncertainty and not knowing, and being conscious of your competence and incompetence (Croskerry, 2002; Croskerry et al., 2013a, 2013b)	Arrogantly thinking you already have all the answers, or alternatively, being paralysed and indecisive in the face of uncertainty	Find a balance between arrogance and indecision so you make judgments without having perfect knowledge: *What do I not yet know? What else do I need to find out? What else do I need to consider? I know I don't know..., so I need more information about ...*
Checking assumptions	Acknowledging potential biases which you may be unaware of, for example about race, gender, culture or socioeconomic status	Overlooking or ignoring your unconscious assumptions	Double-check the hidden reasons behind your decisions: *What am I assuming here? Is this a justified assumption? Who can I ask to check?*

As well as reverse-engineering your expert thinking, it is also useful to reverse-engineer the thinking of those less experienced. Compare the behaviours of those who are good critical thinkers with those who are not. What is it that differentiates them? What are the traps that poor critical thinkers tend to fall into, and what do critical thinkers do to avoid these traps? For example, a common trap for clinical students is they think they must have an immediate answer. If they fall into this trap, they are likely to stick with the first answer that occurs to them, which is called jumping to a conclusion or premature closure (Croskerry et al., 2013a, 2013b).

A quick, intuitive answer can be fine if the clinical situation is not serious, if time is lacking, or if nothing much hinges on the answer, but it is problematic if the situation is serious and important consequences hinge on the answer given. In this latter case, careful consideration is needed. To avoid this trap, critical thinkers first ask themselves: 'What are the consequences of making this decision?' If there are serious consequences involved, then they take more time to consider alternatives before making a judgment. They consider not only whether they are right, but whether they *know* they are right. They carefully articulate the alternatives, and the evidence that supports or excludes each conclusion, and then explicitly justify why they rejected the alternatives in favour of their decision.

See Table 3.2 for examples of some of the fundamental components of critical thinking that we have reverse-engineered. We have articulated a specific thinking task or thinking move, an explicit description of this thinking, and the pitfalls to be wary of. We also use sentences in italics to indicate the questions a critical thinker might ask, and the things they might say. Note that when you reverse-engineer your own thinking moves, you might articulate them in a different way because you are working in a different context.

Think aloud and model the thinking

As well as offering students a concrete description of what critical thinkers do, say and ask, clinical educators also need to show their students how they think critically. They need to model their thinking process (Ajjawi & Higgs, 2008; Korthagen et al., 2006). This can involve think-aloud strategies, where instead of keeping your thinking internalised, you speak it out loud or write it down, so students can explicitly hear or see your thinking (Durning et al., 2011; Reilly, 2007).

Watching an expert question a patient and seeing where they pay particular attention can be very informative, but it doesn't always illuminate the expert's critical thinking. It is even more informative if the expert explains what they are doing and why they are doing it. This is one reason why the 'think-aloud' approach to teaching clinical reasoning is so effective (Norman & Shannon, 1998). The clinical educator could think aloud after they have seen the patient, or in some cases it will be fine to explain the thinking process in front of the patient while the educator is thinking through what to do; for example, if the patient is well known to the educator and is keen to be an active part of the teaching process.

Case study 3.4

Kath is assessing how to look after a patient who has a leg wound, and she articulates her thinking process for her students: 'First, I ask myself "What is going on here?", and my answer is "They have a leg wound that needs a fresh dressing." And I figured this out because the chart says it was x hours since it was last changed, and I know dressings need to be changed at least this often for best healing. Next I ask myself "What are the key things that will help the healing?", and my answer is "Keep it warm and keep it moist, and use a sterile dressing to avoid infection." Next I ask myself "What are the alternatives I could use ...".'

Sometimes a clinical educator makes judgments on the basis of 'fast thinking' (Kahneman, 2011) or 'analytic thinking' (Eva, 2005), whereby they reach a decision quickly and intuitively without being consciously aware of their thinking process (Bargh, 2011). This can be very mysterious for a clinical student, but the educator can still think aloud by explaining how they are deliberately consulting what their experience intuitively suggests is correct. They can also think aloud how they would double-check their intuitions, or how they would think it through if they did not have a clear intuition.

Case study 3.4 (continued)

Kath is thinking aloud in a different clinical situation where she has made a more intuitive, immediate judgment: 'To check my intuition, I might slow down my thinking and justify why I think my intuition is right, and why I have rejected alternatives. If I had no intuition about what to do, I would systematically go through every step of decision-making as I did in the example of dressing a leg wound.'

A related strategy is to encourage your clinical students to ask other clinicians to explain their thinking processes, whenever it is appropriate to do so (and also help them to manage the rebuffs they might get when the clinician is too busy to explain their thinking out loud).

Give frequent and regular opportunities to practise critical thinking

We cannot cultivate critical thinkers by merely imparting information. We want our students to *be* critical thinkers, and this requires them to build the 'conscious habit' or 'habit of mind' of critical thinking (Costa & Kallick, 2000). They have to learn *how* to think critically (the skill), but they also have to practise and build the *habit* so that it is internalised and becomes part of their professional identity (Cruess et al., 2016), and so they will have a disposition towards being critical (Ennis, 1987; Perkins et al., 1993).

To build a habit of critical thinking, students need opportunities to practise critical thinking. So, the third theoretically informed strategy for cultivating critical thinkers is to give frequent and regular opportunities for students to practise critical thinking, which will explicitly build a culture of critical thinking. Once you have identified what a critical thinker does in your clinical context, then ask your students to do this thinking regularly and frequently in meaningful contexts.

Developing the habit of critical thinking starts with the clinical educators leading and guiding their students, but the support they offer should enable students to learn to go on alone (Golding, 2013). As a thinking guide, you start by modelling critical thinking, then you prompt your students to use some of the questions or phrases a critical thinker uses. At first you might ask your students to follow the thinking processes fairly rigidly, but eventually the students will internalise these thinking moves and processes so that they can use them independently and spontaneously without prompting. The following five methods will be useful for you to support your students to effectively practise critical thinking.

Ask for the particular thinking you want

Explicitly ask your students to engage in the thinking you want, using the same sort of prompts identified in Table 3.2, but developed or tailored for your own particular context. Use the name for the thinking you are interested in ('I want you to *justify* your judgment'), and then use the questions and sentence starters as useful scaffolds to enable your students to engage in the thinking themselves. You might ask them the prompt questions ('Why do you think that judgment is correct?'), or invite them to ask themselves ('Why do I think my judgment is correct?'), and then invite your students to respond using the sentence starters associated with this type of thinking ('I think … is correct because …'). These questions and sentence starters are also useful tools for assessing whether the students engage in the thinking: to what extent do they ask these questions or use these prompts? (Delany & Golding, 2014; Golding, 2011).

Case study 3.5

Whenever she can, Jacinda asks her clinical students to articulate their thinking, because she wants this thinking to become habitual for her students. For example, every time her students are going to do something, she asks them 'Why would you do this? Why did you discount the alternatives?' After regularly and frequently asking these questions of her students, she knows they will start to hear her voice in their head asking them 'Why would I do this?' This is how they begin to internalise this thinking. She also assigns a task for her students to complete every day: 'Write about one decision you saw a clinician make. Why did they make this decision? What were the alternatives they could have made, and why did they discount these?'

Ask students to make their thinking visible

You should also ask your clinical students to make their thinking visible while they do their clinical work. The question prompts from Table 3.2 are also effective for this purpose. For example, while you observe your student, or while you are reflecting on what they did, you might say: 'Let's stop you there and pause. Why did you decide to do that? What alternatives did you consider? Why did you reject those alternatives?'

To foster independent thinking in more advanced students, instead of asking them the prompt questions, ask them to identify the questions they need to address: 'In this situation, what questions do you need to ask yourself to consider alternatives and justify your decision?' The students now have to prompt their own thinking, which is how they further internalise the thinking.

Ask for slow thinking

When you ask students to think, and to make their thinking visible, you are giving them the opportunity to think slow rather than fast (Kahneman, 2011). They need the opportunity to slow down their thinking so that they can check what seems obvious, or check the assumptions that they have made and the facts they rely on. Eventually, they will learn to think fast, where many of their judgments seem to happen automatically — this is the nature of developing expertise (Durning et al., 2011; Eva, 2005; Higgs et al., 2008). But to be an expert they need to be able to slow down their reasoning whenever necessary. One way to slow down student thinking is to avoid asking for the final answer or judgment, and instead ask questions to prompt their thinking, like the questions illustrated in Table 3.2: 'What else did you consider? Why do you explore these possibilities? What information helped you to favour this possibility over another?'

Ask for metacognition

A similar approach for enabling students to effectively practise critical thinking is to model and teach metacognition, reflection, self-evaluation and self-monitoring (Flavell, 1979; Perkins, 1995; Zohar &David, 2009). This 'thinking about thinking' is the process we go through to check whether there are errors in our thinking, and the process by which we monitor, evaluate and improve our thinking. When you ask for metacognition from your students, you are asking them to slow down their thinking and make it visible, so it can be examined, evaluated and improved.

Reflection and metacognition are often included as aspects of critical thinking, so learning reflection and metacognition is part of learning to be a critical thinker (Brookfield, 2008; Christensen et al., 2008; Forneris, 2004). But even if these ways of thinking are not counted as critical thinking, they still help our clinical students to notice how they think and to improve their critical thinking.

Case study 3.6

Zach uses the following metacognitive prompts to encourage his students to focus on their thinking. These build on the questions in Table 3.2:

- How did you come to that decision? What else did you consider?
- Why did you do that? Why did you decide that?
- Why did you rule out other alternatives?
- How did you think through this issue? Explain the process, step by step.
- What was going well with your critical thinking? What was not going so well? How can you improve your critical thinking?

Give feedback for each thinking step

We have suggested that clinical learners need regular and frequent opportunities to practise critical thinking. But we do not want them to repeat or rehearse poor thinking or faulty thinking processes, so we also need to give regular and frequent feedback so that they can improve their critical thinking (Boud & Molloy, 2013, and also see Chapter 21).

There are many reasons why a clinical student might go awry in their thinking, but unless you can 'see' their thinking process, you could easily misdiagnose their difficulty. So before you can give feedback, your students have to make their thinking visible, perhaps using the methods described above. Then you can identify the areas of thinking that need more attention, and you can give timely feedback about their thinking — perhaps they need more work on giving reasons or considering alternatives or suspending judgment before making a conclusion. You might point out that they have missed an important step in their thinking, you might give them a simpler version of the thinking to practise, or you might give them simpler tasks upon which to practise the thinking.

Provide conducive environments for cultivating critical thinkers

We need to provide opportunities for our clinical students to practise critical thinking, but for this practise to be effective, it has to be within a conducive educative environment. In the previous sections we talked about more explicit approaches for cultivating critical thinking, but more tacit approaches are also very important (Burbules, 2008). So, the next theoretical strategy for cultivating critical thinkers is to build an educative environment that can tacitly foster critical thinking.

Learners need an environment where it is safe enough for them to practise critical thinking without fear of ridicule or doing harm, but also challenging enough to stretch them. One way to think about this is using the theoretical lens of Vygotsky and the Zone of Proximal Development (Vygotsky, 1978; Wass & Golding, 2014). You need to ask your clinical students to do critical thinking tasks which are just a little too hard for them on their own, but which they can do with support from you or their peers. When students do these tasks regularly and frequently — the tasks that are within their zone of proximal development — they eventually learn to do them independently, and so they learn to be critical thinkers.

Immerse students in a community of critical thinking

Another way to think about this safe but challenging environment is as a community of critical thinking (Golding, 2011). Surround the learners with visible critical thinking; for example, where you and other clinical students and practitioners think aloud regularly and frequently. In such an environment, students tacitly internalise the thinking that they see and hear happening around them: first they hear you engaging in critical thinking, then they start to tentatively try out some of the critical thinking moves ('I think … because …'), and they hear their fellow students doing this as well, and finally it is something they just do naturally.

Putting this another way, students learn to be critical thinkers by being immersed in a community of critical thinkers (Golding, 2011). They learn by participating in the day-to-day culture of clinical critical thinking. This is often explained as professional socialisation into a community of practice (Ajjawi & Higgs, 2008; Clouder, 2003; Egan & Jaye, 2009; Lave & Wenger, 1991; Wenger, 1998), internalisation of social practices (Vygotsky, 1978), or construction of professional identity (Monrouxe, 2010).

One means of professional socialisation into critical thinking is by observing the critical thinking of the professionals, and we have described methods for facilitating this in the theoretically informed strategy of making thinking visible. When students hear their clinical educators think aloud, they learn the words and ways of thinking in the professional community that they are about to join (Blakey, 2016; Golding, 2011). They get introduced to a new discourse community and a new professional culture.

Another means of professional socialisation is to give students frequent opportunities to engage in critical thinking, and to hear their fellow students do the same. This was described in our theoretically informed strategy about providing opportunities to practise critical thinking.

Overall, what we are recommending is a process of externalising the discourse of the critical thinking community, so that clinical students can then be immersed in it, practise it, and finally internalise it. Internalising the discourse of the critical thinking community can also be understood as a process of enabling students to be independent thinkers (see Chapter 9), or as the process of learning from novice to professional thinking (see Chapter 11).

Congruent teaching

A further way to establish an environment favourable for cultivating critical thinking is to employ congruent teaching techniques (Korthagen et al., 2006; Swennen et al., 2008). For example, you cannot cultivate critical thinking by telling your students what they must do, you have to model critical thinking, question them, and ask for their thinking. Inculcation, or telling students what to do, is incompatible with fostering independent critical thinking.

One congruent teaching technique for cultivating critical thinking is to justify and convince students why they need to learn critical thinking, rather than merely telling them. This strategy will also be important to deal with a likely epistemic block to learning critical thinking. Students may think that your job as an educator is to have the answer, and so your attempts to teach them to be a critical, independent thinker and work it out for themselves can meet with resistance: 'Just tell us the answer!' or 'Why are we wasting time discussing this?' Instead, explain why they need to learn critical thinking, why you are asking them to do the thinking work, and why you ask 'why?' all the time.

Thinking-encouraging approach

To create a conducive environment for critical thinking, clinical educators should also take a 'thinking-encouraging approach' (or a thinking-educating approach), rather than being 'answer-focused' or 'outcome-leading' (Golding, 2011). A thinking-encouraging approach is congruent with cultivating critical thinkers, whereas an answer-focused approach is not.

For some clinical educators, a thinking-encouraging approach might mean a big change from 'normal' practice. For example, you need to be concerned whether your students are engaging in critical thinking, rather than whether they have the right answer; and so you ask for further thinking, rather than telling the learners that they have it right or wrong.

> ### Case study 3.7
>
> Amy is trying to cultivate critical thinking in her students, so she pays more attention to their thinking than to their answers, and takes a thinking-encouraging approach. Whatever answer her clinical students give, whether she agrees or not, she asks them to explain their reasons. She asks not only what the answer might be, but why her students think this is the answer, what else they have considered, and why they have discarded the alternatives. Doing this means that her students learn to both examine their thinking and to judge whether they are correct or not, rather than relying on Amy to do their thinking work for them.

If you are only interested in whether your student has the correct outcome or answer (the outcome you judge to be correct), this will be detrimental for cultivating critical thinking, because it reinforces reliance on a teacher and ignores the thinking process. Instead, to cultivate critical thinking, you must shift your focus from the outcomes to the thinking process itself. You should put aside what you judge to be the correct outcome, and assist students to be more skilful at the process of thinking. Rather than asking 'Does my student have the correct answer?', you ask 'What thinking needs to be done next? How would I do this thinking? How can I ask my student to do this thinking?' Table 3.3 illustrates these two approaches.

TABLE 3.3: Comparing an answer-focused approach and a thinking-encouraging approach

Answer-focused approach: Leading the student, but not cultivating thinking	Thinking-encouraging approach: Encouraging and cultivating critical thinking
Clinician: Is it heart failure or asthma? Clinical student: I think it's asthma. Clinician: Yes, you're right.	Clinician (already knowing it is asthma): Is it heart failure or asthma? Clinical student: I think it's asthma. Clinician: How did you come up with that answer? Why do you think it is correct? Clinical student: Well, they had difficulty breathing, so it had to be asthma. Clinician: But heart failure also leads to symptoms of difficulty breathing. How did you rule that out? Clinical student: I don't know. Clinician: Okay. Let's do more work on considering alternatives.

PRACTICAL TIPS

What can you do to cultivate critical thinkers in a clinical setting? Here is a summary of our practical tips:

1. Be explicit about the thinking you want.
   a. Decide what kinds of critical thinking are needed in your clinical practice, and be explicit that this is what you want from your students.
   b. Work with other clinical educators in your course or program, and create a consistent description of critical thinking that all educators and students use.
   c. Using your shared definitions of critical thinking, you might then refrain from using the term 'critical thinking' and instead say what you really mean.
2. Make the thinking visible.
   a. Give a concrete description of the thinking you want, which includes details about what thinkers do, say and ask.
   b. Demonstrate to your students how you do the thinking.
3. Offer your students regular and frequent opportunities to practise critical thinking.
   a. Ask for the different kinds of thinking you want in all your interactions with your clinical students.
   b. Ask your students to slow down and explain their thinking or think aloud.
   c. Ask students to think about, evaluate and improve their own thinking.
   d. Give feedback on your student's performance for each thinking step.
4. Shape the clinical context into an educative environment that supports the development of critical thinking.
   a. Create a community of clinical thinkers where your students will be surrounded by clinicians and other students all articulating their critical thinking.
   b. Have your students participate in this community of critical thinking by practising their own thinking.
   c. Make sure everything you do is consistent with encouraging critical thinking, and will not undermine this aim.
   d. Take a thinking-encouraging approach with your students, rather than being answer-focused. Concentrate on eliciting and improving their thinking, not getting them to the right answer. Focus not just on the right answers, but also on how do your students justify that it is right.

Further research

There are a number of areas where further research would illuminate how to cultivate critical thinking in clinical education. For each of these areas, we also identify questions that practitioners could address as part of informal research about their own practice:

1. We need to research how healthcare professionals think through their professional problems. How do you, in your particular clinical profession, think through your professional problems? What critical thinking is needed in your everyday practice?
2. We need to research how expertise in critical thinking develops, especially in a clinical context. How did you develop expertise in critical thinking? What was your learning path from novice or student to an expert health professional?
3. We need to research the effectiveness of different strategies for cultivating critical thinking. Which strategies for cultivating critical thinking are the most effective for you in your context? What is needed for them to be the most effective? How much time is needed? How regularly or how frequently? Will they work in a year, or do they require several years?

Conclusion

In this chapter we discussed how you may enable your clinical students to be critical thinkers. While 'critical thinking' is a controversial term, and likely to have variations in different allied health professions, and in different contexts, it is essential for clinical decision-making. We suggest that you can foster critical thinking if you are explicit about what kind of thinking you want from your clinical students, and if you think aloud so that your students have a model to emulate. We also suggest that you invite your students to practise their critical thinking by regularly and frequently thinking aloud, following your model, and that you adapt the clinical environment so that it emphasises and encourages critical thinking.

References

Ajjawi, R., & Higgs, J. (2008). Learning to reason: A journey of professional socialisation. *Advances in Health Sciences Education, 13*(2), 133–150.

Alfaro-LeFevre, R. (2015). *Critical thinking, clinical reasoning, and clinical judgment: A practical approach*. St Louis: Elsevier.

Aronson, L. (2011). Twelve tips for teaching reflection at all levels of medical education. *Medical Teacher, 33*(3), 200–205.

Bargh, J. (2011). Unconscious thought theory and its discontents. *Social Cognition, 29*(6), 629–647.

Barnett, R. (1997). *Higher education: A critical business*. Buckingham: Society for Research into Higher Education & Oxford University Press.

Biggs, J., & Tang, C. (2011). *Teaching for quality learning at university* (2nd ed.). Buckingham: Society for Research into Higher Education & Oxford University Press.

Billett, S. (2016). Learning through health care work: Premises, contributions and practices. *Medical Education, 50*(1), 124–131.

Blakey, A. (2016). *What teachers do, how they do it and who they are* (Doctoral thesis, University of Otago, Dunedin, New Zealand).

Boud, D., & Molloy, E. (2013). Rethinking models of feedback for learning: the challenge of design. *Assessment and Evaluation in Higher Education, 38*(6), 698–712.

Brandon, E. (2004). Philosophy as bricolage. In H. Carel & D. Gamez (Eds.), *What philosophy is: Contemporary philosophy in action* (pp. 132–140). London: Continuum.

Brookfield, S. (1987). *Developing critical thinkers: Challenging adults to explore alternative ways of thinking and acting*. San Francisco: Jossey Bass.

Brookfield, S. (2008). Clinical reasoning and generic thinking skills. In J. Higgs, M. Jones, S. Loftus, et al. (Eds.), *Clinical reasoning in the health professions* (3rd ed., pp. 65–75). Amsterdam: Elsevier.

Burbules, N. C. (2008). Tacit teaching. *Educational Philosophy and Theory, 40*(5), 666–677.

Christensen, N., Jones, M., Higgs, J., et al. (2008). Dimensions of clinical reasoning capability. In J. Higgs, M. Jones, S. Loftus, et al. (Eds.), *Clinical reasoning in the health professions* (3rd ed., pp. 101–110). Amsterdam: Elsevier.

Clouder, L. (2003). Becoming professional: Exploring the complexities of professional socialization in health and social care. *Learning in Health and Social Care, 2*(4), 213–222.

Cooke, M., Irby, D., & O'Brien, B. (2010). *Educating physicians: A call for reform of medical school and residency*. San Francisco: Jossey-Bass.

Costa, A., & Kallick, B. (2000). *Habits of mind. Books 1–4*. Alexandria, Va: Association for Supervision and Curriculum Development.

Croskerry, P. (2002). Achieving quality in clinical decision making: Cognitive strategies and detection of bias. *Academic Emergency Medicine, 9*, 1184–1204.

Croskerry, P., Singhal, G., & Mamede, S. (2013a). Cognitive debiasing 1: Origins of bias and theory of debiasing. *BMJ Quality and Safety, 22*, ii58–ii64.

Croskerry, P., Singhal, G., & Mamede, S. (2013b). Cognitive debiasing 2: Impediments to and strategies for change. *BMJ Quality and Safety, 22*, ii65–ii72.

Cruess, R. L., Cruess, S. R., & Steinert, Y. (2016). Amending Miller's pyramid to include professional identity formation. *Academic Medicine*, *91*(2), 180–185.

Davies, M. (2015). A model of critical thinking in higher education. In M. Paulsen (Ed.), *Higher education: Handbook of theory and research* (pp. 41–92). Cham: Springer.

Delany, C., & Golding, C. (2014). Teaching clinical reasoning by making thinking visible: An action research project with allied health clinical educators. *BMC Medical Education*, *14*(1), 20. doi:10.1186/1472-6920-14-20.

Delany, C., Golding, C., & Bialocerkowski, A. (2013). Teaching for thinking in clinical education: Making explicit the thinking involved in allied health clinical reasoning. *Focus on Health Professional Education*, *14*(2), 44–56.

Durning, S. J., Artino, A. R., Jr., Pangaro, L. N., et al. (2011). Context and clinical reasoning: Understanding the perspective of the expert's voice. *Advances in Health Sciences Education*, *45*(9), 927–938.

Egan, T., & Jaye, C. (2009). Communities of clinical practice: The social organization of clinical learning. *Health*, *13*(1), 107–125.

Ennis, R. H. (1987). A taxonomy of critical thinking dispositions and abilities. In J. Baron & R. Sternberg (Eds.), *Teaching thinking skills* (pp. 9–26). New York: WH Freeman.

Eva, K. W. (2005). What every teacher needs to know about clinical reasoning. *Medical Education*, *39*(1), 98–106.

Facione, N., & Facione, P. (1996). Externalising the critical thinking in knowledge development and clinical judgment. *Nursing Outlook*, *44*(3), 129–136.

Facione, P. A. (1990). *Critical thinking: A statement of expert consensus for purposes of educational assessment and instruction* (The Delphi Report: Executive summary). Millbrae, CA: California Academic Press.

Flavell, J. H. (1979). Metacognition and cognitive monitoring. *American Psychologist*, *34*(10), 906–911.

Fonteyn, M., & Ritter, B. (2008). Clinical reasoning in nursing. In J. Higgs, M. Jones, S. Loftus, et al. (Eds.), *Clinical reasoning in the health professions* (3rd ed., pp. 235–244). Amsterdam: Elsevier.

Fook, J., & Gardner, F. (2012). *Critical reflection in context: Applications in health and social care*. Hoboken: Taylor and Francis.

Forneris, S. (2004). Exploring the attributes of critical thinking: A conceptual basis. *International Journal of Nursing Scholarship*, *1*(1, article 9), 1–18.

Golding, C. (2011). Educating for critical thinking: Thought-encouraging questions in a community of inquiry. *Higher Education Research and Development*, *30*(3), 357–370.

Golding, C. (2013). The teacher as guide: A conception of the inquiry teacher. *Educational Philosophy and Theory*, *45*(1), 91–110.

Gordon, M., Murphy, C. P., Candee, D., et al. (1994). Clinical judgment: An integrated model. *Advances in Nursing Science*, *16*(4), 55–70.

Hattie, J. A. C. (2009). *Visible learning: A synthesis of meta-analyses relating to achievement*. Oxford: Routledge.

Higgs, J., Jones, M., Loftus, S., et al. (2008). *Clinical reasoning in the health professions* (3rd ed.). Amsterdam: Elsevier.

Hilsdon, J., & Bitzer, E. (2007). To become an asker of questions. A 'functional-narrative' model to assist students in preparing postgraduate research proposals. *South African Journal of Higher Education*, *8*(21), 1194–1206.

Huang, G., Newman, L., & Schwartzstein, R. (2014). Critical thinking in health professions education: Summary and consensus statements of the Millennium Conference. *Teaching and Learning in Medicine*, *26*(1), 95–102.

Jones, A. (2007). Multiplicities or manna from heaven? Critical thinking and the disciplinary context. *Australian Journal of Education*, *51*(1), 84–103.

Jones, A. (2009). Redisciplining generic attributes: The disciplinary context in focus. *Studies in Higher Education*, *34*(1), 85–100.

Kahneman, D. (2011). *Thinking, fast and slow*. New York: Farrah, Straus and Giroux.

Korthagen, F., Loughran, J., & Russell, T. (2006). Developing fundamental principles for teacher education programs and practices. *Teaching and Teacher Education*, *22*, 1020–1041.

Lave, J., & Wenger, E. (1991). *Situated learning: Legitimate peripheral participation*. Cambridge: Cambridge University Press.

Levi-Strauss, C. (1966). *The savage mind*. Chicago: University of Chicago Press.

McPeck, J. (1981). *Critical thinking and education*. Oxford: Martin Robertson.

Mann, K. V. (2008). Reflection: Understanding its influence on practice. *Medical Education*, *42*(5), 449–451.

Maudsley, G., & Strivens, J. (2000). Promoting professional knowledge, experiential learning and critical thinking for medical students. *Medical Education*, *34*(7), 535–544.

Monrouxe, L. V. (2010). Identity, identification and medical education: Why should we care? *Medical Education*, *44*(1), 40–49. doi:10.1111/j.1365-2923.2009.03440.x.

Moore, T. (2004). The critical thinking debate: How general are general thinking skills? *Higher Education Research and Development*, *23*(1), 3–18.

Moore, T. (2013). Critical thinking: Seven definitions in search of a concept. *Studies in Higher Education*, *38*(4), 506–522.

Norman, G. (2005). Research in clinical reasoning: Past history and current trends. *Medical Education*, *39*(4), 418–427. doi:10.1111/j.1365-2929.2005.02127.x.

Norman, G. R., & Shannon, S. I. (1998). Effectiveness of instruction in critical appraisal (evidence-based medicine) skills: A critical appraisal. *Canadian Medical Association Journal*, *158*, 177–181.

Paul, R. (1993). The logic of creative and critical thinking. *American Behavioral Scientist*, *37*(1), 21–39.

Perkins, D. (1995). *Outsmarting IQ*. New York: Free Press.

Perkins, D., Jay, E., & Tishman, S. (1993). Beyond abilities: A dispositional theory of thinking. *Merrill-Palmer Quarterly*, *39*(1), 1–21.

Reilly, B. M. (2007). Inconvenient truths about effective clinical teaching. *The Lancet*, *370*(9588), 705–711.

Ritchhart, R., & Perkins, D. (2008). Making thinking visible. *Educational Leadership*, *65*(5), 57–61.

Sartori, G. (1970). Concept misformation in comparative politics. *American Political Science Review, 64*(4), 1033–1053.

Swennen, A., Lunenberg, M., & Korthagen, F. (2008). Preach what you preach! Teacher educators and congruent teaching. *Teachers and Teaching: Theory and Practice., 14*(5–6), 531–542.

Vygotsky, L. (1978). *Mind in society: The development of the higher psychological processes*. Cambridge, MA: Harvard University Press.

Wass, R., & Golding, C. (2014). Sharpening a tool for teaching: The zone of proximal development. *Teaching in Higher Education, 19*(6), 671684.

Wenger, E. (1998). *Communities of practice: Learning, meaning, and identity*. Cambridge: Cambridge University Press.

Zohar, A., & David, A. B. (2009). Paving a clear path in a thick forest: A conceptual analysis of a metacognitive component. *Metacognition and Learning, 4*(3), 177–195.

4

Cultivating resilient learners

Clare Delany, Samantha McLeod and Jill Klein

Introduction

Clinical workplaces can be unpredictable and stressful for health professional trainees and students. They are shaped by the changing needs of patients, driven by externally set competencies and expectations (Delany & Watkin, 2009; Rowe et al., 2012), and involve hierarchical relationships between students, supervisors and other colleagues (McAllister & McKinnon, 2009). Such an environment is acknowledged to be stressful for students and junior doctors (Lemaire & Wallace, 2017), especially during times of transition to new placements or new roles (Yaghmour et al., 2017). Clinical learning and practice requires students and practitioners to continually adjust and orient their university-acquired clinical knowledge to the culture, expecations, systems and relationships within clinical situations (Billett, 2001; Egan & Jaye, 2009; Van de Wiel et al., 2011). In addition, the focus of medical and other health professional training, and their associated professional accreditation bodies, is on achieving competencies and emphasising the high-stakes consequences of not being adequately competent. The focus on competency is important for ensuring and maintaining high standards of practice, but it neglects to acknowledge the fallibility and uncertainty which is also a part of healthcare work (Goldberg et al., 2002), or the strengths that students and trainees can bring to the clinical encounter (Delany & Bragge, 2009). As a consequence, health professional students are instilled with ideals of perfection that can be difficult to realise in practice (Scott et al., 2009). They are inclined to individualise their responsibility for mistakes or poor progress, rather than seeing error and setbacks as a potential opportunity for ongoing learning (McGivern & Fischer, 2012).

Resilience for clinical learning

The idea of resilience originated in the disciplines of psychiatry and developmental psychology, based on studies of the personality traits of children who managed to adapt positively and to thrive despite negative life outcomes and experiences (Waller, 2001). These conceptual beginnings led to definitions and descriptions of resilience which emphasised it as a personal quality: an 'adaptive stress resistant personal quality that permits one to thrive in spite of adversity' (Ahern et al., 2008, p 32); an ability to maintain personal and professional wellbeing in the face of ongoing work stress and adversity (Luthar et al., 2000); a protective factor that enhances the ability to manage stress (Kinman & Grant, 2011); and, importantly for this chapter, as a skill that can be acquired through practice.

The development of resilience as an attitude and behavioural response is increasingly promoted as a way to counter negative responses to clinical learning and practice, and, more broadly, as a necessary characteristic to promote lifelong learning in complex, unpredictable and multi-stakeholder clinical environments (Sterling, 2010; Tempski 2012). People who have resilient qualities are more disposed to take on learning challenges, and to persist with learning despite confusion, frustration or setbacks (Wells & Claxton, 2002). In health professional practice, high levels of resilience have been shown to assist in developing a strong sense of professional identity, enabling effective collaboration with others (Adamson et al., 2014; Wald et al., 2015).

In contrast, low levels of resilience can interfere with a person's ability to take in information and to step back and reflect on their own understandings and interpretations (Wald et al., 2015). Students who are stressed or not coping with aspects of their learning are less able to regulate their emotions (Grant et al., 2014), and require more teaching time and educational resources (Lake & Ryan, 2005). They are less inclined to use professional and ethical concepts and reasoning skills to respond to adverse, uncertain or challenging clinical sitations (Wald et al., 2015). Students low in resilience tend to adopt disengaged coping skills, and avoid or deny problems or stressors (Adamson et al., 2014), or they may blame others for their stressors (Delany et al., 2015). These types of responses and behaviours can, in turn, impair the formation of students' professional identity, their sense of personal and professional purpose (Benard, 2004; Wald, 2015), and the attention they give to patient care (Elliott, 2002; Firth-Cozens, 2001a, 2001b; Radcliffe & Lester, 2003; Rompf et al., 1993; Seaward, 2004; Walsh et al., 2010). Building personal resilience is therefore important for students in health disciplines, because it potentially contributes to all stages of their career and standards of practice (Eley & Stallman, 2014).

However responsibility for the development of resilience should not only reside within the individual (Oliver, 2017). Learning and teaching in health workplaces involves a whole community of people (Cruess et al., 2016), and an individual student is buffeted by a range of sociocultural and political forces that shape the clinical workplace. These forces include financial and patient through-put targets imposed by health-funding models, ever-diminishing healthcare resources (staff and direct funding), and local institutional and professional responses to error or perceived stressors in clinical practice (Klein et al., 2017).

Referring to similar forces in higher education, James (2014, p 160) suggests that although learning, teaching and assessment are 'fundamentally individual activities', they are located in an institutional, geographical, political or economic context or setting. This situational understanding of the complex and dynamic influences impacting on clinical learning and teaching is well acknowledged in other chapters in this book. It also has important implications for how clinical educators and institutions can play a role in supporting students to develop higher levels of resilience.

The goals of this chapter are to:
1. define and describe individual dimensions of resilience grounded in psychological theory and applied to the sociocultural environment of clinical education;
2. focus on specific strategies educators can use to both explicitly teach, and to more broadly and proactively cultivate, resilience for clinical learning and future health professional work; and
3. highlight the cultural, political, institutional, curricula and pedagogical arrangements required to take resilience and more broadly health workforce wellbeing seriously.

The chapter begins wth case study 4.1, which includes two perspectives, the first of which provides some details of Sophie, an experienced clinician and clinical educator (in physiotherapy), but her story is applicable to other health professionals. Sophie has recently attended a workshop on resilience for learning. However, she is unsure about how to incorporate the idea of resilience in her everyday education practice. The case also focuses on Win, one of Sophie's final-year physiotherapy students, who has experienced a dip in her confidence after almost failing her previous placement.

After outlining the experiences and thoughts of both the educator (Sophie) and the learner (Win), we describe specific psycho-educational strategies that clinical educators can use to assist students to develop resilient responses to common learning and health practice challenges (*reactive resilience education*). We also highlight the need for broader-based strategies for cultivating a learning environment to more proactively lay the foundations within the workplace that enable resilient characteristics to flourish (*proactive resilience education*).

Case study 4.1

Sophie is a senior physiotherapist who works in a busy respiratory ward in a large tertiary hospital. She has been responsible for supervising and educating second-year physiotherapy students on clinical placement for 8 years. She is also responsibile for mentoring and developing professional development activities for the musculoskeletal group of clinician teachers in the department. Sophie has recently attended a workshop on the role of resilience in clinical learning.

Interview with Sophie

Sophie: 'Next week I have a group of four students arriving for their third of four clinical placements as part of their final-year clinical placements. I would like to use some strategies to build their resilience for learning. I have noticed that some students seem to "bounce back" from setbacks in their clinical placements, and seem to learn from their errors and from the feedback I give them about how they could improve. They are confident and take the initiative to learn from different clinical situations. Other students who have very similar learning experiences seem to lose their confidence, especially after less positive feedback. They seem to withdraw, gradually perform more poorly over the placement, and don't seem to take on the mantle or identity necessary to become a graduate physiotherapist. The workshop I attended on resilience discussed how cultivating and deliberately nurturing resilience was an important part of my role. But there were not many strategies about how to teach or include it in the usual clinical placement learning. And ... I am aware that I don't feel very resilient on some days as I try to cope with my clinical load, administrative tasks and student training requirements.'

Notes from interview with Win

Win is a 24-year-old final-year physiotherapy student. She is from Malaysia, and has received a partial scholarship to complete her physiotherapy degree in Australia. Her parents have taken on extra work to fund the remaining costs for her study. Win has found her last two clinical placements to be very different. In the first placement, her supervisor was both supportive and encouraging, and Win had felt (for the first time) an increasing sense of confidence in her capacity to prescribe appropriate exercises and to conduct assessments of patients within the post-surgical ward in orthopaedics. During this first placement, she began to feel that perhaps she could actually work as a physiotherapist and to make a difference in patients' recovery.

However, in the second placement, in a neurological rehabilitation setting, the centre itself was understaffed and going through a restructure. Her supervisor changed several times. Win found that her supervisors were impatient with the time she took to conduct an assessment of a patient, and they all tended to focus on what she had failed to do, highlighting treatment errors. By the end of this second placement, Win had slipped back to the more familiar state of mind she had been in during her first two years of the physiotherapy program; a feeling of anxiety that she may not be good enough to get through the course, and to work to pay off her loans and work as a physiotherapist, and that maybe she should just join the family business in Malaysia instead, and not continue with her studies.

Theories and dimensions of resilience

Common to definitions of resilience is the idea that positive adaptation acts as a counter to different types of adversity (Adamson et al., 2014). Resilience appears to work as a protective factor to enhance the ability to manage stress associated with adversity (Kinman & Grant, 2011), and, applied to health professional practice, to assist a person to progress along the developmental trajectory of professional identity formation (Howe et al., 2012; Wald, 2015).

Resilience is, therefore, a dynamic construct involving processes of positive adjustments made in challenging life conditions and circumstances (Luthar et al., 2000, p 546). For example, a student may demonstrate resilience in a particular phase of their professional learning or work, but if their personal circumstances change, or the judgments of their peers or educators become less supportive, then they may not maintain the same level of resilience (Day et al., 2006; Delany et al., 2015).

This dynamic idea of resilience also has implications for clinicians as they take on the role of educator. In a four-year longitudinal study of variations in classroom teachers' effectiveness, Gu and Day (2007) identified three factors that affected teachers' capacity to sustain their commitment to education practice, and their resilience to challenges in that role: 1) personal (related to their lives outside school); 2) situated (related to their lives within school); and 3) professional (related to their values and beliefs, and the interactions between these and external policy agendas). A change in one would affect the capacity to manage another (Gu & Day, 2007).

A common misconception is that resilient people are almost always optimistic, or have frequent positive experiences and are free from negative emotions or thoughts. However, in reality resilient individuals tend to expect and move with adversity, accept negative experiences and emotions as equally as positive experiences, and tend to bounce back and grow from difficult challenges (Sarkar & Fletcher, 2014). Dimensions of resilience include a positive and proactive personality, having a sense of control, flexibility and adaptability, achieving balance, and maintaining perspective and social support.

In the school setting, Martin and Marsh (2008, p 55) use the term *academic buoyancy* rather than resilience, and describe this as an 'ability to successfully deal with academic setbacks and challenges that are typical of the ordinary course of school life' (Martin & Marsh, 2008, p 54). These authors identify five dimensions of resilience (5 Cs) which are predictive of individual student resilience (Martin & Marsh, 2008):

1. confidence or self-efficacy;
2. capacity to plan;
3. a sense of control of the learning environment and of learning strategies;
4. composure and low levels of anxiety; and
5. commitment or persistence to study.

Martin and Marsh's 5 Cs focus on the dimensions and characteristics that enable an individual to thrive in their learning and practice journey. Educational strategies which flow from these dimensions include targeted and specific behavioural and cognitive strategies that a student can learn to build their resilience to address specific stressors in their learning and practice. We use and expand upon the 5-Cs framework in our suggestions for supporting the development of resilience in students for clinical learning.

Psycho-education strategies for teaching and cultivating resilience

The education strategies draw from three psychological domains: cognitive behaviour therapy (CBT), sport and performance psychology (SPP), and positive psychology (PP). All three domains are goal-focused, strength- and skills-based, and operate from the premise that cognitive processes (thoughts, beliefs, attitudes, values, images) affect feelings and behavior, which in turn can be monitored and altered through cognitive change (Dobson & Khatri, 2000). The three domains reflect the combination of cognitive, performative and contextual elements of resilience (Miyamoto et al., 2015).

Historically, CBT has been applied in the area of clinical psychology (i.e., mental health), by focusing primarily on eliminating unhelpful patterns of cognitions, behaviours and emotional regulation (Beck, 2011). Some examples of CBT strategies include monitoring and reframing self-talk, goal-setting, activity planning and pacing, relaxation, and communication skills or assertiveness training. A CBT focus emphasises awareness and understanding of the causes of distress, and seeks to match adaptive coping strategies, which include personal control, commitment, composure, and confidence/self-efficacy. These types of characterisitics have also been described as a type of hardiness (Kobasa et al., 1982; Maddi, 2006), mental toughness (Connaughton et al., 2010), or grit (Duckworth et al., 2007; Von Culin et al., 2014), and include a capacity to adopt growth mindsets (Klein et al., 2017; Yeager & Dweck, 2012).

The idea of adopting a growth mindset as a form of CBT derives from mindset theory, which holds that our implicit assumptions about the origins of abilities such as intelligence and talent have a strong impact on how we view setbacks (Dweck et al., 1995). Those with a fixed mindset believe that ability is endowed and static, and thus a setback indicates a lack of ability. Those with a growth mindset view ability as acquired through effort, practice and learning from mistakes, and thus a setback represents an opportunity for development and improvement. Research shows that this fundamental difference in how abilities are viewed has a powerful impact on resilience in the face of adversity (Tabernero & Wood, 1999).

Sports and performance psychology (SPP) is the second psychological domain that is relevant to frame resilience-based education strategies in clinical learning. We suggest that demonstrating competence in skills of assessment, diagnosis, communication, and treatment formulation is a type of performance. Sports and performance psychology focuses on equipping athletes and performing artists to achieve optimal mental wellbeing for the attainment of specific goals, tasks or pursuits under pressure. The techniques include: how to harness concentration for the task; training for specific physiological outcomes of strength and endurance; and deliberate practice and visualisation of a skill or the performance of a specific technique (Balague, 2005; Murphy, 2005). These same goals and techniques are also relevant for clinical skill acquisition and performing clinical tasks in high stakes clinical environments, and therefore applying SPP principles in an academic setting has similar advantages. Some examples of performance enhancement strategies include: realistic goal-setting; stress level or heightened arousal regulation; self-efficacy building (via imagery rehearsal); as well as finetuning of focus, attention and endurance (e.g., graded goals; task-focused rather than outcome-focused).

A third psychological domain relevant to resilience education is positive psychology (PP). Positive psychology emphasises the importance of positive experiences, personal growth, flourishing, and focusing on one's values, strengths or talents and on what one can achieve, rather than psychological disfunction (Linley et al., 2006; Seligman et al., 2000). Using PP as a model for building resilience means: focusing on emotional regulation; mindfulness; identification and acknowledgment of strengths and virtues and achievements; and engagement in passions or pleasurable activities. Although mostly directed towards individual students, PP concepts are also relevant beyond the individual. In the proactive resilience education section below, we identify principles to guide learning goals, and to establish workplace cultures and systems, which incorporate principles of PP, including valuing and showcasing students' strengths, and fostering a supportive learning environment. There is a burgeoning literature on the important role that schools and school learning environments can play to develop the 'whole child' with a balanced set of cognitive, social and emotional skills, so that they are equipped to face the challenges of the twenty-first century (Miyamoto et al., 2015). These same ideals are also being recognised as relevant to health education (Howe et al., 2012).

Reactive resilience education

We describe reactive resilience education as an approach to build resilience, based predominantly in the first two psychological domains — CBT and SPP. It involves assisting students to first recognise their usual responses to adverse situations, and then providing them with skills that assist them to reframe their responses to more positive coping strategies.

Tables 4.1 and 4.2 draw directly from a program of resilience education in physiotherapy (Delany et al., 2015). The program involved a small sample of health professional (physiotherapy) students. Other studies have used similar resilience-promoting interventions (Dyrbye et al., 2010; Wald 2015).

The psycho-education program for physiotherapists was led by a clinical health psychologist (author SM) and educator (author CD). Resilience strategies were introduced to specifically address student stressors and to build practical skills-based resilience. The pedagogical premise of the program was that by developing students' coping skills they would learn how to build a sense of their own self-efficacy, and then learn to use cognitive techniques to be more in control of their own reactions, responses and strategies, to problem-solve and think creatively and purposefully (Padesky & Mooney, 2012). Table 4.1 lists the four steps of the program. The students were first invited to identify stressors they had experienced in their clinical learning, and to discuss their beliefs about, and reactions to, these stressors. They were then given a series of positive coping skills they could use to reframe their reactions (see Table 4.2). The final step was to report back to the group after they had trialled one of the strategies. Six final-year undergraduate physiotherapy students attended four action research sessions led by a clinical health psychologist.

TABLE 4.1: Strategies for an educator to use to identify and match a resilience strategy to address a clinical learning/practice stressor

Building resilience in students	Example
1. Identify stressors Allow students to identify clinical learning stressors, from their perspective	• Have students identify the stresses that they encounter on clinical placement learning • Enhance students' understanding of those stressors by positioning them within the range of possible learning stressors
2. Probe students beliefs and concerns about their stressors, and begin to identify their strengths and coping capacities	• Ask students to identify how they felt when the stress occurred • What are they worried will happen? • Ask students to be specific about their concerns • Ask students to identify how they cope with similar stresses in other areas of their life
3. Match student stressor with positive coping strategy	• Invite students to nominate a positive coping strategy (see Table 4.2), which matches and potentially counters their beliefs and concerns and feelings • Ask students to indicate how they will use this strategy in their clinical placements
4. Evaluate the impact	• Provide a debrief opportunity to enable students to discuss which strategy they used and the impact it had on their learning experience

The seven resilience strategies (7 Cs) (see Table 4.2) used in the program were drawn predominantly from CBT and performance psychology, and built on the 5 Cs proposed by Martin and Marsh (2008). Box 4.1 provides some examples of phrases used within the program to probe students' descriptions of stressors, and to raise students' awareness of the reactions, beliefs and values they were expressing when describing their stressors and responses. Increasing their awareness and capacity to recognise their responses, and to understand their genesis, encouraged students to consider how they could change their habitual responses to stress and anxiety triggers. Over the six-week research period, students' initial descriptions of stressors as 'problems' outside their control, which had resulted in poor thinking and communication, low confidence and frustration, changed to a focus on how they managed and recognised learning challenges as normal, or at least as expected elements of the clinical learning environment. The program outcomes provided some evidence for the idea that replacing or reframing stressful challenges using positive coping strategies offers a potentially powerful tool to build self-efficacy and cognitive control, as well as greater self-awareness as a learner and future health practitioner (Delany et al., 2015).

Proactive resilience education

However, as outlined in the introduction, if resilience is taken to be a multidimensional and dynamic construct that is impacted on by relationships, work cultures and individual self-efficacy, then it may not be enough for educators to merely give students information about resilience and strategies to practise (Oliver, 2017). To promote and broadly cultivate positive coping strategies for students and trainees, educators will need to not only be cognisant of the range of specific (internal) dimensions of resilience and their relevance for different types of adversity, but they will also need to explicitly acknowledge the interrelationships between internal (personality-based) and external (workplace-based) factors, including their own impact as role models as resilient practitioners. As Gu and Day (2007, p 1302) state: 'it is unrealistic to expect students to be resilient if their teachers who constitute their primary source of role models do not demonstrate resilient qualities'.

Drawing on PP principles, we suggest that clinical educators need to acknowledge the challenges inherent in clinical learning, and deliberately nurture positive learning experiences designed to build more general reserves of psychological resilience for future adverse events (Sterling, 2010). Fredrickson (2001) uses the term 'broaden and build', and suggests that it is possible to cultivate more durable resilience through the

TABLE 4.2: Explicit strategies for developing resilience: using 7 Cs

7 Cs (dimensions of resilience)	Examples of resilience strategies	Specific cognitive and behavioural actions
Cognitive control	• Locus of control • Growth vs fixed mindset • Mindfulness/arousal • Monitoring	• Be aware of your response to an adverse event (learning or practice): shift the interpretation from blaming a lack of knowledge to seeing an opportunity for learning • Be aware/mindful of your level of stress. Notice your breathing, emotional feeling, capacity to think clearly (too stressed means you will not be able to access your knowledge or think clearly) • Strategies to control anxiety: *Deep breathing/relaxation/time-out/communicate*
Coping	• Prepare for setbacks • Pleasurable activities/exercise, diet, sleep	• Be prepared rather than surprised when you meet external challenges in clinical placement • Develop some coping skills, such as pleasurable activities to balance; log your achievements in other areas; keep each clinic in perspective as one clinical placement out of many
Composure	• Emotional regulation • Arousal monitoring • Centring • Breathing • Mindfulness	• Use controlled breathing and mindfulness regularly so that you can access them in challenging learning situations
Confidence	• Link to long-term career goals • Vision • Identify peak performance • Log achievements • Coping statements based on strengths and past experiences	• Maintain your own confidence by logging past achievements and keeping an eye on your larger goals, rather than being dependent on others
Communication	• LADDER script (Davis et al., 2008) • 'I' statements	• Remember to focus on achieving one rung of your career ladder at a time. All professionals keep learning in their area. It is not realistic that you are perfect after 1–2 clinical placements • Be aware of your needs and your responses, and use 'I' sentences
Coordination	• Time management • Process vs outcome • Pacing	• Focus on the process of treating a patient (what are their needs), rather than focusing on the outcome of the treatment (your mark or assessment)
Commitment	• Mapping goals	• Keep long-term goals in mind — to graduate as a physiotherapist rather than to achieve a perfect mark in a clinical placement

---

Box 4.1: Examples of phrases educators can use to encourage resilient thinking approaches

Practical approach

Composure

- You seem angry/frustrated/nervous/worried.
- Lots of students find this situation to be challenging.
- I notice by your breathing that you seem anxious.
- How do you feel when you are feeling confident — is it different to this?

Cognitive control

- Can you describe what you are mainly concerned about?
- What is your main worry?
- What do you believe will happen?
- What do you need to do for this patient now?
- What do you need to focus on?
- How stressed do you feel?

Confidence

- Can you think about the last time you managed to organise several tasks?
- Can you tell me all of the tasks you need to do? Is it possible to break them down into chunks?
- We want you to thrive in this job.
- Can you visualise where you will be in two days/months/years?

Coordination

- Can you identify your main goals for this week/month/year?
- How do these goals relate to your longer-term career goals?
- What do you need to do to get there?
- Can you visualise yourself achieving your goals?

Commitment

- Can you identify your main goals this week/month/year?
- How do these goals relate to your longer-term career goals?

Source: Beck (2011), Benard (2004), Wells (2002).

---

mechanism of experiencing positive emotions (within learning experiences). As a result, she observes that learners can 'transform themselves, becoming more creative, knowledgeable, resilient, socially integrated and healthly individuals' (Fredrickson, 2004, p 1369).

This broader approach to cultivating resilience represents a type of proactive education that recognises the pervasive influence of the learning environment, including the hidden curriculum, where informal processes — such as the observation of other professionals' behaviour, values and attitudes — can influence students' professional skills and outlook (Hafferty & Franks, 1994, p 861). Using strategies drawn from positive psychology, the idea is to actively cultivate a visible and positive learning environment and curriculum, which deliberately builds self-confidence and professional identity through positive relationships with colleagues and peers, and active participation in the learning environment (Delany and Bragge 2009; Wald, 2015).

The approach of taking positive experiences of learning seriously relies on viewing a student's personal welfare to be as important as learning experiences designed to develop specific disciplinary competencies. Barnett (2015) has previously described a similar educational idea when discussing the role of higher education more generally: to give students the space to become themselves, and to bring their understandings to bear on situations so that they develop the capacity for critical insight into their own actions, and their identity as a practitioner who is able to positively cope. Hargreaves (1998, p 835) also captures the essence of this more holistic approach to education practice in the following account of good teaching (in higher education):

> Good teaching is charged with positive emotions. It is not just a matter of knowing one's subject, being efficient, having the correct competencies, or learning all the right techniques. Good teachers are not just well-oiled machines. They are emotional, passionate beings who connect with their students and fill their work and their classes with pleasure, creativity, challenge and joy.

The challenge proposed by these ideas is both simple and complex. It requires educators to support and build positive learning experiences for students, not by focusing on their capacity to perform successfully (through tests of competence), but through a broader cultivation of positive learning and work environments. Focusing on building positive relationships and getting to know students and their needs sounds simple, but in the context of hierarchical and competency-driven clinical work environments and pressures, it can be challenging to achieve. Table 4.3 lists principles for developing confidence and positive learning experiences for students. It is based on a previous study of educators' and students' conceptions of what makes a good teacher (Delany & Bragge, 2009). In that study, a key difference that emerged between students' and educators' perspectives of their role was their respective descriptions of how to support learning within clinical placement settings. The clinical educators' conception of their teaching role was to impart structured knowledge to students in response to knowledge deficits. In contrast, the students proposed alternative practical and relational ways to build their knowledge. Their conception of learning involved building relationships with colleagues and learning through positive and supportive learning experiences. The BUILD framework sets out five principles that aim to broaden the educational focus from ensuring specific competencies are met and skills are attained (both of which are important), to also nurturing resilience and supporting sustained wellbeing.

TABLE 4.3: Building resilience through positive learning experiences: the BUILD framework

Education principle	Interpretation
BUILD confidence in students	This principle identifies the need to actively build students' esteem or confidence within the clinical learning placement. This requires a focus not only on students' weaknesses, but also a preparedness to recognise and name students' strengths and possible contributions to the community of health practitioners.
UNDERSTAND students' perspectives	Each student brings their own interpretation or perspective to the learning environment. Therefore, to more effectively engage with students and to encourage them to take on responsibility for planning and self-regulation, there needs to be a commitment to understanding their individual perspective and learning needs.
INSIST on reflection within and about learning	Students are active learners and can identify, through reflection, learning strategies that assist their learning needs. To tap into students' knowledge and understanding, and to reinforce their capacity to contribute to their own learning, clinical education processes and structure should insist on and explicitly value active and regular reflection as a key component of the education process.
LIST strategies for students to actively learn new skills	This includes not only strategies performing set disciplinary competencies, but also broader strategies, such as the importance of collaborating with colleagues and building relationships.
DECIDE on actions to promote each student's clinical skill learning	Acknowledge students' strengths, and develop learning goals in a collaborative and mutually respectful manner.

Adapted from C. Delany & P. Bragge. (2009). A study of physiotherapy students' and clinical educators' perceptions of learning and teaching. *Medical Teacher, 31*(9), e402–e411.

Key messages from the psychoeducation program

The key feature of both the reactive and the proactive resilience education strategies described above are that they are multidimensional. Learning to be resilient is similar to the concept of learning to be a health professional or a teacher (see Chapter 22). It is a cognitive, emotional, sociocultural process which occurs over time, and relies on positive reinforcement, and on learning and teaching relationships built on trust (Higgs & McAllister, 2007). Educators, for their part, need an awareness of how dimensions of resilience (composure, cognitive control, confidence, coordination and commitment) can be modelled and introduced to students. But more broadly, as Eley and Stallman (2014) suggest, educators need to be brave enough to allow students the space and opportunity to learn skills of self-management, planning and self-regulation. This cannot be achieved in clinical workplaces by telling students how they should respond. Instead, it requires modelling of resilient responses, and the deliberate creation of environments where students feel safe to be more open, reflective and emotionally able to change (Eraut & Hirsh, 2010). To influence clinical education environments in this broader way, educators will also need professional development support from their institutions and colleagues, to align both visible and hidden elements of the clinical learning environment.

Learning to be resilient can be transformative, as students are facilitated to open up their thinking to new and previously unfamiliar or inaccessible ways of processing and responding to their learning and practice experiences (Delany et al., 2015; Meyer & Land, 2003). For educators to incorporate resilience-building strategies into their clinical placement education, they will need to assist students to recognise the intrinsic skills and capacities they have to respond 'positively' rather than 'negatively' to the stressors of clinical placement learning. This will require teachers to assist students to work through the 'self-recognition' phase, and then have them 'practise' the resilience skills, and finally 'evaluate' its impact on their learning and performance.

Case study 4.1 (continued): How might this information assist Sophie with planning for clinical education?

Sophie decides to incorporate the four steps (Table 4.1) of identifying a source of stress and then matching that stressor and student response to the stressor into her education practice. In her first introductory tutorial, Sophie plans to set aside 15 minutes to introduce the idea of resilience for learning, and she prepares a handout with the 7 Cs (Table 4.2). She plans to ask each student to nominate a stressor from a previous or current placement, and then ask them to choose a resilience strategy that could be relevant in their current placement.

Sophie also plans to make time to speak with each student separately, to find out more about their past experiences, the highs and lows in their learning, and their future plans. Finally, Sophie plans to consciously focus on a positive aspect of each students' performance early in the placement, to provide a positive substrate for their progress.

Back to Win

Although Win was feeling apprehensive and disillusioned when arriving for this clinical placement, she was surprised and relieved when her supervisor, Sophie, made some time in the first tutorial to discuss some common stressors in clinical learning, and asked each of the students to discuss their experiences. Win felt herself relax a little when listening to fellow students discuss their experiences, and she realised she wasn't the only one to have had ups and downs in her level of confidence about her capacity to be a physiotherapist. Win chose to trial a simple resilience response of building her *composure* by monitoring her breathing when assessing patients. Through talking through her responses, she realised that she would often hold her breath and become highly anxious when a supervisor was observing her techniques with patients.

When Sophie arranged a time to have a coffee with her, Win also felt really pleased. It felt to her like Sophie was treating her as a physio colleague, and not just a student to assess and to find faults. She already felt more confident in this placement, and was looking forward to learning and working with patients.

PRACTICAL TIPS

Jo has been an emergency physician for 25 years, and always receives excellent feedback from her students. One of the recurring themes of this feedback is that students come away from the placement saying they feel more confident about their practice, both in emergency settings and more generally for their future practice.

Interviewer: You have been a clinical teacher for the past 25 years, and your students always give good feedback about their time with you, and amazingly they almost always mention feeling more confident. What is your philosophy of teaching? How do you manage to have this effect?

Jo: Over the years I have developed a number of strategies in my teaching. I purposely set out to build *confidence* in my students. I have observed, and I know from my reading, that if students are nervous or anxious (*composure*), they do not perform well.

So my first teaching tip is to focus on myself. One of the most strategic teaching activities I use is to make sure I can demonstrate how to stay composed and how to *communicate* with colleagues, and always setting out the logic of my decision-making. When I first started teaching, I would focus most strongly on what I needed to teach students, but over time I've found I get much better results by first focusing on my own practice and modelling my processes of thinking and responding. It is a cliché, but students learn from how I do things.

My second teaching tip is to clarify the *goals* of emergency medicine work; that is, the real goals of practice in this area of the hospital. In the emergency department, the goals are not only to examine patients and to diagnose their problems; it is all about homing in on the most pressing problem, and deciding whether they stay in emergency, can go home or need to be referred on for tests or as an inpatient. Students need to know these practical goals, so they can prepare themselves for that sort of thinking and action. Giving them this insider knowledge is a really important way for them to become part of this practice community.

I always start with a session on 'the real goals of practice here', and I ask them whether they have encountered this sort of practice in their other learning experiences, how they managed it, what they found challenging, and why and how they learnt to overcome those challenges. Getting students to start out by problem-solving any potential challenges gives them *confidence* from the beginning.

My third teaching tip is to ask the students about their future goals and interests. I have learnt to do this over time, because I think it helps to ground students and remind them of why they are here. It means when they do have a stressful day, they can put this in perspective in relation to their long-term goals (PP — meaning and purpose).

So my teaching tips aren't really tips about what to do, they are more about my approach to *communicating* with students, with the goal of bringing out their own thoughts and beliefs about their learning. Bringing these inner attitudes and thoughts about learning is a must if I am to have any chance of meaningfully influencing their learning path.

Conclusion

In this chapter, we introduced the concept of resilience, and discussed how it is crucial to enable a student and practitioner to thrive in their chosen health profession, and avoid developing anxieties about performance or finding themselves burnt out with little energy or drive to continue. Using two voices — the educator and the student — we introduced a combination of explicit education strategies and techniques to build resilience. We also highlighted the importance of attending to the implicit messages given when educating students: those that suggest a narrow interest in performance and competencies, and those that demonstrate confidence and respect for the learner's capacities to develop skills, knowledge and professional attitudes.

An important message from this chapter is that, like any skill, the skill of learning to be resilient requires practice, and students need opportunities to trial different responses. They need reinforcement of their efforts through modelled resilience, encouragement in the form of having attention given to their experiences as a learner, and positive acknowledgment of their future capacity to join a profession as a colleague.

References

Adamson, C., Beddoe, L., & Davys, A. (2014). Building resilient practitioners: Definitions and practitioner understandings. *British Journal of Social Work*, 44(3), 522–541. doi:10.1093/bjsw/bcs142.

Ahern, N. R., Ark, P., & Byers, J. (2008). Resilience and coping strategies in adolescents — additional content. *Paediatric Care*, 20(10), 32–36.

Balague, G. (2005). Anxiety: From pumped to panicked. In S. M. Murphy (Ed.), *The sport psychology handbook* (pp. 73–92). Champaign, Il: Human Kinetics.

Barnett, R. (2015). A curriculum for critical being. In M. Davies & R. Barnett (Eds.), *The Palgrave handbook of critical thinking in higher education* (pp. 63–76). New York: Palgrave MacMillan.

Beck, J. S. (2011). *Cognitive behavior therapy: Basics and beyond* (2nd ed.). New York: Guilford Press.

Benard, B. (2004). *Resiliency: What we have learned*. San Francisco: WestEd.

Billett, S. (2001). Knowing in practice: Re-conceptualising vocational expertise. *Learning and Instruction*, 11(6), 431–452.

Connaughton, D., Sheldon, H., & Jones, G. (2010). The development and maintenance of mental toughness in the world's best performers. *The Sport Psychologist*, 24(2), 168–193.

Cruess, R., Cruess, S. R., & Steinert, Y. (2016). Amending Miller's pyramid to include professional identity formation. *Academic Medicine*, 91(2), 180–185.

Davis, M., Eselman, E., & McKay, M. (2008). *The relaxation and stress reduction workbook* (6th ed.). Oakland: New Harbinger Publications.

Day, C., Stobart, G., Sammons, P., et al. (2006). *Variations in teachers' work, lives and effectiveness: Final report for the VITAE Project, DfES*. (Research Report RR743). Nottingham: DfES Publications. http://dera.ioe.ac.uk/6405/1/rr743.pdf.

Delany, C., & Bragge, P. (2009). A study of physiotherapy students' and clinical educators' perceptions of learning and teaching. *Medical Teacher*, 31(9), e402–e411.

Delany, C., Miller, K. J., El-Ansary, D., et al. (2015). Replacing stressful challenges with positive coping strategies: A resilience program for clinical placement learning. *Advances in Health Sciences Education*, 20(5), 1303–1324. doi:10.1007/s10459-015-9603-3.

Delany, C., & Watkin, D. (2009). A study of critical reflection in health professional education: 'Learning where others are coming from. *Advances in Health Sciences Education*, 14(3), 411–429.

Dobson, K. S., & Khatri, N. (2000). Cognitive therapy: Looking backward, looking forward. *Journal of Clinical Psychology*, 56(7), 907–923.

Duckworth, A. L., Peterson, C., Matthews, M. D., et al. (2007). Grit: Perseverance and passion for long-term goals. *Journal of Personality and Social Psychology*, 92(6), 1087.

Dweck, C. S., Chiu, C.-Y., & Hong, Y.-Y. (1995). Implicit theories and their role in judgments and reactions: A word from two perspectives. *Psychological Inquiry*, 6(4), 267–285.

Dyrbye, L., Power, D., Massie, F., et al. (2010). Factors associated with resilience to and recovery from burnout: A prospective, multi-institutional study of US medical students. *Medical Education*, 44(10), 1016–1026.

Egan, T., & Jaye, C. (2009). Communities of clinical practice: The social organization of clinical learning. *Health*, 13(1), 107–125.

Eley, D., & Stallman, H. (2014). Where does medical education stand in nurturing the 3Rs in medical students: Responsibility, resilience and resolve? *Medical Teacher*, 36(10), 835–837.

Elliott, M. (2002). The clinical environment: A source of stress for undergraduate nurses. *Australian Journal of Advanced Nursing*, 20(1), 34–38.

Eraut, M., & Hirsh, W. (2010). *The significance of workplace learning for individuals, groups and organisations*. (SKOPE Monograph 6). Oxford & Cardiff: SCOPE. http://www.skope.ox.ac.uk/wp-content/uploads/2014/12/Monogrpah-09.pdf.

Firth-Cozens, J. (2001a). Interventions to improve physicians' well-being and patient care. *Social Science and Medicine*, 52(2), 215–222.

Firth-Cozens, J. (2001b). Medical student stress. *Medical Education*, 35(1), 6.

Fredrickson, B. L. (2001). The role of positive emotions in positive psychology: The broaden-and-build theory of positive emotions. *American Psychologist*, 56(3), 218.

Fredrickson, B. L. (2004). The broaden-and-build theory of positive emotions. *Philosophical Transactions of the Royal Society B: Biological Sciences*, 359(1449), 1367–1377.

Goldberg, R. M., Kuhn, G., Andrew, L. B., et al. (2002). Coping with medical mistakes and errors in judgment. *Annals of Emergency Medicine*, 39(3), 287–292.

Grant, L., Kinman, G., & Alexander, K. (2014). What's all this talk about emotion? Developing emotional intelligence in social work students. *Social Work Education*, 33(7), 874–889.

Gu, Q., & Day, C. (2007). Teachers resilience: A necessary condition for effectiveness. *Teaching and Teacher Education*, 23(8), 1302–1316. doi:10.1016/j.tate.2006.06.006.

Hafferty, F. W., & Franks, R. (1994). The hidden curriculum, Ethics teaching, and the structure of medical education. *Academic Medicine*, 69(11), 861–871.

Hargreaves, A. (1998). The emotional practice of teaching. *Teaching and Teacher Education*, 14(8), 835–854.

Higgs, J., & McAllister, L. (2007). Being a clinical educator. *Advances in Health Sciences Education*, 12(2), 187–200.

Howe, A., Smajdor, A., & Stöckl, A. (2012). Towards an understanding of resilience and its relevance to medical training. *Medical Education*, 46, 349–356. doi:10.1111/j.1365-2923.2011.04188.x.

James, D. (2014). Investigating the curriculum through assessment practice in higher education: The value of a 'learning cultures' approach. *Higher Education*, 67(2), 155–169.

Kinman, G., & Grant, L. (2011). Exploring stress resilience in trainee social workers: The role of emotional and social competencies. *British Journal of Social Work*, 41(2), 261–275. doi:10.1093/bjsw/bcq088.

Klein, J., Delany, C., Fischer, M. D., et al. (2017). A growth mindset approach to preparing trainees for medical error. *BMJ Quality and Safety*, 26, 771–774. doi:10.1136/bmjqs-2016-006416.

Kobasa, S. C., Maddi, S. R., & Kahn, S. (1982). Hardiness and health: A prospective study. *Journal of Personality and Social Psychology*, 42(1), 168.

Lake, F., & Ryan, G. (2005). Teaching on the run tips 11: The junior doctor in difficulty. *Medical Journal of Australia*, 183(9), 475.

Lemaire, J. B., & Wallace, J. E. (2017). Burnout among doctors. *BMJ (Clinical Research Ed.)*, 358, j3360. doi:10.1136/**bmj**.j3360.

Linley, A., Joseph, S., Harrington, S., et al. (2006). Positive psychology: Past, present, and (possible) future. *Journal of Positive Psychology*, 1(1), 3–16.

Luthar, S. S., Cicchetti, D., & Becker, B. (2000). The construct of resilience: A critical evaluation and guidelines for future work. *Child Development*, 71(3), 543–562.

McAllister, M., & McKinnon, J. (2009). The importance of teaching and learning resilience in the health disciplines: A critical review of the literature. *Nurse Education Today*, 29(4), 371–379.

McGivern, G., & Fischer, M. D. (2012). Reactivity and reactions to regulatory transparency in medicine, psychotherapy and counselling. *Social Science and Medicine*, 74(3), 289–296.

Maddi, S. R. (2006). Hardiness: The courage to grow from stresses. *Journal of Positive Psychology*, 1(3), 160–168.

Martin, A. J., & Marsh, H. W. (2008). Academic buoyancy: Towards an understanding of students' everyday academic resilience. *Journal of School Psychology*, 46(1), 53–83.

Meyer, J., & Land, R. (2003). *Threshold concepts and troublesome knowledge: Linkages to ways of thinking and practising within the disciplines.* (Occasional Report No. 4). Edinburgh: University of Edinburgh.

Miyamoto, K., Huerta, M. C., & Kubacka, K. (2015). Fostering social and emotional skills for well-being and social progress. *European Journal of Education*, 50(2), 147–159.

Murphy, K. R. (2005). Why don't measures of broad dimensions of personality perform better as predictors of job performance? *Human Performance*, 18(4), 343–357.

Oliver, D. (2017). When 'resilience' becomes a dirty word. *BMJ (Clinical Research Ed.)*, 358, j3604. doi:10.1136/bmj.j3604.

Padesky, C. A., & Mooney, K. A. (2012). Strengths-based cognitive-behavioural therapy: A four-step model to build resilience. *Clinical Psychology and Psychotherapy*, 19(4), 283–290.

Radcliffe, C., & Lester, H. (2003). Perceived stress during undergraduate medical training: A qualitative study. *Medical Education*, 37(1), 32–38.

Rompf, E. L., Royse, D., & Dhooper, S. S. (1993). Anxiety preceding field work: What students worry about. *Journal of Teaching in Social Work*, 7(2), 81–95.

Rowe, M., Frantz, J., & Bozalek, V. (2012). The role of blended learning in the clinical education of healthcare students: A systematic review. *Medical Teacher*, 34(4), e216–e221.

Sarkar, M., & Fletcher, D. (2014). Psychological resilience in sport performers: A review of stressors and protective factors. *Journal of Sports Sciences*, 32(15), 1419–1434.

Scott, S. D., Hirschinger, L. E., Cox, K. R., et al. (2009). The natural history of recovery for the healthcare provider 'second victim' after adverse patient events. *Quality and Safety in Health Care*, 18(5), 325–330.

Seaward, B. L. (2004). *Managing stress: Principles and strategies for health and wellbeing* (3rd ed.). Boston, MA: Jones and Barlett.

Seligman, M. E. P., & Csikszentmihalyi, M. (2000). Positive psychology: An introduction. *American Psychologist*, 55(1), 5–14.

Sterling, S. (2010). Learning for resilience, or the resilient learner? Towards a necessary reconciliation in a paradigm of sustainable education. *Environmental Education Research*, 16(5–6), 511–528.

Tabernero, C., & Wood, R. E. (1999). Implicit theories versus the social construal of ability in self-regulation and performance on a complex task. *Organizational Behavior and Human Decision Processes*, 78(2), 104–127.

Tempski, P., Martins, M., & Paro, H. (2012). Teaching and learning resilience: A new agenda in medical education. *Medical Education*, 46(4), 345–346.

Van de Wiel, M. W., Van den Bossche, P., Janssen, S., et al. (2011). Exploring deliberate practice in medicine: How do physicians learn in the workplace? *Advances in Health Sciences Education*, 16(1), 81–95.

Von Culin, K. R., Tsukayama, E., & Duckworth, A. L. (2014). Unpacking grit: Motivational correlates of perseverance and passion for long-term goals. *Journal of Positive Psychology*, 9(4), 306–312.

Wald, H. S. (2015). Professional identity (trans) formation in medical education: reflection, relationship, resilience. *Academic Medicine*, 90(6), 701–706.

Wald, H. S., Anthony, D., Hutchinson, T. A., et al. (2015). Professional identity formation in medical education for humanistic, resilient physicians: Pedagogic strategies for bridging theory to practice. *Academic Medicine*, 90(6), 753–760. doi:10.1097/acm.0000000000000725.

Waller, M. A. (2001). Resilience in ecosystemic context: Evolution of the concept. *American Journal of Orthopsychiatry*, 71(3), 290.

Walsh, J. M., Feeney, C., Hussey, J., et al. (2010). Sources of stress and psychological morbidity among undergraduate physiotherapy students. *Physiotherapy*, 96(3), 206–212.

Wells, G., & Claxton, G. (2002). *Learning for life in the 21st century: Sociological perspectives of the future.* Oxford: John Wiley and Sons.

Yaghmour, N. A., Brigham, T. P., Richter, T., et al. (2017). Causes of death of residents in ACGME-accredited programs 2000 through 2014: Implications for the learning environment. *Academic Medicine*, 92(7), 976–983.

Yeager, D., & Dweck, C. (2012). Mindsets that promote resilience: When students believe that personal characteristics can be developed. *Educational Psychologist*, 47(4), 302–314.

5

Ethics education in clinical learning contexts

Clare Delany, Rosalind McDougall,
Lynn Gillam and Carolyn Johnston

Introduction

Health professionals are expected to graduate with a capacity to recognise the ethical dimensions of their professional practice, to be able to weigh up competing views about ethically appropriate options through critical and methodical reflection, and to make morally justifiable decisions (Hope et al., 2008; van den Hoven & Kole, 2015). To facilitate the development of these skills and dispositions, ethics education has traditionally focused on providing students with some combination of knowledge of the biomedical ethical principles underpinning health practice (Beauchamp & Childress, 2001), the types of virtues and character traits necessary for ethical reflection and practice (Oakley, 2007), and approaches for analysing ethical challenges applied to (often) hypothetical case examples (Delany et al., 2009; Edwards & Delany, 2008). This combination of knowledge and thinking skills is commonly delivered via lectures about biomedical ethical principles, or through opportunities to analyse cases (Donaldson et al., 2010; Gordon & Evans, 2013; Jensen & Richert, 2005; White & Taft, 2004). A key presumption of these approaches to teaching ethics is that students will use this formal ethics knowledge, and their experience of thinking and writing about ethics, to recognise and address ethical issues as they arise in their future clinical work.

However, university-based ethics education grounded in normative concepts, principles and professional duties, and delivered to students by a specialist ethics educator, has been questioned for not adequately preparing health practitioners for the ethical landscape they face in their everyday work (Delany et al., 2017; Mattick & Bligh, 2006). For example, teaching students that deliberation about ethics in practice requires the top-down application of principles and abstract reasoning and justification based only as 'cognitive work' may alienate students from their own moral intuition, perspectives and emotional responses to ethically challenging situations, which can act as a trigger for further ethical reflection (Gillam et al., 2014; van den Hoven & Kole, 2015). These concerns about ethics education resonate more broadly with the pedagogical idea that the more structured and teacher-led the learning processes are, the less likely students are to develop as self-regulated and independent learners (Lucieer et al., 2016; Premkumar et al., 2013). Another challenge to the usefulness of formal learning and teaching approaches to professional ethics relates to the differences between the controlled university 'ethics case' and ethics cases that arise in the workplace. In clinical workplace contexts, established cultures and routines may undermine the ethical ideals taught at university, or at least make it difficult for students and clinicians to speak up or act according to ethical principles (Hafferty & Franks, 1994; McDougall, 2009).

Case studies 5.1 and 5.2 are two previously published and analysed examples involving a medical student and a junior doctor. Each case highlights an ethical challenge common to these learning and practice contexts. In this chapter we extend the ethical analysis of these cases to include the potential role of the clinical educator who may be supervising or be responsible in some way for organising the trainee's clinical placement learning. How could a clinical educator assist students to process this experience? What teaching strategies could a clinician use to convert this ethical concern into a learning opportunity for students?

There is ongoing debate in the health professional ethics education literature about how to adequately prepare or motivate students to develop a level of interest, confidence and literacy in ethical deliberation for clinical practice (Johnston & Mok, 2015; Self et al., 1996). The potential gap or mismatch between knowledge derived from formal ethics education, on the one hand, and the experience of encountering and responding to ethical challenges illustrated in the two case studies, on the other hand, raises a key 'ethics education' question:

What pedagogy and teaching methods can clinician educators use to bridge the gap between formally taught ethical principles and professional ideals, and the everyday ethical challenges that students and trainees encounter in their clinical work?

Case study 5.1: A medical student (context: rural hospital in India)

The patient was an 80-year-old man who spoke no English and had come to the clinic from the countryside. The chief of medicine was performing a rectal examination to rule out prostate cancer when he said, "Wow! This is Big. Get your gloves on and feel this!" One by one all seven of us inserted our fingers into his rectum. I don't know if any of the others were as disturbed by this event as I was.

I saw an elderly man, embarrassed by what he was being subjected to, and to whom nothing had been explained … I knew I needed the experience in the procedure but no one had explained anything to the patient much less asked for his consent. Who was really benefiting from the multiple examinations? (Kushner & Thomasma, 2001, p 25)

Case study 5.2: A junior doctor

Twice in the last week I've had to do pregnancy tests on unwilling girls with abdomen pain. The second time was harder. She came in with her girlfriend. And so at the time when I'd asked her, she said 'well, you know, this is my partner'.

But then my registrar told me 'no, just do the pregnancy test then discharge her once you know that she's not pregnant'. Which is what I did. We'd taken the blood already for the other tests. But it was just not the right thing to do.

What I should have done is gone back and told her that we had to do a pregnancy test. Then if she wanted to vehemently disagree, I could document that she had refused the pregnancy test then that would have been alright. But in the end we did it and it was negative and so she went home.

I think that probably I only did it the way I did because I was pretty confident that she wouldn't be pregnant. So I wouldn't be caught! So that's 4am logic for you. Doing a pregnancy test without consent is something I reflectively oppose but I hadn't considered how easy it seems to just do the test when it's 4am and you want to get a well patient home. (McDougall, 2009, pp 203–204)

Reproduced from McDougall, R. (2009). Combating junior doctors' "4 am logic": a challenge for medical ethics education. *Journal of Medical Ethics, 35*(3), 203–206 with permission from BMJ Publishing Group Ltd.

In this chapter, to address concerns that formal, principle-based and didactic ethics teaching may not adequately prepare students for the ethical dimensions of their clinical learning and future practice, we suggest that ethics education within clinical placement, should more closely mirror and leverage students' authentic experiences to prepare them for their future clinical practice as independent ethical agents. This means that clinical educators have a role in taking seriously and seeking to address students' clinical experiences of dissonance or conflict between what they believe is the right thing to do and what they may observe others do in the workplace. This extends the role of clinicians and clinical educators from clinical practice supervision and education to ethics education and support (McKneally & Singer, 2001).

Clinical educators are uniquely placed to incorporate ethics content and skills into their role, because they are able to identify ethical dimensions of clinical judgments and patient care as they occur. They can take advantage of the teachable 'ethically important moments' which (in the human research context) have been described as 'difficult, often subtle, and usually unpredictable situations that arise' (Guillemin & Gillam, 2004, p 262). As role models for trainees, clinical educators have daily opportunities to assist students to recognise, think about and respond to *ethically important moments* in the clinical setting. They can assist in exposing the so-called 'hidden curriculum' — the influence of specific contexts, relationships and hierarchies, and values that act in the background, and that contribute to ethically challenging situations in the workplace.

This chapter is written for clinical educators who may not have prior training, formal qualifications or specific expertise in teaching ethics. The teaching strategies we describe are distilled from clinical ethics consultation processes — formal processes for considering and resolving ethical challenges and complexities, usually embedded in the hospital work context. Clinical ethics consultations (CEC) are increasingly common in hospitals, and represent a service and process that students are likely to encounter in clinical practice, at least in large health institutions. Clinical ethics consultations aim to resolve conflict, facilitate communication and ease moral distress in healthcare, all directed towards the action of delivering safe and ethically appropriate healthcare. They therefore represent an important arena in which the ethical dimensions of clinical care are addressed in practice. As will be explained below, ethics consultations address real ethical concerns as they arise in clinical practice. They involve ethical deliberation: a process to reach some form of resolution of the ethical issues, and decide on an ethically appropriate response. This means they provide a useful framework to guide clinicians and clinical educators in both modelling and more purposefully teaching students and trainees. Importantly for clinician/educators, the deliberative processes used in CECs do not (necessarily) require a deep and authoritative knowledge of medical ethics and philosophy. They require a willingness to take the ethical dimensions of clinical practice seriously, a capacity for thoughtful reflection, and skills in questioning students with the educative goal of assisting them to articulate and explore their ethical concerns and different perspectives.

In this chapter we describe two clinical ethics consultation examples with the goal of identifying concrete, practical and accessible ethics teaching strategies, and underpinning ethics education pedagogy for clinical educators (with or without formal ethics education qualifications). The first is a CEC service for clinicians within a paediatric public hospital in Australia. The second is a clinical ethics committee formed specifically for students in a medical program in the UK practice.

Clinical ethics consultations: goals and processes

An ethics consultation can occur via an individual ethicist consulting to a clinician/and or patient, or via a clinical ethics committee — usually a multidisciplinary group consulting via a collaborative meeting process with clinicians and/or patients. In the United States, clinical ethics services are an integral component of hospital accreditation (Donaldson et al., 2000). In Australia, the United Kingdom and Europe, clinical ethics committees are not mandated, but there is growing interest in their development (Doran et al., 2014; Fournier et al., 2009; McNeill, 2001; Slowther et al., 2001). There is a range of different types of clinical ethics deliberation models within formal consultation services (Jonsen et al., 2006; Molewijk et al., 2008).

In clinical ethics consultations, ethics knowledge is not passed on from textbooks, professional rules or didactically from ethics experts. Instead, the process of ethical deliberation is modelled by the clinical ethicist and through group consultation and discussion. The modelling of how to think about ethical concerns occurs via ground rules of interaction, which are set either at the beginning or during the meeting. More broadly, the opportunity to 'have the meeting' sends a powerful message about the value of devoting time and resources to discussing ethical issues. A dedicated CEC opens up a space for discussion. These processes of communication and interaction within a group of clinicians sends a set of significant meta-messages about ethical reasoning, which are not exclusively focused on substantive ethical values and principles pertinent to an ethical problem, but demonstrate the value of engaging in a conversation and a collaborative way of thinking about ethical challenges.

We argue that these processes have fundamental educational value, because they enable students and clinicians to gradually improve their ethical reasoning through the opportunity to participate in discussions (Delany & Hall, 2012; Newson, 2015), and to gain experience in seeing recurring patterns of ethical analysis. This is similar to the process of developing expertise in clinical reasoning, where, with practice and experience, clinicians are able to look beyond the cluster of systems and identify a pattern, which then leads to greater understanding of a clinical problem, and diagnosis and clinical management (Norman, 2005).

Clinical ethics consultation examples

A children's bioethics centre

The authors are involved in providing CEC consultation within the Children's Bioethics Centre (CBC) at the Royal Children's Hospital in Melbourne, Australia. The explicit goal of the CBC is as a consulting service for clinicians. This approach differs from CEC services in North America (Kesselheim et al., 2010) and Canada (Gaudine et al., 2010), where families and patients are directly involved. However, the model at the Royal Children's Hospital has allowed a unique and sustained focus on the ethics support required by clinicians, and insight into the educational value of their participation.

At the CBC, clinical ethics consultations are conducted via a Clinical Ethics Response Group (CERG). The CERG comprises a multidisciplinary committee made up of approximately 20 doctors, nurses and allied health practitioners, in addition to ethicists, and pastoral care and legal representatives. Any clinician within the hospital can refer a case to the CERG. The role of the clinical ethicist leading the discussion is to facilitate discussion and ensure that the ethical question emerges clearly, all concerns are discussed, relevant ethical concepts are explored and the group reaches a resolution within the (usually hour-long) meeting (Gold et al., 2011). Box 5.1 outlines the stated purpose and processes followed in CERG consultations.

Box 5.1: Royal Children's Hospital Clinical Ethics Response Group — the purpose and processes of clinical ethics case meeting

The purpose of the clinical ethics case meeting is to conduct a thorough ethical analysis of the case at hand. The goal is not to make specific decisions for clinicians. We may give specific advice about appropriate ethical actions, depending on the discussion. We will attempt to:

- articulate the nature of the ethical issue/s or question/s involved;
- identify the range of possible options for proceeding from this point;
- identify and weigh up the ethical pros and cons of each option;
- identify options which are clearly ethically appropriate, or not.

And in the hour we have available, we will attempt to:

- be comprehensive;
- think critically;
- identify and consider seriously the full range of possible views and positions.

The discussion which occurs within the CERG consultations has been documented in several studies (Delany & Hall, 2012; McDougall & Notini, 2016). While the ethical deliberation and discussion implicitly draws from principles of moral philosophy, the focus of the discussion is on patient outcomes, and involves a systematic approach to considering and understanding the interests of others (McDougall, 2014), using a combination of knowledge of ethical theory, concrete questioning and conceptual analysis. Table 5.1 identifies how fundamental ethical principles form the background to a series of specific and practical questions. The formal ethical principles listed in Table 5.1 may not be explicitly raised in the discussion, at least not frequently and not as a starting point. Instead, the aims of the discussion are to develop a thorough understanding of the ethical concern being raised, including to determine who is involved, and/

or whether the ethical challenge arises from disagreement between the clinician and the family, or between clinicians, about what is in the best interests of a child (Gillam et al., 2015). To facilitate this type of critical thinking, a semi-structured discussion format is used, where questions are posed (often by the ethicist) to draw out the practical, clinical, psychological and cultural details that frame and possibly shape the nature of the ethical issue (see Table 5.1).

TABLE 5.1: Ethics principles and guiding questions in paediatric clinical ethics consultations

Principle	Some key questions
Promoting the best interests of the child • Minimise harms/ risks • Maximise wellbeing/benefit	• What is *life like* for this child? • How does this child *feel*? • What would the child's life be like after the proposed intervention? • What would the child's life be like if the intervention wasn't done? • Are there any other options that could get at least some of the benefits, and perhaps avoid some of the harms/risks? • What is the long-term outlook for the child?
Respecting the parents as decision-makers • Consider both mother and father • Views of both count, even if legal requirement is for the consent of only one parent	• What have the parents been told, and what do they believe/think/ understand? • Have they been told clearly how serious the situation is for the child, what is likely to happen to their child? • Have they been given different messages by different staff? • Have they been given a clear recommendation, with the reasons explained? • What do the parents want? What are they trying to achieve for their child? • What sort of role do the parents want to play in the decision-making? • Do the parents agree with each other? • Who else is significant in the parents' decision-making? • What would be the effects on the child of going through with what the parents want? • What would be the effect on parents, child and family of going against the parents' decision? • Is the parents' decision within the zone of parental discretion? • Has communication with the parents become 'stuck' — are there now entrenched positions? • Are there any new strategies or approaches to break the impasse? • Have the parents considered what their child knows and wants?
Respecting the child and child's growing autonomy	• What has the child been told, and what do they understand/think? • What does the child want (in terms of medical treatment, and more broadly)? • If the child is refusing or resisting treatment, do we know why? • Is the child worried about something? • Do the parents know what the child wants, and vice versa? • If the parents and the child disagree, do we know why? • Can the parents and the child be assisted to communicate with each other? • To what extent does the child want to be involved in making decisions? • Is it possible that the child is a mature minor? • Has there been a formal assessment of the child's competence, and if not, could this be done? • What might happen if the child is treated against their wishes?

This sometimes involves going around the table for each person to give their initial view at the start, or their considered view near the end. It also involves acknowledging that identifying and analysing ethical dimensions of practice in this way is a different process to ward-based clinical case presentations, where key clinical features are emphasised and diagnostic certainty or the presentation of evidence underpinning prognoses are required. In contrast, the questioning and discussion in CECs involves asking awkward or 'clinically naïve' questions that probe clinical assumptions or routine practices, which may otherwise go unexamined within clinical teams steeped in routine ways of practising. Committee members are also encouraged to take on the role of devil's advocate — actively looking for arguments against a consensus view. To achieve this more open discussion, it may be necessary to explicitly set up the ground rules of discussion, and to purposefully cultivate and model questioning techniques, respect for a range of perspectives, and genuine curiosity about processes and reasons behind clinical practice decisions.

In many cases, a single ethically appropriate response emerges from the discussion. In other discussions, it becomes apparent that there may be more than one ethically justifiable action to take. The meeting discussion and outcomes are summarised by the ethicist, and are later documented in a brief summary of the meeting and sent to the clinicians. It is then up to the clinician and the team to decide how to implement the outcomes of the discussion within their clinical practice.

A specific educational goal of CECs at the CBC is to contribute to the ethics capability of all those attending, where ethics capability includes developing dispositions to think critically about an ethical concern, and to identify and consider seriously a full range of possible views and positions. We suggest there is educational value in clinician educators using a similar process of questioning and reflecting on ethical dimensions of everyday clinical situations as a form of ethics education within clinical placements. Importantly, these types of discussions will encompass ethical issues arising not only between a single practitioner and a patient, but also within the broader interprofessional team.

In the second CEC example, the clinical ethics consultation process is replicated at a student level. This represents a more focused and direct learning tool to encourage students to think ethically about real clinical situations. It is both practical and reflective.

A student-led clinical ethics committee

The Student Clinical Ethics Committee (SCEC) was established by author Carolyn Johnston (CJ), at King's College London (UK) in 2010, and at the time was perhaps the first of its kind. The educational rationale for developing this committee was initially to provide an opportunity for medical students to engage in ethical reasoning concerning real clinical scenarios, those in fact that are experienced by the students themselves during their clinical training.

As Advisor in Medical Ethics and Law at GKT School of Medical Education, CJ delivered ethics and law teaching across the medical curriculum, in line with the General Medical Council's Outcomes for Graduates (General Medical Council, 2015), and drawing on the Institute of Medical Ethics' core content of learning (Stirrat et al., 2010). Through her previous work with the UK Clinical Ethics Network, and as a member of three trust-based clinical ethics committees in London, she recognised the value of interdisciplinary discussion of ward-based ethical dilemmas. The aim of establishing the SCEC was to support students in some of the challenging situations they experienced, and as a means of translating student learning into practical application.

Process of the SCEC

The SCEC was established through discussion with a committed core group of medical students (Johnston et al., 2012). Meetings were held monthly during the academic year, provided that a student had referred a case for discussion. The meetings were extracurricular, and took place in the early evening after teaching, to maximise the attendance of students on clinical placements who may have to travel to campus. The invitation to attend meetings was initially extended only to medical students; however, to mirror the interdisciplinary case discussion carried out by trust-based CECs, this was later expanded to include nursing and midwifery students, and those taking the MA in medical ethics and law at King's College. A maximum of 25 places were allocated for each meeting, in order to promote the ability of all students to engage in the discussion. In fact many students attended meetings regularly, which created a 'memory' of prior experiential learning. The discussion was facilitated by a Chair (a member of faculty with a background in philosophy, and a member of a trust-based CEC), who introduced the case and identified the ethical questions to be addressed.

The cases discussed in the SCEC meeting were referred by students themselves: the experiences they had encountered in clinical practice, which they found troubling and of concern to them. The student discussed the ethical questions to be addressed with CJ, following which a referral form, comprising the case summary, questions to be addressed and suggested pre-reading, was circulated to the students attending. The purpose of the discussion was solely educational, and this was made clear to the clinician with the care of the patient, whose agreement was sought.

Originally a framework for discussion, was used (see Box 5.2) and this was drafted with the core group of students who established the SCEC, and was later revised through various iterations. For example, some of the questions are similar to those listed in Table 5.1, and encouraged participants to probe the practical features of the situation, but others tended to be formulaic and over time they were no longer used, as they tended to stifle rather than promote reflective and critical thinking. The Chair shaped the discussion, encouraged all of the students to express their views, and ensured that key ethical issues — autonomy, beneficence, harm, etc — were addressed, and indeed understood in the context of the discussion.

Box 5.2: Framework for discussion — Student Clinical Ethics Committee

1. Summary of case
2. What are the clinical and other relevant facts?
3. Who is involved in the decision/what are their perspectives?
4. What are the possible outcomes in this case, and the practicality of these options?
5. What does law/guidance say about this option?
6. What are the morally significant features of each option?
    i. Patient preferences, including religious and cultural factors
    ii. Patient capacity (the ability to believe, understand and retain information) (what are we assessing capacity of?)
    iii. Best interests (quality of life, long-/short-term interests, stakeholder interests?)
    iv. Non-maleficence/harm
    v. Justice/equity
7. What are the duties of the health professionals involved?
8. What are the consequences of this option?
9. What are the pros and cons of the option?
10. Conclusion

A range of cases from diverse clinical specialties were discussed, including: the use of electroconvulsive treatment for an elderly, frail patient who wished to die and was refusing treatment; the propriety of detention for assessment and treatment of a young woman, increasingly socially isolated, who washed obsessively; a family's request not to inform their grandmother, who did not speak English, that she has a terminal diagnosis; and the role of a doctor to make further enquiries about potential domestic abuse in respect of a homosexual man who presented to a fracture clinic.

The originality of the cases referred, and the complexity of the interprofessional discussion, really engaged the students. Two further features of the student-led cases were: 1) that they raised ethical concerns, which may not ordinarily be raised in more formalised ethics teaching; and 2) they provided a forum, which validated and to some extent normalised, similar ethical concerns and experiences encountered by other students. For example, in one of the cases described in detail in Johnston et al. (2014), the students grappled with whether a homeless man with a (self-reported) risk of suicide should be admitted to hospital (i.e., provided with an overnight bed). The student who bought the case for discussion was uncertain about whether the man, with nowhere to go and at a potential (however small) risk of major psychiatric harm and certain physical discomfort, should be asked to leave the emergency department without further intervention. The case raised a number of complex and interrelated issues about: responding to patient vulnerability when it was self-reported rather than objectively assessed; hospitals' roles to protect people or to 'house' people when they have nowhere else to go, and the impact on resources. As discussed in Johnston et al. (2014), the case also resonated with students' experiences in other contexts, and provided some acknowledgment that these ethical dimensions of their practice were common, complex and not necessarily resolved through the application of standard biomedical ethical principles.

Students valued the forum of the SCEC in which to discuss real cases in such depth, many noting that there was no other opportunity to do so. The learning has been disseminated to the wider student body through online modules and as case examples in teaching sessions, and many of the case discussions have been written up for publication, with the referring student as co-author (Johnston et al., 2016).

However, there were some limitations of the SCEC model as an ethics education learning strategy. It is an extracurricular opportunity, and enables only a minority of students to engage in this experiential learning. Ideally, such a format could be embedded in the curriculum as a teaching methodology, although this would require significant time and logistical support. Despite this, considerable benefits have been demonstrated. The fact that many former students who attended SCEC meetings have gone on to become members of trust-based CECs is testament to the lifelong learning embedded through such a process. They are able to thus draw on their expertise to enable an ethics infrastructure in the clinical setting.

Clinical ethics consultations as a form of ethics education

The two examples of CEC services described above have different purposes. The first example, an established service operating within a hospital, aims primarily to resolve ethical challenges and find a way forward in specific cases. We suggest the process of deliberation and multidisciplinary involvement has valuable educational spin-offs. The second example is solely designed for ethics education purposes. In this section, we further discuss these educational processes and spin-offs.

The first educational feature is that CECs represent a dialogical process (derived from and informed by discussions between the people directly involved). We suggest that participating in dialogue with others (peers and other colleagues from different disciplines) is an essential activity for learning health ethics. Dialogue in CECs refers to the opportunity to discuss an ethical concern and to hear the views and perspectives of other people (Burbules & Rice, 1991). The ground rules for discussion are explained and modelled, and explicit value is given to being curious about and probing alternative perspectives about an ethical problem.

Educational philosophy sheds further light on the processes and possible impact of dialogue where values and differing moral perspectives are discussed. Burbules and Rice (1991) use the term 'dialogue across difference'. They suggest a key benefit of participating in *dialogue across difference*, for students and others in an education context, is the development of a particular type of epistemic knowledge, which includes greater understanding of an issue, enhanced skills in problem-solving and deliberation, and increased awareness of how and why one view may differ from another.

This perspective enables students and clinicians to construct a deeper sense of professional moral identity, by being challenged to consider routine assumptions that typically frame daily decisions about meeting patients' and families' needs. Pursuing and maintaining dialogue across difference is also likely to foster dispositions and practices of communication that are relational in character, and that enhance relationships between people within the CEC and, importantly, beyond that sphere into the clinical context, for the benefit of patients.

A further educational feature of CECs is that they represent and emerge from authentic clinical activities. They are grounded in everyday clinical encounters and the ethical concerns that emerge directly from clinicians' and students' personal experiences and emotional reactions, and the specific circumstances of learning and working in clinical environments. Ethics consultations therefore acknowledge a dimension of clinical practice that is often 'hidden' or in the shadows in comparison to the dominant clinical outcomes and clinical evidence focus of hospital work. Making time for an ethics discussion with other colleagues reinforces the idea that ethical aspects of clinical practice have value and are worth thinking about. In addition, CECs provide a process for how to consider the views of others, and how to use this knowledge to develop a deeper understanding of an ethical issue. The outcome being an understanding that ethical problems are not necessarily resolved by taking and arguing for a position or a particular moral stance. Table 5.2 lists key CEC processes matched to educational outcomes.

TABLE 5.2: Clinical ethics consultation processes linked to ethics education

Clinical ethics consultation processes involve:	Ethics education outcome
Making time for a sustained discussion about an ethical concern	A direct antidote to the insidious harms of the hidden curriculum (Hafferty & Franks, 1994; McCammon & Brody, 2012; Sperry, 2004), where ethical issues and challenges either are not discussed, or are decided by those with authority
Cutting across usual clinical team groupings and hierarchies	A concrete way to achieve goals of interprofessional practice (Irvine et al., 2002) by listening to and hearing the perspectives of peers and colleagues from different disciplines
Listening to other views and perspectives about an ethical concern	Raises awareness and contributes to understanding the complexity of workplace-based ethical issues, beyond the label of the ethical rule or principle
An opportunity to contribute a personal/professional view to a diverse group of colleagues	An opportunity to develop some moral agency by framing and justifying an opinion about an ethical issue in a meaningful workplace setting (Edwards et al., 2005; Wald et al., 2015)
A structured conversation to guide (an empirical–ground-up, rather than principled-ethical theory-driven) exploration of an ethical issue	A template for thinking about the ethical dimensions of clinical practice
Modelling a way to figure out ethical complexity using a combination of ethics-based knowledge, concepts, values and practical considerations	A visible and accessible model of ethical reasoning and deliberation
Exposing the inherent uncertainty of clinical practice, and the sometimes partial understandings of an issue or a person's perspective	A realistic and less perfectionist view of clinical practice (Delany et al., 2015; Doyal & Doyal, 2007; Kitto et al., 2004)

What educational theory supports these teaching processes?

Further theoretical and philosophical ideas that strengthen the argument that CECs provide a valuable and sustainable form of ethics education for the clinical workplace are derived from the concept of interpersonal reflective equilibrium, and philosophical ideas of pragmatism and democracy.

Clinical ethics consultation as a form of interpersonal reflective equilibrium

Interpersonal reflective equilibrium (van den Hoven & Kole, 2015, p 148) draws from Rawls's (1971) concept of reflective equilibrium as a method to help people develop moral theory or to arrive at justified moral judgments in particular situations (Rawls, 1971, pp 18–19). Van den Hoven and Kole suggest that an interpersonal element further enriches this concept. The interpersonal component refers to including the (empirically gathered) moral views of peers (students or a range of clinicians) who are embedded in clinical practice (van den Hoven & Kole, 2015, p 150). The model they introduce and justify parallels the learning that occurs in CECs. Through discussion with others, students learn how to both recognise and then attain some conceptual distance and perspective from their own personal views and puzzlement about a complex ethical situation. Van den Hoven and Kole (2015) describe (p 148) three important characteristics of their model, which are also relevant to processes of CECs:

1. It allows for a diversity of both moral and non-moral ingredients (case facts, situational elements, people involved and their circumstance) in the process of moral reasoning and justification, and models a process of working towards a 'shared moral understanding', and demonstrates the importance of shared responsibility for formulating and working towards achieving moral goals. It highlights the importance of dialogue — that is, 'doing ethics' is not just 'thinking about ethics individually'.

2. It assumes that these ingredients are all revisable during the process; demonstrating how ethical principles may need to be interpreted and understood in light of the facts of a case, or that initial intuitions or 'settled moral positions' (Newson, 2015) may need adjusting in light of principles.

3. It assumes that a moral judgment concerning a case will be justified if it is part of the strongest possible coherence of a given set of diverse ingredients.

Clinical ethics consultation as a pragmatic form of ethics education

Pragmatism as a philosophical theory emphasises the practical application of ideas (Gutek, 2014, pp 76, 100). John Dewey's pragmatic theory of inquiry focused on constructing a bridge between science and ethics by describing inquiry as the use of intelligent thought to solve problems naturalistically. This requires people to avoid or suspend reflexive or habitual ways of responding within their environment, and instead to survey a problematic situation and form a plan of action for resolution of the problem (Miller et al., 2000, p 87).

These steps of reasoning and 'intelligent thought' are similar to the steps of clinical reasoning in health practice defined by Norman (2005), as developing and testing hypotheses, by drawing on broad dimensions of knowledge and experience (Norman, 2005). Miller et al. (2000, p 83) suggest that pragmatism in clinical ethics derives from the empirical turn in bioethics and a consequent rejection of:

… theoretical elegance as the measure of good bioethics and health law, and insistence instead on evaluating what meets the needs of individuals in clinical settings …

Discussions in CECs do not occur in abstract principled ways, but highlight ethical bottom lines, which are relevant in specific clinical contexts. Universal ethical values are not sidelined, but rather are placed in the context of ethical issues being perceived in a number of ways, and that there is value in acknowledging these differing perspectives.

Clinical ethics consultation as a democratic form of ethics education

Dewey's conception of moral and philosophical enquiry describes moral judgments as emerging through processes of enquiry where moral principles are used as hypothetical tools or guides in the process of ethical enquiry (Miller et al., 2000, p 89). Ideals of cooperation, discussion, consultation and participation are key constructs to this idea of moral discussion and enquiry. This approach to ethical enquiry aligns closely with models of collaborative and democratic ideals of healthcare delivery, which seek to decrease or compensate for power differentials within clinical encounters. Examples include models of shared decision-making (Charles et al., 1997, 1999); patient-centred care (Zlotnik-Shaul, 2014); making clinical decision-making transparent (Brody, 1989), and conversational models of care (Katz, 1984). The two examples of CEC described in this chapter similarly focus on breaking down hierarchies and providing opportunities for all people to be involved and to voice their perspective. Students' and clinicians' inherent moral knowledge and insight are acknowledged and valued (Verkerk & Lindemann, 2012).

Bringing pedagogy to practice via elaboration and resolution

An understanding of these pedagogical bases changes the goals of, and approaches to, ethics education from a top-down application of principles and abstract reasoning and justification to:
- a focus on fostering sensitivity to the worldview of others;
- generating an overriding commitment to establishing shared or common meanings about health and associated values in healthcare;
- demonstrating acceptance of uncertainty and partial understandings of an issue or a person's perspective;
- preparedness to learn from what another has to say;
- a commitment to building a type of communicative trust where people (students, clinicians and patients) can contribute views to overcome misunderstandings or conflicting views.

Returning to the two case studies raised at the start of the chapter, the key questions we address in this final section are: What is the teaching moment, and how do we make the most of it? Case study 5.1 involves

TABLE 5.3: Ethical principles and questions to encourage articulation of ethical concerns

Principle	Some key questions
Promoting the best interests of the patient • Minimise harms/risks • Maximise wellbeing/benefit	• What do you think this patient was experiencing? • How would this make him *feel*? • What are the benefits of this examination for the patient ? • What are the benefits of this examination for students? • What are the harms of this experience for the patient and for the participating students? • Are there any other options in this particular setting, which could get at least some of the benefits, and perhaps avoid some of the harms/risks? • What is the impact of the chief of medicine conducting this examination?
Respecting the patient's autonomy	• What has this patient been told? • Have they been told about the purpose of the examination? • Have they been told about the purpose of including students in the examination? • Have they been given the option of saying yes or no? • How does this particular clinical setting normally approach patient consent? • In this clinical setting and these circumstances, are there any options for increasing the possibility of showing respect for this patient?

a student expressing concern for a patient's discomfort, wondering about whether the elderly man should have been given more information and choice before having seven students examine him; and wondering whether the patient's discomfort and embarrassment was worth the benefit of learning from this examination. The student's concern tacitly refers to the ethical principles of respect for patient autonomy, beneficence and avoiding harm, and the student acknowledges that there are both benefits and harms arising from this clinical learning scenario. In the discussion of the case in *Ward ethics* (Kushner & Thomasma, 2001), the commentators analyse these concerns using concepts of patient vulnerability (Agich, 2001) and requirements for informed consent (Goldworth, 2001).

Using the same template as Table 5.1, Table 5.3 lists the ethical principles and the types of questions that might encourage this student to articulate their ethical concerns, and to discuss ethically appropriate responses in that situation.

In case study 5.2, the junior doctor faces the issue of testing for pregnancy when the patient has not given consent. Under pressure from a more senior colleague, and confident that the test will be negative, she tests a patient's blood sample for pregnancy without the patient's consent. Ethical concepts such as informed consent, respect for patient autonomy, and beneficence underlie her discussion of the situation. She later reflects that she opposes pregnancy tests without consent, but found it difficult to act in line with that view in the context of a busy department overnight. The case is used to argue that medical ethics education ought to equip students with skills for implementing their ethical decisions in the challenging clinical environments where they work. Similar questions might encourage this student to articulate her ethical concerns, and to discuss ethically appropriate responses in that situation, and how the junior doctor might respond next time.

The ethics questions listed above do not explicitly refer to formal ethical principles. We suggest their educational value derives from an acknowledgment of students' ethical concerns, the opportunity for students to name and bring the ethical problem as they experience it, exposure to ways of talking about and conceptually framing ethical problems, and the fact that their concerns about their own practice, uncertainties and relationships with peers and colleagues were taken seriously. This educational work includes:

- introducing ethical thinking tools to help students about ethical issues;
- using a pragmatic approach, and focusing on what needs doing to address an ethical concern;
- taking a democratic approach that values all opinions and makes a space for contributions.

PRACTICAL TIPS

Based on informal interviews conducted by the authors of this chapter with clinician educators, the following specific strategies were suggested when students encounter or raise ethical challenges:

- Work out whether the student is wanting a resolution to the problem, or is needing a way to think about the problem.
- Try to identify the ethical question that needs an answer.
- Ask questions that encourage the student to describe concrete details about their concern, such as outcomes of treatment, risks and benefits of treatment/examination.
- Ask about the different dimensions of harms and benefits, including physical, psychological, emotional and social, and the relationships that are at stake in the situation.
- Demonstrate genuine curiosity about the students' views and concerns.
- Show that you, as an experienced clinician, are open to be persuaded by others and to change your mind about what matters for a patient and family after hearing alternative perspectives.
- Think of yourself as a role model for how to have an ethical discussion without jumping to and justifying a moral stance too early.

Good things to say in response to a trainee who raises an ethical problem or concern:

- That is an interesting issue that you raise.
- Can you tell me a little more about your concern?
- Can you explain a little more?
- How did that make you feel?
- Your perspective is valuable.
- My usual way of thinking about this is ..., but you have raised some further issues to think about.

Not so good things to say in response to a trainee who raises an ethical problem or concern:

- Don't worry about that.
- The clinical outcome was good, and that is the most important thing.
- It is not up to you to worry about that.
- This type of problem is just commonsense.
- Just focus on what you need to know for the exams.
- This is not your responsibility, don't' worry about it.

Conclusion

The ideals and strategies for ethics education that we have introduced share similar pedagogical features to the educational strategies raised by the authors in this text. For example, we suggest a clinician can take on the role of ethics educator by noticing and taking advantage of learning opportunities for students that: translate (not only identify an ethical issue, but open up ways of understanding) ethical complexity (Chapter 11); make the type of thinking and deliberation used for ethical decision-making visible and accessible to students (Chapter 3); build in key features of the workplace context (Chapter 7); prepare students with practical thinking and communication techniques for dealing with inevitable conflict or competing moral perspectives (Chapter 6); and acknowledge and build on the knowledge and perspectives students bring to a situation, so they incorporate their ethics knowledge and practice into their professional identity (Chapter 8).

Our core message in this chapter is that ethics education can, to some extent, be done by all thoughtful and reflective practitioners who have an understanding of the idea of ethics education that we have put forward here, and who are motivated to use everyday practice as a learning opportunity to extend and enhance patient care.

References

Agich, G. (2001). Commentary. In T. K. Kushner & D. C. Thomasma (Eds.), *Ward ethics: Dilemmas for medical students and doctors in training* (pp. 29–32). Cambridge: Cambridge University Press.

Beauchamp, T., & Childress, J. (2001). *Principles of biomedical ethics* (5th ed.). Oxford: Oxford University Press.

Brody, H. (1989). Transparency: Informed consent in primary care. In J. Arras & B. Steinbock (Eds.), *Ethical issues in modern medicine* (5th ed., pp. 94–100). Mountain View: Mayfield Publishing Company.

Burbules, N., & Rice, S. (1991). Dialogue across differences: Continuing the conversation. *Harvard Educational Review*, 61(4), 393–417.

Charles, C., Gafni, A., & Whelan, T. (1997). Shared decision-making in the medical encounter: What does it mean? (or it takes at least two to tango). *Social Science and Medicine*, 44(5), 681–692. doi:10.1016/s0277-9536(96)00221-3.

Charles, C., Whelan, T., & Garni, A. (1999). What do we mean by partnership in making decisions about treatment? *British Medical Journal*, 319, 780–782.

Delany, C., Gillam, L., & McDougall, R. (2009). Ethics in clinical education. In C. Delany & L. Molloy (Eds.), *Clinical education in the health professions* (pp. 173–186). Sydney: Elsevier.

Delany, C., & Hall, G. (2012). 'I just love these sessions': Should physician satisfaction matter in clinical ethics consultations? *Clinical Ethics*, 7, 116–121.

Delany, C., Richards, A., Stewart, H., et al. (2017). Five challenges to ethical communication for interprofessional paediatric practice: A social work perspective. *Journal of Interprofessional Care*, 31(4), 505–511. doi:10.1080/13561820.2017.1296419.

Donaldson, M., Kohn, L., & Corrigan, J. (2000). *To err is human: Building a safer health system*. Washington, DC: National Academy Press.

Donaldson, T., Fistein, E., & Dunn, M. (2010). Case-based seminars in medical ethics education: How medical students define and discuss moral problems. *Journal of Medical Ethics*, 36(12), 816.

Doran, E., Fleming, J., Jordens, C., et al. (2014). Managing ethical issues in patient care and the need for clinical ethics support. *Australian Health Review*, 39(1), 44–50.

Doyal, L., & Doyal, L. (2007). Moral and legal uncertainty within medicine: The role of clinical ethics committees [Editorial]. *Postgraduate Medical Journal*, 85(1007), 449–450.

Edwards, I., Braunack-Mayer, A., & Jones, M. (2005). Ethical reasoning as a clinical-reasoning strategy in physiotherapy. *Physiotherapy*, 91(4), 229–236.

Edwards, I., & Delany, C. (2008). Ethical reasoning. In J. Higgs, M. Jones, S. Loftus, et al. (Eds.), *Clinical reasoning in the health professions* (3rd ed., pp. 279–289). Boston: Elsevier.

Fournier, V., Rari, E., Førde, R., et al. (2009). Clinical ethics consultation in Europe: A comparative and ethical review of the role of patients. *Clinical Ethics*, 4(3), 131–138.

Gaudine, A., Thorne, L., Lefort, S., et al. (2010). Evolution of hospital clinical ethics committees in Canada. *Journal of Medical Ethics*, 36(3), 132–137.

General Medical Council. (2015). Outcomes for graduates. http://www.gmc-uk.org/education/undergraduate/undergrad_outcomes.asp.

Gillam, L., Delany, C., Guillemin, M., et al. (2014). The role of emotions in health professional ethics teaching. *Journal of Medical Ethics*, 40, 331–335.

Gillam, L., McDougall, R., & Delany, C. (2015). Making meaning from experience: A working typology for pediatrics ethics consultations. *American Journal of Bioethics*, 15(5), 24–26.

Gold, H., Hall, G., & Gillam, L. (2011). Role and function of a paediatric clinical ethics service: Experiences at the Royal Children's Hospital, Melbourne. *Journal of Paediatrics and Child Health*, 47(9), 632–636.

Goldworth, A. (2001). Commentary. In T. K. Kushner & D. C. Thomasma (Eds.), *Ward ethics: Dilemmas for medical students and doctors in training* (pp. 27–29). Cambridge: Cambridge University Press.

Gordon, J. J., & Evans, H. M. (2013). Learning medicine from the humanities. In T. Swanwick (Ed.), *Understanding medical education: Evidence, theory and practice*. Chichester: John Wiley & Sons.

Guillemin, M., & Gillam, L. (2004). Ethics, reflexivity, and 'ethically important moments' in research. *Qualitative Inquiry*, 10(2), 261–280.

Gutek, G. (2014). *Philosophical, ideological, and theoretical perspectives on education*. New Jersey: Pearson.

Hafferty, F. W., & Franks, R. (1994). The hidden curriculum, ethics teaching, and the structure of medical education. *Academic Medicine*, 69(11), 861–871.

Hope, R., Savulescu, J., & Hendrick, J. (2008). *Medical ethics and law: The core curriculum* (2nd ed.). Edinburgh: Churchill Livingstone.

Irvine, R., Kerridge, I., McPhee, J., et al. (2002). Interprofessionalism and ethics: Consensus or clash of cultures? *Journal of Interprofessional Care*, 16(3), 199–210.

Jensen, G. M., & Richert, A. E. (2005). Reflection on the teaching of ethics in physical therapist education: Integrating cases, theory, and learning. *Journal of Physical Therapy Education*, 19(3), 78–85.

Johnston, C., Baty, M., & Elnaiem, A. (2014). King's College London Student Clinical Ethics Committee case discussion: Should a homeless, potentially suicidal man be admitted to hospital overnight for the purposes of addressing a short-term shelter problem? *Clinical Ethics*, 9(2–3), 104–107.

Johnston, C., Baty, M., & Kelly, P. (2016). King's College London Student Clinical Ethics Committee case discussion: An elderly patient wants to go home following inpatient treatment, but it is thought she may be at risk in her own home and her discharge is delayed. *Clinical Ethics*, 11(4), 210–213.

Johnston, C., & Mok, J. (2015). How medical students learn ethics: An online log of their learning experiences. *Journal of Medical Ethics*, 41(10), 854–858.

Johnston, C., Williams, D. C., Lapraik, A., et al. (2012). Setting up a student clinical ethics committee. *Clinical Ethics*, 7(2), 51–53.

Jonsen, A., Siegler, M., & Winslade, W. (2006). *Clinical ethics* (6th ed.). New York: McGraw-Hill.

Katz, J. (1984). *The silent world of doctor and patient*. New York: Free Press.

Kesselheim, J., Johnson, J., & Joffe, S. (2010). Ethics consultation in children's hospitals: Results from a survey of paediatric clinical ethicists. *Paediatrics, 125,* 742–746.

Kitto, S., Chesters, J., Villanueva, E., et al. (2004). Normalising uncertainty in undergraduate clinical transition seminars. *Focus on Health Professional Education, 6*(1), 37–51.

Kushner, T. K., & Thomasma, D. C. (2001). *Ward ethics: Dilemmas for medical students and doctors in training.* Cambridge: Cambridge University Press.

Lucieer, S. M., Geest, J. N. V. D., Elói-Santos, S. M., et al. (2016). The development of self-regulated learning during the pre-clinical stage of medical school: A comparison between a lecture-based and a problem-based curriculum. *Advances in Health Sciences Education: Theory and Practice, 21*(1), 93–104.

McCammon, S., & Brody, H. (2012). How virtue ethics informs medical professionalism. *HEC Forum: An Interdisciplinary Journal on Hospitals' Ethical and Legal Issues, 24*(4), 257–272.

McDougall, R. (2009). Combating junior doctors' '4am logic': A challenge for medical ethics education. *Journal of Medical Ethics, 35*(3), 203–206.

McDougall, R. (2014). Collaboration in clinical ethics consultation: A method for achieving 'balanced accountability'. *American Journal of Bioethics, 14*(6), 47–48. doi:10.1080/15265161.2014.900146.

McDougall, R., & Notini, L. (2016). What kinds of cases do paediatricians refer to clinical ethics? Insights from 184 case referrals at an Australian paediatric hospital. *Journal of Medical Ethics, 42*(1), 586–591.

McKneally, M., & Singer, P. (2001). Bioethics for clinicians: 25. Teaching bioethics in the clinical setting. *Journal of the Canadian Medical Association, 164*(8), 1163–1167.

McNeill, P. M. (2001). A critical analysis of Australian clinical ethics committees and the functions they serve. *Bioethics, 15*(5–6), 443–460.

Mattick, K., & Bligh, J. (2006). Teaching and assessing medical ethics: Where are we now? *Journal of Medical Ethics, 32,* 181–185.

Miller, F., Fins, J., & Bacchetta, M. (2000). Clinical pragmatism: John Dewey and clinical ethics. In F. Miller (Ed.), *Frontiers in bioethics. Essays dedicated to John C Fletcher* (pp. 83–104). Hagerstown, MD: University Publishing Group.

Molewijk, A. C., Abma, T., Stolper, M., et al. (2008). Teaching ethics in the clinic: The theory and practice of moral case deliberation. *Journal of Medical Ethics, 34*(2), 120–124.

Newson, A. (2015). The value of clinical ethics support in Australian health care. *Medical Journal of Australia, 202*(11), 568–569.

Norman, G. (2005). Research in clinical reasoning: Past history and current trends. *Medical Education, 39*(4), 418–427. doi:10.1111/j.1365-2929.2005.02127.x.

Oakley, J. G. (2007). Virtue theory. In R. E. Ashcroft, A. Dawson, H. Draper, et al. (Eds.), *Principles of health care ethics* (2nd ed., pp. 87–91). Chichester: John Wiley & Sons.

Premkumar, K. J., Pahwa, P., Banerjee, A., et al. (2013). Does medical training promote or deter self-directed learning? A longitudinal mixed-methods study. *Academic Medicine, 88*(11), 1754–1764.

Rawls, J. (1971). *A theory of justice.* Cambridge, MA: Harvard University Press.

Self, D. J., Baldwin, D. C., & Wolinsky, F. D. (1996). Further exploration of the relationship between medical education and moral development. *Cambridge Quarterly of Healthcare Ethics, 5*(3), 444–449.

Slowther, A., Bunch, C., Woolnough, B., et al. (2001). Clinical ethics support services in the UK: An investigation of the current provision of ethics support to health professionals in the UK. *Journal of Medical Ethics, 27*(1), i2–i8.

Sperry, L. (2004). Ethical dilemmas in the assessment of clinical outcomes. *Psychiatric Annals, 34*(2), 107–113.

Stirrat, G., Johnston, C., Gillon, R., et al. (2010). Medical ethics and law for doctors of tomorrow: The 1998 consensus statement updated. *Journal of Medical Ethics, 36*(1), 55–60.

van den Hoven, M., & Kole, J. (2015). Distance, dialogue and reflection: Interpersonal reflective equilibrium as method for professional ethics education. *Journal of Moral Education, 44*(2), 145–164.

Verkerk, M., & Lindemann, H. (2012). Toward a naturalized clinical ethics. *Kennedy Institute of Ethics Journal, 22*(4), 289–306.

Wald, H. S., Anthony, D., Hutchinson, T. A., et al. (2015). Professional identity formation in medical education for humanistic, resilient physicians: Pedagogic strategies for bridging theory to practice. *Academic Medicine, 90*(6), 753–760. doi:10.1097/acm.0000000000000725.

White, J., & Taft, S. (2004). Frameworks for teaching and learning business ethics within the global context: Background of ethical theories. *Journal of Management Education, 28*(4), 463–477.

Zlotnik-Shaul, R. (2014). *Patient and family-centred care: Ethical and legal issues.* New York: Springer.

6

Educating for conflict resolution

Haavi Morreim

Introduction

Like many other fields of human endeavour, healthcare has its share of conflict. Teams with diverse backgrounds and training must collaborate closely to care for patients whose needs and goals vary widely. Professionals formerly accustomed to functioning with a high degree of independence must now trust teammates — who often may change from week to week, even day to day — to execute their respective tasks with a high degree of precision and coordination.

In healthcare, conflict can be particularly destructive because the stakes are so high. If a coffee shop barista touches the wrong number on the computer screen you might receive the wrong beverage or pay the wrong price — a minor and usually fixable, if annoying, problem. If a doctor placing an online drug order touches the wrong number in precisely the same kind of error, or if a nurse programing an IV pump likewise makes exactly that same kind of error, someone could die, or land in intensive care, or incur needless pain or expense.

Beyond such clinical practice-oriented errors, it has been estimated that communication problems are 'a root cause in nearly 70% of reported sentinel events, surpassing other commonly identified issues such as staff orientation and training, patient assessment, and staffing' (ECRI, 2009, p 1). In this setting of great consequence and high stress, conflict — a key source of communication problems — can thus threaten patient safety, precipitate adverse outcomes and engender patient dissatisfaction, provider burnout and moral distress. Where professionals do not respect and trust each other, they may decline to share important information; when a patient or family are deemed 'difficult', clinicians may avoid them, perhaps speak more succinctly (or abruptly) than usual or use a confrontational tone of voice — one that perhaps emulates rather than deescalates the negative tone coming from the other side; and when a clinician finds a particular colleague intimidating, they may simply avoid communicating, or talk to someone else instead.

The high stakes of healthcare also involve ethics. Life, death and quality of life are on the line. People of diverse backgrounds may bring widely differing conceptions of what counts as a life worth living or a risk worth taking, and who should be empowered to make such decisions — and what response should be taken by those who are asked to implement a decision with which they may profoundly disagree. In these cases, assistance may be sought from the health service's ethics specialist, where this service is available — an 'ethics consult'. Occasionally the issue focuses on 'moral puzzlement', in which everyone involved is genuinely perplexed about what is the right thing to do. Much more commonly, however, ethics consults are about conflict. As ethics by definition concerns that which is of utmost importance, it follows that in this high-stakes, high-stress environment, ethics-based conflict resolution becomes all the more important.

In this context a major US bioethics organisation, the American Society for Bioethics and Humanities (ASBH), has created a set of recommendations regarding how ethics consults are best undertaken, and what sorts of knowledge and skills should be possessed by those who purport to offer such a service (ASBH Task Force, 2011). Not surprisingly, conflict resolution skills such as facilitation, negotiation and mediation rank high on that list.

In this chapter, I suggest that these same skills are both necessary and useful for clinical educators and trainees in different phases of their learning and teaching experiences. In many cases the ethics consultant's or clinician/educator's best service may not be to provide their own recommendations. Where everyone has credible reasons supporting their own perspective, declaring that 'these people are right and those people are wrong' or 'I prefer A over B' may simply amount to taking sides, while letting the underlying conflict continue to fester. Instead, it may be better to provide the people in conflict with the opportunity to be heard and understood, so that they can come to a reasonable, durable agreement of their own. Such an approach can often enable disputants to have the respectful, problem-solving conversation that finds common ground and a mutually acceptable plan of action. In these conversations the intermediary does not provide the answers; rather, the people in conflict do.

In a similar vein, in 2009 the US Joint Commission on the Accreditation of Healthcare initiated requirements that hospitals 'provide […] a system for resolving conflicts among individuals working in the hospital' (LD.01.03.01 EP-7), and that '[t]he hospital manage […] conflict between leadership groups to protect the quality and safety of care' (LD.02.04.01) (Scott & Gerardi, 2011a; Scott & Gerardi, 2011b; Conard & Franklin, 2010).

In summary, healthcare is often rife with conflict, and the importance of addressing it has become widely recognised. Conflict arises from inherently high stakes and great complexity, from the need for interdependence even as highly trained professionals often value and seek to exercise independent judgment, and from the need for ethically momentous decisions. If healthcare is to achieve its goals of safe, effective, efficient, high-quality care, it would seem essential that the skills of conflict resolution be among those that health professionals learn. And if professionals-in-training should learn them, then so must the faculty who teach them.

In this chapter I use a pair of cases that capture common types of conflict in the clinical setting, then explore various ways in which conflict resolution can be taught. One approach, which emphasises a very practical array of skills and strategies, is a particular focus. Detailed explication of all those skills and strategies is not possible in the setting of a brief chapter, but a few of them are highlighted as they are then brought to bear on the two cases. Both cases highlight conflict between clinicians and patients and illustrate opportunities for learning and teaching conflict management skills. Several formats in which such skills are taught are discussed. Finally, some suggestions for evaluation and research are proposed.

Consider, then, the following pair of cases — real, but for a few modifications to protect privacy.

Case study 6.1

Carl, age 48, had been admitted earlier in the month for gastrointestinal pain and then discharged home, feeling better but with no clear diagnosis (although several important potential diagnoses had been ruled out). A few days later he was readmitted, albeit for soft indications. Several days later, when Carl pegged his abdominal pain at most as a 3 on a scale of 10, the team informed him he would be discharged home that afternoon. Carl objected, insisting that he should feel completely fine before going home. After all, he pointed out, he ended up right back in the hospital shortly after the last discharge. Meanwhile, at this point the case manager, in consultation with the patient's insurer, indicated to the faculty supervising doctor that coverage for additional days' hospitalisation was about to be cut off for lack of 'medical necessity'. The doctor is unsure whether or how to raise this financial question with Carl, who is still insisting that he needs further testing — testing the medical team deems unnecessary, just like his current hospital stay. The supervising doctor in Carl's case sees an exacerbation of conflict brewing ...

Case study 6.2

Alice is a 14-month-old toddler admitted to the neurology floor in a paediatric hospital, for what is probably nothing more than a simple febrile seizure. Although frightening to parents, a febrile seizure is usually just a convulsion that accompanies a fever. Unlike more serious disorders such as epilepsy they are usually harmless one-time episodes not associated with any ominous or ongoing neurological problems. Alice was born premature at 26 weeks, and has had chronic respiratory problems ever since. She is gradually outgrowing her breathing issues but, because of her current infection (probably just a respiratory virus), she is working somewhat harder to breathe, with mild retractions. The nurses on the neuro floor are not accustomed to seeing children with this sort of baseline respiratory function, and Alice's nurse is quite alarmed. Over the past two days she has increasingly insisted to Alice's mother that the child should be transferred to the paediatric intensive care unit (PICU). The second-year resident has now been called at 3 am. He is convinced the child does not need PICU care, but is not sure what to say to Alice's mother, who was recently overheard to say 'the interns know nothing; the residents think they know everything; and then there are the real doctors ...'

Background educational theory

If adequate mechanisms for resolving conflict in healthcare are essential, it follows that the relevant skills should be taught. Books and articles abound, both on negotiation (managing and resolving one's own conflicts directly with another person or group) and mediation (serving as a third-party neutral — someone who is not a partisan in the conflict, and who assists parties in conflict towards resolution of their own design). Prominent books include Fisher and Ury's classic *Getting to Yes* (1991), Moore's *The Mediation Process* (2003) and a host of others (Ury, 1993; Stone et al., 1999; Mayer, 2015). Relevant articles on mediation and negotiation are, not surprisingly, too numerous to mention. Likewise websites abound, offering concepts, skillsets, exercises and even games for teaching conflict resolution to those in corporate workplaces, schools and communities (see the online resources section at the end of the chapter). There are also a wide variety of conflict resolution publications focused specifically on healthcare (Marcus et al., 2011; Morreim 2014a; Morreim 2014b; Morreim 2015; Morreim 2016; Marcus 2002; Gibson 1999; Bergman 2013; Fiester 2011; Fiester 2012; Dubler & Liebman, 2011).

Conflict resolution can be learnt and taught in a variety of ways. One general approach emphasises intellectual and cognitive processes: one must understand what conflict is, where it comes from and what kinds of concepts make the most sense for changing the paths of conflict. One such course, *Clinician–Patient Communication to Enhance Health Outcomes* (see the online resources section), emphasises four Es: engage, empathise, educate and enlist. A careful exploration of these concepts is followed by exercises to help participants apply the concepts to situations and thereby understand and use them better. If offered as a primary mode for teaching conflict resolution, this approach presumes that to change behaviour, we mainly need to educate the mind. Insight brings wisdom, it may be supposed, and with greater understanding we will naturally change what we do in the light of our enhanced discernment.

A different approach, also largely focused on intellect, emphasises understanding one's own personal style, and the other disputants' styles, for engaging in conflict. The Thomas–Kilmann (2010) approach, for instance, identifies five styles: competing, compromising, avoiding, accommodating and collaborating. They are distinguished largely on two axes: assertive versus unassertive, and cooperative versus uncooperative. Those who bring a *competitive* style to conflict tend to be confrontational, assertive and not particularly cooperative towards the overall goal of winning. People who *avoid* conflict are unassertive, yet also uncooperative. They simply don't address the conflict, whether by sidestepping an issue, postponing a discussion or simply leaving when a threatening situation arises. Those who *compromise* reside in the middle. Their goal is a mutually acceptable resolution that at least partly satisfies everyone, by finding some sort of middle ground. *Accommodaters* are also unassertive but more cooperative, as they tend sometimes to neglect their own concerns, engaging in some self-sacrifice and yielding to others' points of view in order to end a conflict. Finally, a *collaborator* will be cooperative and also assertive, in the search to find creative resolutions that maximally address both sides' underlying concerns. Collaborators will explore issues with greater depth than the compromisers (Thomas & Kilmann, 2010; Schaubhut, 2007).

A variation on the same theme — identifying styles for interacting and engaging in conflict — looks at four personality types, in the DISC approach. A person's style can be dominant, influential, steady or conscientious (Discinsights.com, 2017). Each broad type is distinguished on two axes, according to whether the individual is active or passive, task-oriented or people-oriented (Marston, 1970; Marston, 1979; Rohm 1993; see also Changing Minds information in the online resources section). The *dominant* person, for instance, tends to be quite direct, decisive, bottom-line focused and problem-solving — with the potential weakness that they may not always listen to others. The *influential* personality is enthusiastic, talkative, optimistic, creative and a good motivator for others — with the possible weakness that they may not attend adequately to detail or tangible results. A *steady* personality tends to be stable and predictable, even-tempered, dependable, sympathetic and generous — and, as a weakness, may be reluctant to change or to face conflict directly. Finally, the *conscientious* person is inclined to be accurate, detail-oriented, systematic and reality-based — with the potential downside that it may be difficult for these people to verbalise feelings, or be less able to bring flexibility and an ability to see the larger picture.

The overriding theme behind the DISC approach is that the better we understand how someone functions, what motivates versus what deters that person, and the better we understand how we ourselves function, then the better we are equipped to work effectively with each another to reach mutually agreeable resolutions. As with the earlier approaches, improved understanding is seen to move one to action. Insight changes behaviour.

In contrast to a focus on intellectual concepts, or on personality inventories that may enable people to think more deeply about conflict, other approaches describe specific behavioural responses that can more directly enable one to explore, defuse and, ultimately (it is hoped), resolve conflict. The 'crucial conversations' (Patterson et al., 2012) approach, for instance, features ABCs: agree (start with the areas of agreement that often occupy the greatest share of ground between the parties; identify mutually shared purposes); build (use the areas of agreement to reframe areas of disagreement and build a more complete picture of what needs to be discussed); and compare (explore how one's own path differs from the other person's, with an emphasis on creating a complete picture rather than contradicting each other). Relevant skills for those conversations include: sharing one's own facts, story and path; asking for the other person's path as well; speaking in a tentative fashion rather than dogmatically; and encouraging testing, not just of the other person's views, but also of one's own. This approach thus combines intellectual analysis with specific communication skills.

Notwithstanding the value of the foregoing approaches, a person in conflict may not have the opportunity to discern the details of counterparts' personalities. And correctly labelling someone's conflict style does not necessarily tell us what to do in a particular situation. By the same token education, even great insight, does not always change behaviour. Especially in the heat of a conflict, intellectual assertions of fact and rationality cannot always overcome emotions and underlying agendas. Insight does not always stir us to better-quality action when action is difficult.

A different practice-based approach takes an even more granular tactic, focusing on a toolbox of specific skills and strategies and emphasising learn-by-doing. From Aristotle: 'For the things we have to learn before we can do them, we learn by doing them …' (Aristotle 350 BCE). While neither diminishing nor denigrating the value of the other perspectives, this last pedagogical approach looks to a collection of very specific skills and strategies — what, concretely, to do or say in virtually any situation, to elicit hoped-for responses (Moore, 2003). Those techniques include summarising, restating, asking questions (closed-ended, open-ended and clarifying), reframing, appropriate body language and vocal tone including mirroring and modelling, distinguishing overt positions from underlying interests (Fisher & Ury, 1991), and many more.

This practically oriented, skills-based approach to learning and teaching conflict resolution in the clinical setting supposes that skills and strategies are best built by being used and honed in practice, again and again, essentially creating a kind of 'muscle memory' or 'autopilot' in which best practices are more likely to appear and be used, even in the heat of a moment that may not allow for full reflection or intellectual processing. This is the approach used in this chapter, and further details of this teaching method are discussed below.

To see how this sort of conflict resolution might then look in practice and how it might be taught, we now return to the two case scenarios described just above.

Bringing pedagogy to practice: resolving conflict in the case studies

The first case above concerned Carl, a 48-year-old man with abdominal pain who wants to be treated in the hospital. His insurance coverage is about to be cut off on the ground that hospitalisation is no longer medically necessary. Let us assume, for purposes of argument, that the medical team has done a thorough workup and that no further testing or observation would provide reasonable prospect of medical value. Let us also assume that the insurer can legitimately cite medical necessity criteria to justify a decision to end coverage for the current hospitalisation.

Nevertheless, Carl's doctor wonders whether and how to bring this to Carl's attention in a way that will not precipitate conflict or damage their relationship of trust. If the resident simply says 'your insurance won't cover this', Carl may conclude that she is colluding with the insurer to save money by denying him care. And yet if nothing is said, he may end up with a large bill to pay, perhaps leading him to conclude his doctor did not advocate for him sufficiently against the insurer. Or he may feel betrayed simply because the doctor did not care enough to say anything, one way or another.

Based on these factors the optimal resolution may not be to force the financial information on Carl, but rather to explore his potential interest in the issue. Several skills and strategies come to mind. First, a clinician in this type of situation needs to set the stage for the conversation — provide a context that can make it clear to Carl that the focus is on his own interests. This strategy is called *managing expectations*: let people know, ahead of time, what to expect, thereby diminishing the possibility of unpleasant surprises. Here, the clinician might move the conversation in the desired direction by discussing how Carl is feeling, asking about his concerns about going home, and indicating that such transitions are often challenging.

Towards that end, an associated strategy in this case might be to *normalise*: when people see that something is normal, familiar and that many other people have similar experiences or interests — that the person's situation or concerns are 'normal' — they are often more comfortable discussing something that might otherwise be uncomfortable. Here, the clinician might note to Carl that, these days, a lot of people in the hospital worry about whether they will have an unhappy surprise, in the form of a large bill that may be difficult to pay. They don't always say it, but many patients wonder about it.

Having set the stage in this fashion, the clinician might then *ask for permission*: asking for permission is an act of genuine respect towards the patient, by returning to him some of the control that is so often muted in the healthcare setting. Thus, after noting that many people are concerned about costs, the clinician might add that sometimes those costs are generated when an insurer decides that inpatient care is no longer needed. Then she can ask Carl whether he would like to be notified if his own insurer seems to be moving in that direction. If so, the team will gladly comply. If he would prefer not to think about finances at this time — an equally legitimate choice, when one is ill — the team will assuredly honour that as well.

The conversation can proceed from there, depending on how Carl responds, with the goal of enhancing worthwhile communication and, quite likely, preventing conflict in the process. Indeed, it could promote a more meaningful conversation about the role of inpatient versus outpatient care for his abdominal pain. Such a result is not guaranteed, of course, because these situations are often fraught with many unseen layers and hidden agendas. But if it leads to a better discussion about Carl's concerns and fears, this sort of conversation can be productive on many levels.

Conflict deriving from a lack of insurance coverage for a hospital stay is particularly pertinent in the US context. However, the key messages from this case, relevant across many other healthcare settings, is the need to recognise, plan for and actively manage differing values and communication and clinical decision conflicts, through specific communication strategies.

The second case above concerned a 14-month-old who, as a prematurely delivered infant, has had respiratory problems since birth — a little exacerbated by her current illness, but not alarmingly so. A nurse who is unaccustomed to caring for such children is concerned and urges the mother to demand transfer to the PICU. The resident is in an awkward position. The mother clearly trusts the nurse, who spends far more time at the bedside. And the resident is admittedly still in training, not yet vested with the credibility of a more senior doctor.

In the actual case the resident's response to the mother was to assert: 'She's a nurse … I'm the doctor. The PICU is not medically indicated for Alice at this time. If at some point I think she needs it, I won't hesitate to transfer her at that time. There now — do you have any other questions?'

A preferable approach would start, not with flat counter-assertions to overturn the nurse's statements, but rather with *active listening*: the resident could invite the mother to describe her concerns, and ask her to explain what she finds particularly worrisome about Alice's condition. The conversation will feature plenty of questions, including *open-ended questions* and *clarifying questions*, both to understand the mother's concerns, and to ensure that she feels heard and respected. In that context, *drilling down for details* can be very useful: helping the mother to describe as precisely as possible what she's worried about, as opposed to making assumptions about those concerns, will enable the resident to respond in ways that actually address those concerns, rather than skirting or missing what is most important in her eyes.

In the process, a useful skill is *affect labelling*: observing the emotion(s) the mother is displaying, and naming it aloud. Often, a person in a strong emotional state will not feel heard when the conversation remains on a strictly factual plane. Acknowledging the underlying feelings can go a long way towards building the level of communication that, in turn, can promote resolution. Thus, the resident might say 'as you hear such different things from the people caring for Alice … that's probably pretty confusing. And maybe scary. Does that capture some of what you're experiencing right now?' Throughout, *building trust* with her is imperative for resolving conflict successfully. Listening carefully helps to establish a more solid human connection with people in conflict, often a prerequisite for achieving successful resolution. A similar set of skills would, of course, be brought to other conflicts embedded in the situation, such as that between the nurse and the resident.

Teaching conflict resolution for healthcare

So how does one learn and teach this? Several levels of intensity are available. In my own work, the most in-depth training involves several days. Day one combines some didactic material with a variety of brief practice scenarios. A spectrum of conflict resolution platforms is introduced, from negotiation to coaching, facilitation, mediation and arbitration, helping participants to understand better what sorts of conflicts appear in their own lives and work. Thereafter, a collection of specific skills and strategies is presented. They include summarising, restating, asking questions (closed-ended, open-ended and clarifying), reframing, appropriate body language and vocal tone including mirroring and modelling, distinguishing overt positions from underlying interests, and many more.

Importantly, and in accordance with the pedagogical approach of 'learning by doing', in day one, participants periodically work, mainly in pairs, to practise those skills and strategies in scenarios that capture conflicts commonly found in healthcare. These are labelled 'practice scenarios' rather than 'role plays' because the latter tends to suggest two or three people at the front of the room, acting out a situation while everyone else watches and critiques. Instead, my approach makes sure everyone is directly involved in every exercise. Learning happens best when a person is 'in the moment' of a realistic conflict with another person and must somehow find the right response, using the right words, inflection and gestures. These practices are designed to reflect the real conflicts that arise during healthcare and, at the same time, invite participants to use — again and again — the specific skills they are being taught. Thus, as each pair does each exercise, one person might be 'the doctor' while the other is 'the patient'; or one might be 'the nurse' while the other is 'the spouse'. Extensive debriefing of each scenario is then followed by the next set of skills and strategies as they are introduced and put into practice, a few at a time.

On days two and three the training is virtually wall-to-wall practice-and-debrief. Here, the practice scenarios are mainly mock mediations that place participants in groups of three to five people instead of in pairs. One person serves as the mediator while other group members play one of the other participants in the situation, with each having their own private information. Because everyone is either a mediator or another character in every mock mediation, several mediations are running simultaneously. In one case the mediator might help quarrelling parents come to a decision about what is best for their child. In another scenario the mediator may help the daytime nursing supervisor to work through the issues with a night-shift supervisor who seems not to be doing their job. Cases become more complex as participants become more experienced. Each mediation runs for 45 minutes, followed by extensive debriefing.

As noted, in mediation one person serves as a neutral, a non-partisan who helps those in conflict to listen to each other and collaborate to define and resolve their differences. Mediation serves as the platform on days two and three for several reasons. Admittedly, most participants will not actually become mediators when they complete the training. Nevertheless, we learn a great deal about conflict, and how to resolve it, from watching other people fight, from helping them to clarify their thinking and expression, and from controlling our own temptation to dive into the fracas, take sides and tell everyone what they should do. The mediator must figure out, right in the moment, how to ask a question that will help people figure out for themselves what, really, is the problem; how to acknowledge and sometimes redirect another person's emotions; how to take a moment of apparent impasse and help people move towards collaborative problem-solving.

During days two and three, each person serves as the mediator at least twice across eight to ten different cases. Other times they serve as one of the people in conflict. This, too, is instructive as we use empathy to appreciate why a person thinks, feels and acts the way they do.

Mediation is also a useful platform because, using multi-party scenarios, it requires us to juggle a variety of different perspectives at once. And because mediation is a way to assist others' negotiations, and sometimes privately to coach one or more of the parties in conflict, it relies on other kinds of conflict resolution such as negotiation and coaching.

Finally, although many participants will not become mediators as such, a number of them actually will need to provide mediation-type services from time to time. As discussed above, those who provide ethics consultation services quickly discover that most consults are about conflict, not moral puzzlement. Hence one's best service in many of those cases is to facilitate a conversation between people in conflict, to help them come to their own best resolution. Often, if the consultant simply favours one side over another, little is actually resolved. Across more than three decades of doing ethics consults, not once have I heard a clinician, patient or family member say 'Gosh, the ethics expert thinks my view on this situation is wrong — so surely I must be mistaken, and I need to change my mind about this!' Not once.

In many hospital settings, clinicians themselves are required to adopt or incorporate aspects of these more formal mediator or clinical ethicist roles. In case conferences and family conferences, for instance, patients, families and clinicians meet to address uncertainties and sometimes disagreements about the most appropriate care, going forward. Therefore, this same intensive workshop-style training would also be relevant for their ongoing professional development as clinicians and educators.

Briefer training events can also provide skills, strategies and practice. For example, I provide a full-day 'Communications Bootcamp' training for first-year residents including nurses in a one-to-one ratio. This training focuses mainly on conflict resolution in the one-on-one negotiation situation (i.e. one's own conflicts) rather than on multi-party mediation. Still, the basics are the same. During the morning some didactic lectures teach an array of skills and strategies, a few at a time and interspersing them with various practice scenarios. During the afternoon, participants work with various partners in a number of more complex scenarios. The scenario may feature clinician–patient, clinician–family, clinician–team, etc. Also, as the doctor sometimes plays the nurse, and vice versa, each type of professional has the opportunity to gain insight into the other's perspective. Debriefing discussions, as with the three-day training, are extensive and crucial to the learning process.

Even briefer trainings are half-day or less, with a somewhat smaller 'toolkit' of skills and fewer, briefer practice scenarios. Nevertheless, they can be of considerable value as an introduction to conflict resolution and collaborative problem-solving.

Finally, learning and teaching these types of skills need not be confined to formal workshops. It can also come on the spot, through real-life cases. For instance, it can come through one-on-one coaching to help faculty colleagues who are figuring out how best to manage a conflict, or to prevent one from occurring, or to explicitly model and teach trainees.

Evaluation and research

Based on the foregoing discussion, skills and strategies for resolving conflict can indeed be learnt, practised and honed. Avenues for evaluation and further research can be explored on two levels. On a micro level are discussions about how best to evaluate individuals and whether training has helped them to be more successful in managing conflict. More broadly on a macro level this includes how best to make such training more widely available, and whether such training can reduce the level and destructiveness of conflict in healthcare overall.

At the micro level, research would involve discerning whether an individual learner has acquired reasonable proficiency in using various skills and strategies of conflict resolution and, more specifically, whether that person has become adept at resolving conflicts in the day-to-day clinical setting. The challenges are real. Direct observation of someone while they are working on a real conflict could be intrusive on participants' privacy and disruptive of the process itself, simply by virtue of the observer's presence. Nevertheless, certain kinds of in-person opportunity may be available. In the legal context, mediation of lawsuits permits 'shadowing' and co-mediating, to provide new mediators the opportunity to see a real mediation in process, and then to undertake one's own mediation under the direct tutelage of an experienced mediator. Similar opportunities could be created in the clinical setting, particularly in teaching hospitals where clinical educators can actively model conflict resolution strategies and provide trainees with opportunities to practise them in supported environments.

Still, it can also be challenging to evaluate the success, or not, of a real-life instance of conflict management. It may not always be clear what counts as an outcome in the first place, or what would be a 'success' in clinical conflict resolution. If the conflict evaporates because the dispute was about treatment choices and the patient got better on their own, is that 'successful conflict resolution' or simply good fortune? Other times, a patient's worsening medical condition might erase the benefits of an agreement genuinely embraced by all — for example, where everyone agreed it would be worthwhile to try a brief period of artificial ventilation but then the patient had another stoke and died. Finally, somewhat analogous to psychotherapy, counselling or other disciplines involving interpersonal relationships, conflict resolution does depend at least partly on interpersonal chemistry. The same person might do very well with one person or group, and not as well with someone else. With limited opportunities for live observation, it could be difficult to discern the extent to which one is observing the person's skill level, versus a complex nexus of interpersonal chemistry overlaid by background issues.

More traditional evaluations include written exams. Although multiple-choice questions have well-known limits, a computer-based, interactive series of questions surrounding various scenarios, each set triggered by responses to the previous one, might provide greater depth of analysis than the typical multiple-choice question. Beyond this, thoughtfully conceived essay questions can provide a broader opportunity for someone who is learning conflict resolution skills to show depth and breadth of ability to bring various skills and strategies to explore a conflict and work towards resolution.

In-person examination is arguably optimal for evaluating skills and their strategic use. Where any kind of skill is required, as beyond simply intellectual recall of facts, written tests of recall, analysis and judgment will not necessarily exhibit those skills. Thus, for instance, the United States Medical Licensing Examination (USMLE) for doctors has recognised that written questions cannot suffice to test whether a medical student can establish rapport with patients, elicit key medical history, provide information in lay language and form a partnership for decision-making. Hence, the USMLE Step 2 exam includes a day-long, in-person component. The student spends 15 minutes each with 12 'standardised patients' (actors trained to behave as real patients). After each encounter the student is allowed 10 minutes to write a note appropriately listing history, physical findings, diagnostic impressions and management plans.

Nevertheless, for conflict resolution skills a formal, in-person exam — for example, an oral exam featuring professional actors in exam-designed scenarios — would probably be costly and could feel, and be, a little extreme if the goal is simply to help faculty and trainees to learn these skills. Hence, the more productive focus might be to create workshops as described above, and to expand opportunities for collaborative learning and mentoring.

At the macro level, research would need to focus partly on how to broaden the availability of such training, and additionally on whether such training can reduce the level and destructiveness of conflict in healthcare overall. The latter question requires complex social science methodology. Credible research design would require: (a) defining what will count as 'conflict'; (b) determining how to measure the kinds and levels of conflict within a given institution; and (c) controlling for a wide variety of variables, as one then attempts to discern whether conflict training has, at that institution, been causally active in changing the level of conflict.

The former question, namely how to broaden the availability of training in conflict management, encourages us to construct what might be called the 'business case' for it. As noted above, communication problems are 'a root cause in nearly 70% of reported sentinel events, surpassing other commonly identified issues such as staff orientation and training, patient assessment, and staffing' (ECRI, 2009, p 1). Conflict is a key source of poor communication, as people at odds with one another tend not to communicate with each other adequately. Patient safety and medical errors, and with them the hazards of medical malpractice litigation, are thus a central focus of the business case for conflict resolution training. Additionally, unresolved conflict can cause provider burnout, staff turnover, department-level dysfunction, patient and family dissatisfaction, and a dysfunctional culture generally. Good business, as well as good care, requires addressing these effectively.

PRACTICAL TIPS

The key practical tips which can be used by clinical educators in their own clinical practice, and/
or explicitly modelled to learners, are listed below.

- Use *active listening* by inviting patients/learners/colleagues to describe their concerns. Listening carefully helps to establish a more solid human connection with people in conflict, and is often a prerequisite for achieving successful resolution.
- Ensure these discussions include plenty of questions, including *open-ended questions* and *clarifying questions* with the goal of understanding the other person's concerns, and to ensure that they feel heard and respected.
- Focus on *drilling down for details* to assist the other person to describe as precisely as possible what they are worried about. This will avoid making assumptions about those concerns, and will enable you to respond in ways that actually address those concerns, rather than skirting or missing what is most important in the other person's eyes.
- Use *affect labelling* — observing the emotion(s) the other person is displaying, and naming it aloud. Acknowledging the underlying feelings can go a long way towards building the level of communication that, in turn, can promote resolution.
- It is imperative to work at *building trust* as a condition of managing conflict successfully.

Conclusion

Conflict plays a large role in healthcare. The stakes are enormous. The work is complex and requires a high level of teamwork, even as highly trained professionals need to exercise independent judgment, and even as patients and families do not always envision the same goals and means as their providers. Competent conflict management is thus essential to patient safety, patient and provider satisfaction, organisational efficiency and effectiveness, and a host of other important parameters.

Good conflict management comes more naturally to some people than to others, yet it can indeed be taught. A large body of skills and strategies can be helpful. Critical to the learning process, however, is the opportunity for supervised practice and debriefing. Simply learning a concept is insufficient. One cannot gain proficiency without opportunities to use that skill, discuss whether the practice went well and how it might be improved, and then try it again. Clinical educators are in a prime position to promote these opportunities via modelling and actively scaffolding trainees' learning and by lobbying for explicit training. Eventually, with good training and follow-up coaching, proficient skills can simply emerge on their own when needed.

Online resources/further reading

Online conflict resolution training examples:
- http://conflict911.com/resources/Exercises_and_Training_Activities_To_Teach_Conflict_Management/
- www.edcc.edu/counseling/documents/Conflict.pdf
- www.helpguide.org/articles/relationships/conflict-resolution-skills.htm
- www.creducation.net/resources/CR_Guidelines_and_10_CR_lessons_FCPS.pdf
- www.crnhq.org/content.aspx?file=66138%7C373821
- http://study.com/academy/lesson/teaching-conflict-resolution-to-adults.html

Institute for Healthcare Communication:
- Clinician-Patient Communication to Enhance Health Outcomes: http://healthcarecomm.org/training/faculty-courses/clinician-patient-communication
- Faculty course (Train-the-Trainer): http://healthcarecomm.org/wp-content/uploads/2014/05/CPC-TTT-course-overview-_5-6-14.pdf

Discinsights.com — DISC personality types:
- http://changingminds.org/explanations/preferences/disc.htm

References

ASBH Task Force. (2011). *Core competencies for healthcare ethics consultation* (2nd ed.). Chicago: ASBH.

Bergman, E. (2013). Surmounting elusive barriers: The case for bioethics mediation. *The Journal of Clinical Ethics*, 24(1), 11–24.

Conard, J. R., & Franklin, J. F. (2010). Addressing the art of conflict management in healthcare systems. *Dispute Resolution Magazine*, 16(3), 15.

Discinsights.com. (2017). *DISC theory and DISC personality traits*. Available at: https://discinsights.com/disc-theory/. (Accessed 22 November 2017).

Dubler, N., & Liebman, C. (2011). *Bioethics mediation: a guide to shaping shared solutions*. Nashville: Vanderbilt University Press.

ECRI. (September, 2009). *Healthcare Risk Control: Supplement A, at 1*. Available at: www.ecri.org/PatientSafety/RiskQual16.pdf.

Fiester, A. (2011). Ill-placed democracy: Ethics consultations and the moral status of voting. *The Journal of Clinical Ethics*, 22, 363–372.

Fiester, A. (2012). Mediation and advocacy. *The American Journal of Bioethics: AJOB*, 12(8), 10–11.

Fisher, R., & Ury, W. (1991). *Getting to yes: negotiating agreement without giving in* (2nd ed.). New York: Penguin Books.

Gibson, K. (1999). Mediation in the medical field. *The Hastings Center Report*, 29(5), 6–13.

Marcus, L. J. (2002). A culture of conflict: Lessons from renegotiating health care. *Journal of Health Care Law and Policy*, 5, 447–478.

Marcus, L. J., Dorn, B. C., & McNulty, E. J. (2011). *Renegotiating health care: resolving conflict to build collaboration* (2nd ed.). San Francisco: Jossey-Bass.

Marston, C. (1970). *Motivating the 'what's in it for me?' workforce*. Hoboken, NJ: John Wiley.

Marston, W. (1979). *The emotions of normal people*. Minneapolis: Persona Press, Inc.

Mayer, B. S. (2015). *The conflict paradox: seven dilemmas at the core of disputes*. San Francisco: John Wiley & Sons.

Moore, C. W. (2003). *The mediation process: practical strategies for resolving conflict* (3rd ed.). San Francisco: Jossey Bass.

Morreim, E. H. (2014a). Conflict resolution in health care. *Connections*, 18(1), 28–32.

Morreim, E. H. (2014b). In-house conflict resolution processes: Health lawyers as problem-solvers. *The Health Lawyer*, 25(3), 10–14.

Morreim, E. H. (2015). Conflict resolution in the clinical setting: A story beyond bioethics mediation. *The Journal of Law, Medicine & Ethics: A Journal of the American Society of Law, Medicine & Ethics*, 43, 843–856.

Morreim, E. H. (2016). Story of a mediation in the clinical setting. *The Journal of Clinical Ethics*, 27, 42–49.

Patterson, K., Joseph Grenny, J., McMillan, R., et al. (2012). *Crucial conversations: tools for talking when stakes are high* (2nd ed.). New York: McGraw-Hill.

Rohm, R. (1993). *Positive personality profiles*. Atlanta, GA: Personality Insights Inc.

Schaubhut, N. A. (2007). *Technical brief for the Thomas-Kilmann conflict mode instrument*. Available at: www.cpp.com/Pdfs/TKI_Technical_Brief.pdf.

Scott, C., & Gerardi, D. (2011a). A strategic approach for managing conflict in hospitals: Responding to the Joint Commission leadership standard; Part I. *Joint Commission Journal on Quality and Patient Safety*, 37, 59–69.

Scott, C., & Gerardi, D. (2011b). A strategic approach for managing conflict in hospitals: Responding to the Joint Commission leadership standard; Part II. *Joint Commission Journal on Quality and Patient Safety*, 37, 70–80.

Stone, D., Patton, B., & Heen, S. (1999). *Difficult conversations*. New York: Penguin Books.

Thomas, K. W., & Kilmann, R. H. (2010). *Thomas-Kilmann conflict mode instrument profile and interpretive report*. Available at: www.cpp.com/en-US/Products-and-Services/TKI.

Ury, W. (1993). *Getting past no*. New York: Bantam Dell.

Section 2

Education approaches within clinical learning contexts

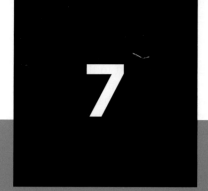

7

The influence of workplace context on learning and teaching

Joanna Bates, Rachel Ellaway and
Christopher Watling

Introduction

Embedded in the real-life work of healthcare, clinical education is inevitably shaped by the different clinical contexts within which it takes place. The healthcare contexts for workplace learning are increasingly diverse; they may be rural or urban, they may be hospital or community-based, they may involve elderly people as patients or newborn babies, and they may involve different mixes of ethnicity, socioeconomic status, and disease and injury profiles. The contexts for clinical education define much of the learning that is possible within them (Billett, 2016; Dornan, 2012). For instance, context can shape learner attitudes (Dornan et al., 2014), it can create opportunities for professional identity development (Creuss et al., 2014), it can motivate learners (Mann et al., 2009), and it can afford authentic opportunities for learners to apply their skills and knowledge (Dornan et al., 2014).

Context can also present challenges. For instance, learners are regularly required to adapt to new contexts, particularly when rotating between training locations (Bernabeo et al., 2011; Miles et al., 2015; Teunissen & Westerman, 2011). Learners who are struggling to adjust to different settings may miss some learning opportunities, avoid others (Atherley et al., 2016), and generally fail to thrive (Attrill et al., 2015; Teunissen & Westerman, 2011). As the diversity of contexts for clinical learning expands and the numbers of learners being rotated through these increasingly heterogeneous training contexts increases, the challenges learners face also increase. Even similar-seeming workplace contexts may differ in significant yet largely unnoticed ways (Ellaway & Bates, 2015). Given that clinical educators generally do not move as often as their trainees do, they may struggle to support their trainees to navigate this shifting landscape.

Clinical workplaces are complex and unpredictable (Durning et al., 2010; Fenwick, 2012; Plsek & Greenhalgh, 2001; Stacey, 2007), not least because their main focus is on providing care rather than on education. Clinical educators are often unsure how to help incoming learners to adjust to their workplace contexts, or how to make the best use of the learning opportunities that these contexts afford. This uncertainty is in part due to their becoming so used to their everyday working contexts that they no longer notice the idiosyncracies or dynamics. Nevertheless, clinical educators need to understand both the affordances of their clinical workplace and its distinctive features to be able to provide meaningful and effective learning experiences for their trainees.

In this chapter, we aim to help clinical educators to better understand and make more effective use of their clinical workplace contexts for teaching. We begin with a case study that describes the experience of Sandy (a community-based clinical educator) and Sean (her clinical trainee). Sean is struggling to make sense of this unfamiliar clinical workplace context, and Sandy is struggling to understand Sean's challenges in adapting to his new circumstances. From this, we systematically describe clinical workplace contexts to help educators to understand their own clinical workplaces. We build on these insights by drawing on aspects of sociocultural learning theory to explore how and what it is that learners learn from the clinical workplace contexts in which they find themselves. We then describe different pedagogical strategies that clinical educators can use to enhance the ways in which their trainees can learn from their clinical workplace contexts. Finally, we return to the case study to re-examine the contextual learning opportunities Sandy and Sean can now draw on.

Case study 7.1

The context

Our case study is framed by the transition of a learner from a tertiary-care downtown teaching hospital to a rural generalist context, to illuminate both the struggles and the potential in using the clinical context effectively for teaching and learning.

The clinical educator

Sandy Morton is a family doctor in Valleyfield, a mining town with a population of 23,000. The town has 10 family doctors, 4 general specialists and an 18-bed hospital. The town borders a large Indigenous protected area, and Sandy has a mixed practice of young workers with physically demanding and often dangerous jobs, Indigenous patients and long-time residents. The town is 300 kilometres from the city of Langdon where the main medical school campus is based, and Sandy is a clinical educator for Langdon trainees taking their required rural clinical experience in Valleyfield. Although relatively new to clinical teaching, Sandy has had several senior students placed with her, and these placements went well. However, she is struggling with Sean. Sean arrived over a week ago for an 8-week mandatory rural clinical placement. He has shown little interest in engaging in the care of her patients, and he appears to lack confidence in how to interact with them. Sean has also avoided doing shifts in the emergency room, even though previous learners found the emergency room an exciting environment in which to try out their skills. Sandy eventually calls the program coordinator in Langdon to find out whether Sean has had problems on other clinical placements. She is told that there have been no issues to date, although this is his first clinical placement outside the city.

The clinical learner

Sandy has correctly identified that Sean is struggling. Indeed, Sean feels as though he has landed on a different planet. In his previous clinical placements, he was a member of a team, with a peer group of fellow students and with postgraduate trainees who were a few years senior to him, which meant that he rarely interacted directly with his clinician educators. However, in Valleyfield there is no one to ask for advice, and everyone around him is too busy providing care to have time for teaching seminars and formal rounds. The patients Sean is used to were hospitalised with life-threatening illnesses, and he usually referred these patients to the army of specialists and subspecialists in the Langdon teaching hospital. As a result, he has no idea how to approach the care of patients with ongoing chronic illnesses — patients who seem to know more about their conditions than he does, and who regularly challenge his advice. And the patients themselves are different. He recalls that he learned about Indigenous cultures in school, but he hasn't ever actually treated an Indigenous person and is uncertain about how he should do so. Sean feels lost and unable to find his feet, and he is constantly unsure of what to do or how to be an effective member of the team or even a clinical learner in this setting.

Background educational theory

Clinical educators need to understand their particular clinical workplace context(s), because different contexts afford different opportunities for learning and teaching (Billett, 2001, 2016; Cruess et al., 2014; Eraut et al., 2004). Achieving this understanding may be challenging, however. Workplace contexts are like the 'dark matter' in the universe of learning and teaching; they are difficult to perceive by those habituated to them (Dewey et al., 2008). Indeed, the idiosyncrasies of clinical workplaces are often perceived most readily by the learners who are new to them. In this section, we unpack the notion of context by using six interacting patterns of clinical training contexts (Bates & Ellaway, 2016; Ellaway & Bates, 2015) (see Figure 7.1).

- *Patient patterns:* Clinical workplaces allow learners to interact with patients, practise their skills on them, and learn from them (Dornan et al., 2014; Teunissen & Wilkinson 2011). To educators, particularly those who have spent some time in their current practice context, one patient may seem much like any other, providing educational opportunities based primarily on their presenting symptoms or differential diagnoses (Asgarova et al., 2017; Epstein, 2007; de Jong et al., 2013). Learners moving between contexts, however, may have to adapt to very different patient populations. For instance, patients may differ in age, they may present with life-threatening illnesses or mild chronic conditions, or they may come from particular religious or ethnic groups with very different ideas about health and healthcare. Skills developed in the context of one patient population often need to be adapted, sometimes quite considerably, in order to be effective for different patient populations (Truong et al., 2014). Indeed, the only common feature may be the need for healthcare.

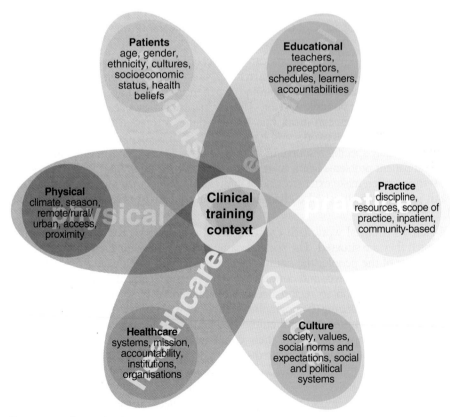

Figure 7.1: Patterns of context

Rachel Ellaway Joanna Bates. 6 context patterns flower v2. ResearchGate 2018: Available from: https://www.researchgate.net/publication/324259674_6_context_patterns_flower_v2. Accessed April 4 2018. DOI 10.13140/RG.2.2.15866.59844

- *Practice patterns:* The dynamics of clinical practice differ according to context. There may be differences in the services offered, the scopes of practice of those offering them, and the ways in which care is provided (or withheld) (White et al., 1961). Patterns of interprofessional practice may shift who does what. For example, a rural setting with few specialists or treatment resources requires a much broader scope of practice for healthcare providers than a more urban practice context. The pace of care may be leisurely and reflective, or fast-paced and unpredictable.

- *Educational patterns:* Health professional education systems define who the clinical learners and teachers are, what they should (and should not) do as learners and teachers, and when they should do it. For instance, the opportunity (or lack thereof) of formal faculty development offerings and expectations shapes the educational pattern of different training contexts. Other variables include differences in admissions, policies, curricula, promotion and educational culture (Brosnan & Turner, 2009). Education systems also define the stage at which learners are placed in clinical workplace contexts and for what reasons. For instance, midwifery learners completing a final clinical practicum will have different experiences to residents completing an obstetrics rotation, even though they are sharing the same workplace context. In some settings, learners have to adapt to many different clinical teachers, each with their own style and expectations (Goldszmidt et al., 2015), whereas in other contexts they may work with the same few teachers over an extended period of time. The availability and degree of supervision, and the presence or absence of peer learners, further shape the pattern of clinical education.

- *Institutional patterns:* Healthcare institutions (such as clinics and hospitals) differ in terms of their organisation, their funding, their rules and regulations, and their expectations. For instance, workplace learning contexts in institutions that are closely tied to university-based health professional programs are more likely to have formal structures and policies to accommodate learners than those that are not. Furthermore, the availability of inhouse diagnostic tests, treatment options, and subspecialists can influence the way that care is delivered and the very perception of 'good care'. Clinics and hospitals in rural towns inevitably lack some of these resources, but in contrast may be better connected with their communities.

- *Geography:* Clinical workplace contexts can vary according to their physical geography, climate and time of year. For instance, training in a remote site that encounters seasonal tropical storms or blizzards may afford quite different learning experiences depending on whether transportation to a tertiary-care centre is possible or not. The geographical distance between the academic centre and different training sites can mean that learners doing a rotation at some sites are more isolated from their social support networks and have less access to academic supports than learners at other sites. Geographically-specific resource industries, such as forestry and mining, influence the kinds of patients and patient problems learners are exposed to. Certain geographical contexts, such as rural and remote settings, often make extensive use of information and communication technologies (ICT) and telehealth services, which can also change the learning experiences and opportunities these contexts afford.

- *Societal patterns:* Clinical workplace contexts are also shaped by the communities they serve and within which they are situated. The societal pattern of context is enacted through the values, beliefs and behaviours of the people, the nature of their interactions with each other and with healthcare, and the expressions of power and compassion. For instance, clinical workplaces differ from country to country or from region to region because of differences in their broader societal contexts. At a more local level, changing demographics (such as the influx of refugees into a community), access to particular technologies, and cultural generational differences can all impact on the clinical workplace. Patient populations and their concomitant disease profiles often cluster in specific geographical areas. For instance, genetic diseases may be more common in some communities than others, or complex chronic multi-morbidities may be more common in areas with greater social deprivation.

Although not exhaustive, we have found that these six patterns reflect the main recurring differences between clinical training contexts. As useful as they are for mapping out the learning landscape, we should not assume that these patterns are completely separable. For instance, patients will tend to reflect their community's culture; educational practice will be shaped by the availability of services and by local approaches to medical practice; and patient presentations will to some extent reflect environmental challenges (such as season and climate). A single element (such as a clinical service or a demographic characteristic) may also relate to more than one pattern, and elements within a single pattern will often interact with each other as well as across patterns (Bates & Ellaway, 2016). It is also important to note that these patterns and the elements within them tend to be in a permanent state of flux. Some changes may happen rapidly, such as a multiple vehicle crash affecting an emergency room workplace (Durning et al., 2010), whereas other changes may happen less abruptly, such as the adoption of new policies and procedures (Stacey, 2007). Indeed, some changes may happen very slowly, possibly over years, such as the widespread adoption of new technologies or the ageing of a population (Lewin, 1999). Smaller cycles may often occur within longer ones, each shaping the other. For instance, a community that is slowly growing or shrinking will continue to experience seasonal change in its healthcare context.

While the patterns of the clinical workplace are complex, interactive and evolving, the six patterns can be used as a lens to illuminate the workplace context.

Context and theories of learning

How does learning occur?

Sociocultural theories of learning can provide insights into how clinical workplace contexts can shape the learning that takes place within them (Monrouxe & Rees, 2009). These theories model learning as a social process, constructed through the interactions of learners with others in a particular context, such as a clinical workplace. Healthcare institutions (as healthcare communities) have their own distinct ways of working (Wenger, 1998; Wenger-Trayner et al., 2014). These differences may be reflected in a local hospital's policies and procedures, in a clinic's hours of operation and ways of keeping patient records, or in a practice's ways of organising patient appointments. These 'ways of getting things done' are typically encompassed within formal policies, practice guidelines, and accreditation structures, but play out differently in different clinical workplaces.

When someone new arrives in a particular context, it takes time for them to find their way to participate fully in the practices of the community. These incomers are what Lave and Wenger term '*legitimate peripheral participants*' (Lave & Wenger, 1991; Wenger, 1998). The learner is 'legitimate' because they are allowed to be there; they are 'peripheral' because they are not yet able to participate fully in the activities of the community; and they are a 'participant' because learning occurs through participation in the activities of the community. With clinical learners, the learner is not only an incomer, but is usually also a novice, working towards a level of expertise. The learner is guided into a fuller participation by clinical educators and other members of the healthcare team (Dornan et al., 2014; Teunissen & Dornan, 2008). By learning through participation, the learner is gradually drawn further into the community's work, participating more effectively and gradually taking on more autonomy. Members of a practice community acknowledge and accept the learner's developing competence as contributing to the activities of the community (Wenger, 1998). And, as a community acknowledges the learner's developing competence through their ability to participate in the activities of the community, the learner forms and refines their professional identity, developed from their legitimate and increasing participation in the community (Wenger-Trayner et al., 2014).

For learners to be integrated into a professional community, they are to some extent socialised to its values, and they will adopt its customs, its attitudes, and its ways of working (Brosnan & Turner, 2009). Context is particularly influential in the development of attitudes and values (see Table 7.1). Participation in the work of a practice community supports 'informal learning' — the learning that emerges from doing, rather than the learning that emerges from classroom teaching or codified knowledge (such as books) (Eraut, 2000, 2004). Informal learning often occurs without conscious recognition of what is being learned, and, as a result, learners tend to accumulate 'tacit knowledge' through such learning. And it is precisely this tacit knowledge that clinicians and their learners draw on (often without thinking) in order to accomplish many of their tasks. This use of tacit knowledge can free up the individual to use their cognitive capacity to address more complex problems — problems that require particular attention and focus. Prior informal learning and current tacit knowledge are fundamental enablers for clinicians to function effectively in any given clinical workplace.

TABLE 7.1: Different levels and forms of contextual dependence for different forms of learning*

	Level of contextual dependence		
	Low	Medium	High
What is best learned or developed	Knowledge	Behaviour	Attitudes
	Skills	Discrimination	Identity
Nature of (in) dependence	Knowledge and skills can be learned or developed in one context and translated to other contexts	Behaviours related to medical competencies and the ability to discriminate between alternative paths of action need to be learned or developed in particular kinds of contexts, but can transfer to other similar contexts	Individual attitudes and the resulting behaviours and the development of physician identities can be highly dependent on the contexts within which they were developed and will continue to influence future practice

Note: This reflects broad tendencies rather than absolute dependencies.
Adapted from J. Bates & R. H. Ellaway. (2016). Mapping the dark matter of context: A conceptual scoping review. *Medical Education, 50*(8), 807–816.

Context impacts learners

Health professions education programs use clinical placements to develop learners' professional knowledge, skills and attitudes. Typically, learners move from the formal university setting into clinical workplaces, and then move from one clinical workplace to another (Wenger-Trayner et al., 2014). Wenger-Trayner characterises the individual's movement from setting to setting as an individual trajectory across a landscape of practice (Wenger-Trayner et al., 2014). When learners move from one clinical workplace context to another, they not only become a legitimate peripheral participant in the new workplace, they also find their tacit knowledge less useful for their new setting than for their old. The more differences there are between workplace contexts, the less a learner's tacit knowledge from one context is likely to be useful in the others. For example, a learner moving from a respiratory rotation to an orthopaedics rotation, even if they are in the same hospital, is likely to have a different patient profile, with different lengths of stay, different schedules of therapy, and different expectations about the role of the learner and what learners are expected to focus on and accomplish.

On the other hand, the learner can draw on their tacit knowledge about the policies, resources and values of the hospital as a whole. Learners can also draw on their developing understanding of what it means to be a clinician (Eraut et al., 2004). By comparison, a learner moving from a clinical discipline in one setting to a different clinical discipline in a completely new setting may find that virtually all of their tacit knowledge no longer applies, and as a result the learner may struggle to figure out how 'things are done here'. The more change there is, the more disruption the learner is likely to experience. Indeed, a learner moving from a pathology rotation in a large academic centre to a community-based general surgery rotation at a distance from the main centre may need to adapt to changes in virtually every pattern of context; even their own sense of professional identity may be challenged. The more differences there are between rotation contexts, the more work the learner has to do in order to transition successfully, both practically and emotionally (Wenger-Trayner et al., 2014).

No matter the educational intent, moving between contexts requires that learners adjust their approaches to learning and practice. Moving to a new clinical workplace, even within the same hospital, can take much energy and attention, and often provokes uncomfortable feelings in learners, including anxiety, stress, frustration, intimidation and fear (Bernabeo et al., 2011). Moving to a completely new clinical workplace can carry even more burden: the time and cost of having to relocate, and the loss of personal supports and opportunities for personal life. Learners may feel uncertain of their role and responsibilities in the new workplace (Atherley et al., 2016; Howe & Kumar, 2017), and they may struggle with logistics, such as *where* to find equipment or forms, or *who*, *how*, and *when* to contact others for help. (Attrill et al., 2015; Miles et al., 2015). In effect, every small task can take effort, which may interfere with their ability to learn.

Context, competence and capability

Educators often think about competence as something that an individual acquires, and that, once owned, is something that can be transferred between different clinical workplace contexts (Sfard, 1998). In contrast, sociocultural learning theory describes competence as something developed and embedded within a community, rather than being owned by an individual. A corollary to the concept of competence being constructed within a specific setting is the idea that competence cannot be transferred across different contexts: performing the same role in different settings requires further learning and adaptation (Eraut et al., 2004). Indeed, 'competence is contextual, reflecting the relationship between a person's abilities and the tasks he or she is required to perform in a particular situation in the real world' (Epstein, 2007, p 387). For clinical learners, competence is inseparable from the settings in which their learning occurs. It exists in the moment, and reflects an interplay of contextual factors. In other words, 'competence is a moving target' (Eraut et al., 2004, p 264).

Why not then embed clinical learners in a single clinical workplace to develop their skills? The practice, in health professions education, of moving learners through a range of contexts has evolved for a very sound reason. Competence developed within one setting is not enough to train a modern clinician; they need 'capability' (Fraser & Greenhalgh, 2001) — the ability to deal with unpredictable and complex environments. Hase and Kenyon (2003, p 2) have asserted that:

> ... capable people are more likely to be able to deal effectively with the turbulent and complex environment in which they live by possessing an 'all round' capacity centred on the characteristics of: high self-efficacy, knowing how to learn, creativity, the ability to use competencies in novel as well as familiar situations, possessing appropriate values and working well with others.

The development of capability is dependent on clinical learners' participation in multiple different clinical settings.

Opportunities in clinical workplaces

In clinical education, the affordances of a clinical workplace are the opportunities it presents for learners to engage with, participate in, and learn from it (Billett, 2001). It is not enough for the potential for action to be there; affordances must be perceived in order to be used effectively by clinical educators and learners. However, teachers and learners may perceive clinical workplace affordances quite differently (Billett, 2001; Teunissen & Wilkinson, 2011). Moreover, the affordances of a clinical workplace can vary according to a learner's discipline or level of training. For instance, a senior clinical learner in surgery will tend to perceive (and therefore be able to engage with) the affordances of an operating room in different ways from a junior medical student (Billett, 2016). Furthermore, learners are not passive players in their engagement with workplace affordances; rather, they have agency in determining how to engage with a clinical workplace affordance (Billett, 2011), and that agency can be encouraged and guided. The affordances provide situated opportunities for learners, with the community itself becoming the learning resource: this leads to learning of different kinds that takes place in many different ways (Mann, 2011). In spite of this variability in the affordances of a clinical workplace, clinical educators can identify stable affordances for learning in their workplace (see Table 7.2).

Once a clinical educator has identified the affordances of their particular clinical workplace, they can start to establish a contextual curriculum for it (Billett, 2006a; Strand et al., 2015). The contextual curriculum identifies specific affordances of the clinical workplace for learning, and identifies the learning that is possible. This contextual curriculum will need to be adjusted over time to track the ways in which the clinical workplace shifts and changes in order to maintain the focus on providing effective learning experiences. The contextual curriculum will also need to be adapted to different learners' motivations and agency, as well as to differing levels of learner expertise and confidence. An example of creating contextual learning from affordances in the clinical workplace is shown in Table 7.2.

Learners impact context

So far we have focused on the impact of clinical workplace contexts on learners. However, clinical workplaces are dynamic learning ecologies, where changes in one part of the system can change other parts (Fenwick, 2012). Not only are individual learners changed through their participation in a clinical workplace, they also change the workplace through their participation in its work and its culture. For instance, the regular presence of learners can lead to the establishment of learning routines, such as scheduled rounds, or to changes in service routines, such as who is on first call (Dionysiou & Tsoukas, 2013). These adaptations,

TABLE 7.2: Understanding your clinical workplace context and its affordances for teaching and learning

Context pattern	Question	Examples of answers	Resulting learning affordance
Practice	What is your practice setting?	Young community with transient workers	Opportunity to engage with differing cultural and socioeconomic patient demographics, particular focus on workplace injuries and obstetrics
	What is your scope of practice?	A broad generalist scope; I do more than my colleagues in the cities	Opportunity to expand professional identity
	What other professions do you work with?	I work closely with nurse practitioners	Opportunity for interprofessional learning
Education	How do I train my clinical learners?	They are with me 24/7 — I am their full-time clinical educator	Opportunity to role model and discuss resilience and life balance
	Are there other clinical learners around?	No, mostly just my learner	Opportunity to support independence
	Are there formal teaching sessions?	Not yet	Opportunity to build interprofessional teaching rounds
Patients	What kinds of patients do you encounter?	I have a large ethnic population	Opportunity to learn cultural competence, to adjust communication skills to a new patient group
Geography	How do patient presentations or services change according to season?	We have an influx of tourists during the summer	Opportunity to diagnose and treat problems when follow-up is limited
	What is possible and not possible because of your location?	In the winter patients can't get in for an appointment because of snow	Opportunity to use telemedicine
Culture	How do local values and beliefs shape the way patients present?	People here tend to wait until they are really ill before they access medical care	Opportunity to engage with health promotion and community health as well as individual patient complaints
Organisation	What are the local rules and expectations regarding service provision?	Everyone here does a voluntary extra shift each week, and nobody leaves until all of the day's business has been completed	Opportunity to demonstrate commitment and professionalism

in turn, will impact on the teaching of other learners in that context, as well as the disposition of the clinicians and the organisation as a whole towards medical education. Even a disruptive or problem learner in a particular context will require the clinical educators around them to change their behaviours to more directly support the learner or to limit any harms they might do. In this way, clinical workforce contexts are constantly changing, and adapting on the fly to new situations (Durning et al., 2010).

Making sense of a dynamic system

In healthcare, we mainly think of actions and outcomes as linked in linear and understandable ways: when given this drug, the patient will respond in these predictable ways. Clinical workplaces do not act in this way (Fenwick, 2012), not least because of the reciprocal relationship between learners and context — each affecting the other — that means that learning outcomes may be difficult to program or predict. Complex adaptive systems like clinical workplaces are, by their nature, unpredictable (Lewin, 1999); small changes in clinical educators, learners or patients may create major disruptions (both positive and negative) in group function, while seemingly much larger changes may have little impact. Complex adaptive systems theory calls this frustrating phenomenon *non-linearity* (Mennin, 2010). At a practical level, non-linearity means that clinical educators may not be able to predict how learners, clinical educators and the clinical workplace will organise themselves, nor what learning will emerge from this interaction. A significant learning outcome, such as a shift in learner attitudes, can arise from what appears to be a very small clinical workplace event.

Equally, what may seem like a major change might have little impact on the functioning of the group. At a practical level this means that, while clinical educators can and should plan their teaching in advance to some extent, a lot of their teaching practice needs to be responsive to the emerging and non-linear nature of their learners' performance in a particular context. Not only may changes in the clinical workplace impact the learner and clinical educator, but the performance of individuals working in the same context is dynamically connected. The learning and behaviours of the individuals working within a particular workplace context is to some extent 'entangled' (Scott & Orlikowski, 2014). In other words, the learning and behaviours of any one individual learner cannot be entirely separated from that of those they interact with. At a practical level this means that clinical teachers need to be aware of the ways in which both their healthcare team and their learners can help or inhibit the learning of those around them. Clinical educators can reflect on their own role in the team, and guide learners in recognising and responding to these entanglements.

Given the dynamic system properties of clinical workplaces, clinical teachers have to be constantly aware of the changing affordances, entanglements and processes of their clinical setting (Durning & Artino, 2011). They are engaged not just in facilitating the training of individual learners, but in configuring and reconfiguring the workplace learning context as a whole, to create affordances for and respond to the needs of those working within it.

Educational strategies to enhance learning in the clinical workplace

Having outlined theories of learning that shine a light on how the context of the clinical workplace can both facilitate and inhibit learning, we next consider educational strategies that clinician educators can use to enhance learning.

Supporting integration and participation

Armed with an understanding of the important sociocultural dimensions of learning and the dynamic nature of the clinical workplace, we now ask the question: How can clinical educators support learners' integration into and participation in the clinical workplace? In her work on how newcomers can be 'onboarded' into an organisation, Bauer has identified three phases of the process, each of which requires careful attention: 1) orientation, 2) role clarification, and 3) commitment and full engagement (Bauer & Erdogan, 2011). In phase 1, formal orientations, mentorship and shadowing can help an individual transition into a new organisational context. This phase is also influenced by the individual's attributes and behaviours. Learners should be encouraged to be proactive in this orientation phase, asking questions, seeking feedback, and developing relationships with others. In phase 2, the focus is on helping the learner to understand the institutional culture and values, and how to be accepted by people within the organisation. In phase 3, the focus shifts to facilitating the learner's integration into the organsation through demonstrating ongoing commitment and high levels of performance. This model of organisational socialisation, adapted for clinical education (see Figure 7.2), has been shown to be highly effective in helping clinical learners to adapt to new clinical workplaces (Atherley et al., 2016; Dornan et al., 2014; Houghton, 2014; Teunissen & Westerman, 2011). Clinician educators can support their learners by attending to the work of each phase: orienting learners when they first arrive, subsequently clarifying role expectations, and ultimately welcoming learners as junior colleagues.

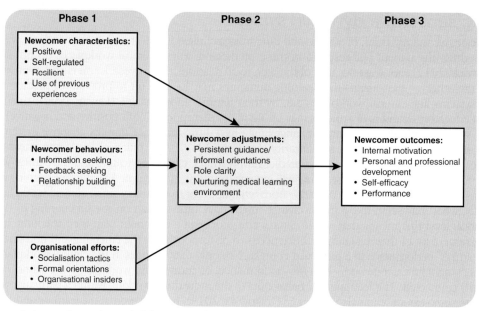

Figure 7.2: Adaptation of model for organisational socialisation for a clerkship transition
Source: *A. E. Atherley, I. R. Hambleton, N. Unwin, C. George, P. M. Lashley, & C. G. Taylor (2016). Exploring the transition of undergraduate medical students into a clinical clerkship using organizational socialization theory.* Perspectives on Medical Education, 5(2), 78–87.

Clinical educators can support the participation of their learners in other ways beyond formal orientation and informal socialisation. After all, the clinical teacher is not a passive observer of their learners' engagement in the clinical workplace. There are a number of specific educator strategies that can enable the clinical learner to progress towards fuller participation in the clinical workplace (Billett, 2002a, 2002b, 2016). For instance, one effective strategy is to deliberately introduce the learner to the clinical workplace, and then support their increasing participation (Sheehan et al., 2005). Deliberate role modelling by the clinical educator is another useful initial strategy to support participation, especially when a learner is grappling with unfamiliar situations (Benbassat, 2014). Observing a clinical educator communicate with a patient, or refer a patient to another healthcare professional, can provide learners with the language and skills they need to rehearse before participating more fully in these clinical activities.

Role modelling is particularly effective in teaching clinical learners about behaviours in situations that they find challenging. To optimise learning, the learner should be provided not only with opportunities to observe the relevant behaviours, but also with opportunities to debrief the situation with their clinical teacher; this approach makes the learning accessible to the learner when they need to draw on it (Eraut 2004; Teunissen & Wilkinson 2011; Yardley et al., 2012).

Contextualising the curriculum

The clinical educator is usually working from a predefined set of goals or objectives for their learners. These goals tend to be highly generic, and are intended to be realised in many different clinical workplace contexts. The clinical educator can review these goals with the learner, identifying how and where the learner can meet the goals in the current clinical context. This approach helps to contextualise these otherwise generic goals, and provides the learner with an understanding of how, when and why they should engage in the current workplace context to further their learning. This interaction can also help to open up conversations between clinical educators and their learners about any contextual challenges to which they may be struggling to adjust. Examples of how to contextualise learning goals in this way are provided in Table 7.3.

The clinical educator is unlikely to be the only direct source of teaching. The clinical learner is often surrounded by other members of the healthcare team, and these team members (often from other professions) can be a rich source of informal learning for the clinical learner (Noble et al., 2017). Moreover, different workplace contexts will offer differing learning opportunities that may not map to a specific program goal

TABLE 7.3: Examples of contextualising program goals and objectives

Domain	Objective	Clinical workplace affordance	Contextualised objective
History-taking	Take a complete history	High proportion of Iindigenous patients, opportunity to learn about care of Indigenous patients	Take a complete history from an Indigenous patient
		Clinic for refugees and recent immigrants	Use interpreters effectively
Physical examination	Complete a physical examination of the cardiovascular system	High volume of IV-drug-using patients	Determine murmurs of subacute bacterial endocarditis (SBE)
		High volume of obstetrical care	Practise a cardiovascular examination in a newborn
Management	Management of an acute abdomen	General surgical service	Follow a patient with acute abdomen from the emergency department to surgery and postop
		Remote community	Diagnose a patient on clinical indicators, and decide whether to transport to a secondary-care-level hospital
Professionalism	Demonstrate professional boundaries with patients	Patients with psychiatric illnesses	Demonstrate effective professional boundaries with challenging patients
		Rural community	Demonstrate effective professional boundaries with patients who you see in the community
Interprofessional care	Develop skills in interprofessional teamwork	Team approach to stroke rehabilitation	Work effectively with a interprofessional team with a stroke patient
		Connection to remote community	Work effectively with the nurse practitioner in the remote community
		Palliative care team and specialised ward	Work with the palliative care team to follow and help to manage a dying patient

or objective. The clinical educator can explore these opportunities with the clinical learner, and enable the learner to engage in an individualised experience aligned with their own goals. Clinical educators can also encourage their learners to be open to the unexpected; different contexts offer unplanned learning possibilities that may have a lasting influence on learners, sometimes shaping their future career trajectories. In this way the clinical educator can help to align the opportunities of the clinical workplace and the intentions and needs of the learner (Billett, 2002b).

Given that much of the learning in the clinical workplace is shaped by context, the role of the clinical educator is to identify these affordances and guide the learner towards better and more meaningful participation in their current context. This may involve reviewing the learning goals, identifying the affordances of the setting that may be relevant to those goals, and empowering and guiding the learner in their engagement with those affordances.

Fostering reflection

Clinical educators can draw on another key educational strategy: fostering reflection and developing reflective capacity in their learners. Reflection refers to 'those intellectual and affective activities in which individuals engage to explore their experiences in order to lead to a new understanding and appreciation' (Boud et al., 1985, p 19). Reflection can also allow the learner to articulate the tacit knowledge that arises from their informal learning, and to differentiate between the way things are done in one setting and the ways in which they are done in another, and thereby to learn how to adjust their behaviours to new clinical workplaces (Eraut 2004; Harris & Delany, 2013). Reflection deepens learning, (Yardley et al., 2012), and so formal opportunities for learners to engage in reflection about their experiences with their clinical educators can foster transformative learning from the clinical workplace.

Reflection can also enable the clinical learner to grapple with the hidden curriculum (Holmes et al., 2015), with their own values and attitudes (Asgarova et al., 2017), and with their developing professional identities (Cruess et al., 2014). Holmes et al. (2015) propose a specific set of reflective competencies for clinical learners as they engage with the clinical workplace: understanding their motivations to conform to external pressures in the workplace; becoming aware of these pressures in the moment; analysing their experiences with trusted clinical educators or peers; and contemplating and committing to a personal set of values and behaviours.

Despite a growing interest in developing clinical learners' reflective abilities, there is as yet little clear evidence as to how exactly to do this (Sandars, 2009). However, it is evident that with time, a safe place, and a trusted and engaged clinical educator, learners can strengthen their reflective capacities (Mann et al., 2009). Clinical educators can explore with their learners what they are experiencing in the clinical workplace, and engage them with questions intended to provoke reflection (Delany & Watkin, 2009; Harris & Delany, 2013; Holmes et al., 2015; Sandars, 2009). Examples of such questions are provided in Table 7.4.

Following a session of reflective learning, the clinical educator can identify specific clinical situations in which to prime awareness generated from the reflective session in the clinical trainee (Schön, 1983). Promoting reflection does not have to always be a lengthy session: asking learners to reflect on an aspect of the clinical workplace, such as the roles of different health professionals prior to a clinical shift, can prime the learner to notice and learn from an aspect of the clinical setting (Seymour & Watt, 2015).

Back to the case: from theory to practice

We can reprise our exemplar case by drawing on the theories and approaches we have considered in this chapter.

Sandy now realises that her workplace context, so normal for her, may be different from other contexts, and that she has made assumptions about Sean's preparedness for her setting. She considers that Sean may have had little or no experience with rural settings, with the healthcare provided within these settings, or with the ways that these and other factors are shaping his professional development. Sandy sits down with Sean over dinner to sort out the issues in his placement. Using the patterns outlined above, she first asks about his previous experience with rural healthcare, with Indigenous patients, and with a high-volume workplace focused on attending to patients in a timely manner.

Given time and a caring listener, Sean is able to explore his previous experience and consider its impact. He explains that he has never lived or even stayed in a rural area before. His clinical workplace experience to date has been in the context of a large tertiary-care urban teaching hospital with every specialist just down the hall. He has experience with patients from a range of multicultural backgrounds, but virtually no experience with Indigenous patients. He just doesn't know how to deliver care effectively. His immediate thought is often to refer the patient to other services, but that entails a long trip for the patient. How would his clinical educator handle the problem?

Sandy explores Sean's previous experiences with him — with rural settings, with Indigenous patients, with broad or generalist scopes of practice, with care delivery in resource-restricted settings, and so on. With each example that Sean offers, Sandy is able to articulate the different contextual factors in her setting that are challenging Sean's ability to perform adequately in this context. Sandy now sees her role as supporting Sean in adapting his previous competent performance to this new workplace context, and then building on it.

Before developing strategies to enable Sean to participate fully in the clinical workplace, she first addresses his sense of dislocation. She invites Sean to accompany her in attending several community events, and

TABLE 7.4: Questions designed to provoke reflection in the clinical learners about learning arising from the clinical workplace context

Question	Provoke reflection about	Examples of learner responses
What kinds of patients did you interact with in your previous setting?	Social, cultural, ethnic, religious backgrounds; disease prevalence	'Most of my patients were too sick to talk to me, and most of them couldn't speak English anyway — they came from many different immigrant backgrounds.'
How are the patients you are seeing now different from your previous patients?	Identifying a new or different patient group	'There are a lot of Indigenous patients here; I learned about them in school, but I don't have any experience actually caring for them.'
What do you need to learn in order to feel competent with these patients?	Learning needs; resources	'I have only been in hospitals; I don't know how to manage chronic illnesses like diabetes and heart disease.'
How is the health system here similar to or different from what you are used to?	What is 'normal'; how dependent they have become on a particular set of circumstances	'I had every specialist I could want just down the hall.'
Are there professions you are used to having as members of your healthcare team?	Dependence on others to provide interprofessional care	'We always had a social worker as part of the team; we would refer patients to her, and the patients would be supported after discharge. I don't know how to do that.'
How did you learn in your last setting?	How generic learning goals or outcomes can be achieved in different ways	'I was the only learner, so I was with my clinical educator all the time. I got used to doing things his way.'
Who would usually see this kind of patient in follow-up in your previous setting?	How providers and patients can access services in very different ways according to context	'I was in a family practice setting; there weren't many specialists, so we would follow the patients. The specialists were there just to provide advice.'
Are you used to seeing homeless or indigent patients?	Social determinants of health and illness	'I have never seen indigent patients. Should I get Social Services involved?'
We can only get patients airlifted out during daytime. How have you managed critically ill patients before?	Particular challenges faced both by patients and caregivers in particular contexts	'I have never transferred a patient out.'

she connects him to a local hiking group, thereby enabling him to develop informal social connections and a feeling of belonging.

Sandy next directs Sean to do a literature review on working with Indigenous patients. As Sandy and Sean discuss what he has found out, they both realise that he needs more grounding in the history and culture of the Indigenous people he will be serving. Sandy purchases two books to serve as references on these issues, not only for Sean, but also for other learners in the future. She arranges for Sean to shadow the nurse practitioner who provides primary care on the traditional lands, and lets the nurse practitioner know that Sean wants to develop his skills in working with Indigenous patients.

Sandy asks one of the nurses in the emergency department to train Sean for a day, to orient him to when laboratory tests and X-rays can be done, what tests are available on-site, how patients get referred and transferred to the main urban hospital, and what the specialists expect to have referred to them. Drawing on his experience, Sean creates an orientation manual, ensuring that the next learner who arrives at Valleyfield without prior experience in a rural community can adapt to the context more quickly.

Sean is not planning to practise in a rural setting; rather, he hopes to become a consultant surgeon. Sandy arranges for him to scrub in with the local general surgeon one day a week. Over the course of the placement, Sean does more and more in the operating room, as there are no surgical postgraduate trainees to compete with the first assistant position. Sean also spends time with surgical patients, both before and after their surgeries, even doing home visits. His work with the nurse practitioner enables him to feel comfortable caring for Indigenous patients who are booked for surgery.

By the end of the 8-week rotation, Sandy feels that Sean has met the goals and objectives of his placement, as they relate to her setting. Sean has become an enthusiastic participant, highly motivated by his own goals, and is making use of the learning opportunities in the workplace.

Future evaluation and research

As much as there is substantial evidence and theory to guide clinical educators in using their clinical workplace context as a teaching and learning tool, there is still much that we do not know. For instance, we do not always know how or why clinical educators and learners perceive and engage in the affordances of their workplace differently. We know that there is individual variation in the perception of workplace affordances, but we do not yet know why that is so. Nor do we understand the benefits and problems arising from this individual variation. Although it is clear that learners need to encounter some different clinical contexts during their training, it is less clear how much variation is needed, nor is it clear at what stages in their training these changes should be encountered. More needs to be known about the differences between clinical workplaces, the ways that teachers and learners engage with them, and the ways in which they can be configured to afford better opportunities for learning. We need to understand how learners integrate the many different ways of investigating and managing illness in the different contexts they encounter. More attention to context in health professions education scholarship is needed, both in response to the growing diversity of training contexts and to reflect the challenges of perception, affordance and entanglement in clinical workplace contexts.

PRACTICAL TIPS

Before the placement starts

- Reflect carefully on your own context; being a useful guide to learners requires you to understand your context's distinct features.
- Meet with your healthcare team to explore their insights into the clinical workplace affordances.
- Identify resources that the learners can use to adjust more quickly to your clinical workplace context: books, videos, and cultural competence orientations.
- If you have a specific patient population or healthcare organisation that the learners have not been exposed to previously, alert your healthcare team to the need to orient learners.
- Examine the objectives and goals for the clinical placement, and draft a list of potential experiences available in your workplace for the learners to meet those objectives.

When the placement begins

- Set aside time to welcome and orient your learners. Learners arriving at a new clinical workplace first need to feel welcomed and expected; they must feel they are legitimate participants in your healthcare setting.
- Introduce the other team members in the clinical workplace to the learner, explain their roles and introduce the clinical learner as a new member of the team. The roles of the other team members may be quite different in different clinical workplaces.
- Provide an overview of how the clinical workplace functions — the context, the patients, the scope and the processes.
- Identify resource limitations in your context, and strategies for addressing them.
- Explain how you are going to teach, how supervision will work, and who the learner should approach with questions. While this is an important strategy with all clinical placements,

trainees who are transitioning from another workplace context may have assumptions based on their experience in the previous setting. For example, are there formal rounds, or will patients be discussed when care decisions are made?

- Find out what workplace contexts the learner has experience with. This will help you to compare and contrast with the learner how things are done in different settings.

During the placement

- Acknowledge the uncertainty and anxiety of the learner. Clinical learners often mask their feelings of anxiety and stress in order to appear confident and competent to their clinical educator. Help the learner to accept their feelings as part of the transition process, and to develop skills to adjust to new clinical workplaces.
- Encourage questions. If there is not time to address questions that arise, deal with them at the end of the day.
- Embed discussions of context in real clinical work; for example, addressing the needs of an individual with an uncommon medical condition in a small community may spark discussions about scope of practice, the threshold for specialist referral, and the use of technology to access support.
- Ask how the learner has managed a patient problem in their previous context. Discuss the differences between this approach and your approach, and the underlying contextual reasons for those differences.
- At regular intervals, set aside protected time for you to debrief with your learner. Find out what is different and challenging in this particular clinical workplace. Critical reflection will help the learner to integrate into your clinical workplace.
- After a learner has watched you talking with a patient, or making a clinical decision, explain your actions if they are affected by the workplace context you are in.
- Encourage the learner to explore and experience the community outside of their clinical role.
- Keep discussions of different contexts respectful.

At the end of the placement

- Meet with your learner to debrief their experience of your clinical workplace. If you find out how your clinical workplace is different from other workplaces and what the learner was able to learn, you will be better prepared for the next clinical learner.

Conclusion

In this chapter, we have introduced the importance of the clinical workplace context for learning in health professions education. We have discussed how shifting across different settings can disrupt the confidence and performance of a learner. We have outlined the learning theories that can make sense of the learning that occurs from the workplace context, and we have set out pedagogical approaches for the clinical educator that can support this learning.

An important message from this chapter is that the context of the clinical workplace impacts on learning by providing opportunities for participation in practice. Each clinical workplace is different, and learners will engage not only according to the expectations of the setting, but also according to their perceptions of the setting and their own learning needs and wishes. The role of the clinical educator is to support guided participation, drawing the learners over time further into the specifics of practice in each clinical workplace they encounter. Capability in health professions practice develops through the accumulation of specific context-bound learning and practice experiences. Clinical teachers can increase their teaching effectiveness by becoming aware of, competent in, and responsive to the role of context in the preparation of tomorrow's doctors.

References

Asgarova, S., MacKenzie, M., & Bates, J. (2017). Learning from patients: Why continuity matters. *Academic Medicine, 92*(11S), S55–S60.

Atherley, A. E., Hambleton, I. R., Unwin, N., et al. (2016). Exploring the transition of undergraduate medical students into a clinical clerkship using organizational socialization theory. *Perspectives on Medical Education, 5*(2), 78–87.

Attrill, S., Lincoln, M., & McAllister, S. (2015). International students in speech-language pathology clinical education placements: Perceptions of experience and competency development. *International Journal of Speech-Language Pathology, 17*(3), 314–324.

Bates, J., & Ellaway, R. H. (2016). Mapping the dark matter of context: A conceptual scoping review. *Medical Education, 50*(8), 807–816. doi:10.1111/medu.13034.

Bauer, T. N., & Erdogan, B. (2011). Organizational socialization: The effective onboarding of new employees. In S. Zedeck, H. Aguinis, W. Cascio, et al. (Eds.), *APA handbook of I/O psychology* (Vol. III, pp. 51–64). Washington, DC: APA Press.

Benbassat, J. (2014). Role modeling in medical education: The importance of a reflective imitation. *Academic Medicine, 89*(4), 550.

Bernabeo, E. C., Holtman, M. C., Ginsburg, S., et al. (2011). Lost in transition: The experience and impact of frequent changes in the inpatient learning environment. *Academic Medicine, 86*(5), 591–598.

Billett, S. (2001). Learning through work: Workplace affordances and individual engagement. *Journal of Workplace Learning, 13*(5–6), 209–214.

Billett, S. (2002a). Toward a workplace pedagogy: Guidance, participation, and engagement. *Adult Education Quarterly, 53*(1), 27–43. doi:10.1177/074171302237202.

Billett, S. (2002b). Workplace pedagogic practices: Co-participation and learning. *British Journal of Educational Studies, 50*(4), 457–481.

Billett, S. (2006). Constituting the workplace curriculum. *Journal of Curriculum Studies, 38*(1), 31–48.

Billett, S. (2011). Subjectivity, self and personal agency in learning through and for work. In M. Malloch, L. Cairns, K. Evans, et al. (Eds.), *The SAGE handbook of workplace learning* (pp. 60–72). London: Sage.

Billett, S. (2016). Learning through health care work: Premises, contributions and practices. *Medical Education, 50*(1), 124–131.

Boud, D., Keogh, R., & Walker, D. (1985). Promoting reflection in learning. In D. Boud, R. Keogh, & D. Walker (Eds.), *Reflection: Turning experience into learning* (pp. 18–40). London: Kogan Page.

Brosnan, C., & Turner, B. S. (Eds.), (2009). *Handbook of the sociology of medical education*. London: Routledge.

Cruess, R. L., Cruess, S. R., Boudreau, J. D., et al. (2014). Reframing medical education to support professional identity formation. *Academic Medicine, 89*(11), 1446–1451.

de Jong, J., Visser, M., Van Dijk, N., et al. (2013). A systematic review of the relationship between patient mix and learning in work-based clinical settings. A BEME systematic review: BEME Guide No. 24. *Medical Teacher, 35*(6), e1181–e1196.

Delany, C., & Watkin, D. (2009). A study of critical reflection in health professional education: 'learning where others are coming from. *Advances in Health Sciences Education: Theory and Practice, 14*(3), 411–429.

Dewey, J., & Boydston, J. A. (Eds.), (2008). *The later works of John Dewey, 1925–1953. Volume 7,: 1932, Ethics.* Carbondale, IL: Southern Illinois University Press.

Dionysiou, D. D., & Tsoukas, H. (2013). Understanding the (re) creation of routines from within: A symbolic interactionist perspective. *Academy of Management Review, 38*(2), 181–205.

Dornan, T. (2012). Workplace learning. *Perspectives on Medical Education, 1*(1), 15–23.

Dornan, T., Tan, N., Boshuizen, H., et al. (2014). How and what do medical students learn in clerkships? Experience based learning (ExBL). *Advances in Health Sciences Education: Theory and Practice, 19*(5), 721–749.

Durning, S. J., & Artino, A. R. (2011). Situativity theory: A perspective on how participants and the environment can interact. AMEE Guide No. 52. *Medical Teacher, 33*(3), 188–199.

Durning, S. J., Artino, A. R., Jr., Pangaro, L. N., et al. (2010). Perspective: Redefining context in the clinical encounter: Implications for research and training in medical education. *Academic Medicine, 85*(5), 894–901.

Ellaway, R. H., & Bates, J. (2015). Exploring patterns and pattern languages of medical education. *Medical Education, 49*(12), 1189–1196.

Epstein, R. M. (2007). Assessment in medical education. *New England Journal of Medicine, 356*(4), 387–396.

Eraut, M. (2000). Non-formal learning and tacit knowledge in professional work. *The British Journal of Educational Psychology, 70*(1), 113–136.

Eraut, M. (2004). Informal learning in the workplace. *Studies in Continuing Education, 26*(2), 247–273.

Eraut, M., Maillardet, F., Miller, C., et al. (2004). *Learning in the professional workplace: Relationships between learning factors and contextual factors.* Paper presented at the annual conference of the American Educational Research Association, San Diego, 12 April.

Fenwick, T. (2012). Complexity science and professional learning for collaboration: A critical reconsideration of possibilities and limitations. *Journal of Education and Work, 25*(1), 141–162.

Fraser, S. W., & Greenhalgh, T. (2001). Complexity science: Coping with complexity: Educating for capability. *British Medical Journal, 323*(7316), 799.

Goldszmidt, M., Faden, L., Dornan, T., et al. (2015). Attending physician variability: A model of four supervisory styles. *Academic Medicine, 90*(11), 1541–1546. doi:10.1097/acm.0000000000000735.

Harris, A., & Delany, C. (2013). International medical graduates in transition. *The Clinical Teacher, 10*(5), 328–332. doi:10.1111/tct.12021.

Hase, S., & Kenyon, K. (2003). Heutagogy and developing capable people and capable workplaces: strategies for dealing with complexity. In *Proceedings of the Changing Face of Work and Learning Conference.* Edmonton, AB: University of Alberta. https://www.researchgate.net/profile/Stewart_Hase/publication/37359136_Heutagogy_and_developing_capable_people_and_capable_workplaces_strategies_for_dealing_with_complexity/

links/5475c2bb0cf29afed612b37c/Heutagogy-and-developing-capable-people-and-capable-workplaces-strategies-for-dealing-with-complexity.pdf. (Accessed 30 January 2018).

Holmes, C. L., Harris, I. B., Schwartz, A. J., et al. (2015). Harnessing the hidden curriculum: A four-step approach to developing and reinforcing reflective competencies in medical clinical clerkship. *Advances in Health Sciences Education: Theory and Practice, 20*(5), 1355–1370.

Houghton, C. E. (2014). Newcomer adaptation': A lens through which to understand how nursing students fit in with the real world of practice. *Journal of Clinical Nursing, 23*(15–16), 2367–2375.

Howe, P. W., & Kumar, K. (2017). A qualitative exploration of anesthesia trainees' experiences during transition to a children's hospital. *Pediatric Anesthesia, 27*(3), 263–270.

Lave, J., & Wenger, E. (1991). *Situated learning: Legitimate peripheral participation.* Cambridge: Cambridge University Press.

Lewin, R. (1999). *Complexity: Life at the edge of chaos.* Chicago: University of Chicago Press.

Mann, K. (2011). Theoretical perspectives in medical education: Past experience and future possibilities. *Medical Education, 45*(1), 60–68.

Mann, K., Gordon, J., & MacLeod, A. (2009). Reflection and reflective practice in health professions education: A systematic review. *Advances in Health Sciences Education: Theory and Practice, 14*(4), 595–621.

Mennin, S. (2010). Self-organisation, integration and curriculum in the complex world of medical education. *Medical Education, 44*(1), 20–30.

Miles, S., Kellett, J., & Leinster, S. J. (2015). Foundation doctors' induction experiences. *BMC Medical Education, 15*(1), 118.

Monrouxe, L. V., & Rees, C. E. (2009). Picking up the gauntlet: Constructing medical education as a social science. *Medical Education, 43*(3), 196–198.

Noble, C., Brazil, V., Teasdale, T., et al. (2017). Developing junior doctors' prescribing practices through collaborative practice: Sustaining and transforming the practice of communities. *Journal of Interprofessional Care, 31*(2), 263–272.

Plsek, P. E., & Greenhalgh, T. (2001). The challenge of complexity in health care. *BMJ (Clinical Research Ed.), 323*(7313), 625–628. doi:https://doi.org/10.1136/bmj.323.7313.625.

Sandars, J. (2009). The use of reflection in medical education. AMEE Guide No. 44. *Medical Teacher, 31*(8), 685–695.

Schön, D. (1983). *The reflective practitioner: How professionals think in action.* New York: Basic Books.

Scott, S. V., & Orlikowski, W. J. (2014). Entanglements in practice: Performing anonymity through social media.

MIS Quarterly, 38(3), 873–894. doi:10.25300/MISQ/2014/38.3.11.

Seymour, P., & Watt, M. (2015). The professional competencies toolkit: Teaching reflection with flash cards. *Medical Education, 49*(5), 518.

Sfard, A. (1998). On two metaphors for learning and the dangers of choosing just one. *Educational Researcher, 27*(2), 4–13.

Sheehan, D., Wilkinson, T. J., & Billett, S. (2005). Interns' participation and learning in clinical environments in a New Zealand hospital. *Academic Medicine, 80*(3), 302–308.

Stacey, R. D. (2007). *Strategic management and organisational dynamics: The challenge of complexity to ways of thinking about organisations.* London: Pearson Education.

Strand, P., Edgren, G., Borna, P., et al. (2015). Conceptions of how a learning or teaching curriculum, workplace culture and agency of individuals shape medical student learning and supervisory practices in the clinical workplace. *Advances in Health Sciences Education: Theory and Practice, 20*(2), 531–557.

Teunissen, P., & Dornan, T. (2008). The competent novice: Lifelong learning at work. *BMJ. British Medical Journal, 336*(7645), 667.

Teunissen, P. W., & Westerman, M. (2011). Opportunity or threat: The ambiguity of the consequences of transitions in medical education. *Medical Education, 45*(1), 51–59. doi:10.1111/j.1365-2923.2010.03755.x.

Teunissen, P. W., & Wilkinson, T. (2011). Learning and teaching in workplaces. In K. Mann, A. Scherpbier, J. Spencer, et al. (Eds.), *Medical education. Theory and practice* (pp. 193–209). Edinburgh: Churchill Livingstone.

Truong, M., Paradise, Y., & Priest, N. (2014). Interventions to improve cultural competency in healthcare: A systematic review of reviews. *BMC Health Services Research, 14*(1), 99.

Wenger, E. (1998). *Communities of practice: Learning, meaning, and identity.* Cambridge: Cambridge University Press.

Wenger-Trayner, E., Fenton-O'Creevy, M., Hutchinson, S., et al. (2014). *Learning in landscapes of practice: Boundaries, identity, and knowledgeability in practice-based learning.* London: Routledge.

White, K. L., Williams, T. F., & Greenberg, B. G. (1961). The ecology of medical care. *New England Journal of Medicine, 265*(18), 885–892.

Yardley, S., Teunissen, P. W., & Dornan, T. (2012). Experiential learning. AMEE Guide No. 63. *Medical Teacher, 34*(2), e102–e115.

8

Professionalism, identities and embodiment
Supporting the internalisation of professionalism through addressing the hidden curriculum

Malissa Shaw, Paul Crampton, Charlotte Rees and Lynn Monrouxe

The doctor laughed at the patient's questions and comments even though the patient was worried and his concerns were real concerns to him. The doctor told him he had two options: carry on taking the clopidogrel [antiplatelet medication] and bleed to death [during the removal of a colonic polyp, a small lump of cells that grow on the lining of the colon]; or do not have the colonic polyp removed and get cancer. The patient was understandably scared about being given this decision to make by himself … the patient should have been treated better by the doctor who should have explained the risks [of each option] and helped the patient to make the decision. The doctor should not have laughed at the patient's comments and questions. It was very rude of him to do so. It still annoys me that the doctor spoke to the patient in such a way. And to think that he may talk to and treat other patients the same way.

(Sarah, fifth-year UK medical student)

Introduction

Professionalism matters in healthcare: it is the cornerstone of safe and effective patient care (Monrouxe & Rees, 2017). Professionalism means different things to different people, in different cultures and across different time periods (Chandratilake et al., 2012; Jha et al., 2015; Monrouxe et al., 2017). Despite its diversity, the study of professionalism has recently accelerated as educators contemplate how to instil notions of professionalism in their learners (Cruess et al., 2016), and prepare them to reflect on experiences of professionalism dilemmas such as that narrated by Sarah, above. Becoming a professional is a process that entails learners internalising and coming to identify with the norms and values of healthcare professionals, as well as rejecting those that are not appropriate (Monrouxe, 2016). Central to this process is the development of professional identities: who one is and who one wants to become (Monrouxe, 2016). A social constructionist perspective interprets identities to comprise multiple, intersecting understandings of the self (Monrouxe, 2015; Tsouroufli et al., 2011) that are influenced by an intertwining of both external and internal factors (Monrouxe, 2009, 2016; Rees & Monrouxe, 2010). Key to the internalisation of professional identities is the concept of *embodiment*, in which experiences and knowledge become ingrained in oneself through practice and reflection, impacting not only on how one acts but also on who one is — one's identity (Burkitt, 1999; Johnson, 1989, 1991).

Narratives and storytelling, such as those presented in this chapter and beginning with Sarah above, facilitate the exploration of learners' embodiment of professionalism and their identity transformation, and how educators can assist learners along this journey. The narratives presented in this chapter come from a 10-year program of research with over 4000 healthcare learners from four countries (the United Kingdom, Australia, Taiwan and Sri Lanka), and the collection of over 2000 oral and written narratives of professionalism dilemmas (Monrouxe & Rees, 2017). All narratives have been edited and paraphrased for comprehension and clarity, but the original meanings have been maintained. All names are pseudonyms.

In this chapter, the interweaving of professionalism, identities and embodiment is considered in the quest to support the internalisation of professional identities through addressing the hidden curriculum. The chapter begins by exploring the theoretical constructs of professionalism, identities and embodiment, to understand what is meant by these terms, how they are formed during clinical placements, and how they interrelate to one another. Then these theoretical propositions are brought to life through an illustrative narrative case (case study 8.1) that begins to unpack the complex interplay at work. The following section outlines a number of strategies that educators could adopt to facilitate learners' embodiment of professional identities through addressing the hidden curriculum, again using an illustrative case (case study 8.2). Finally, the interconnectedness of theory and the learning strategies are highlighted in case study 8.3, and the chapter is concluded. By the end of this chapter it is intended that educators will be better able to understand and use the concept of embodiment to improve *their* educational, supervisory and clinical practice.

Theoretical background: professionalism, identities and embodiment

In this section, the key theoretical issues around the teaching and learning of professionalism, the formation of identities and the concept of embodiment are presented. Underlying these theoretical issues are the processes of the hidden curriculum, socialisation and first-hand experiences and reflection.

Professionalism, the hidden curriculum and learners' dilemmas

Professionalism is the cornerstone of ethical, safe, respectful and dignified healthcare practice (Monrouxe & Rees, 2017). These wider norms of ideal practice form the foundation for learners' development of more specific understandings of what constitutes appropriate professional conduct. In the broadest sense, healthcare professionalism includes the 'means by which individual doctors fulfil the … profession's contract with society' (Hafferty, 2016, p 55). Parallel to healthcare practice in general, understandings of healthcare professionalism are not objective, but rather vary across cultures, people and time (Chandratilake et al., 2012; Jha et al., 2015; Monrouxe et al., 2011; Monrouxe et al., 2017). Given the dynamic and cultural-specific nature of professionalism, it is through diverse ways of facilitating learning that professionalism norms and values become inculcated in learners.

In the past decades, professionalism teaching has been incorporated into the formal curriculum of healthcare education institutes (Hafferty & Castellani, 2009). The formal curriculum includes that which is specifically 'stated, intended, and formally offered and endorsed' (Hafferty, 1998, p 404), and involves explicit teaching and assessment intentions. These commonly occur through planned classroom educational activities, but may actually be present anywhere across healthcare education. Notions of professionalism learning are also present in informal and hidden curricula. The informal curriculum involves 'serendipitous or opportunistic learning that takes place through teacher–learner interactions' (Monrouxe & Rees, 2017, p 33). The hidden curriculum, on the other hand, generally concerns the 'unwritten social and cultural values, rules, assumptions and expectations' (Wear & Skillicorn, 2009, p 452) that are embedded within healthcare practices, educational curricula and even the architectural layout of learning and clinical spaces.

As learners become socialised into the profession, they assimilate these obscured structural and institutional aspects of healthcare education, which can contribute positively or negatively to learners' professional development (Hafferty, 2016; Monrouxe & Rees, 2017).

Unlike the formal curriculum, both informal and hidden curricula focus on what is learned rather than what is taught. Therefore, practices and perspectives that are learned through informal and hidden curricula, such as during clinical placements, may go unnoticed by healthcare educators. Furthermore, although distinctions are made here between these three educational realms, they are interconnected and all feed into learning. Despite developments to professional identity formation that may accompany clinical placements, the structural forces underlying practices observed or participated in during such placements may not always coincide with the ideals of professionalism taught during formal curricula.

Indeed, the hidden curriculum is often theorised through perceptions of disconnectedness (Hafferty & Castellani, 2009): most commonly, the disconnection is between what is taught in the formal curriculum and the practices, values and sentiments that learners may witness, experience and thus internalise in the clinical environment (Monrouxe & Rees, 2017). In such settings, learners may witness or participate in events that they think are unprofessional, unethical or *wrong* — so called *professionalism dilemmas* (Christakis & Feudtner, 1993; Ginsburg & Lingard, 2011; Hendelman & Byszewski, 2014; Ho et al., 2017; Monrouxe et al., 2015; Rees et al., 2014; Rees & Monrouxe, 2011). Monrouxe and Rees (2017) suggest that learners can experience identity confusion (or struggles) when what they encounter during clinical placements does not correspond with their formal professionalism education. In other words, when learners observe professionalism lapses among their educators, such lapses present professionalism dilemmas to them in the form of barriers to their own professionalism and professional identity development.

Identities and their construction

Identities are generally held to be developed through an interaction between individuals' minds/bodies (i.e. psychosocially) and external influences (i.e. the social world; Jenkins, 2008). Theoretical perspectives on the development of identities differ in terms of the respective emphasis they place on the psychological and social worlds (Monrouxe, 2009, 2016). Identity theories can therefore be considered along a continuum: from being psychologically (i.e. internally) strong and socially (i.e. externally) weak, to being psychologically weak and socially strong (Smith & Sparkes, 2008). This chapter draws on the social constructionist perspective of identities, which heavily emphasises the social and interactional (external) components in the construction of one's identities. In other words, from this perspective, identities are formed through acting and interacting in the world. Thus, identities are dependent on the environment within which people interact and the individuals with whom they interact (Coulter, 1979; Jenkins, 2008). It is through these external influences, such as informal and hidden curricula — and individuals' interpretations of them — that individuals' understandings of their multiple, intersecting identities are formed and expressed (Tsouroufli et al., 2011). From this perspective, identities are active and transformative.

Through interactions with others, individuals continually seek to perform, to claim and to assert their identities: 'we seek to *be* and *be seen to be*' by others in light of the ideal image of oneself (Monrouxe, 2010, p 44). Being a habitual routine, this performative expression of one's identity is often an unconscious process, influenced by what Bourdieu has labelled *Habitus*: behaviours and thought processes learned through *socialisation*, or growing up in a particular context with established norms and values (Bourdieu, 1990). Socialisation — the process of internalising societal norms, values and expected behaviours and roles — begins at birth, and continues to transform who people are as their lives develop (Jenkins, 2008). Individuals undergo a process of secondary socialisation when joining a new group, such as becoming a healthcare professional. During this process, aspects that appear unusual, irregular or discordant to an outsider become commonplace and taken for granted as individuals come to internalise group norms and identify with the group (Mavor et al., 2017; Tajfel & Turner, 2004). In the healthcare setting, learners' identities are co-constructed (and at times constrained) through social interactions and language exchanges with healthcare professionals, patients and peer learners (Monrouxe & Rees, 2015). These discursively constructed identities are interwoven with the dominant social perspectives and institutional factors of what it means to be a doctor (Monrouxe, 2009).

Identities, and the dominant and subtler interactional factors that influence their formation, can be explored through conversations, narratives and storytelling (Monrouxe, 2016) to illuminate how learners make sense of their experiences, themselves and others (Rees et al., 2013). Johnson (1989, pp 374–375) explains that narratives express 'bodily reality', as they elucidate individuals' 'perceptions, feelings, experiences, and actions', and include their awareness of the 'patterning and flow' of their experiences as they internalise and make sense of them. Through focusing on the meaning within narratives as voiced through the narrators' understanding of events (Labov & Waletzky, 1967), rather than the events themselves, individuals can explore embodied experiences of identity construction and the factors that influence such processes.

Embodiment

Following Hafferty (2016), in order to be socialised into any profession, new members must come to identify with and internalise the particular norms and values of that profession: a transformation that is more profound than adopting specific competencies (i.e. behaviours, knowledge and skills). Another way to think about the internalisation of professional identity is through the concept of *embodiment*: the internalisation of experience and understandings that happen within oneself.

Embodiment theory is not solely concerned with the physical body, but rather the connection of the mind and the body. Embodiment entails viewing one*self* as an integrated being (i.e. mind *and* body) who comes to know the social world they inhabit through bodily sensations and experiences (Johnson, 1991). This integrated understanding of the self (or of identities) considers how identities are influenced by experiences, interactions, emotions, cultures and one's presence in the physical world (Burkitt, 1999). Further, it is through an individual's bodily interactions with their environment that knowledge is developed and is in constant transformation (Johnson, 1991). Knowledge in this instance refers to processes of sense-making and understanding that happen through personal experiences and social interactions (Sfard, 1998). Here, knowledge is an active, changeable entity, rather than a fixed or static one (Dewey, as cited in Johnson, 1991). Embodiment theorists call this form of understanding *experiential* or *embodied knowledge*. Personal experiences become embodied knowledge through repetition and reflection: through these 'cyclic patternings' (Johnson, 1989, p 369) of meaningful experiences, embodied knowledge comes to be rhythmically known through one's body. Indeed, research on the role of simulated patient encounters in learners' socialisation highlights how healthcare practices must be repeatedly 'rehearsed quite literally in the flesh in order to become part of the medical student' (Underman, 2015, p 183). Reflecting on such experiences and practices is also integral to the creation of embodied knowledge. As individuals reflect on their embodied experiences, the consequences that may accompany them and their influences on the self, they come to make sense of their significance in a way that may scaffold deeper learning opportunities.

When considering how identities come to be embodied, it is essential to remember that identity construction is a process and that learners' embodiment of professional identities will occur at different rates during their healthcare training, and may be influenced, both positively and negatively, by diverse experiences. This can be seen clearly in the following dilemma narrated by Hui-Wen, a fifth-year Taiwanese medical student, who narrates the identity struggles she experienced as she observed her teacher losing patience with a patient with bipolar disorder (see case study 8.1).

Case study 8.1: Hui-Wen's dilemma and an interpretation — how professionalism dilemmas impact on learners' embodiment of professional identities

Hui-Wen: ... The patient has bipolar disorder and she is now experiencing a switch phase, so she's moving from depressed mood to manic mood, and she sensed that. When she came she said she hadn't slept last night, so she's a bit not that clear. So she talks really slow, which is why I took history for like an hour, because it's hard, I had to wait for her response ... But the teacher's opinion is that, he said, 'No, she is now going to have manic, um, she's going to be into the manic state, so there are too many thoughts in her mind and that's why she couldn't speak fluently.' And then he asked her if that was correct. And she was like, 'No, it's because yesterday I didn't sleep and I feel drowsy now.' But the teacher just stuck to the flight of ideas things, and he lost his patience [with]in about five minutes [of interviewing her] ... he said, 'No, this is intolerable, there's too many things going on in her head and she can't put them clearly, and it's circumstantial. It's obvious, it's going to be manic attack, so prescribe drugs and send her away.'

Interviewer: So did he get quite angry with the patient? What did he do? Raise his voice, or just ...

Hui-Wen: He didn't raise his voice, he just showed his impatience, and he thought that it was good to do that. He thinks being [emotionally] neutral is not actually professionalism. He thinks he should be a mirror, reflecting and showing the patient how other people next to her will feel. He thinks that *that* is professionalism. He can reflect that and he can think neutrally 'What is the diagnosis?' I mean this is kind of too hard for me ... but it's, he has to reflect ...

Interviewer: So ... You see this happening and you don't feel that it is appropriate. Do you think that when you are a doctor ... how do you think you'll behave?

Hui-Wen: But what I think is each doctor has their own theory, and if this is not harming the patient or it is not harming most, I think they have their reason to do that. And if ... so I can't, I don't know how to be a doctor like that, I can't either. Maybe afterwards [after more experience] I can, but it's just like a choice. What kind of doctor, what kind of interaction you would like to have with your patient? It's something new, but I think he has his reasons, being a mirror reflecting. Sometimes it might be helpful.

Interviewer: So you didn't say anything because of this?

Hui-Wen: Yeah, because, I was taken aback because I never heard of this theory, being a mirror ... He didn't act out, but he just showed his impatience, and he told us, 'I'm impatient, because ...'

Interpretation: While on a clinical placement, Hui-Wen observes a doctor (her teacher) disregarding the patient's description of her current mental status, and displaying impatience with the patient while Hui-Wen takes the patient's medical history. While Hui-Wen suggests that the doctor appeared to lack empathy in her narrative, she nevertheless interprets the doctor's behaviour as professional, largely because of his seniority and because of the explanation he offers for his actions: that he disagrees with doctors acting like neutral (non-emotional) bystanders in their interactions with patients. Hui-Wen's professionalism dilemma therefore appears to negatively affect her understanding of healthcare professionalism. As Hui-Wen explains to the doctor (her teacher), being emotionally *neutral* is not professional. Instead, he believes that the professional doctor should *react* to patients in the same way that others would react to the patient.

Through providing a rationale for the doctor's conduct, based on the doctor's own justification, Hui-Wen fails to uphold the principals of patient-centred care taught to her as part of the formal curriculum. Hui-Wen experiences inconsistencies between what she observes as professionalism during her clinical placement and her own embodied identity. This disconnect causes her to struggle with *her* interpretation of professionalism: expressing her claim that it is hard for her to present herself as a 'mirror', but maybe with more practice she will be able to do so. In Hui-Wen's narrative she reproduces the notion that experience/practice may lead to the embodiment of a new identity (and the behaviours that correspond with it). However, what she aims to embody contradicts ideal professionalism norms, for example, set out through professionalism codes from regulatory bodies. This example clearly demonstrates how identities are co-constructed through narratives and social interactions, and raises concerns about what norms and values displayed through educators' practices learners are embodying.

Embodied identities and educational strategies

Understanding identity formation and embodiment as processes that take place through formal, informal and hidden professionalism curricula, suggests a number of educational strategies that could be adopted by educators in their quest to support the embodiment of professional identities among learners. Despite various educational strategies to facilitate this embodiment process, learners do not always internalise positive notions of professionalism. For example, some learners may merely come to *act* in a professional fashion, rather than *becoming* professionals (Monrouxe et al., 2011). Therefore, the following section outlines three strategies:

1. addressing curricula inconsistencies and the negative impact of the hidden curriculum;
2. promoting learners' active, first-hand experiences of observing and participating in the clinical setting;
3. facilitating opportunities for learners to reflect on the hidden curriculum and their identity formation.

The first strategy concerns the importance of educators and learners acknowledging and addressing the inconsistencies between formal, informal and hidden curricula, and recognising the negative impact the hidden curriculum can have on identity construction. The second strategy addresses the centrality of learners' active, first-hand experiences of observing and participating in clinical settings. Finally, the third strategy covers the importance of educators facilitating opportunities for learners to reflect on and make sense of their clinical experiences and their impact on learners' identity formation, in addition to also encouraging clinical educators to reflect on their own practice and educational strategies. While these strategies are initially presented separately below, they are obviously interconnected, as is illustrated at the end of the chapter.

Strategy 1: Address curricula inconsistencies

In an ideal world, what is taught about professionalism conduct (the combination of not only professional behaviour but the embodiment of professional norms and values) and identity in the formal learning environment should reflect what is experienced through informal and hidden curricula during clinical teaching and in the structures and cultures of the healthcare workplace. However, certain social norms and structural forces are difficult to eliminate. Hafferty and Castellani (2009) claim that what is learned through the hidden curriculum is generally analysed by scholars as having a negative affect on learners. Indeed, learners themselves recognise this: 'There's always … a gap between what you get taught and what you see … and the further you get into the programme I think the more acceptable that gap sometimes gets … you start justifying it, you know?' (excerpt from a narrative by an Australian fourth-year medical student, 'Christine': Monrouxe & Rees, 2017, p 44). This quote is aligned with the earlier discussion about experience and embodiment, as it is through (repeated) experiences of professionalism lapses that learners may come to internalise such practices as acceptable despite formal teaching to the contrary.

Therefore, in addition to teaching professionalism through the formal curriculum during pre-clinical placements, educators should work towards intertwining both the taught curriculum with its hidden counterparts by helping to make visible and address hidden curriculum issues within the formal education of healthcare learners (Neve & Collett, 2014). In acknowledging the hidden curriculum with learners, educators facilitate them to become conscious of its various potential consequences. In doing so, learners will be better able to recognise the negative aspects of the hidden curriculum once they enter the clinical setting. Formal discussions about the ways in which the hidden curriculum can negatively affect professionalism, and the potential negative consequences for healthcare, will better prepare learners to follow their own initiatives and perhaps even challenge professionalism lapses. Consequently, educators should strive towards empowering learners, not only to recognise the negative impacts of the hidden curriculum on themselves, but to also resist, directly or indirectly, such organisational factors that impact on their professionalism and professional identity formation. Repeated resistance to professionalism dilemmas, such as challenging perpetrators and raising concerns, should help to facilitate the embodiment of professional identities, benefiting learners, colleagues and patients. However, in making this recommendation it is vital, as part of learners' empowerment, that structures and systems are put in place to support learners who do hold firm to their professional selves to ensure that they are not victimised for raising concerns (see http://www.gmc-uk.org/guidance/29517.asp for an example of further information).

Strategy 2: Promote learners' active, first-hand experiences

As emphasised by embodiment theory, it is through (repeated) bodily experiences and reflection that individuals come to embody particular knowledge and practices, including one's perceptions of the self; that is, their identity. Research conducted with doctors in the United Kingdom by Nettleton and colleagues (2008) suggests that the lack of opportunity provided through the current curricula both to observe in the clinical setting and to actually *perform* medical practice is reducing the abilities of young doctors as healthcare knowledge (including the formation of professional identities) becomes less embodied. Clinical and practical knowledge for healthcare professionals becomes embodied through 'senses of sight, sound, touch, smell … and more general senses, such as "feeling that a situation makes sense", having a "gut feeling" or a sense of salience' (Gordon, 1988, p 269). In other words, learners require experiential learning that emphasises hands-on experience and active engagement in clinical practices for healthcare knowledge and professional identities to become embodied. This includes not only observing in the clinical setting, as is commonplace, particularly during early clinical experiences as early as the first year in healthcare education, but also physically taking the role of practitioner-in-training by the end of the final year.

Experiential learning, supported through both formal and informal curricula, will assist learners to acknowledge the norms, values and ethical practices that they are taught in the classroom, and to observe how these aspects of professional practice can be applied in the clinical setting. During clinical rounds, educators can further learners' understanding of professionalism by asking them how they would handle a particular situation, what abilities they already have to address the issue, and what experiences they feel they are missing to address a similar situation in the future. Verbal discussion while observing or participating in clinical practice will help learners better engage the situation, and embrace how the situation makes them react both professionally and emotionally. Furthermore, supporting learners to repeatedly engage in clinical practice will enable them to recognise that such values and norms can be enacted in various ways and applied to diverse clinical situations. For instance, the way a healthcare professional displays empathy may vary depending on the characteristics of the patient and the patient's ailment, and such an understanding of particular situations is gained through practice. Knowledge developed through practice not only supports the application of that knowledge to a specific scenario, but, as it becomes embodied (and even second-nature), that knowledge can be adopted to fit various scenarios. Therefore, educators who have curriculum development responsibilities should advocate for early clinical experiences for learners in healthcare schools, with their level of active participation in patient care increasing up to the time of graduation. However, this will require educators to only involve learners in clinical practices that are appropriate for their level of competence, and to supervise learners when they are participating in patient care activities for which they are not yet competent (Monrouxe & Rees, 2017).

Strategy 3: Facilitate opportunities for reflection

In order for professional identities to become embodied in learners, they must be given opportunities to reflect on their clinical experiences, to make sense of them and explore how they impact on their understandings of self. Relating to the concept of narrative identities, educators can help facilitate learners' embodiment of professionalism through incorporating conversational activities into learning that prompts learners to reflect on who they are now and who they want to be. Such narrative activities could be implemented early on in the degree program through small-group clinician-led workshops, where learners openly discuss their own beliefs of right and wrong with peers, and how these relate to their personal and professional identities. As learners progress through their education continuum, such peer meetings could incorporate discussions about interactions with patients and healthcare professionals, including professionalism dilemmas they have personally experienced, and the impact of them on their developing identities. The more opportunities learners have for reflection within the formal curriculum, 'the less likely it is that student understandings of professionalism will be negatively influenced by the hidden curriculum. This may be partly a result of the embodied nature of knowing that emerges from such sense-making activities' (Monrouxe et al., 2011, p 600).

When learners do ponder in silence over the professionalism dilemmas they have experienced, as in Hui-Wen's case presented in case study 8.1, they may appropriate such practices and unethical morals into their identity as healthcare professionals. Conversely, through ample opportunities for guided reflection and discussion of professionalism dilemmas, learners can strengthen their understandings of professional conduct and their ideal images of themselves as healthcare practitioners. This can be seen clearly in case study 8.2, where Daniel, a third-year Australian medical student, narrates observing the professionalism lapses of his educators, which helped him reflect on the type of doctor he wants to be.

Learners should be encouraged by educators to explore the complexities of professionalism dilemmas and how they made them feel (as individuals, as healthcare learners, as future healthcare professionals), how they think the dilemmas made patients feel, and how they think the situations could have been avoided or better addressed. Furthermore, when provided with pedagogical spaces to explore lived clinical experiences within safe, formal educational environments, learners should become, with time, better equipped with the skills and confidence to recognise and reflect on professionalism lapses both on their own and in peer-groups external to the educational setting. Such reflection may serve as peer support and a form of empowerment as learners assist each other in their professionalism development. Enabling learners to reflect on their experiences through narratives may facilitate changes to their practice to counter problematic aspects of their experiences.

Learners' reflection however should not only be encouraged through oral narratives in group situations alone. Indeed, various means for reflection exist to address learners' diverse approaches to learning. Although educators should be encouraged to create safe environments where all learners feel comfortable sharing their experiences and emotions, not all learners will feel comfortable doing so in public settings. Therefore, in addition to group activities, educators could encourage learners to keep an audio or written diary of their clinical experiences and how their experiences made them feel, as a means of reflection. This may be used as a tool to then guide future discussions in which learners construct their own professionalism and professional identity formation.

Finally, educators might reflect on what professionalism and the hidden curriculum means for them, and share these personal understandings and experiences of professionalism with learners. As discussed above, identities are co-constructed through communication and social interactions. Given this, educators, and healthcare professionals in general, should be conscious of the ways in which they present their understandings of professionalism, and how they do or do not promote professionalism in their clinical and educational practice. This may include, for instance, considering how they demonstrate patient-centredness and empathy during, for example, bedside teaching with real patients. Through educators displaying patient-centred tendencies, learners will observe how to 'empower patients within an educational setting' and will begin to cultivate 'their own identities as patient-centred professionals internally and relationally' (Monrouxe, 2016, p 45).

Case study 8.2: Daniel's dilemma and an interpretation — how educational strategies (active engagement and reflection) can facilitate embodiment

Daniel: I was tempted to become a dobber [report the behaviour] once in the emergency department because … after I was asked to do an examination on an intellectually disabled man who was uncommunicative and … totally paralysed … he just had cellulitis [infection of the skin and the soft tissue underneath] that potentially had developed into osteomyelitis [infection of the bone] of his olecranon [bony point of the elbow]. And I was asked to examine him, and when I came back … and gave my findings … I also reported that his eye was productive of yellow pus and looked quite red and inflamed … and the resident said, 'I didn't hear you say that', again, 'I didn't hear you say that', and I said, 'You didn't hear me say what? About the arm or about the eye', and she went, 'D-d- shhh.' She said, 'I'm giving him antibiotics for his arm, and I'm, we're, sending him back to the home.' … She obviously did not want to put herself out to go and get an ophthalmology review or … you know go assess the patient because he clearly wasn't valuable enough to her, to treat him wholly.

Interviewer: And so you nearly … 'dobbed', did you say?

Daniel: … I didn't go and tell anybody, but I, I pushed her further. I said, 'He has this: what are you going to do for it? Are the antibiotics that you're giving him going to help for that or potentially treat it?' But I … didn't write anything down in the notes at that stage, I wasn't doing that sort of thing; again it was my second rotation in week five of being there … But I went home absolutely disgusted … But I did do something with somebody who had a motorbike accident and had a plastics review because of extensive bleeding in the hand, and the plastics registrar came down, looked at it, went, 'Move it around a bit.' The patient responded, 'It is a bit sore', and then the plastics registrar looked at me and said, 'Can you just … Well, I'm just going to dress this, so can you clean it up?' So I said, 'How about I clean it up, and then I'll dress it? What dressing do you want on it?' The hand looked quite manky and gross … and she agreed … When I was cleaning, I was convinced that I could feel foreign bodies in different parts of the hand, and it was my job to wrap him up so he could be shipped out, and I said to one of the bosses, 'This is what I've been doing on this patient. I'm not happy to dress it and send him out, because I'm convinced there's foreign bodies in his hand.' And at that point the previous plastics consult hadn't looked at any imaging, but they called another plastics consult down, and sure enough he had big chunks of glass and rock left in his hand. And I was glad I did that, because I actually felt like … you know, that that could really cause that kid damage in his hand. But who's to say that the … intellectually disabled man might not have lost his eye … I don't know if it was how long I'd been there at that point. That I'd had more time to feel more comfortable with people, but I feel a bit gutted that I wasn't prepared … to go and stand up for someone who … absolutely couldn't stand up for themselves. But I did it for the other guy … because I was actually concerned about the functionality of his hand. But why wasn't I concerned about the functionality of this other guy's eye?

Interpretation: Daniel narrates two professionalism dilemmas that he encountered during his emergency department placement. He acknowledges both incidents as sub-optimal, constructing both as unethical treatment of the patients concerned, demonstrating that Daniel has a clear sense of what professionalism looks like. In the first experience, Daniel claims that he (indirectly) resisted the professionalism lapse of the doctor (ignoring the patient's infected eye) by questioning her further about whether her proposed management would also treat the patient's eye. Despite such questioning, Daniel explains that the doctor 'did not want to put herself out' in terms of getting an ophthalmology review, suggesting that her actions were both unprofessional and selfish.

While Daniel describes the doctor's behaviour as 'disgusting', he did not report the incident, which he clearly regrets, claiming in his narrative how disappointed he felt with himself. In reflecting on the event and narrating his experience as he did, it is clear that Daniel does not want to be *that* kind of doctor.

However, Daniel reports having been more proactive during the second dilemma, as he not only offered to clean and dress the man's injured hand, but also later voiced his concern that there were still foreign bodies in the man's hand that needed to be removed. Daniel narrates how taking this initiative made him feel glad that he was able to help the patient, as he felt concerned for the patient's wellbeing. But, when reflecting on the incident, he claims it also resulted in him questioning his intentions when he did not speak up for the first patient. In Daniel's narrative, he partially answers this query for himself: because he had spent little time on the placement when he interacted with the first patient. As already discussed, embodying new practices and identities is a transitional process that requires time. The more time Daniel spent in his placement, including additional time spent observing the clinical environment and practising *being* a doctor-in-training, that the better Daniel was able to act in the latter case. Indeed, Daniel indicated that, given his additional experience, he started to feel more comfortable. Comfort is associated with confidence, in that as one becomes more comfortable in a situation their understanding of the situation and the abilities they have in that situation also become clearer. Developing confidence is essential to the healthcare socialisation process (Hafferty, 1988), and can help facilitate the embodiment of professional identity (Underman, 2015, p 182).

Daniel's sustained questioning of his previous inaction when confronted with the first professionalism dilemma, even after having positively responded to the second dilemma, suggests that Daniel had internalised this initial lack of action in a way that made him reflect on how he views himself as a healthcare professional. Thus, experiencing these professional dilemmas and reflecting on them appears to have helped facilitate Daniel's embodiment of his professional identity.

Integrating professionalism, identities and embodiment to address the hidden curriculum

The three educational strategies outlined above (i.e. acknowledging the impact of the hidden curriculum, active engagement in repeated clinical placements, and making sense of both active and emotive experiences through reflections) together can assist learners to incorporate workplace-based professionalism experiences into developing their embodied professional identities (see Figure 8.1). As individuals make sense of events happening in their surroundings through reflecting on personal experiences and interactions, they come to develop an embodied form of knowledge. This embodied knowledge influences their sense of self and ultimately their identities. This then completes the circle, from first-hand experiences of professionalism dilemmas in clinical placements, to reflecting on experiences and dilemmas in order to make sense of the situation and embody their significance.

During the early stages of healthcare education, learners will develop fundamental understandings of professionalism and identity (both professional identity and their personal understandings of themselves) through the formal curriculum. The educational strategies discussed here (labelled in Fig. 8.1 as 'Address hidden curriculum', 'First-hand experience', and 'Reflection') will help learners to further their understandings of professionalism, and make-sense of the professionalism dilemmas they encounter in real healthcare settings. Furthermore, through narrative reflection on experiences, sentiments and (re)actions to such experiences, learners will come to transform their identities within this sense-making process.

However, when foregoing the suggested educational strategies, it is likely that learners will struggle to embody professionalism, as they will not have reflected on their experiences, and therefore may *act* like professionals but not actually *become* professionals. Likewise, as in the case of Hui-Wen (case study 8.1), failing to explore and reflect on professionalism dilemmas may negatively impact on learners' identity formation. Finally, case study 8.3 explores how limited time — a key structural element of the hidden curriculum outlined in both narratives above — can affect educators' professionalism, and how, in turn, making time for reflection may help learners recognise better the hidden curriculum and its potential impact on their embodiment of professional identities (and that of others).

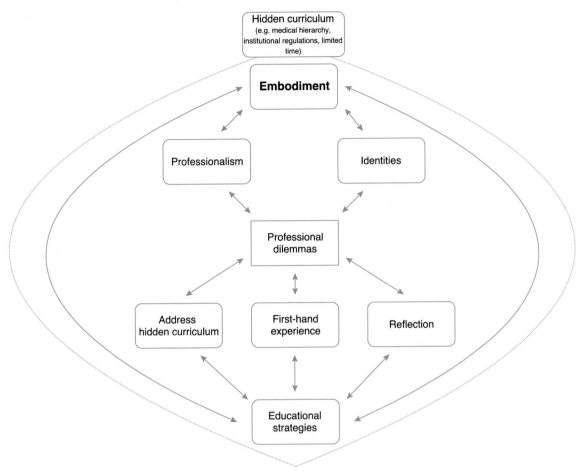

Figure 8.1 A model to support learners' embodiment of professional identities through addressing the hidden curriculum

Case study 8.3: Supporting the embodiment of professional identities through addressing the hidden curriculum

Interpretation: In the examples of professional dilemmas discussed in case studies 8.1 and 8.2, insufficient time and resources likely contributed to the doctors' questionable decisions. For example, not taking the time to take a complete history and listen thoroughly to the patient (case study 8.1), not taking the time to get the ophthalmology referral and not taking the time to examine the images of the patient's hand (case study 8.2). It is not known whether insufficient time was what led to the three doctors neglecting their patients' healthcare needs, but such structural constraints may come to be internalised and produce a perception of perpetual limited time, which may alter a doctor's professional identity as they come to find it acceptable to make diagnoses based on quick decisions and limited data. Moreover, this structural lack of time was directly embedded in Daniel's own words ('he could be shipped out') as he discussed the immediate need to send the patient on his way so that Daniel could move on to other tasks. This reiterates the embeddedness of this particular structural constraint within healthcare professionals' understandings of healthcare practice, and how susceptible learners may be to internalising such perceptions during clinical placements.

Daniel's and Hui-Wen's reflections on their experiences will not necessarily alter the structural practices built into the clinical setting and, thus, learned through the hidden curriculum. However, through sense-making activities, these hidden structures (e.g. time availability) can be partly addressed. Sense-making can be facilitated through formal education that directly acknowledges the existence of such (hidden) structural factors and the impact they may have on clinical practice. This curriculum should discuss the various structural barriers that learners may confront, and suggest strategies for addressing each, such as: 1) transforming their practice to better serve the patient's needs; and 2) directly raising concerns with healthcare professionals about the professional's own practice or learners' practices. Furthermore, curricula is needed that will facilitate learners to reflect on their clinical experiences — including experiencing barriers to ethical, moral and effective practice — through educator and peer-led small group discussions. Through reflexive discussions, learners can be encouraged to discuss: what they have experienced during clinical placements; what, if any, professionalism dilemmas they have encountered; how they addressed the dilemmas; and if they did not address the dilemma, how they would do so retrospectively. Sharing such experiences in a group setting will bring further awareness to structural barriers and how they can be addressed, allowing learners to develop first-hand from the experiences of their peers. By recognising how factors such as time affect practice or the practice of others, awareness is raised about the existence of such structures. This is the necessary first step to help empower learners to alter their behaviour and alert educators to how they could change their practice to better reflect professionalism ideals.

Conclusion

This chapter has explored how cultivating a learner's professional identity is a process that involves the embodiment of specific norms, values, ethical codes and practices, and knowledge, factors that represent the cornerstone of all healthcare professions, and influence a learner's sense of self; that is, their identity. The analysis of two narratives (case studies 8.1 and 8.2) considered the impact that inconsistencies between formal, informal and hidden curricula, often experienced as professionalism dilemmas, can have on learners' understandings of professionalism and their own professional identities, resulting in identity struggles about their own developing practices as proto-healthcare professionals.

In summary, educators should aim to promote learners' embodiment of professional identities by addressing the hidden curriculum through the three interconnected educational strategies discussed previously: addressing curricula inconsistencies, promoting learners' active, first-hand experiences, and facilitating opportunities for the reflection of both learners and educators. Thus, educators must strive to promote an embodied sense of professionalism among learners that reflects not only ideal healthcare attitudes and practices, but also a sense of identity that is connected to learners' personal ethics, values and motivations. It is through this complex interconnected process that a learner can be supported to transform from *acting* like a healthcare professional to embodying professionalism and actually *becoming* a professional.

PRACTICAL TIPS

1. Reflect on how professionalism is taught and learned at your institution, taking into account the formal, informal, and hidden curricula. What are the strengths and weaknesses of these curricula?
2. During formal teaching, directly address the impact that the informal and hidden curricula may have on learners' professionalism identity formation. Directly discuss issues that may arise during learning activities, and explore with learners the significance of this impact on their learning and their professional identity formation. Through such discussions and role-playing activities, learners can become empowered to resist the professionalism lapses that they experience during clinical practice.
3. During clinical practice and observation, ask learners to hypothesise about how they would react in certain professionalism lapse situations, what skills they have to address such situations, and what experiences they would need to address similar situations in the future. Discuss how they reacted to certain situations, both professionally and emotionally, and how such experiences impact on their sense of self.

4. Encourage learners to reflect on who they are, how they see themselves, and how they think others see them. Ask them about why they want to be a healthcare professional, and how they imagine themselves working in the healthcare environment. Explore what facilitators and barriers learners have encountered in regards to developing their professional identity.
5. Support learners to discuss positive and negative clinical experiences they have had, and how such experiences impact on their sense of self.
6. Share authentic personal understandings and experiences of professionalism lapses, identity any confusion you have experienced, and discuss with them your reasons for being a healthcare professional. These could include both positive and negative experiences that have shaped your indentity as a healthcare professional.
7. For further practical tips, see Chapter 5 in Monrouxe and Rees (2017).

References

Bourdieu, P. (1990). *The logic of practice*. Cambridge: Polity Press.

Burkitt, I. (1999). *Bodies of thought: Embodiment, identity and modernity*. London: Sage Publications.

Chandratilake, M., McAleer, S., & Gibson, J. (2012). Cultural similarities and differences in medical professionalism: A multi-region study. *Medical Education, 46*(3), 257–266. doi:10.1111/j.1365-2923.2011.04153.x.

Christakis, D. A., & Feudtner, C. (1993). Ethics in a short white coat: The ethical dilemmas that medical students confront. *Academic Medicine, 68*(4), 249–254.

Coulter, J. (1979). *The social construction of mind: Studies in ethnomethodology and linguistic philosophy*. London: Macmillan Press.

Cruess, R. L., Cruess, S. R., & Steinert, Y. (2016). *Teaching medical professionalism: Supporting the development of a professional identity*. Cambridge: Cambridge University Press.

Ginsburg, S., & Lingard, L. (2011). 'Is that normal?' Pre-clerkship students' approaches to professional dilemmas. *Medical Education, 45*(4), 362–371.

Gordon, D. R. (1988). Clinical science and clinical expertise: Changing boundaries between art and science in medicine. In M. Lock & A. Young (Eds.), *Biomedicine examined* (pp. 257–295). Dordrecht: Kluwer Academic Publishers.

Hafferty, F. W. (1988). Cadaver stories and the emotional socialization of medical studies. *Journal of Health and Social Behavior, 29*(4), 344–356.

Hafferty, F. W. (1998). Beyond curriculum reform: Confronting medicine's hidden curriculum. *Academic Medicine, 73*(4), 403–407.

Hafferty, F. W. (2016). Socialization, professionalism, and professional identity formation. In R. L. Cruess, S. R. Cruess, & Y. Steinert (Eds.), *Teaching medical professionalism: Supporting the development of a professional identity* (2nd ed., pp. 54–67). Cambridge: Cambridge University Press.

Hafferty, F. W., & Castellani, B. (2009). The hidden curriculum: A theory of medical education. In C. Brosnon & B. S. Turner (Eds.), *Handbook of the sociology of medical education* (pp. 15–35). New York: Routledge.

Hendelman, W., & Byszewski, A. (2014). Formation of medical student professional identity: Categorizing lapses of professionalism, and the learning environment. *BMC Medical Education, 14*, 139.

Ho, M.-J., Gosselin, K., Chandratilake, M., et al. (2017). Taiwanese medical students' narratives of intercultural professionalism dilemmas: Exploring tensions between Western medicine and Taiwanese culture. *Advances in Health Sciences Dducation: Theory and Practice, 22*(2), 429–445. doi:10.1007/s10459-016-9738-x.

Jenkins, R. (2008). *Social identity* (3rd ed.). New York: Routledge.

Jha, V., McLean, M., Gibbs, T. J., et al. (2015). Medical professionalism across cultures: A challenge for medicine and medical education. *Medical Teacher, 37*(1), 74–80. doi:10.3109/0142159X.2014.920492.

Johnson, M. (1989). Embodied knowledge. *Curriculum Inquiry, 19*(4), 361–377.

Johnson, M. (1991). Knowing through the body. *Philosophical Psychology, 4*(1), 3–18. doi:10.1080/09515089108573009.

Labov, W., & Waletzky, J. (1967). Narrative analysis: Oral versions of personal experience. *Journal of Narrative and Life History, 7*(1–4), 3–38.

Mavor, K. I., Platow, M. J., & Bizumic, B. (Eds.), (2017). *Self and social identity in educational contexts*. New York: Routledge.

Monrouxe, L. V. (2009). Negotiating professional identities: Dominant and contesting narratives in medical students' longitudinal audio diaries. *Current Narratives, 1*(1), 41–59.

Monrouxe, L. V. (2010). Identity, identification and medical education: Why should we care? *Medical Education, 44*(1), 40–49. doi:10.1111/j.1365-2923.2009.03440.x.

Monrouxe, L. V. (2015). When I say … intersectionality in medical education research. *Medical Education, 49*(1), 21–22. doi:10.1111/medu.12428.

Monrouxe, L. V. (2016). Theoretical insights into the nature and nurture of professional identity. In R. L. Cruess, S. R. Cruess, & Y. Steinert (Eds.), *Teaching medical professionalism: Supporting the development of a professional identity* (pp. 37–53). Cambridge: Cambridge University Press.

Monrouxe, L. V., Chandratilake, M., Gosselin, K., et al. (2017). Taiwanese and Sri Lankan students' dimensions and discourses of professionalism. *Medical Education*, *51*(7), 718–731. doi:10.1111/medu.13291.

Monrouxe, L. V., & Rees, C. E. (2015). Theoretical perspectives on identity: Researching identities in healthcare education. In J. Cleland & S. J. Durning (Eds.), *Researching medical education* (pp. 129–140). Hoboken, NJ: John Wiley & Sons.

Monrouxe, L. V., & Rees, C. E. (2017). *Healthcare professionalism: Improving practice through reflections on workplace dilemmas*. Oxford: Wiley Blackwell.

Monrouxe, L. V., Rees, C. E., Dennis, I., et al. (2015). Professionalism dilemmas, moral distress and the healthcare student: Insights from two online UK-wide questionnaire studies. *BMJ Open*, *5*(5), e007518. doi:10.1136/bmjopen-2014-007518.

Monrouxe, L. V., Rees, C. E., & Hu, W. (2011). Differences in medical students' explicit discourses of professionalism: Acting, representing, becoming. *Medical Education*, *45*(6), 585–602. doi:10.1111/j.1365-2923.2010.03878.x.

Nettleton, S., Burrows, R., & Watt, I. (2008). Regulating medical bodies? The consequences of the 'modernisation' of the NHS and the disembodiment of clinical knowledge. *Sociology of Health and Illness*, *30*(3), 333–348. doi:10.1111/j.1467-9566.2007.01057.x.

Neve, H., & Collett, T. (2014). *Revealing the hidden curriculum to medical students: Insights from threshold concept theory*. Paper presented at the Fifth International Biennial Threshold Concepts Conference, Threshold Concepts in Practice, Durham University, UK, 9–11 July 2014. http://www.ee.ucl.ac.uk/mflanaga/abstracts/TC14Abstract32.pdf. (Accessed 17 April 2017).

Rees, C. E., & Monrouxe, L. V. (2010). 'I should be lucky ha ha ha ha': The construction of power, identity and gender through laughter within medical workplace learning encounters. *Journal of Pragmatics*, *42*(12), 3384–3399. doi:10.1016/j.pragma.2010.05.004.

Rees, C. E., & Monrouxe, L. V. (2011). Medical students learning intimate examinations without valid consent: A multicentre study. *Medical Education*, *45*(3), 261–272. doi:10.1111/j.1365-2923.2010.03839.x.

Rees, C. E., Monrouxe, L. V., & McDonald, L. A. (2013). Narrative, emotion and action: Analysing 'most memorable' professionalism dilemma. *Medical Education*, *47*(1), 80–96. doi:10.1111/j.1365-2923.2012.04302.x.

Rees, C. E., Monrouxe, L. V., & McDonald, L. A. (2014). 'My mentor kicked a dying woman's bed …' Analysing UK nursing students' 'most memorable' professionalism dilemmas. *Journal of Advanced Nursing*, *71*(1), 169–180. doi:10.1111/jan.12457.

Sfard, A. (1998). On two metaphors for learning and the dangers of choosing just one. *Educational Researcher*, *27*(2), 4–13.

Smith, B., & Sparkes, A. C. (2008). Contrasting perspectives on narrating selves and identities: An invitation to dialogue. *Qualitative Research*, *8*(1), 5–35.

Tajfel, H., & Turner, J. C. (2004). The social identity theory of intergroup behavior. In J. T. Jost & J. Sidanius (Eds.), *Political psychology: Key readings in social psychology* (pp. 276–293). New York: Psychology Press.

Tsouroufli, M., Rees, C. E., Monrouxe, L. V., et al. (2011). Gender, identities and intersectionality in medical education research. *Medical Education*, *45*(3), 213–216. doi:10.1111/j.1365-2923.2010.03908.x.

Underman, K. (2015). Playing doctor: Simulation in medical school as affective practice. *Social Science and Medicine*, *136–137*, 180–188. doi:10.1016/j.socscimed.2015.05.028.

Wear, D., & Skillicorn, J. (2009). Hidden in plain sight: The formal, informal and hidden curricula of a psychiatry clerkship. *Academic Medicine*, *84*(4), 451–458.

9

Scaffolding for progressive independence in workplace contexts

Mark Goldszmidt and Lorelei Lingard

Introduction

Clinical learners require support in their progressive independence (Franzone et al., 2015; Kashner et al., 2010; Kennedy et al., 2005). The characteristics of the clinical placements, learners and educators all play important and overlapping roles in shaping how, and the extent to which, progressive independence is supported (Billett, 2002). The notion of scaffolding — the provision of a variety of supports to clinical learners to bridge the gap between required performance and independently achievable performance — provides a useful metaphor for exploring clinical placements, clinical educator supervisory strategies, and their intertwined relationship in support of learner progressive independence. While there are many relevant theories that relate to this topic, the two that we will be focusing on are sociomateriality and rhetorical genre theory. Both were selected for their complementarity and ability to draw teachers' attention to powerful features of the workplace learning setting that they may not currently consider explicitly: namely, material features such as physical layouts, electronic records and team schedules, and genres such as case review.

In exploring the topic of scaffolding for progressive independence, we will use a case study of an inpatient internal medicine clinical teaching unit where we have explored this topic extensively. In this setting, a mix of clinical trainees ranging from third-year medical students to fifth-year residents participate in the interdisciplinary care of patients with moderate to high acuity. The need to deliver high-quality, safe and efficient care may be in tension with educational deliverables in this setting, a tension well recognised in the literature (Hoffman & Donaldson, 2004). Our overarching purpose in the chapter is to make visible how scaffolding for progressive independence can be used to support both high-quality care and learner education.

Case study 9.1

Carl and Yvonne are newly hired phsyicians in an academic teaching hospital. Over coffee one afternoon, they begin a conversation that they will likely revisit many times over the next few years. Over the next few weeks, each for their first time, they will have the chance to be taking on the role of consultant physician, hereafter referred to as the 'clinical educator', on one of the three internal medicine inpatient teaching teams at their hospital. Each of these teams includes a mixed group of clinical learners: two to three senior medical students, two to three first-year residents, one second-year resident, and one third-year resident. During their conversation, Carl and Yvonne focus on the difficulty of balancing the inherent tensions of their clinical and teaching roles. In particular, they are worried about how they will balance the provision of patient care with the supervision of learners. Like many, they wonder how they will balance getting the work done with ensuring a good learning experience. As part of the discussion, they compare some of their role models who have been in practice for many years and are well respected by their peers.

They start with Dr M

Working with Dr M is really fun. Dr M is easy to get along with, and you get a real sense that Dr M trusts the senior resident. Feedback is universally one of praise for the team. Dr M typically shows up for morning rounds, but lets the senior resident run things. After rounds, Dr M 'gets out of the way' so that the team can get their work done. Dr M believes that the best way to learn is by doing. While both agree that Dr M is well liked and that it was fun being a learner on Dr M's team, they are less sure that they would personally feel comfortable supervising the team as Dr M does. The clinical context has changed a lot in the past few years, and the demand to move large volumes of increasingly sick patients through the healthcare system safely seems somewhat at odds with Dr M's approach.

With this in mind, they then discuss Dr D

Dr D is frequently in early, and has often pre-seen all of the new patients. Morning rounds are very efficient, and even include time for a 30-minute didactic teaching session. Due to Dr D's efficiency and strong work ethic, the team's patient load is often lower than for other teams. To ensure quality of care and flow within the system, Dr D often discharges patients first thing in the morning, and always personally dictates the discharge summary. While both agree that Dr D is a fantastic clinician who provides high-quality patient care, they do wonder if Dr D's style is one that sufficiently supports learner development.

With this in mind, they turn their discussion to Dr E

Working with Dr E can, at times, be a bit intimidating. While Dr E sets very high expectations of the learners, Dr E does a lot of work to support them: Dr E always seems to know what is going on with every learner on the team, but does not do the work for them; Dr E uses each admission to teach the team about how to conceptualise and care for the complex patients they are admitting; Dr E regularly meets with both senior and junior learners to explore how things are going, and to provide feedback. Both agree that there are many positive attributes to Dr E's approach, but they wonder how to do it; a lot of Dr E's work was invisible to them when they were in training, and they are still not sure how Dr E stays on top of everything.

Theories, definitions and dimension of scaffolding for progressive independence

Scaffolding

The definition of scaffolding we are working with originated in developmental psychology. In his essays on development, Lev Vygotsky described the highly popularised notion of the zone of proximal development (ZPD) (Vygotsky, 1978). The ZPD represents the difference between what a learner can perform with and without assistance. *Scaffolding*, a term first used in relation to the ZPD by Wood and colleagues (Wood et al., 1976), represents the ways in which learners are assisted to practise at the level required by the workplace in which they are placed. Through scaffolding, learners can work within their ZPD — a locus widely accepted as being optimal for learning — while also being supported to bridge the difference between their current abilities and those required by their clinical placements. Over time, as a learner's abilities increase, they not only require less scaffolding, they themselves begin to participate in the scaffolding of more junior learners (Lave & Wenger, 1991). Scaffolding can therefore involve multiple levels of learners each receiving and providing scaffolding.

Following on the developmental psychology origins of scaffolding, it is tempting to focus on how clinical educators provide scaffolding, and many useful studies have done so (Dunphy & Dunphy, 2003; Dunphy & Williamson, 2004). However, emerging research suggests that scaffolding is not only about what people do. Rather, this research suggests that the materialities of our workplaces are intricately entangled with the people within them, and that this entangled whole powerfully shapes learning and practice (Billett, 2002; Fenwick, 2014, 2016). In the next sections, we will describe how a sociomaterial approach provides a unique perspective for exploring these complex relationships, and how the insights gained can help Carl and Yvonne use scaffolding effectively in their new roles as consultant physicians and clinical educators.

The importance of the sociomaterial

During his first week as the clinical educator on the inpatient internal medicine team, Carl noticed that, despite his best intentions of conducting ward rounds with the team at patient bedsides, nearly every case review had taken place in a conference room.

This section will summarise two principles from sociomaterial theory as they relate to clinical teaching:
1. Not only people but also materials matter.
2. People and materials assemble in particular ways to create practice.

Sociomateriality is an umbrella term used to describe a set of related approaches (Goldszmidt, 2017). Actor network theory, cultural historical activity theory, and complexity theory are just a few of the approaches that have been pulled together under this term (Fenwick et al., 2011). While each has its own unique history, sociomaterial approaches all share a decentring of humans as the focus of attention (Fenwick et al., 2011). These approaches are a shift away from attending to social practices, and towards attending to the complex 'entangled' relations that exist between social and material forces and the practices that 'assemble' around them (Fenwick, 2014). Sociomaterial approaches counteract our natural tendency to look at people and materials separately, and they undermine our assumptions that we can improve practice by just changing people *or* materials. Attention to both is necessary for understanding scaffolding for progressive independence.

Materials refer to just about everything. In clinical workplace settings, they include tangible things like buildings, rooms, beds, doors, computers, and patient charts, and they also include less tangible things like policies and schedules. Because materials are so inextricably bound up in all human activity, from a sociomaterial perspective they are considered to be 'constitutively entangled' — or just 'entangled' (Orlikowski, 2007). In observing any form of practice, what we see are the 'assemblages': the way the social and material came together to produce a particular thing instead of something else.

Admission case review in the inpatient setting of the hospital where Carl and Yvonne work is a good example for exploring the ideas of entanglements and assemblages. As happens in many institutions (Gonzalo et al., 2014; Ramani et al., 2003), admission case review at their hospital almost universally takes place in one of the team conference rooms. In exploring the question of why case review most consistently assembles as a discussion around a table in a conference room, and not at a patient bedside where many educators argue it should take place (Gonzalo et al., 2014; Ramani et al., 2003), we can look at the types of entanglements that exist. Some of the entangled sociomaterials in this assemblage include time, the number of patients admitted to hospital each day, the number of members of the team, the size of patient rooms, contact precautions, and concerns about undermining clinical learners in front of their patients. For those trying to push clinical teams back to the bedside, the challenge involves more than changing the minds or skills of clinical teachers and learners. The challenge requires tinkering with people and materials, observing how they assemble, and then trying again (Fenwick, 2014).

The introduction of longitudinal integrated clerkships (LIC) are an excellent, larger-scale example of how complex sociomaterial entanglements assemble around scaffolding for progressive independence. Although not described from a sociomaterial perspective, Walters and colleagues' review of LIC beautifully describes the multiple material entanglements that have assembled over the past several decades to create LIC in multiple schools around the world (Walters et al., 2012). Example materials leading to their creation have included: a dearth of rural experiences, rural workforce shortages, scheduled discontinuity of educational experience, patient care discontinuity, and tertiary case mix inadequacies. As this list suggests, many of the materials are entangled within social constructs, like student-centredness, patient-centredness, humanism and social accountability. For example, a dearth of rural experiences takes on added importance when schools begin to consider their social mandates and population needs.

Looking more closely, we can also see that many of these entanglements are premised on the assumption that longitudinal experiences will also offer better scaffolding, and therefore more opportunities for progressive independence. And, research has shown that in many instances the assemblage resulting from changing the materials of rotation scheduling towards a longitudinal primary-care experience produces positive results (Walters et al., 2012). Reported successes have included better or equivalent exam scores, greater patient-centredness, and improved interprofessional collaboration (Walters et al., 2012). There are, however, many schools where the entanglements have not assembled to produce these positive outcomes (Walters et al., 2012). Not having an immersive clinical experience in paediatrics and psychiatry, for example, can assemble to produce clinical learners uncomfortable in dealing with these patient populations.

When LICs assemble to produce progressive independence, learners increasingly add value to the clinical practice through their development of increased independence, and satisfaction from clinical educators is high. By contrast, when they do not assemble in this way, over time clinical educators begin to resent the loss of income that arises as a result (Walters et al., 2012). The point is that materials matter! And, despite many apparent similarities between settings, how materials assemble with the social to produce practice often differs in fundamental ways (Bates & Ellaway, 2016).

The importance of genre

Like many clinical educators, Yvonne considers case review to be an invaluable tool for supporting patient care and teaching. She has previously been taught not to interrupt clinical learners during their case presentations. But, on her first day as the clinical educator on team, she believes she must have interrupted her clinical learners at least four times each per reviewed case.

This section will summarise two principles from genre theory as they relate to clinical teaching:

1. Genre is not just structure, it also embodies purpose.
2. By their very nature, genres scaffold. However, genres need to be supported by clinical educators if they are to optimally support our purposes.

As one of the 'materials' that dominates clinical and education practice, communication warrants special attention. Communication practices in the workplace occur in highly standardised ways. These standardised practices, which arise in response to recurring situations, can be referred to as *genres*. Genres can be written, electronic or oral forms of communication. In clinical practice, these can include things like a case review with a learner following their clinical encounter with a patient (an oral genre) or their consultation note (a written genre). Of course, we don't all do things in exactly the same way. The nuanced differences that we each employ within a genre are referred to as *repertoires*.

From a rhetorical genre theory (RGT) perspective, genres are not just thought about in relation to their descriptive properties (e.g. the features of a good consultation note). Rather, they are considered to be a form of social action that allows people to do work in the world, and it is through our genre repertoires that we have access to choices about how to influence what work gets done. During case review, for example, an interruption to the learner's presentation to ask them to present the medications in relation to each of their medical problems has at least two social actions: 1) it helps the consultant be sure that the learner can attend to the medication list in a meaningful way and 2) it signals to the learner what to do differently next time. The interruption itself is part of a repertoire of strategies that different consultants use to achieve particular social actions. Other examples of genres that clinicians work with every day are patient interviews, admission notes, clinical case reviews, progress notes and discharge summaries.

Genres do not function in isolation. Rather, they exist in sets each supporting the other: patient interviews lead to admission notes and case reviews, which themselves inform the data that clinical learners collect during their interviews. By thinking about our communication practices from an RGT perspective, we can make visible important aspects of our collaborative and scaffolding practices. As Miller wrote in her seminal work on RGT, 'what we learn when we learn a genre is not just a pattern of forms or even a method of achieving our own ends. We learn more importantly, what ends we may have.' (Miller, 1984, p 165). That is, by understanding our shared genres, we are able to explore our shared purposes and the strategies or repertoires that may be used to achieve them.

In clinical placements, purposes are typically dual: not just clinical or educational, but some combination of the two (Kesselheim & Cassel 2013; Sanfey et al., 2011; Sholl et al., 2017; Turner et al., 2016). To understand genre purpose, consider the following question: Have you ever participated in a case review with a clinical learner where, like the example above, you have had to interrupt them to correct the way they were presenting the case? Maybe it was their sequence of starting with the physical findings rather than the history. Maybe it was that they omitted key elements that you expected to hear. Beneath these structural errors, however, the more fundamental problem likely was that their genre errors were undermining the case review's purpose of supporting shared clinical reasoning. You could not effectively reason along with them through the patient's case as you heard the presentation, because the order was wrong or key pieces of information were missing (Lingard et al., 2003). One of the purposes of oral and written genres in clinical contexts is to support collaborative efforts to diagnose, treat and manage patient requests. Together, these genres share the purpose of progressively helping the team to define and refine their understanding of the problems a patient is facing, and the plans for addressing these; this process has been referred to as *progressive collaborative refinement* (Goldszmidt et al., 2014).

By their very nature, genres scaffold (Schryer, 2011). Even when clinical teachers are not around, genres teach learners to collect particular types of information, to develop differential diagnoses, and to create plans for their patients. The structure of the oral case presentation, for instance, tells learners that certain data are required. Similarly, the existence of a progress note tells clinical learners that a written daily update is required. In these ways, genres teach learners what purposes they should have and what they should value.

Such scaffolding through genre is largely implicit and can be very powerful (Schryer, 2011; Schryer et al., 2003). However, as many of us have likely experienced, genres also need explicit support from clinical educators to help learners optimally take up their purposes (Cadieux & Goldszmidt, 2017). Depending on the clinical educators' own case review and feedback repertoires, they may be more, or less, prepared to provide that explicit support. Scaffolding for explicit genre understanding should involve meaningful discussion of the genres and the repertoire options available, to ensure they achieve their intended purposes. Interruptions of learners during case review, for example, need to include explicit attention to violations of genre purpose as the reason for interruption. Similarly, critiques of learners' documentation also need to explain the underlying violations.

Without explicit discussions with clinical learners about why they should modify their genres in a particular way, misinterpretation may arise. The learner may hear critique of their structural errors without understanding the underlying purpose violations those structural errors produce, and they may 'correct' their genres based on teachers' feedback in unproductive and potentially detrimental ways (Lingard & Haber, 1999; Lingard et al., 2003). For example, the explicit correction to skip the presentation of the social history during admission case review could be interpreted by learners to mean that social history data is not important, when what the feedback intends is that it is less central during admission case review than at others times (Lingard & Haber, 1999; Lingard et al., 2003). Providing explicit and robust genre feedback requires a vocabulary: in the example above, for instance, this could mean explicit attention to how the relevance of social history changes as genre purposes change (from admission case review, through progress notes and discharge summary) throughout a patient's hospital stay. While many of us have a sense of some of the possibilities available through genre for achieving our purposes, for the most part we are limited by our own experiences and a lack of vocabulary for discussing this topic. In the next section, we will review some of the empirical work that can inform both our own personal use of genre in clinical teaching settings, and the feedback we offer to our learners.

Strategies for scaffolding for progressive independence

In this section, building on the theoretical perspectives of sociomateriality and rhetorical genre theory, we explore strategies for *scaffolding for progressive independence* — here defined as 'a process of progressively independent delivery of patient care by a trainee, associate with a decreasing level of supervision by clinical teachers' (Kennedy et al., 2005). In the interest of clarity, we will try to explore these scaffolding strategies by focusing, in turn, on the characteristics of the learners, the educators and the clinical placements. In each section, however, we will attempt to highlight some of the constitutive entanglements among the three.

Clinical learners

Scaffolding is a simple educational idea, but it is complicated to enact in clinical settings. Its success relies heavily on creating an assemblage that has learners feeling that service and learning go hand in hand (Sanfey et al., 2011). When learners see their role as making up for workforce shortfalls, not surprisingly they devalue service learning. By contrast, when service learning is associated with meaningful interaction with clinical educators, it is more highly valued (Sanfey et al., 2011). Therefore, as Sholl and colleagues point out, you know there is a problem with the informal teaching in settings where formal teaching is valued more highly (Sholl et al., 2017). Observing how the work is carried out by clinical learners also provides important insights. It provides insight into the quality of the work, and it provides insight on the perception learners form of the value of the work to their learning (Cadieux & Goldszmidt, 2017). In a study of clinical documentation and patient care follow-up, those learners who approached their roles as a collaborative, patient care-related task viewed it as important for both learning and service. By contrast, those who approached the task more superficially appeared to value it less.

PRACTICAL TIP

Successful scaffolding for progressive independence involves helping learners to strive towards the right goals — in particular, to become progressively independent in their ability to meaningfully contribute to quality patient care in relation to the intra- and interprofessional team with whom they work.

Successful scaffolding for progressive independence also involves helping learners to strive towards the right goals — in particular, to become progressively independent in their ability to meaningfully contribute to quality patient care in relation to the intra- and interprofessional team with whom they work (Cadieux & Goldszmidt, 2017; Lingard, 2012). This does not mean that they do not strive towards being individually competent. Rather, it directs our attention to the potential overshoot that may arise from the current rhetoric around competence (Lingard, 2009), which may lead them to assume that they will be judged primarily based on how independent they are. According to clinical educators, the 'sweet spot' involves progressively becoming a valuable collaborator on the team (Cadieux & Goldszmidt, 2017). It also involves diligence, which teachers define as 'the extent to which trainees [learners] take a comprehensive approach to generating a problem list, pay careful attention to detail (e.g. ensuring the past medical history and medication list are accurate and up to date) and persistently pursue information that is unclear or incomplete' (Cadieux & Goldszmidt, 2017). It is therefore essential that scaffolding helps learners to recognize these nuances in clinical practice.

Table 9.1 is an example from one internal medicine inpatient clinical placement of the types of practices more and less effective clinical learners do when performing clinical documentation and patient care follow-up. Notably, these practices themselves involve entanglements. For example, doing effective follow-up care involves diligently reviewing existing documents, both electronic and paper-based, finding time to interact with other members of the interdisciplinary team, and navigating, at times, unclear genre expectations. Strategies for getting learners to strive in the right direction can involve many different modifications. Examples can include observing learners and providing feedback, modifying assessments to reflect expectations, sharing Table 9.1 with them or, given institutional differences, using Table 9.1 as a template for making institution-specific handouts. Other important strategies will be discussed in the next sections on clinical educators and clinical placements.

Clinical educators

PRACTICAL TIP

Clinical educators can play an important role not only in supporting but also undermining scaffolding for progressive independence. Any strategy for enhancing scaffolding therefore also needs to consider the entanglements that can lead to undermining it.

TABLE 9.1: Selected examples of the least-effective and the most-effective practices of clinical learners as they perform patient follow-up and documentation tasks

Situation	Least-effective practices	Most-effective practices

Reading practices	• Selective reading practices, including:
	  • the most recent progress note and laboratory values
	  • neglects notes written by nursing and other allied health providers
	• Dependent on other team members to advise on active issues to follow-up on
	• Searches for specific information requested by the team
		• Comprehensive reading practices including:
		  • admission documents
		  • notes from nursing and other allied health providers
		  • previous team progress notes
		  • overnight orders
		  • clinical documentation from previous encounters
		• Seeks out individuals to verbally discuss the patient and receive updates (nurses, allied health, senior medical resident)
		• Looks for progression, patterns and trends of issues over time
		• Screens for and anticipates potential complications and/or side-effects of current and proposed treatment
		• Reviews active issues and medications when trying to determine the cause of abnormal investigations or physical findings

Patient encounter	• Does not utilise chart review prior to seeing the patient to guide the clinical encounter • Conducts generic history and physical exam regardless of active issues or patient familiarity	• Pre-reads the patient chart and reviews new labs to identify actives issues to address at the bedside • Conducts a focused history and physical exam pertaining to active issues and patient complaints
Composing practices	• Responds to abnormal lab values without necessarily understanding/ identifying a cause • Documents physical exam findings that were not personally observed, but were previously noted • When covering a peer's patient, defers responsibility of advancing patient care until the team member returns • Does not investigate or follow-up on unclear information	• Reviews and refines active issue list • Seeks out missing or unclear information to clarify • Double-checks the accuracy of previously documented information • Independent study of the literature and review of patient cases, to address knowledge gaps before seeking assistance • Consolidates information from various sources into a comprehensive problem-based note that reflected refinement of active issues in the context of the patient's chronic problems

Continued

TABLE 9.1: Selected examples of the least-effective and the most-effective practices of clinical learners as they perform patient follow-up and documentation tasks — cont'd

Situation	Least-effective practices	Most-effective practices
Textual features	• Includes all issues into a single SOAP (subjective, objective assessment plan) note • Uses the same format for all patients regardless of clinical complexity	• Problem-based documentation with a separate SOAP or equivalent headings for each active issue • Documentation reflects progressive collaborative refinement of active issues
Informal notes	• Inconsistent approach for keeping track day to day • Takes notes on their patients only • Record information in case they are 'pimped'* by the team	• Writes key information from morning review for their own patients as well as those being cared for by other members of the team • Uses personal notes with checkboxes on patient list to keep track of completed tasks and reminders for the day • Keeps an additional set of notes on each patient they are following, listing chronic and active problems, medications, results of key investigations and other pertinent information to track progress over time

*The term 'pimped' refers to the learners' perspective that consultants or other senior team members ask them questions to catch them out or embarrass them rather than to collaborate.
Source: D. C. Cadieux & M. Goldszmidt. (2017). It's not just what you know: Junior trainees' approach to follow-up and documentation. *Medical Education, 51*(8), 812–825. doi:10.1111/medu.13286. Reprinted with permission of John Wiley & Sons

Many clinical educators combine at least three distinct but overlapping roles in relation to clinical placements: 1) direct patient care; 2) clinical supervision of clinical learners as they provide patient care; and 3) teaching (Goldszmidt et al., 2015). To carry out these roles, clinical educators combine activities that are visible (*frontstage*) to their team, such as patient care and teaching rounds, and activities that are not visible (*backstage*), such as reviewing the results of investigations in the privacy of their offices, or seeing patients on their own (Kennedy et al, 2007). While some groups of clinical educators have managed to separate the roles of patient care provider and clinical teacher, most are required to find ways to balance them (Sholl et al., 2017). By necessity, this means compromise. As part of a recent study, we identified four styles that clinical educators in internal medicine appear to use to navigate their multiple roles and the frontstage and backstage activities, and compromises that this navigation may lead to (Goldszmidt et al., 2015).

Table 9.2 describes the four identified styles. We have already described three of the four; Carl's and Yvonne's three respected clinical educators Drs D, E and M each, respectively, represented direct care, empowerment and minimalist. We did not describe the fourth style of mixed practice. As seen in the table, each style has a set of key strategies that are used to meet the multiple competing demands. Each style also represents a response to the sociomaterial realities of practice, and is predicated on a set of assumptions about clinical learners and those realities of practice. While all of the styles likely have strong proponents and clinical educators within each may be well liked by learners, they are not equal with regard to effectively scaffolding for progressive independence.

In comparing the styles, all except the minimalist style respond to the increasing demands by hospitals and healthcare systems to enhance patient safety while also maintaining patient flow within the system. Their greatest differences, therefore, are the strategies they use to carry out the work, and the assumptions that underlie them.

TABLE 9.2: Clinical educator in internal medicine style descriptions in relation to their key strategies, what they are responding to, and their underlying assumptions

Style name		Description
Minimalist	Key strategies	Using this style requires a great deal of trust in the senior clinical learners on the team. For the most part, minimalist clinical educators let the senior resident do all the patient care supervision and teaching on the team. While there is an acknowledgment that more work needs to be done when the team has a less effective senior resident, the key strategy is to grant autonomy first and see what happens.
	Response to	Unlike the other three styles, the minimalist style responds to the need to do other work while on-call for the clinical-educator role.
	Assumptions	Senior learners (typically third-year residents) are capable of running the team, and optimal learning takes place when learners are granted independence. Patient care and teaching in the inpatient setting competes with other outside activities.
Direct care	Key strategies	Using this style involves owning the role of care provider. Direct care clinical educators spend a considerable amount of time in direct patient care. This is often done backstage, making the specifics of what they are doing less visible to learners. To save time, case review typically takes place in a conference room. Teaching also takes place in the conference room. While clinical learners are given their own patients, much of the work is done or re-done by the clinical educator. Learning is by doing, but without ultimate responsibility for getting the work done.
	Response to	Rising patient volumes, increasing patient complexity, time constraints and pressures to discharge patients, large numbers of learners and the need to ensure safe and high-quality patient care.
	Assumptions	Teaching and patient care compete for time, clinical learners cannot be relied on to ensure safe and high-quality care, freeing up learners from being responsible for patient care can allow them to more safely learn by doing.
Empowerment	Key strategies	Using this style involves focusing oversight activities on empowering clinical learners to play the primary role of providing direct patient care. Concerns over team competency lead to activities where team members jointly share information about patients. Heavy emphasis is placed on clinical documentation to ensure quality of care even when the primary learner responsible for a patient is absent. Teaching and patient care are highly integrated. Case review often involves anticipation to empower clinical learners in their provision of follow-up care. While clinical educators may provide direct patient care, they take great pains to ensure that their learners know what they have done and why.
	Response to	The need to support clinical learners' progressive independence while also responding to rising patient volumes, increasing patient complexity, time constraints, and pressures to safely care for and discharge patients.
	Assumptions	Teaching and patient care can effectively be combined in meaningful ways that support patient safety and learners' progressive independence. Progressive independence can only be truly achieved when learners feel a sense of responsibility and ownership for their patients.

Continued

TABLE 9.2: Clinical educator in internal medicine style descriptions in relation to their key strategies, what they are responding to, and their underlying assumptions — cont'd

Style name		Description
Mixed practice	Key strategies	Using this style involves invoking multiple teaching strategies. Which strategy is used depends on the assessed competence of the clinical learners on the team. When time is constrained or learners are less competent, direct patient care will be provided by the clinical educator. Teaching topics are often triggered by learning gaps identified during patient care; however, they may be seen as an opportunity to touch broadly on a topic rather than to empower the team in the provision of patient care to the specific patient where the gap was identified.
	Response to	Rising patient volumes, increasing patient complexity, time constraints, and pressures to discharge patients, large numbers of learners and the need to ensure safe and high-quality patient care.
	Assumptions	Teaching and patient care compete for time, clinical learners cannot always be relied on to ensure safe and high-quality care. The clinical educator role involves assessing where learners are at, and teaching to those needs while also ensuring safe and effective patient care.

The minimalist style offers independence, but at a cost. The cost potentially includes patient safety and learner education. Notably, one of its assumptions — that clinical learners can effectively learn from unsupervised practice — is not well supported by the literature (Scallan, 2003; Sholl et al., 2017).

The direct care style — those consultants who take on more of the doing of the day-to-day clinical work — certainly models safe and effective practice, and addresses clinical learners' concerns about excessive service requirements (Sanfey et al., 2011). However, its key strategies may undermine overall team effectiveness, as clinical learners may be called on to make decisions or provide information without realising that the clinical educator has different plans in mind. By potentially taking the sense of responsibility away from the learners, the direct care style may also undermine progressive independence. This is especially true if the clinical educator uses *backstage* strategies, where the work they are doing is less visible and accessible to the team. As described by Piquette and colleagues, if the direct care provision is done frontstage, there are still strategies that can be used to scaffold for progressive independence (Piquette et al., 2015). These strategies could include thinking aloud, the delegation of subtasks such as administering the sedation prior to a procedure, or directly guiding a learner through the doing of a task. However, even with the use of these frontstage strategies, concerns over clinical learners' sense of patient ownership remain.

By contrast, the empowerment style responds to many of the same concerns with a set of strategies that appear to more consistently scaffold for both progressive independence and safe and effective patient care. For example, even when a learner might need to be talked through a task, an empowerment style consultant will start by asking the learner how they plan to approach the task, before offering any of their own suggestions.

The mixed practice style is much harder to place due to its flexibility. It likely represents a middle ground that is highly dependent on how it is carried out. Again, if backstage work is used for oversight but not direct patient care, it is more likely to support safe and effective care without undermining progressive independence.

In summary, clinical educators have many competing demands which they respond to by adopting a particular style of practice. While each style has a tacit logic behind it, learners are not consistently made aware of these logics. Furthermore, each style is not equal with regards to supporting the progressive independence of learners. Supporting clinical educators in their scaffolding efforts requires explicitly acknowledging the underlying realities of practice, and then sharing strategies for addressing those that also support progressive independence.

Characteristics of clinical placements

The materialities of practice related to clinical placements assemble to undermine or support scaffolding in multiple ways. In this section, we will focus on three examples of materials and genres that can be tinkered with in support of scaffolding: physical spaces, schedules, and oral and written genres.

PRACTICAL TIPS

There are many ways clinical educators can attend to the materialities of practice to support scaffolding.

1. Try moving some of your case review discussions out of the conference room and over to the bedside.
2. Consider whose job it is to take notes during case review, and ensure that they recognise that it is their job and that they have the right tools available (i.e. the chart).
3. Play with the genres of communication, and try to build up learners' repertoires of possibilities for the common communication challenges they face.
4. Try playing with schedules; consider who is where, when and with whom and what they are doing.

While most clinical educators have little control on the physical spaces available to them, they can attend to how scaffolding for progressive independence assembles depending on how they use those spaces. For example, if case review typically takes place in a conference room, consider moving to the bedside for review. Or review one case at a time, visiting the patient's bedside between reviews. While the numbers of learners on the team and time constraints may appear to preclude this, the assumption that it cannot be done is untrue. It does, however, require tinkering, and it does not always have to be done one way or the other.

As well, think about what materials are available during case review. Is the patient chart present or absent? Whose responsibility is it for documenting in the chart during or after review? Are they making effective notes to allow them to come back and fully capture what was decided? Each of these things can have an impact on patient care and on learning.

Consider also how physical spaces play a role in shaping backstage and frontstage clinical educator activities, and try tinkering with what is being done. Some clinical educators will spend time in their offices, away from patient care areas, using electronic medical records to place orders on their patients from afar. Instead, they could make notes of the things they are hoping the team will attend to and, during meetings with the team later in the day, confirm that the team dealt with each. Clinical learners who discover that the work is being done behind their backs have the potential to withdraw from their own responsibility. By contrast, those who know that the clinical educator is monitoring but giving them the opportunity to step up will be more likely to strive to do so.

There are many types of schedules and many ways that schedules can impact on scaffolding for progressive independence. At the macro level, rotation schedules dictate the length of time clinical learners rotate through a clinical placement. Research by Bernabeo and colleagues on rotation transitions suggests that shorter rotation lengths can contribute to an assemblage producing greater attention to efficiency than to meaningfully supporting patient care and personal development (Bernabeo et al., 2011). Similarly, micro-level scheduling — on-call schedules, daily schedules of formal teaching, informal teaching, and patient care time — can impact on the development of progressive independence (Dresselhaus et al., 1998; Guarisco et al., 1994; Mooradian et al., 2001). The greater the continuity of care, the more clinical learners can take ownership of their patients. The greater the fragmentation of continuity, the more others need to take on the role of owning care provision. Tinkering with scheduling can lead to meaningful changes from a scaffolding perspective, but will require buy-in from the many stakeholders involved.

As previously discussed, genres play a major role in scaffolding. Unless attended to explicitly, genres tend to work invisibly (Devitt, 2004). When clinical educators are aware of the key premises of genre introduced above, they can access a whole new set of scaffolding strategies. The first strategy involves expanding repertoires. This could involve tinkering with repertoire and observing the impact of different choices on scaffolding. Paying attention to the use of interruptions and the types of detours they cause is just one of many examples of what this could look like (Goldszmidt et al., 2012). Another form of tinkering with repertoires involves observing for the impact of different genre choices on engaging the whole team versus individuals on the team; ideally, effective case review leads to the whole team knowing the patient and not just the admitting learner and the clinical educator. This form of scaffolding plays itself out over days rather than in the moment. A second strategy could involve more explicit feedback to clinical learners on their own repertoires. Feedback on case presentations, for example, could teach clinical learners about the SNAPPS model:

- **S**ummarise the case;
- **N**arrow the differential;
- **A**nalyse the differential;
- **P**robe the preceptor;
- **P**lan management; and
- **S**elect an issue for self-directed learning.

The SNAPPS model has been shown to result in greater learner-driven teaching (Wolpaw et al., 2012). Similarly, feedback on clinical documentation practices can better scaffold learners in their provision of patient care (Cadieux & Goldszmidt, 2017).

In summary, attention to sociomateriality and genres offers clinical teachers a number of strategies to enhance scaffolding for progressive independence. While we have organised these strategies into three sections — clinical learners, clinical educators and clinical placements — we have also tried to emphasise how these are inexorably entangled with each other.

Case study 9.1 (continued): Bringing pedagogy to practice

Coming back to Carl and Yvonne, let us now revisit their questions and see whether we can offer them some ideas about how they can best support the scaffolding of their learners for progressive independence. To do so, we will simulate a conversation between them and one of us (Mark), a clinician with 17 years of experience working in that setting.

Carl: Which supervisory style do you use?

Mark: I always try to use an empowerment style. For me, it is the only style that consistently supports both patient care and the development of progressive independence.

Yvonne: What about the mixed practice style? In many ways, that one seems to be a better match to much of the other existing literature on teaching in the clinical setting.

Mark: First, let me say that because I favour the empowerment style my perspective may be a bit coloured. I do think that many of the identified styles can lead to good teaching. In particular, the mixed practice model seems to offer a lot of flexibility to the supervisor. However, if one of the genre purposes is scaffolding for progressive independence, the mixed practice style does not as consistently appear to work towards this. For example, when reviewing a case, there are numerous issues that arise that could be taught about; the empowerment-style clinical educator will consistently choose one that also will support the team in caring with some independence for this patient.

Carl: But what about teaching evaluations? I get the sense that learners don't always like receiving the type of feedback needed for the empowerment style to work.

Mark: That's a great question. It really draws attention to the fact that learner-based evaluations aren't sufficient for evaluating clinical teachers. While I want to be able to connect with all of my learners and have them immediately get it, I do recognise that, for some, it may take more time than the two weeks I get to work with them on team to start to appreciate what is being offered. Ideally, evaluations of our teaching should also involve evaluating our outcomes — both clinically and educationally. I suspect that there are very few institutions that are able and willing to invest in this way. However, I think that the empowerment style also involves strengthening the relationship with learners, and that is something they recognise and can legitimately assess. It also involves going more often to the patient's bedside, which many learners do appreciate. We may need to adapt our teaching evaluations to better capture such dimensions of effective clinical teaching.

Yvonne: In the chapter, you have written about sociomateriality. How would you recommend that we incorporate this into our day-to-day clinical teaching?

Mark: This is not an easy question to answer. In part, it is because what we do is heavily influenced by the institution we work at. Let me therefore start by suggesting a few diagnostic questions that you could ask of your own institutions that will attune you to sociomateriality and genre. You can begin by asking how people and materials typically assemble. In particular, focus on progressive independence and collaborative refinement. When you look at clinical learners over the course of their rotation with you and your colleagues, do they consistently demonstrate the development of progressive independence? What are the entanglements that appear to most contribute to this? Which ones undermine it? Similarly, look for how the genres and other materials of practice assemble with the people to support or undermine collaborative refinement. Next, actively work with your colleagues both intra- and interprofessionally to try to tinker with things.

For example, at my institution we moved our afternoon case review out of the conference room and into the hallways, and we changed the genre of review to better include our nursing colleagues. We now make an overhead announcement indicating which hallway we are starting rounds in. As we meet up with each nurse, we check which patients we are sharing, and discuss those ones as a group before moving on to the next nurse. While it has not solved all of our collaboration problems, it has made a very big difference. Nurses are now more privy to the plans and are able to contribute to them. When we forgot to order things we discussed on rounds, they can easily follow up. And, when we place a different order than we said we would, they more easily catch those errors. They also have an opportunity to meaningfully contribute to the developed plans — sometimes they quash ideas that are not achievable, and at other times they suggest things the physician team had not considered.

We still struggle with the number of learners that we have to round with. Some have tried splitting the team in half to do this, but the distribution of learners with patients does not easily follow where patients are geographically situated. We have, however, been working with the admission bed planners to better locate our patients geographically, so that a consistent set of nurses can look after all of our patients. This can make the difference between trying to collaborate with 6 versus 12 nurses each day. We also now have our clinical learners pre-dictate their discharge summaries; that is dictate prior to the patient leaving the hospital instead of after they have already left the hospital. This has allowed us to provide more real-time feedback that can still be acted on, and it empowers the clinical learners to do discharge education. I have found that providing feedback on one to two discharge summaries is typically all it takes for the clinical learners to be able to consistently produce first drafts that are ready to be signed.

Carl: You alluded to a few genre-related suggestions above, like the discharge summaries. Are there any other ways that you use genre to scaffold and support progressive independence?

Mark: I have several genre-related strategies that I consistently use. 1) I have handouts for how to do admission notes, progress notes and discharge summaries that are based on the best practices that we have learned work to support the genres' purposes (see Figs 9.1 and 9.2). 2) When we do case review, we always have the chart with us, regardless of whether we are in the conference room or at the bedside. And, we have someone other than the presenter making a clinical note that summarises the assessment and plan, so that there is less risk of error from the presenter trying to recall it later. We also negotiate the titles around each problem list item. This typically means coming up with creative titles that best describe our understanding of the problem and that signal to the next reader what they need to do. For example, we will title a problem 'atrial fibrillation with rapid ventricular response on warfarin with high INR' instead of just 'atrial fibrillation'. As you can see, the title itself provides the scaffolding, telling the clinical learner that they need to address the rate control and the high INR. 3) I regularly review learners' clinical notes and provide feedback on them. Typically, that feedback involves a conversation where I get them to look at the note and ask the questions: 'Let's look at the past few notes. How are they supporting collaborative refinement? Would the next person to care for this patient understand our thinking to date? Is there anything else you could do to improve on that?' 4) During evening handover to the on-call overnight team, I also explicitly ask them to show me their system for keeping track. Depending on what they use, I will often end up showing them some of the strategies we have identified that more effective clinical learners use. Regardless of what you want to call it, the strategy of having a 'to do/did list' — that is, a list to keep track of what you were supposed to report back to the team about, or what you got called to deal with that you then use to report back to the team with — is just another genre, but it is surprising how few learners get taught it. Most seem to learn it by trial and error.

Continued

Inpatient Documentation

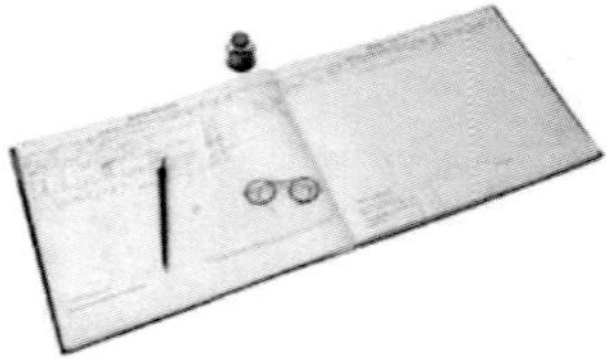

In this document, you will find the answers to many of your inpatient related documentation questions:

I. How should I write up my <u>admission</u> notes?
II. How should I write up my <u>follow-up</u> notes?
III. Special Circumstances (goals of care orders and procedure notes)

Note: Information on how to dictate a D/C summary can be found in a separate document title: *"Discharge Planning and the D/C Note"*.

Prepared by:
Mark Goldszmidt MD, PhD, FRCPC
<u>Mark.Goldszmidt@Schulich.uwo.ca</u>

Last updated Sept. 2016

II. How should I write my <u>follow-up</u> notes?

The following is meant as a guideline for deciding when to write a note and what to include in that note. You may alter the format to suit your own style as long as it contains the same type of information.

i. How often should I write a note?
- All patients do not need a full daily note. For many patients, especially those awaiting tests or with no active problems, this ends up taking up a lot of your time with little real patient benefit.

ii. Do my notes contain the right amount and type of information?
- One good trick for assessing the quality of your notes is to pretend that you don't know the patient and that you have been called to assess them for acute SOB. Can you use the most recent notes to understand what has been going on and the team's plans for this patient?

iii. The Summary note:
This format should be used for the following situations.
- Picking up a patient for the first time.
- When you have not seen them for a few days (i.e. on the Monday if you were not on call all weekend).
- Prior to the weekend when you are not on call that weekend.
- When there is a change in your patient's medical status (i.e. deterioration, new problem etc.)

Format:
Start off with a brief summary of the patients stay so far, followed by a list of the active medical problems. Then, for each active problem, do a separate SOAP style note

For example:
Mr./Mrs. _____ is a _____ y.o. who was admitted _____ days ago with _____ (chief complaint) which we have since diagnosed as _____. His/her stay has been complicated by _____.
His/her active problem list includes:
1.
2.

Re: "title for problem #1"
Subjective: This essentially is the follow-up history with regards to this problem. If the problem is CHF, it relates to orthopnea, PND, SOB, SOBOE etc.

Re: title for problem #2"
Subjective: "

Objective: This refers to your pertinent physical and investigations. It is best to combine these into one section rather than by problem

Assessment and Plan:
Again, separate these by problem title
Problem #1 Assessment: Has the diagnosis or ddx. changed? How well are we managing this problem?
Problem #1 Plan: What is the ongoing plan for this problem?

iv. Problem specific/Update note
This one is easy. Start off with a statement like. See note dated _____ for full details. Then, state the problem you will be addressing (Re: _____) with this note and use the SOAP format to write the note.

III. Special Circumstances (DNR orders and procedure notes)

i. Goals of Care Orders:
- All goals of care orders (e.g., DNR) should be reviewed with the senior resident and or attending on the team
- The type of discussion and the people involved in the discussion needs to be well documented in the chart

ii. Procedure Notes
- All procedures need to be documented in the chart
- The note should include what procedure was performed, indications for the procedure, what discussion was had with the patient and/or their family prior to the procedure (consent), who performed it, how was it performed, who supervised it and the preliminary findings.
- If the procedure was attempted unsuccessfully, this also needs to be documented.

IV. Addendum
For all of these, don't forget:
- Always sign your note.
- Always document the date and time of your note.
- Consider putting your pager number next to your signature.
- Remember the person on call...make it legible!
- Consider getting info from outside sources (i.e. call F.D. or specialists involved in patients care in the community etc.)

Figure 9.1: Front and back images of fold-up handout on inpatient documentation
These handouts support scaffolding by providing explicit guidance on the genres of clinical documentation.

I. How should I write-up an Admission Note

The following is meant as a sample only. Individual styles may vary.

I.D.: Mr. X. is a ___ y.o male who lives in London with his wife. He works as a...

Reason for Admission/chief complaint:
He was referred by ___ for ___

Active Problem List
List the most important headings on the problem list

Source:
Include if the source is not the patient or the history does not seem to be reliable

Past Medical History (this is one of the most important sections)
Use titles and then detail in subsections. For example
1. CAD:
   a. Anterior MI 1997 complicated by CHF
   b. Inferior MI 1998
   c. Triple CABG 1998: no chest pain since then or Class II angina since (see HPI). Etc.

Past Surgical History
1. ___: 1998
2. ___: 1997, complicated by ...

HPI/Active Problems
Use the headings from your active problem list
1. **Re:** ___
(these headings are not symptom based, they are Problem/System based. i.e. Re Chest pain means: discuss all relevant symptoms pertaining to this differential diagnosis; don't discuss SOB and Chest pain as separate problems unless you think that they are unrelated i.e. Angina and COPD)
-First paragraph (introduction of patient problem up until arrival to see you)
At baseline, he is ___ **(this sentence about baseline level function is very important for patients with chronic illness.)** One week PTA (prior to admission/arrival) he began to develop ___ this subsequently progressed such that ___. He finally presented to hospital ...

-**Subsequent paragraph(s)**
The rest of the HPI has two purposes:
1) Problem Solving: Demonstrate your thinking process with regards to determining the diagnosis and ruling out alternative diagnoses. This would include describing the symptoms in details and elaborating on pertinent +ve and -ve risk factors.
2) Decision Making: Once you have an idea of what is the likely diagnosis, you may need further information to help you determine how to manage the patient (i.e. Severity/prognosis, risk modification, improve symptoms (effect on function), decisions regarding further interventions (patients expectations of health care... for example if they would never consider bypass surgery, why perform an angiogram....) etc.
Note: These two processes are usually integrated together.
2. **Re:** ___
This is usually a secondary active problem which may be relevant but is not the chief complaint. It takes on its most important role with patients with multiple significant medical illnesses or in a clinic setting.

Allergies: NKDA or list each medication and indicate type of reaction, many people say they are allergic but mean intolerant of so specify.
1. Penicillin: Anaphylaxis
2. Codeine: GI upset
Meds: List with dosages etc. "See admission orders" is not acceptable since this list is often used for patient teaching on discharge.

ROS: A Review of systems should almost always be done but rarely does much of it need to be documented. The real purpose of the ROS is to be sure you have not missed something important in your history and to help you to better understand your patient.

Family History:

Current Life situation (social)
In internal medicine, this can be a crucial piece of information as it helps with discharge planning etc.

Physical Exam:

Results of Investigations

Summary:
Summarize the pertinent patient history. For example: Mr. ___ is a 65 y.o. male who presents with a history of prolonged C/P 5 days PTA with increasing SOBOE, PND and orthopnea since. He has new ECG findings consistent with a recent MI in the septal region and his CXR is consistent with CHF. His background history is significant for stable Class II angina and poorly controlled Type II DM.

Assessment and Plan:
1. Main Problem
   a. DDX #1
   b. DDX #2
   c. DDX #3
2. Secondary Problem
3. Other problems that need to be monitored such as DM etc.

Example:
1. **SOB, orthopnea and PND**
   Assessment:
   a. Worsening CHF because of medication non-compliance and anemia:
   This is the most likely because history, ...symptoms and ...physical etc.
   b. Acute MI
   This is also a reasonable possibility because
   c. Pulmonary embolism
   Although this is possible, it is less likely because...
   c. COPD exacerbation
   I think that this is unlikely because...

   Plan:
   List the main points of your plan (i.e. control CHF with IV lasix, topical nitro, consider adding ACE when stable....Echo to determine underlying etiology. If evidence of underlying ischemic cause, consider...)

2. **Hypokalemia**
   Assessment:
   a. Diuretic use
   This is the most likely because...
   b. Diarrhea
   Although this is possible, he is only having four BM per day and therefore it is not likely, it may be a contributor
   Plan: Start K replacement and send stool for C. Diff, C& S etc.

Figure 9.1., cont'd

Discharge Planning and the D/C Note

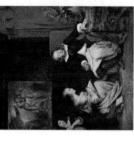

Milton dictating 'Paradise Lost to his Daughters

Discharge planning and the D/C note represent a very important aspect of inpatient care. This teaching brochure has been designed to help guide you through the process.

Prepared by:†
Mark Goldszmidt MD, MHPE, FRCPC
Mark.Goldszmidt@Schulich.uwo.ca

† Last updated Sept. 2016

Abbreviated Dictation Format

Introduction: Identify self, role, date, patient name, PIN # and their D.O.B.

Copies to: Chart, Family physician, other specialists (first and last names)

DATE OF ADMISSION:
DATE OF DISCHARGE:

I. MOST RESPONSIBLE DIAGNOSIS:

II. I.D.: Mr. Doe is a

III. ACTIVE PROBLEMS LIST:

1. _____ etc.
2.

IV. OTHER PAST MED/SURGICAL HISTORY

V. RE: "TITLE FOR ACTIVE PROBLEM #1"

(Include abbreviated HPIs, course in hospital and functional status at time of D/C for each active problem)
RE: "Title Active problem #1"
RE: "Title Active problem #2" etc.

VI. SUMMARY OF INVESTIGATIONS

VII. MEDS AT TIME D/C & ALLERGIES

VIII. RECOMMENDATIONS & FOLLOW-UP

- Dictate by problem (*I. Re Diabetes:*)
- State final opinion of what problem is
- Plans for managing problem:
  o Current/Planned therapies
  o Planned/Pending investigations
  o What patient/family have been told
  o Who will provide follow-up and what they will be doing

Also indicate
  o Disposition (nursing home, home etc.)
  o Services Arranged (home care etc.)
  o Results of Goals of care discussions

---

responsible diagnosis"). Be sure to dictate new headings for each one:

New paragraph "RE: CHF" new line …
Try to keep paragraphs relatively brief (i.e. 3-5 sentences/paragraph).

For each **Active Problem** be sure to include:

- Synopsis of original presentation including only pertinent +ves and –ves from the history, physical and investigations. **(Complete history and physical does not belong here!)**
- Course in hospital for that problem *including functional status* and pertinent *physical findings* at time of D/C. Also include results of any consultations or relevant results (labs, echo, CT, PFT etc.).
- **Note:** For 2° problems, this may be brief

VI. **Summary of Investigations (optional)**
Only include major investigations like echos, CTs etc.

VII. **Discharge Meds:**
Goal is to have one list of meds that clarifies how they have changed since admission. It should only include Prn's that they will be using at home:

1. Metoprolol 25 mg bid (↑ from 12.5 mg bid)
2. lasix 20 mg bid (↓ from 40 mg bid)
3. Plavix 75mg OD (new) …
In addition, lisinopril and celebrex were D/C'd

Note: Do not include a separate list of admission meds.
Do mention drug allergies (including the reaction type).

VIII. **Recommendations & Follow-up:**
This is the most important section so take your time here. For each problem, give it its own section and go in the same order you used above.

1. RE DM:
2. RE CHF:

For each, be sure to clarify:

☐ What the problem is:
  o Diagnosis, severity and prognosis (if relevant)

☐ Plans for managing problem:
  o Current therapies
  o Planned therapies
  o Planned/Pending investigations
  o What has been discussed with the patient/family (Goals of Care, resuming activities, lifestyle changes, monitoring issues (sugars, daily weights etc.) and prognosis (when relevant)
  o Who will provide follow-up, what they will be doing and why for example:
    "Because of the risk of hyperkalemia and worsening renal dysfunction, we have asked the family doctor to re-check electrolytes in two weeks"‡

Also be sure to indicate:
  o Disposition (nursing home etc.)
  o Services arranged (CCAC etc.)
  o Results of Goals of care discussions

Good luck and happy dictating,

[signature]

‡ For things you expect others to do, ask the transcriptionist to **"Bold that"**

Figure 9.2: Front and back images of fold-up handout on discharge notes

D/C Checklist

Discharge planning begins at the time of admission. However, if not already done, don't forget to do the following:

1. Day before D/C

☐ Contact patient's family doctor and/or pertinent specialists (if relevant).

☐ Fill out forms:

☐ Plan Scripts keeping in mind the following:

  o No change to their prior medication regimen- reconcile but do not provide new script

  o If changing doses – in the comments section indicate that this is a change from the prior dose (e.g. increased from prior dose of...)

  o Don't forget to use the **limited use codes** when required.

  o **If pre-hospitalization meds have been stopped, you will need to hand-write these onto the electronic script at the time of discharge (HUGO does not allow discontinue scripts**

  o Don't provide scripts for PRN meds unless truly indicated

☐ Discuss D/C plans with patient and/or their families.

  o What happened in hospital

  o Changes in meds

  o What to expect

  o Complications to watch for and what to do if they occur

☐ Inform/arrange for home care (CCAC) etc. when appropriate.

2. Day of D/C

☐ Do any tasks not already done.

☐ Review **scripts** with senior.

☐ Ensure that appropriate **follow-up** has been arranged and that the patient is aware of these plans. This includes the need for follow-up tests or to review pending tests.

☐ **Dictate** the D/C summary
  -Must be done **within 24 hours**

Note: Patients who have **died** also need a death! If you are on call when this occurs, and you are not just cross-covering, as a courtesy to your team mates, please dictate the summary (the charts are often difficult to track down afterwards). If not, let the team senior know the next morning so they can ensure that it gets done

Dictation

1. Prior to Dictating:

☐ Be sure that you are clear on the discharge plans for the patient (you may need to discuss these with the senior prior to dictating your note).

☐ Make a list of all the names (first* and last) of physicians who should receive a copy of this note (attending, family physician, any specialists who were involved in their care while they were in hospital or who follow them on an outpatient basis). Also include a copy to places like their nursing home.

☐ Find a quiet place to dictate

☐ Remind yourself to "speak slowly" and spell key words (esp. physician last names, drug names and doses etc.)

2. Starting your dictation

Identify self, role, date, patient name, PIN # and their D.O.B.:
  "this is John Smith PGY1 dictating for Dr. M. Goldszmidt on April 1st 2015. This is a dictation on Mr. John Doe, PIN # 1234567, DOB 05/01/69)".

Identify all physicians who should receive a copy of the D/C summary. Be sure to include their **first name/initial as well as their last name!** Also indicate:

Date of Admission:
Date of Discharge:

3. Dictation Format†

I. Most Responsible Diagnosis

II. Patient Identification
Mr. Doe is a 66 yo who was admitted from home where he lives with his wife...His active problem list includes:

III. Active Problems list
(1)CAD with CHF 2) Acute on Chronic renal failure 3) Type II DM etc.)
This is not all past medical problems, only active ones. It may include social issues such as inability to cope and complications arising in hospital etc.

IV. Past Medical/Surgical History
Include a full list of their past history. Some of these may be same titles as the active problems.

V. RE____
(A.k.a. History of Active Problems dealt with in hospital) For this series of sections, start with most important active problem (usually same as "most

* For transcription services to mail/fax it out, you need at least a first initial. If you have a fax number as well, include it in the dictation. This is especially important for out of town physicians. For these, you may even want to indicate in what city they practice

† When dictating the first heading, indicate that you wish them to put all headings in "ALL CAPS". Also, say *"new heading"* for each new section.

Figure 9.2, cont'd

Yvonne: One of the things I have been wondering about is how to stay on top of everything and use an empowerment style. I can see how tempting it would be to just use a direct care style. Certainly, it would be more efficient, which might leave more time for formal teaching.

Mark: You are right. I feel like the way I try to carry out the empowerment style does takes a lot of time, and I try not to book anything else when I am on the inpatient unit. However, I think it is time well spent. Typically, it takes me three days working with a team to get most of them functioning in support of collaborative refinement. Part of the key, I think, is being sure the clinical learners feel a sense of ownership of their patients. That means I cannot go around and do stuff for them backstage; the moment I do that, they begin to feel redundant. It is also something I need to teach the senior residents. In the first few days, it always feels more efficient to just do the work. However, the second they start to feel like they don't have to worry because you will just do it, you've lost them. Then you are stuck doing the work for the entire time you are on team. What I do instead for my backstage activities is make notes on all of the things that I have identified that I want to be sure they have attended to, like correcting the low potassium or adjusting the dose on one of the patient's medications, and then I know that during the afternoon case review I will listen for it having been done. That of course doesn't always work, and sometimes you need to go do things yourself. When that happens, I always try to the work frontstage and bring them with me, or find them and let them know what I have done.

Carl: How do you keep track of everything and stay on top of the patients? You mentioned making notes about things that you want to be sure got done during the day, like adjust meds or treating laboratory abnormalities, but what about the big picture?

Mark: From a genre perspective, there are two types of notes, formal and informal. Formal notes are the ones that go in the chart, informal notes are the ones we keep for ourselves to help us get the work done. While we have not published on this yet, what we have noticed is that everyone uses them to help stay on track. Like the other genres, there are different repertoires that people have for doing this. The one we have noticed that seems to work best is having some form of cue-card that the clinical educators keep on each of their patients. Things they write on them include a list of the patient's past medical history, the active problems list and other big-picture items like the pending echocardiogram or the temporary medications that are on hold. When I do follow-up case review, I always take out my card to be sure that we don't forget things like restarting that held drug or pulling the urinary catheter that we temporarily placed.

Yvonne: Last question. We've talked a lot about the inpatient setting. Any advice for us about case review in the ambulatory setting?

Mark: For that question, I would turn to the work done by my Australian colleague, Dr James Brown. Again, what we are looking for is progressive independence. As much as possible, I would encourage you to 'manage with' rather than 'managing for' or 'managing through'. If your clinical learners feel like the patients are theirs, they just seem to up their game. For more junior clinical learners in the ambulatory setting, you do have to sometimes 'manage for' but even then, I try to get them to go as far as they can on their own and give them feedback about what it would take to go further. Of course, it is also easier to 'manage with' when you work with the same learner more than once — another entanglement involving scheduling — a material — and social practices.

Conclusion

In this chapter, we introduced the concept of scaffolding for progressive independence. We then introduced two theories that we have found particularly powerful in providing novel insight into the complexity of scaffolding: sociomateriality and rhetorical genre theory. By introducing sociomateriality, we hope to have offered clinical educators new perspectives for viewing clinical placements and the people/material entanglements that exist within them. We also hope that by looking at what assembles from these entanglements, clinical educators will feel more empowered to tinker until the assemblages better support our dual missions of clinical education and patient care.

We also introduced rhetorical genre theory. It is our hope that a better understanding of genre will help educators to consider how they use genre, and identify strategies for being more proactive. These can include broadening and playing with their own repertoires to see which ones better support our dual purposes, and supporting their clinical learners as they develop and broaden their own repertoires.

References

Bates, J., & Ellaway, R. H. (2016). Mapping the dark matter of context: A conceptual scoping review. *Medical Education, 50*(8), 807–816. doi:10.1111/medu.13034.

Bernabeo, E. C., Holtman, M. C., Ginsburg, S., et al. (2011). Lost in transition: The experience and impact of frequent changes in the inpatient learning environment. *Academic Medicine, 86*(5), 591–598.

Billett, S. (2002). Toward a workplace pedagogy: Guidance, participation, and engagement. *Adult Education Quarterly, 53*(1), 27–43. doi:10.1177/074171302237202.

Cadieux, D. C., & Goldszmidt, M. (2017). It's not just what you know: Junior trainees' approach to follow-up and documentation. *Medical Education, 51*(8), 812–825. doi:10.1111/medu.13286.

Devitt, A. J. (2004). *Writing genres.* Carbondale: Southern Illinois University Press.

Dresselhaus, T. R., Luck, J., Wright, B. C., et al. (1998). Analyzing the time and value of housestaff inpatient work. *Journal of General Internal Medicine, 13*(8), 534–540.

Dunphy, B. C., & Dunphy, S. L. (2003). Assisted performance and zone of proximal development in surgery. *Australian Journal of Educational and Developmental Psychology, 3*, 10.

Dunphy, B. C., & Williamson, S. L. (2004). In pursuit of expertise. Toward an educational model for expertise development. *Advances in Health Sciences Education: Theory and Practice, 9*(2), 107–127.

Fenwick, T. (2014). Sociomateriality in medical practice and learning: attuning to what matters. *Medical Education, 48*(1), 44–52.

Fenwick, T. (2016). *Professional responsibility and professionalism.* London: Routledge.

Fenwick, T., Edwards, R., & Sawchuk, P. (2011). *Emerging approaches to educational research: Tracing the sociomaterial.* Abingdon: Routledge.

Franzone, J. M., Kennedy, B. C., Merritt, H., et al. (2015). Progressive independence in clinical training: Perspectives of a national, multispecialty panel of residents and fellows. *Journal of Graduate Medical Education, 7*(4), 700–704. doi:10.4300/JGME-07-04-51.

Goldszmidt, M. (2017). When I say … sociomateriality. *Medical Education, 51*(5), 465–466. doi:10.1111/medu.13149.

Goldszmidt, M., Aziz, N., & Lingard, L. (2012). Taking a detour: Positive and negative effects of supervisors' interruptions during admission case review discussions. *Academic Medicine, 87*(10), 1382–1388.

Goldszmidt, M., Dornan, T., & Lingard, L. (2014). Progressive collaborative refinement on teams: Implications for communication practices. *Medical Education, 48*(3), 301–314.

Goldszmidt, M., Faden, L., Dornan, T., et al. (2015). Attending physician variability: A model of four supervisory styles. *Academic Medicine, 90*(11), 1541–1546. doi:10.1097/acm.0000000000000735.

Gonzalo, J. D., Heist, B. S., Duffy, B. L., et al. (2014). Identifying and overcoming the barriers to bedside rounds: A multicenter qualitative study. *Academic Medicine, 89*(2), 326–334. doi:10.1097/acm.0000000000000100.

Guarisco, S., Oddone, E., & Simel, D. (1994). Time analysis of a general medicine service: Results from a random work sampling study. *Journal of General Internal Medicine, 9*(5), 272–277.

Hoffman, K. G., & Donaldson, J. F. (2004). Contextual tensions of the clinical environment and their influence on teaching and learning. *Medical Education, 38*(4), 448–454.

Kashner, T. M., Byrne, J. M., Henley, S. S., et al. (2010). Measuring progressive independence with the Resident Supervision Index: Theoretical approach. *Journal of Graduate Medical Education, 2*(1), 8–16. doi:10.4300/JGME-D-09-00083.1.

Kennedy, T. J., Lingard, L., Baker, G. R., et al. (2007). Clinical oversight: Conceptualizing the relationship between supervision and safety. *Journal of General Internal Medicine, 22*(8), 1080–1085.

Kennedy, T. J., Regehr, G., Baker, G. R., et al. (2005). Progressive independence in clinical training: A tradition worth defending? *Academic Medicine, 80*(10 Suppl.), S106–S111.

Kesselheim, J. C., & Cassel, C. K. (2013). Service: An essential component of graduate medical education. *New England Journal of Medicine, 368*(6), 500–501. doi:10.1056/NEJMp1214850.

Lave, J., & Wenger, E. (1991). *Situated learning: Legitimate peripheral participation.* Cambridge: Cambridge University Press.

Lingard, L. (2009). What we see and don't see when we look at 'competence': Notes on a god term. *Advances in Health Sciences Education: Theory and Practice, 14*(5), 625–628.

Lingard, L. (2012). Rethinking competence in the context of teamwork. In B. Hodges & L. Lingard (Eds.), *The question of competence: Reconsidering medical education in the twenty-first century* (pp. 42–69). Ithaca, NY: Cornell University Press.

Lingard, L., & Haber, R. J. (1999). What do we mean by 'relevance'? A clinical and rhetorical definition with implications for teaching and learning the case-presentation format. *Academic Medicine, 74*(10 Suppl.), S124–S127.

Lingard, L., Schryer, C., Garwood, K., et al. (2003). 'Talking the talk': School and workplace genre tension in clerkship case presentations. *Medical Education, 37*(7), 612–620.

Miller, C. (1984). Genre as social action. *Quarterly Journal of Speech, 70*, 151–167.

Mooradian, N. L., Caruso, J. W., & Kane, G. K. (2001). Increasing the time faculty spend at the bedside during teaching rounds. *Academic Medicine, 76*(2), 200.

Orlikowski, W. J. (2007). Sociomaterial practices: Exploring technology at work. *Organization Studies, 28*(9), 1435–1448. doi:10.1177/0170840607081138.

Piquette, D., Moulton, C.-A., & LeBlanc, V. R. (2015). Model of interactive clinical supervision in acute care environments. Balancing patient care and teaching. *Annals of the American Thoracic Society, 12*(4), 498–504. doi:10.1513/AnnalsATS.201412-565OC.

Ramani, S., Orlander, J. D., Strunin, L., et al. (2003). Whither bedside teaching? A focus-group study of clinical teachers. *Academic Medicine, 78*(4), 384.

Sanfey, H., Cofer, J., Hiatt, J. R., et al. (2011). Service or education: in the eye of the beholder. *Archives of Surggery*, *146*(12), 1389–1395. doi:10.1001/archsurg.2011.292.

Scallan, S. (2003). Education and the working patterns of junior doctors in the UK: A review of the literature. *Medical Education*, *37*(10), 907–912. doi:10.1046/j.1365-2923.2003.01631.x.

Schryer, C. (2011). Investigating texts in their social contexts: The promise and peril of rhetorical genre studies. In D. Starke-Meyerring, A. Pare, N. Artemeva, et al. (Eds.), *Writing in knowledge societies* (pp. 31–52). Fort Collins, CO, & Anderson, SC: WAC Clearinghouse and Parlor Press.

Schryer, C. F., Lingard, L., Spafford, M., et al. (2003). Structure and agency in medical case presentations. In C. Bazerman & D. R. Russell (Eds.), *Writing selves / writing societies: Research from activity perspectives* (pp. 62–96). Fort Collins, CO: WAC Clearinghouse.

Sholl, S., Ajjawi, R., Allbutt, H., et al. (2017). Balancing health care education and patient care in the UK workplace: A realist synthesis. *Medical Education*, *51*(8), 787–801. doi:10.1111/medu.13290.

Turner, T. L., Fielder, E., & Ward, M. A. (2016). Balancing service and education in residency training: A logical fallacy. *JAMA Pediatrics*, *170*(2), 101–102. doi:10.1001/jamapediatrics.2015.3816.

Vygotsky, L. S. (1978). *Mind in society: The development of higher psychological processes*. Cambridge, MA: Harvard University Press.

Walters, L., Greenhill, J., Richards, J., et al. (2012). Outcomes of longitudinal integrated clinical placements for students, clinicians and society. *Medical Education*, *46*(11), 1028–1041. doi:10.1111/j.1365-2923.2012.04331.x.

Wolpaw, T., Côté, L., Papp, K. K., et al. (2012). Student uncertainties drive teaching during case presentations: More so with SNAPPS. *Academic Medicine*, *87*(9), 1210–1217.

Wood, D., Bruner, J. S., & Ross, G. (1976). The role of tutoring in problem solving. *Journal of Child Psychology and Psychiatry*, *17*(2), 89–100.

10

Coaching clinical learners

Stephen Trumble

'The interesting thing about **coaching** *is that you have to trouble the comfortable, and comfort the troubled.'*

(Dr Ric Charlesworth AO, former medical practitioner, federal politician, hockey Olympian, state cricket captain, and coach of the multiple Olympic- and World Cup-winning Australian Women's Hockey team)

Introduction

As with other cities where sport has acquired the status of a religion, Melbourne's winter newspapers are filled every Monday with damning critiques of each Australian Football League team's coach. Never mind that the sport is hardly known beyond these shores, the city holds its collective breath each time one of these coaches is appointed or, more frequently, sacked. It's as if the success of the team is wholly dependent on the individual coach rather than the players.

This chapter considers a model of coaching clinical learners that is far removed from the celebrity coach of professional sport. While they have some points in common, the successful clinical coach stands quietly beside their learner and helps them to notice aspects of their performance that they want to improve. It's not about the coach; it's about the learner.

Cast your mind back to a time when you were coached. How did it feel to have someone commit to helping you to achieve your goals? Someone who, in an atmosphere of trust and respect, helped you make just a small adjustment to your technique that vastly improved your performance? That's coaching. It's not just about helping élite athletes to achieve superlative performance; it's also about there being some aspect of a clinician's everyday work that requires an external perspective in order for changes to be made that will lead to improvement.

We've all been coached. The first memory to come to mind might be from childhood, fondly remembering a patient parent running along behind your wobbling bicycle and encouraging you to pedal harder, despite your delicious terror. Or you may have played sports at high school, turning to your coach to help you improve your technique and achieve higher levels of performance on the track or field. Or you might recall incidents during secondary school, when a committed teacher made a personal connection with you and inspired you to go beyond your current level of competent work to achieve better results. The external observation and encouragement provided by coaches is welcomed in many aspects of life where we seek to improve our performance, and yet it is only recently being recognised as an effective strategy in education for the health professions. While the role of 'clinical supervisor' is well-recognised in ensuring patient safety during the learner's journey towards competence, the role of 'clinical coach' in challenging the learner to strive for improvement is less acknowledged.

Coaching for competitive success in business has become commonplace for executives. The International Coach Federation (ICF), a worldwide, not-for-profit membership organisation, defines coaching as 'partnering with clients in a thought-provoking and creative process that inspires them to maximize their personal and professional potential' (International Coach Federation, 2017a). Parallels for health professionals are clear, with shared concepts of learning partnerships, the generation of insights to performance, and a drive to be the best they can be.

The core competencies used by the ICF in credentialling coaches revolve around establishing a firm contract between coach and 'coachee', building a relationship based on trust, communicating effectively, facilitating results through increased awareness, trialling new approaches that align with the agreed plan, and continually revisiting goals for which the person being coached remains accountable (International Coach Federation, 2017b). In a 2010 review, Grant and colleagues described coaching as '… a collaborative relationship formed between coach and coachee for the purpose of attaining professional or personal development outcomes which are valued by the coachee' (Grant et al., 2010, p 126). Common to both this definition and the ICF's definition is the concept of coaching as being centred on a relationship in which the coachee retains responsibility for both setting and achieving the goals that matter to them, with the coach facilitating this process.

Coaching aligns well with clinical supervision as part of the breadth of the health educator's role. The frequently-used definition by Kilminster and colleagues of clinical supervision as 'the provision of guidance and feedback on matters of personal, professional and educational development in the context of a trainee's experience of providing safe and appropriate patient care' (Kilminster et al., 2007, p 3) appropriately places it within the context of ensuring patient safety, with the learner's striving to achieve their goals always coming second to what's best for the patient. Unlike élite sport, clinical practice is not about 'winning at all costs', and the educator-coach needs to always prioritise the quality of the patient's experience and outcomes.

Kilminster's definition also acknowledges that effective supervision addresses all aspects of the learner's development, not just a narrow area of their performance. What distinguishes the clinical educator as a coach rather than merely a supervisor is their engagement in a trusting relationship with the learner that is aimed at progression towards the best in patient outcomes, rather than just overseeing a competent performance.

While the role of the clinical educator-as-coach can be distinguished from their role as supervisor, there is a lack of clarity as to what differentiates a coach from a mentor (Bachkirova & Kauffman, 2009; Ferrar, 2004; Passmore & Gibbes, 2007). The overall intent of both, of course, is to facilitate change in the individual. Clutterbuck (2008) notes that both involve giving advice that is variably directive and aimed at assisting the learner to achieve their goals, while suggesting that coaching tends to focus on a specific aspect of performance while mentoring takes a broader view of the individual's development. Salter (2014) acknowledges that the roles frequently overlap, and that the one person may use skills from both domains. She also found that, while a shared professional background is not always central to an effective coaching relationship, a mentor is usually an experienced practitioner of the same discipline as the mentee.

Clark and colleagues (2006) describe mentoring in primary medical care as 'regular guidance and support offered by a more experienced colleague' (p 113), although this definition does not specify the interpersonal connection that usually distinguishes effective mentoring. Mentors are often portrayed in literature as caring, parental figures (in fact, the original Mentor in Homer's *Odyssey* stood in for Odysseus as a father-figure for his son, Telemachus, while Odysseus was trying to find his way home) (Homer, 2014), whereas good coaches tend to be less parentally encouraging and more outcomes-focused. Coaches don't have to be liked or admired, but they do need to be respected and trusted.

A 2015 systematic review of surgeons being coached in order to achieve better operative performance showed positive influences on their skills and attitudes, as well as some links to improved patient outcomes (Min et al., 2015). A coaching program for paediatric residents resulted in more reflection and goal-setting, and better-quality feedback (Rassbach & Blankenburg, 2017).

Surgeon and author Atul Gawande, reflecting on his own experiences of choosing to be coached in the operating theatre by a respected peer, describes the coach as one who observes and then breaks down performance into its critical individual components; who speaks with credibility, makes a personal connection and is not self-interested (Gawande 2011). He felt that while he was already a very good surgeon, he needed someone else to help him find a way to be even better.

Gawande also points out that the coach need not be as proficient in the clinical activity as the person they are coaching. Rather, their valued skills lie in their ability to create a relationship that engenders trust and a readiness to change (Augustijnen et al., 2011; Boyce et al., 2010; Dagley 2010).

This chapter presents the clinical educator in the role of coach: observing the learner's performance and providing focused feedback to assist them to achieve the goals for which they are striving. Central to the model is a personal commitment to these goals being realised that is shared by both the learner and the educator. Although the roles are interwoven, it is this commitment that perhaps best distinguishes the coach from the supervisor. By walking alongside the learner rather than standing ahead as an admirable mentor figure or pushing from behind as a task-driven supervisor, the clinical educator-coach builds a trusting, outcomes-orientated relationship that allows them to motivate and challenge the learner to achieve their personal best.

Case study 10.1 illustrates a learner-centred model of coaching in which the educator engages in active listening, goal-setting, direct observation and focused feedback, to encourage the learner to improve their performance. The structured coaching models used by the educator are explained later in the chapter.

Case study 10.1

Part 1: Cautious Chris and precious Pat

Therese has been a general practitioner in a large rural town for many years. She is a passionate teacher, and welcomes learners of all levels and health disciplines into her clinic, bearing most of the burden for teaching and supervision after her practice partner declared himself burnt-out following a succession of 'difficult trainees'. At times, Therese acknowledges that she, too, is close to burning out when she finds herself resenting the excessive time and effort that some trainees need.

Two GP registrars (medical graduates who have completed at least two years in hospital-based training following medical school) arrived in Therese's clinic yesterday for six-month placements. As she prepares for their first teaching sessions, Therese reflects that they couldn't be more different. Chris seems hesitant, lacking in confidence and reluctant to take on responsibility, whereas Pat has already been labelled by the reception staff as being brash and over-confident.

'Cautious Chris and Precious Pat,' joked Therese's colleague over their morning coffee. 'What a pair!'

Therese regarded him coolly over the rim of her cup. 'Yes, well, I don't think we should be judging them on their first day. And calling them names is bullying, in my book ... We're better than that. I'd like to see just how good they want to be, and then help them to achieve that.' Her firm bite into a buttered scone dissuaded him from further comment, and they sat in silence for a few moments while Therese reflected that prejudging the two young doctors was the best way of ensuring their failure. Still annoyed with her colleague, Therese felt her resolve harden to make a proper commitment to coaching Chris and Pat to excellence. If they're up for it.

Therese decides that she will spend the next morning observing Chris, and then she'll sit in with Pat in the afternoon. With her long experience, and as a veteran of multiple supervisor training courses, Therese has developed a range of approaches to dealing with challenging supervisory situations. In both cases, she plans to adopt a learner-centred coaching model of clinical education that's worked well for her in the past, including what she's learnt as the 'AERO' model for structuring feedback:

- **A**ffective: prompt the learner to describe how they *feel* about their performance.
- **E**ffective: ask them what they did that was most effective.
- **R**eflective: challenge them to consider their performance and what they would do differently next time.
- **O**bjective: Only then, offer objective observations as to how they can better achieve their goals.

Therese expects that each learner will need a different approach: Chris seems to lack confidence while Pat's apparent over-confidence will need tempering. At least she has a decent period of six months to work with them both; she's not expecting overnight results.

Part 2: The morning with Chris

When Chris arrived in the clinic at the beginning of the week, Therese had engaged in a discussion with him in which they established that his immediate learning goal was to improve his skills in defining and prioritising the patient's agenda. He ruefully admitted that he had felt overwhelmed in outpatient clinics by the number of problems that patients would lay out, and that he preferred his previous emergency department rotations where he could focus in on their immediate reason for presentation. He acknowledged a background awareness that he could have been a better ED registrar had he considered patients in their whole context, but he found it difficult to manage so many pieces of data presented haphazardly.

Therese sits quietly and watches Chris struggling to manage several older patients with complex presentations, and, at the end of a particularly 'messy' interaction with a patient on multiple medications, she takes him to a private room and begins the AERO model by asking him how he feels about the consultation. When Chris says that he feels awful because he knows he didn't meet all of the patient's needs, she empathises with him ('Yes, I could see that you felt frustrated'), and then brings him back to considering the task at hand by asking what he did that actually worked well. Chris seems surprised that Therese could consider that there were any points in the consultation at which he'd been effective, but he thinks for a moment and then says that at least he 'safety-netted' the patient by arranging for her to return the next day with all of her medications for review.

Therese acknowledges this as an important patient safety strategy, and then moves Chris into the reflective stage of her model, by asking him what he might do differently tomorrow. He ponders again, and then tentatively suggests that he might focus the consultation on reviewing the patient's need for each medication, rather than trying to solve the wide range of other, less urgent problems confronting her. The bagful of medications could be an anchoring point for the consultation, he suggests. Therese agrees that this would be an excellent way to proceed, and then moves to the final step by asking Chris whether he would like her views on how he could better achieve this goal. They spend a few moments discussing ways of reducing polypharmacy in older patients, and approaches to simplifying medication regimens. She feels that she has appropriately coached Chris to focus in and deliberately practise one element of his performance until he is ready to take on more. In turn, Chris feels supported, validated and able to trust Therese. As the weeks pass, he finds himself calling patients in from the waiting room with genuine pleasure and curiosity, rather than dread.

And, to Therese's satisfaction, the waiting room is always full of older patients wanting to see 'that very thorough young doctor'.

Part 3: The afternoon with Pat

By contrast, Therese's observation of Pat during the afternoon session makes her realise that they need to engage differently than she did with Chris. Pat appears to lack interest in the problems patients present, and only deals superficially with issues raised. Therese can see that using the AERO model to focus in on one observed facet of Pat's performance is not going to be much use until they both acknowledge that change is needed. Therese goes to her mental coaching playbook and decides to 'stop the play' and confront Pat. She decides to use a second model, ALECS, which requires her to:

- **A**cknowledge there's a problem that they both need to deal with.
- **L**isten actively to the learner's side of the story.
- **E**mpathise with what the learner says in order to build trust.
- **C**hallenge the learner in order to generate insight as to the need to change.
- **S**upport the learner to make the change and achieve their goals.

When Pat dismisses a mother's concern about her child's fever, Therese seizes her opportunity. She politely intervenes and provides the mother with the information and reassurance that she needs. After the patient has gone, Therese closes the door and states that she believes there is a problem with Pat's consulting style that they need to discuss: 'I'm interested in your comment to Caleb's mother that she was worrying about nothing. She looked quite upset. What made you decide that, and to express it in that way?'

Pat seems taken aback, and tries to justify the approach used as being in the best interests of the child and her 'overly anxious' mother. But Therese is resolute and continues to gently but firmly challenge Pat's assertions. She makes sure that Pat can see that she is not being judgmental, but rather is reflecting her performance back to her so that she can see that it is not as good as she appears to think. Eventually, Pat confesses that she is not entirely sure about her career path, as she had really wanted to pursue a more procedural specialty like surgery or anaesthetics, but that competition for training posts was too great.

After listening actively, Therese briefly empathises with Pat's situation ('I can see you feel disappointed with the way things have worked out'), but then challenges her again by reminding her that she is now training for general practice, and that she is not performing adequately; she will fail in her GP training if she doesn't change her approach. Not to mention the risk of doing harm to patients. Pat's cheeks flush hotly, and she opens her mouth to deliver a sharp retort; Therese returns a steady gaze.

Pat drops her eyes and says nothing. Therese senses that their coaching relationship has reached a critical point, and deliberately switches her approach from challenging Pat to offering a supportive way forward. To do this, she needs to know what Pat's internal motivations are, and how she can best use them to coach her towards a goal that has true meaning for her. In the few minutes before the next patient arrives, she extracts from Pat a vehement declaration that nothing is more important to her than getting the best clinical outcomes.

'OK,' says Therese, 'we definitely have that as a common goal. And I'm fully committed to helping you achieve the best for your patients. And for yourself. I'd like to see the next patient myself, while you observe and then give me feedback on what I do that works best in addressing the patient's agenda. We can alternate for the rest of the afternoon.'

At the end of the session, Therese can tell that Pat has been unsettled by her confrontational approach. 'Good,' she thinks to herself. 'She needed to be made a bit uncomfortable, and it was the right opportunity to give her a jolt. I'm her coach, not her friend.'

Therese decides to build their coaching relationship through another round of the ALECS model. She *acknowledges* the tension between them, and *listens* to Pat talk about how she's feeling. She *empathises* when Pat says she's upset that Therese could consider her clinical approach to be dismissive and possibly harmful. Therese then *challenges* Pat by providing clear examples of when that was exactly what happened, and offers to *support* her in changing her approach.

They talk for a while about the cultures and customs of different healthcare specialties, before agreeing that the senior clinicians whom each can identify as being excellent all use a patient-centred approach, regardless of their discipline. Pat reluctantly acknowledges that exquisite procedural skills and a caring, empathic consulting style are by no means mutually exclusive: they combine to create the best patient experience.

Therese encourages Pat to consider the positive aspects of her work as a general practitioner, and offers to support her in developing her consulting skills and deeper engagement with her patients. Over the next few weeks, through role-modelling and discussion of interesting cases, she motivates Pat to take more interest in her patients and their problems, and to be genuinely curious about the complexities they present. She also arranges for Pat to spend more time with her practice partner, who has a more procedural practice, with Pat assisting in anaesthetics, surgical procedures and obstetrics.

By actively coaching Pat to change her clinical approach with repeated episodes of feedback, Therese watches Pat develop the self-regulatory skills necessary to become a highly competent and caring practitioner. At the end of her six-month placement, Pat is firmly set on advanced training for a career in a rural area where she can practise her procedural skills while delivering holistic, compassionate care as part of a community.

Background educational theory

While Therese (the clinician in the case study) is probably unaware of the educational theories underpinning her coaching of her two learners, the approaches she used are well-aligned with best practice in clinical education. Deliberate practice, learning from experience, and balancing challenge with support are all well-recognised components of the way clinical learners become competent. By making a personal commitment to improving their performance, Therese stepped beyond a simple supervisory role and acted as a coach.

The differences between coaching, mentoring and supervising are not always distinct in the clinical context, but that doesn't really matter to clinical educators, most of whom will find themselves intuitively using elements of all three roles at different points of their interactions with learners. The goal of the clinical educator is to assist the learner to become a competent practitioner in their chosen discipline and, should the learner be suitably motivated, to move beyond basic competence to become the best they can be. Coaching is all about taking the simple process of a learner acquiring clinical competence and accelerating it. Fortunately, the theories that underpin the acquisition of clinical competence and the motivation for doing so are pleasingly accessible.

Focused reflection on experience

Informed by classical educational theorists Dewey and Piaget, Kolb's 1984 theory of experiential learning builds on earlier work by Lewin (1946) and describes learners undergoing cycles of reflecting on an experience, theorising as to what worked well (or otherwise) and why, and then experimenting with modified approaches to achieve the same or better outcome next time (Kolb, 1984). (See Fig. 10.1.)

Problems arise, however, when the learner's appraisal of their own performance from their position deep within the experience is flawed (Kruger & Dunning, 1999; Mann et al., 2011). Eva and Regehr (2008) have summarised the literature to show that we humans are hardwired to be overly optimistic about our own abilities, and that external feedback is necessary if we are to gain an accurate assessment of how we are performing. It is here (in facilitating the learner's reflective observations) that the clinical educator's role as the learner's coach becomes clear, ensuring that their reflections are based on accurate data and are free of the cognitive biases with which we protect our egos (Archer, 2010; Bok et al., 2013; Perrella, 2017).

As a supervisor, the clinician can observe the learner's performance and ensure that it is adequate. As a coach, the clinician draws the learner's attention to the areas most in need of improvement. The coach also plays a valuable role in helping the learner to identify ways of rectifying any deficiencies that they do recognise. Eva and Regehr make it clear that clinical learners may well be able to monitor their own performance and determine when they are straying beyond their safe limits, but that assessing which strategies would best improve their performance going forward is a different matter. This is where the coach is well placed to offer the learner objective support in deciding those strategies.

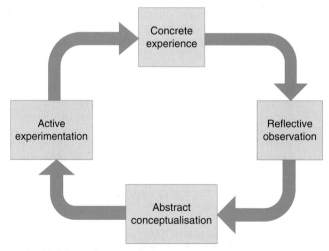

Figure 10.1: Kolb's experiential learning cycle

Source: David Kolb. Experiential Learning: Experience as the Source of Learning and Development. *2nd Edition. Upper Saddle River NJ: Pearson Education 2015*

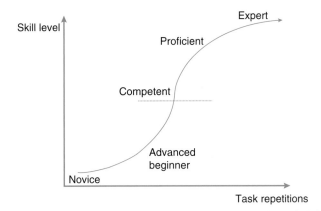

Figure 10.2: Adaptation of Dreyfus and Dreyfus's five-stage model of skills acquisition
Source: *Derived from H. L. Dreyfus & S. E. Dreyfus. (1988).* Mind over machine. *New York, NY: Free Press, pp 21–36.*

Deliberate practice

Originally derived from work with groups as diverse as pilots and chess players, Dreyfus and Dreyfus (1988) published a model of skills acquisition in adults in the 1980s that has been widely adapted to education for the health professions, most fully in nursing by Benner (1984). Benner's early adoption of the Dreyfus model met some criticism for suggesting that expertise was situationally dependent rather than being transferable between contexts, and for being unclear on the meaning of intuition and the power it carries in clinical practice (Cash, 1995; English, 1993; Hargreaves & Lane, 2001). Peña (2010) has questioned the wholesale applicability of the Dreyfus model to the acquisition of clinical problem-solving skills, noting that a rich interplay of implicit and explicit domains of knowledge continues to influence the decisions of even expert clinicians. Nevertheless, the clinical educator will recognise the progress of learners from a novice state where a task is performed with careful deliberation to that of the expert who practises much more fluidly and exercises prudent wisdom in deciding the approach to take. (See Fig. 10.2.)

The gradient of the curve in Fig. 10.2 — that is, how quickly the learner moves from being an incompetent novice to being considered competent at the task and then going on to become expert (and maybe even on to mastery) — depends on a range of intrinsic and extrinsic factors. While the learner's capabilities and motivation to improve are central, the role of the clinical supervisor is to monitor the learner's performance and assist earlier achievement of competence and hence improved patient safety. The learner will usually find their own path to competence following enough repetitions, but the supervisor acting as a coach may accelerate the process and take the learner beyond competence. This is not to suggest that the coach should drive the learner recklessly; rather, the coach ensures that the learner's rate of progress is maximised at all times by ensuring optimal learning conditions, particularly in terms of giving the learner enough support for them to venture safely beyond their comfort zone, and enough challenge to make them need to do so.

Achieving goals by balancing challenge and support

Being coached is not a cosy experience. The person being coached is really giving permission to the coach to make them uncomfortable in order to help them achieve a difficult goal.

Returning to your reflections on your own experiences of being coached, it is likely that you were more inclined to invite and respond to feedback on performance in an area in which you were internally motivated to achieve excellence. If you hated swimming and only wanted to learn enough skills not to drown, then any coach who tried to drill you in preparation for élite competition would have encountered a reluctant participant. If competitive success in the pool was an achievement to which you aspired, however, you will have welcomed your coach's relentless tweaking of your technique during countless early-morning repetitions, no matter that it required extreme effort on your part. Pushing a learner to master a task to which they have no personal commitment is less about coaching and more about pushing. No athlete is going to improve in their sport unless they are invested enough to make the effort required. Similarly, the clinical learner who seeks to improve their performance needs enough self-efficacy to feel committed to doing the necessary work, and needs skills in self-regulation of their learning so as not to depend on others for all motivation and direction (Hattie & Timperley, 2007).

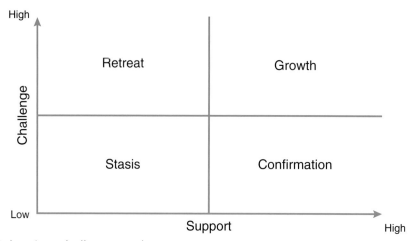

Figure 10.3: Balancing challenge and support
Source: *L. A. Daloz. (1999).* Mentor: Guiding the journey of adult learners. *San Francisco: Jossey-Bass, p 208. With permission of John Wiley & Sons.*

Committing to improved performance — and accepting the guidance of a coach in achieving it — requires a dynamic balance of several factors. In the context of being guided through potentially difficult stages of growth as a professional, this balance has been well described by Daloz (1999) as the provision of a carefully judged mix of challenge and support, while holding to a vision of where the learner wants to go. In coaching mode, the clinical educator is continually monitoring the learner's needs and adjusting their input to suit. The tentative learner needs lots of support to confirm that they are safe, before they will be open to a higher level of challenge. A clinical placement that provides too much challenge without enough support is likely to overwhelm the learner and make them retreat from the task; in the worst cases they might withdraw altogether. Conversely, there is little stimulus for development in a learner who remains in a placement that lacks challenge but in which they are given repeated supportive messages, confirming what they're already competent to do.

In Daloz's model (see Fig. 10.3), the educator dynamically and frequently adjusts their balance of support and challenge until the coaching relationship is strong enough that both can be maximised, allowing the learner not just to achieve competence in a supervised task but to grow towards their vision of best performance. As a coach, the educator cannot remain fixed in place and apply a set level of supervision. Even during a single encounter, the agile educator-coach continually monitors the learner's needs in order to deliver the right mix of challenge and support for that learner at that moment in those circumstances. To do this requires free-flowing, two-way communication between the educator-coach and their coachee, with the coach continually demonstrating that they are listening to the coachee and understanding their perspective. In other words, the coach is being empathic.

The strength of the coaching relationship — and its resilience when things get difficult — is the learner's experience of the coach's empathy (Jowett et al., 2012; Kilminster & Jolly, 2000; Subramaniam et al., 2015). The educator-coach who listens actively to their learner, and who acknowledges the personal meaning of the learner's experience, is well on the way to building a supportive, trusting relationship within which significant amounts of challenge can be deployed to drive improved performance.

The unempathic educator who attempts to adopt a coaching role by increasing the learner's level of challenge without a concomitant increase in support (both emotional and practical) or any acknowledgment of the learner's perspective may be indistinguishable from a bully. Despite a recent focus on the prevalence of bullying and harassment in healthcare (Barber, 2012; Lamberth, 2015; Ling et al., 2016; Patterson, 1999; Venkatesh et al., 2016), many clinical workplaces continue to harbour bully-supervisors who make the disingenuous claim that they are a 'tough coach', or that they are merely setting high standards for their trainees to ensure peak performance and optimal patient safety. The fact that these trainees are driven to hide their errors, not seek advice, and even to retreat from the workplace is testament to these supervisors' lack of emotional intelligence and insight to their own behaviour (Granstra, 2015; Shannon, 2015; Tingle, 2013).

Both parties to the successful coaching partnership should be aware of the 'professional intimacy' that characterises such relationships, with both acknowledging that they have gone beyond mere supervision. The empathic educator coaches by demonstrating to the learner that any discomfort they might cause by drawing attention to a gap between the learner's performance and the required standard is carefully calibrated to have maximum benefit without causing harm. If the educator has communicated their understanding of the learner's needs adequately, the learner should recognise that the educator is acting in their best interests and strive to resolve the uncomfortable dissonance between how they see themselves and the perspective their coach has shown them.

Coaching with feedback

If empathy is a vitally important skill in building a trusting relationship within which coaching can be effective, then the clinical educator's most important coaching tool to use within that trusting relationship is feedback. And as with all powerful tools, feedback will be ineffective — or even harmful — if used incorrectly (Carless et al., 2010). While they might not recognise being coached as part of their clinical careers, healthcare learners are often no strangers to receiving feedback from coaches in other parts of their lives. Watling and colleagues investigated the experiences of medical learners also being coached in music and sports, and noted that the feedback most valued by the learners was characterised by being specific, timely, actionable and credible (Watling et al., 2014).

In their seminal meta-analysis of the effects of feedback interventions on performance, Kluger and DeNisi (1996) found that more than a third of the interventions they studied actually decreased performance, particularly those that uncomfortably shifted the learner's attention to themselves rather than the task they were performing. Hattie and colleagues (1996) also identified that shifting learners' attention away from the objectives of their task and onto themselves weakened the impact of feedback. Praise and rewards were similarly ineffective. LaDonna and colleagues (2017) encourage a coaching style in which feedback is demonstrably divorced from assessment, and acknowledges that the learner's performance may be hampered by being observed. Boud and Molloy (2013) stress the importance of feedback that shows the learner a way forward to improvement. These insights help to explain why the frequently used 'sandwich' or 'hamburger' model of feedback provision is largely ineffective. Nestling the 'meat' of the feedback between two sugary buns of praise just distracts the learner from embracing constructive comments while they try to process a pair of unrelated compliments.

The challenge for the clinical educator who decides to emphasise their coaching role, therefore, is to provide feedback that focuses on the outcomes the learner is trying to achieve while not ignoring the transformational process they are going through as they develop their identity as a health professional. The delivery of quality healthcare is more than just the competent performance of a series of tasks, which is why the competencies that describe what a health professional actually does include personal and behavioural attributes rather than just clinical skills (Epstein & Hundert, 2002). The effective coach makes feedback personalised without allowing it to become personal.

Several models of feedback provision are well-described in healthcare education, and the clinical educator is free to choose the one that suits them or, better, to employ the model or mix of models that best meets the learner's needs. The most basic model is the simple feedback loop in which information about an observed performance is communicated to the learner, who then is expected to change their approach to emphasise positive aspects and to remediate deficiencies. Deeply embedded within both engineering theory and Kolb's cycle of experiential learning, this loop has been described by Boud and Molloy as 'Feedback Mark 1' (Boud & Molloy, 2013, p 701), and has been criticised for not giving the learner responsibility for regulating their own learning. Encouraging the learner to identify their own areas for improvement is inherent in most models of feedback.

Pendleton's Rules are frequently cited as a guide for providing feedback to healthcare learners. They encourage the learner to go first in describing what they did well, before the observer/s offer their positive views. The learner then states what needs improvement and the observer/s do the same (Pendleton et al., 1984). Perhaps uncharitably, we could consider that this approach is an 'open sandwich of feedback', with a 'good' message always preceding a 'bad' one. This regimented approach of first focusing on what the learner did well and then on what they need to improve still makes the conversation about the teacher's agenda rather than the learner's, albeit one in which the learner is invited to self-assess before others give their opinion. Silverman's model resembles Pendleton's but is more explicitly driven by the learner's agenda to achieve specific outcomes (Silverman et al., 1996). Common to most approaches to providing effective feedback is challenging the learner to engage with their performance by identifying the aspects on which they are most prepared to focus in order to improve their chances of achieving their goals.

Boud and Molloy describe their preferred model of 'Feedback Mark 2', which is less dependent on others to communicate information about the learner's performance. It encourages the engaged learner to actively seek insights to their performance (rather than just being told what others have observed), so that the health professional coach can engender a culture of self-regulation and agency in which the trainee has true responsibility for their learning. Implicit within this model is a gradual weaning of the coach's input as the trainee assumes this responsibility and becomes self-sufficient. This carefully judged process involves frequent conversations between the coach and coachee rather than a monologue or — worse — a diatribe that is not responsive to the learner's stage of readiness.

The clinical educator-as-coach stands ready, then, to use learner-centred, outcomes-orientated feedback skills to challenge their learners to strive for their personal best within a trusting, supportive relationship (Johnson et al., 2016). The case study demonstrates this role in action.

Bringing pedagogy to practice

Case study 10.1 (continued)

Therese finished her weekly teaching day feeling quite exhausted. Having spent the morning observing Chris and sharing the afternoon session with Pat, she felt as though she'd done three days' work in one. She took a moment before going home to write up her journal and reflect on what she had achieved. As she jotted down her thoughts, it struck her that she'd employed two quite different models of coaching with her trainees. The similarity between the two, however, was an empathic, learner-centred approach that made the trainees do most of the heavy lifting, and left her feeling satisfied with what she'd achieved and less likely to burn out as a supervisor. By helping each learner to focus on the one key element of their performance that they agreed they needed to improve (amongst multiple), she felt she'd done a good day's work.

Whether she was conscious of it or not, Therese used a number of core pedagogical strategies in her coaching of the two junior doctors. Asking questions to determine the limits of her trainees' ability and then focusing her work at that leading edge has its origins as far back as Socrates in the fifth century BC. Neither learner was likely to respond well to a clinical educator/coach who just told them what she thought rather than seeking their perspective. In both cases, Therese accompanied her learners on their journeys around Kolb's cycle, augmenting their reflections on their concrete experiences with her carefully judged, probing questions. By standing alongside them as they reviewed their performance, she was able to challenge their misinterpretations of the data, helping them to recognise what they'd done that had worked well and should be further developed, or creating dissonance between their self-assessment and what had actually happened.

Thinking back to her **AERO** model of providing feedback to Chris, Therese recognised the importance of prompting him to make an emotional connection to his work:

Affective: 'How do you *feel* about that consultation, Chris?'

She also saw that it was important for him to identify those parts of his performance that were actually achieving the purpose of the health interaction; after all, that's what he was there for:

Effective: 'So what did you do that *worked well*?'

Therese could see that there was no point in letting Chris move on to the next patient only having identified what he'd done well. But she also knew that he was most likely to work hard on issues that he identified himself:

Reflective: 'Well then, what do you think you'll *do differently* next time?'

It wasn't easy sitting back and letting Chris do all the talking when Therese had so much she wanted to say, but she knew there was no point giving him a barrage of direction before he'd completed his own reflection. And only then could she offer him her objective perspective on how to best achieve his goals (or objectives).

Objective: 'So you'll focus on reducing her polypharmacy? Sounds like a plan. Would you like to hear what *I* observed that should help you get there?'

These steps of providing feedback from the AERO model of learner-centred coaching are outlined in Table 10.1.

TABLE 10.1: The AERO model of learner-centred coaching

Step	Description	Purpose	Examples
1. **A**ffective	An **affective** question that asks the learner to consider their emotional response to their performance	The learner is required to reflect on their performance and to take responsibility for it through an emotional connection	*'How do you feel about that?'* *'How was that?'* *'Feeling OK … ?'*
2. **E**ffective	A question as to what the learner thinks they did that was **effective** in contributing to a good patient outcome	The learner is required to identify at least one aspect of their performance that was effective and so is worth building on	*'What did you do that was most effective?'* *'What worked well?'*
3. **R**eflective	A question that prompts the learner to be **reflective** in reviewing their own performance	The learner is required to analyse their performance and identify areas on which they are prepared to commit to improving	*'What might you do differently next time?'* *'What needs to change?'* *'Where should we focus?'*
4. **O**bjective	The coach seeks permission to provide their **objective** viewpoint, in order to help the learner achieve their **objectives**	The learner is required to check that they have completed their guided self-appraisal and are now ready to receive external input	*'Would you like to hear my thoughts on how to better reach your goals?'* *'I saw a couple of things we could discuss …'*

There was no question in Therese's mind that Chris's excessive caution and anxiety about making a mistake was a barrier to his development as a clinician. She found that she had to consciously take herself back along the 'Dreyfus curve of competence' to remember what it felt like when she first entered the unfiltered world of general practice as a registrar. She was able to recall the envy with which she'd watched her supervisors displaying the *phronesis* ('prudent wisdom') of the expert GP, blithely yet safely cutting corners as they followed the patient's agenda, while she'd plodded on with the laborious, algorithmic approach of the novice. Exhausting! As Chris's coach, Therese had to find the right balance for him between being supported to change his approach, while seeing compelling enough reasons to be motivated to do so.

In Pat's case, Therese had realised that she'd needed to reverse the balance between support and challenge as described by Daloz. Her first coaching task was to make Pat aware that there was a gap between her self-appraisal and the way she was truly performing. Then it was time to check in and make sure that they were working towards the same goal. There's no way Therese was going to invest her meagre time in coaching Pat if they didn't share a common vision.

Therese hadn't enjoyed having to confront Pat so directly, but it's what she'd had to do in order to give Pat insight to her situation. Reflecting on her ALECS model (see Table 10.2), Therese was glad she'd called a time-out by *acknowledging* there was a problem that she and Pat had to work on together rather than conspiring to ignore. Fortunately, by *listening* and *empathising*, she'd been able to create enough trust in the relationship that it could withstand that degree of *challenge*, and *supporting* Pat to improve her performance had given both of them a sense of progression towards their shared goal.

In each encounter with Chris and Pat after that first day, Therese had made it a routine to check in with them as to how they were feeling about their work, what they felt was going well for them and where they felt they could make improvements. Only then would she offer her objective observations as to what might help them to achieve their goals. As the term progressed, Therese was pleased that her coaching was able to become progressively more subtle. And at the end of each encounter, she always invited them to give her feedback on her performance as their supervisor. What had she done that they had found most effective in assisting them towards their goals? After all, a coach's performance is judged by the performance of those they coach.

At the farewell dinner organised by the clinic staff at the end of Chris and Pat's placements, Therese's practice partner took her aside and congratulated her on proving him wrong: both junior doctors were

TABLE 10.2: The ALECS model of relationship-centred coaching

Step	Description	Purpose	Examples
1. **A**cknowledge	A firm statement acknowledging that there is an issue that needs to be dealt with	Intentionally disruptive, this statement is intended to focus attention	'Before we go any further, there's something we need to discuss.' 'I'm not comfortable with the way that went.'
2. **L**isten	Having set the agenda for discussion, the coach now invites the learner to give their perspective first	Rather than telling the learner what they're thinking, the coach gains more by listening actively	'What do you see as the reasons for what happened?' 'I'm interested in your thoughts …'
3. **E**mpathise	The coach makes an empathic statement to show that the learner's perspective has been heard and understood (if not necessarily endorsed)	An empathic statement at this point builds trust and forms the pivot around which the coaching conversation can move to the next stage	'I can see that those things have been difficult for you.' 'I understand that nothing's as easy as it seems.' 'You've clearly got a lot on your plate …'
4. **C**hallenge	The coach clearly describes the challenges to the learner's success and the consequences of not addressing them	With the relationship established, the coach generates insight that change is needed if the learner is to achieve their goals	'The problem is that you're not on track to achieve your goals.' 'There are some changes you'll need to make if you want to succeed.'
5. **S**upport	The coach offers support to assist the learner to overcome these challenges	Having created dissonance for the learner, the coach shows the learner that they are willing and able to support them in resolving it	'… and I'm willing to do what I can to help you succeed.' 'Would you like to discuss some options?'

showing signs of becoming excellent GPs. And he remarked that she made it look so easy. After all, every time he saw her in a feedback session with either trainee, they were doing all the talking. She just sat there listening.

Shaking her head ruefully as she left the dinner, Therese reflected that nothing about the past six months had been particularly easy. Every minute that she was in 'coach mode' with her trainees had been spent analysing their needs and continually adjusting the balance of support and challenge she offered them. Confronting them on their assumptions, reassuring them on their uncertainties, always striking the right balance, her role as coach had been anything but passive.

Coaching in diverse learning and teaching contexts

Much has been made in this chapter of the importance of establishing a trusting relationship within which to coach a clinical learner. Unfortunately, the very structure of the healthcare system can make it difficult to have more than a fleeting or short-term contact with individual clinical learners. The six-month placements enjoyed by Therese in the case study, complete with paid one-to-one teaching sessions, must be the envy of many readers. Rather than retreating from supervisory roles, however, busy clinicians are encouraged to embrace coaching models that can bring about significant improvements for learners even with brief encounters.

Short-term contacts

When contacts with clinical learners are brief and infrequent, trust needs to be built rapidly. The clinician who can demonstrate that they are not only an expert at their clinical craft, but also care about the learner's progress, is likely to find themselves trusted as a supervisor and thus able to coach the learner forward. This can be achieved quite rapidly by adopting the learner-centred, genuinely interested approaches described in this chapter.

While supervisors may express frustration at not being able to observe their learners' progress over time, in some ways this model of coaching resembles the relatively brief, episodic encounters that clinicians have with their patients. Improvements can be seen even if contact is not frequent or necessarily ongoing, and this style of empathic encounter can take less time than more old-fashioned interactions.

What might distinguish the expert clinical coach in this situation from the everyday clinical supervisor is the former's realisation that dumping a year's worth of feedback on the learner in a couple of weeks is going to do more harm than good. While it is imperative to keep the patient safe, of course, and critical issues need to be dealt with first, the real coaching skill lies in deciding which two or three aspects of the learner's performance are the most easily addressed with the greatest effect. A well-targeted piece of coaching in a single afternoon — perhaps making use of models such as AERO when things are going well, or ALECS when they aren't — may well have greater consequence than multiple episodes of mute observation.

Team coaching

Another aspect of modern healthcare that can compromise coaching relationships is the sharing of roles within a clinical team. Supervisory responsibility is usually shared between a number of different clinicians within the team. In these situations, the clinical educator may consider themselves part of a coaching panel, where clear communication is necessary between members of the panel to ensure that the learner is receiving consistent messages that lead them to continual growth, rather than backtracking and revisiting old ground. Again, the parallel with patient care is obvious: no clinician would hand over a patient without adequate communication about diagnosis, current management, and future planning. In the same way, the coaching team must ensure that their learners are handed over with clearly communicated information on their observed performance and plans for the next steps.

Learners may doubt the authenticity of feedback delivered by one supervisor on behalf of another, especially when the content is challenging, so feedback on clinical performance is best delivered by the clinician who witnessed or who was responsible at the time of the learner's encounter.

A clear benefit of team coaching is the ability to recruit a 'specialist coach' to step in and focus very tightly on a specific area. Just as a pro footballer might benefit from time with a kicking coach, or a singer with a breathing expert, so the clinical learner might benefit from a session with a coach renowned for their communication skills, for example, if that is an identified area of need.

Disparate disciplines

Situations arise where the educator taking a coaching role with a clinical learner is from a different disciplinary background. Although having clinical credibility may be important in some cases, it is the educator's coaching skills that are vital in providing the learner with the framework they need to improve their performance. As in brief encounters, the coach in this situation needs to deliberately build trust with the learner early in the relationship before focusing on areas for improvement.

Remote coaching

Although modern telecommunications and social media have done much to reduce geographical isolation, a relationship-centred approach to coaching clinical learners can struggle when the learner is remote from the coach. As with any relationship, connections and feelings of trust may be stronger following at least one face-to-face meeting. At other times, regular scheduled communication sessions and a clear protocol for contact in specific circumstances can convey the degree of support necessary for a remote learner to perform safely and with growth.

The patient comes first

Students preparing for healthcare careers come to understand that their learning will always take second place to patient needs. From groups of medical students who miss tutorials because their clinical teacher was delayed in theatre to the student nurse who is moved aside by their supervisor during a tricky procedure, they have to accept that there will sometimes be times when a judgment is made to prioritise patient care over student learning.

In most situations, however, the clinician who has made the commitment to coaching their learners, rather than just supervising their work, is able to find a way to act in the patient's best interests without neglecting their students' learning. Tutorials can be rescheduled, and there are ways of intervening in a patient-care procedure that doesn't make the learner feel incompetent and rejected. Increasing the level of support available to the learner, for example, or guiding them through the more difficult parts of the procedure, is likely to encourage them to learn more than being physically pushed aside.

Coaching the learner you don't like

We don't like everybody we meet, be they colleagues, patients or other people with whom we have to interact. And yet we manage to sustain relationships with all of them, to some extent or another.

The emotional connection of a coaching relationship with a healthcare learner whom you dislike can be difficult to establish and maintain. Recognising antipathy early in the relationship, acknowledging it and talking it through is a valuable professional skill that can engender enough trust and respect for coaching even when interpersonal warmth is lacking. On other occasions, it may be necessary to agree that the relationship is not going to develop to the point where it will be robust enough to support coaching, and so agree to maintain a more orthodox supervisory relationship while seeking other people to provide coaching. An open, honest discussion about this being in the best interests of all involved is vital.

Our preconceived opinions about learners can change. Sometimes we are quick to make personal judgments based on little information or under the influence of our unconscious biases and stereotypes, including those related to race and gender.

Coaching the learner who is really in difficulty

The struggling learner warrants careful consideration as to the reasons for their poor performance. Rather than dismissing them as being incapable of performing the role, the prudent clinical supervisor goes into diagnostic mode to determine any underlying cause of impaired performance. Mental or physical health problems, dependence issues, personal pressures at home or work, and loss of motivation are all commonly encountered. Using the ALECS model can be an effective way of identifying the problem and engaging the learner in accepting coaching to help solve it.

Few things are more challenging in clinical education than working with a learner who, in the absence of any remediable factor, is inherently not suited to the healthcare career for which they are preparing. All too often, educators avoid these difficult situations and the unsuitable learner progresses through their training through a combination of ineffectual intervention and 'failure-to-fail'. While blending the coach and 'selector' roles can lead to difficulties with role ambiguity, it is vital that the clinical coach who is presented with clear, valid evidence that the learner is not fit to practise and is unable to become so, acts on this evidence by holding one or more difficult conversations with the learner. In the best of circumstances, the coach is able to present evidence that helps the failed learner gain insight to the inappropriateness of the path they are currently trying to follow. More commonly, however, the clinical coach has to draw on other aspects of their training as a healthcare professional to remain empathic yet resolute and steadfast in counselling the learner onto a different career path.

Potential directions for evaluation and research

The intense professional relationship that can develop between clinical educators and those they are training will be familiar to most of us, although they have yet to be empirically analysed. The elements of effective feedback that are the central tools within the coaching relationship have been well-described, but more work is required to demonstrate the effectiveness of coaching within real-world clinical settings.

Those who deliver professional development to clinicians on their teaching skills will be familiar with the sceptical expressions that pass across their audience members' faces when they are exhorted to spend more time coaching their learners. In the reality of busy clinical services, time spent providing feedback is seen as time away from patient care. Distilling the core elements of the coaching relationship that are believed to have the greatest effect on learning (such as commitment to goals, active listening, probing with questions, and focused feedback with specific suggestions) for deployment in the clinical workplace requires a reframing of the supervisor's role beyond mere observation. More research is needed to determine how best to integrate these components of coaching within clinical care, so that clinical learning and teaching are tuned for sustainable efficiency in the busy workplace, as well as for effectiveness and appropriateness.

PRACTICAL TIPS

Two factors are central to the success of the clinician who chooses to adopt a coaching role with a learner: the trusting relationship they create, and the way they interact within that relationship. Two practical approaches to feedback provision are suggested here that are designed to enhance trust through active listening, in much the same way that empathic clinicians interact with their patients.

The first approach is intended for day-to-day use when things are going well. It casts the coach in the role of the Socratic facilitator of learning, using questions to encourage the trainee to analyse their own performance, and to identify their own strategies for improvement to which they can commit. This AERO method (Table 10.1) draws from well-established models such as Pendleton (Pendleton et al., 1984) and Cambridge-Calgary (Silverman et al., 1996) to present a learner-centred, outcomes-orientated approach that can be deployed efficiently within the workplace. Somewhat counter-intuitively for both learners and teachers, it casts the teacher in the role of an active listener rather than the deliverer of news. It deliberately casts the clinical educator into the role of a coach who can only help their coachee to reach their goals if the coachee takes responsibility for doing the work. Not that the clinician-coach's role is in any way passive; the agility required to continually find the focal point for the learner's improvement requires a nimble mind and close attention.

A word of caution on the use of the AERO model: the prudent coach does not ask their learner 'So, how do you feel about that?' after every single observed clinical activity. Such repetitive behaviour deserves the exasperated eye-roll it will receive. A sincere enquiry into how the learner is feeling can take many forms without being stereotypical and obvious. And the question doesn't need to be asked every time.

The same prudent coach is also alert to discordances between what the learner says and what the coach has perceived. A learner who declares themselves well-satisfied with a performance that was clearly substandard, and who can see no areas for improvement, is going to need much more time spent in the 'objective' area than the learner who has good insight.

Insight, unfortunately, is not a universally-held attribute. As was seen in the case study, sometimes the coach needs to confront their learner with hard evidence of their unsatisfactory performance before they can shift to a more learner-driven approach such as AERO.

The second model (presented in Table 10.2), ALECS, is for such occasions. It is designed to be disruptive and to clear the way for a firm, trusting relationship into which appropriate measures of challenge and support can be introduced once the relationship is robust enough.

As with all models, the judicious user should adapt these suggestions to suit their personal style, that of their learners and the situations in which they find themselves. As a general structure, however, they may be useful in conducting coaching conversations that are effective and efficient.

Some brief online modules in which experienced educator-coaches give their views on clinical teaching and feedback can be undertaken through the EXCITE (Excellence in Clinical Teaching) program from the University of Melbourne (EXCITE, 2013).

Conclusion

Many clinical educators reading this chapter will have come to the conclusion that there is nothing particularly revolutionary about taking a coaching approach to the development of healthcare learners. After all, building a trusting, resilient relationship within which hard work can be done by both partners to achieve mutually-agreed goals is the essence of what we do as clinical practitioners. We accompany our patients on their healthcare journey, supporting them when necessary, while also challenging them to make the changes they need to in order to be healthy.

We don't accept minimum outcomes in healthcare; we continually encourage our patients in being as healthy as they can be. But, in both therapeutic and educational relationships, the responsibility for setting goals and providing the energy to achieve them sits best with the 'coachee'. Our role as a coach is to provide this individual with an objective yet intensely committed perspective on how they are tracking, and achievable suggestions on how to improve their trajectory.

This chapter has attempted to describe the clinical-educator-as-coach as a trusted colleague who commits to helping the learner improve their performance by stepping back and using effective feedback skills to make the learner notice what needs to change. And then assisting the learner to implement their own path to improvement. Not all clinical educators will find themselves well-suited to the coaching role, and not all learners will respond to coaching. What sets it apart from other strategies used in healthcare education, however, is that coaching is tightly centred on the needs of the individual as a developing professional. Part of this comes from a deliberate shift in the approach of the educator-coach: always framing their communication as being not what the coach wants to say, but what the learner needs to hear if they want to do better.

This chapter opened with a quotation from Australian Olympian, doctor and master coach, Dr Ric Charlesworth, who paraphrased the German humanitarian Dietrich Bonhoeffer by saying that '… the interesting thing about coaching is that you have to trouble the comfortable, and comfort the troubled'. Finding just the right mix of challenge and support to drive change entails far more listening than talking on the part of the coach, with most of the effort in identifying strengths and weaknesses being expended by the coachee. It also means that strategies for improvement are identified by the learner, meaning that they are more likely to be pursued.

Coaching is by no means a passive role, but nor is it overbearing. The effective clinical educator-coach is ever active in providing their learners with a trusted, respected and goal-orientated perspective on their performance that the learner cannot gain on their own. And maybe that is the key attribute that distinguishes the clinical coaching role from routine clinical supervision: the learner recognises that their educator-coach is neither a sour armchair critic nor a cavorting cheerleader. They are a committed, competent professional who cares about the learner doing the best job they can.

References

Archer, J. C. (2010). State of the science in health professional education: Effective feedback. *Medical Education, 44*, 101–108.

Augustijnen, M., Schnitzer, G., & Van Esbroeck, R. (2011). A model of executive coaching: A qualitative study. *International Coaching Psychology Review, 6*(2), 150–164.

Bachkirova, T., & Kauffman, C. (2009). The blind men and the elephant: Using criteria of universality and uniqueness in evaluating our attempts to define coaching. *Coaching: An International Journal of Theory, Research & Practice, 2*(2), 95–105.

Barber, C. (2012). Use of bullying as a management tool in healthcare environments. *British Journal of Nursing, 21*(5), 299–302.

Benner, P. (1984). *From novice to expert:Excellence and power in clinical nursing practice*. London: Addison-Wesley.

Bok, H. G., Teunissen, P. W., Spruijt, A., et al. (2013). Clarifying students' feedback-seeking behaviour in clinical clerkships. *Medical Education, 47*(3), 282–291.

Boud, D., & Molloy, E. (2013). Rethinking models of feedback for learning: The challenge of design.

Assessment and Evaluation in Higher Education, 38(6), 698–712. doi:10.1080/02602938.2012.691462.

Boyce, L., Jackson, R., & Neal, L. (2010). Building successful leadership coaching relationships: Examining impact of matching criteria in a leadership coaching program. *Journal of Management Development, 29*(10), 914–931.

Carless, D., Salter, D., Yang, M., et al. (2010). Developing sustainable feedback practices. *Studies in Higher Education, 36*(1), 1–13.

Cash, K. (1995). Benner and expertise in nursing: A critique. *International Journal of Nursing Studies, 32*(6), 527–534.

Clark, P., Jamieson, A., Launer, J., et al. (2006). Intending to be a supervisor, mentor or coach? Which, what for and why? *Education for Primary Care, 17*, 109–116.

Clutterbuck, D. (2008). What's happening in coaching and mentoring? And what is the difference between them? *Development and Learning in Organizations: An International Journal, 22*(4), 8–10.

Dagley, G. (2010). Exceptional executive coaches practices and attributes. *International Coaching Psychology Review, 5*(1), 63–80.

Daloz, L. A. (1999). *Mentor: Guiding the journey of adult learners*. San Francisco: Jossey-Bass.

Dreyfus, H. L., & Dreyfus, S. E. (1988). *Mind over machine*. New York, NY: Free Press.

English, I. (1993). Intuition as a function of the expert nurse: A critique of Benner's novice to expert model. *Journal of Advanced Nursing*, 18, 387–393.

Epstein, R. M., & Hundert, E. M. (2002). Defining and assessing professional competence. *Journal of the American Medical Association*, 287(2), 226–235.

Eva, K., & Regehr, G. (2008). 'I'll never play professional football' and other fallacies of self-assessment. *Journal for Continuing Education in the Health Professions*, 28, 14–19.

EXCITE (Excellence in Clinical Teaching). (2013). *University of Melbourne*. <https://edtech.le.unimelb.edu.au/login/excite/>.

Ferrar, P. (2004). Defying definition: Competences in coaching and mentoring. *International Journal of Evidence Based Coaching and Mentoring*, 2(2), 53–60.

Gawande, A. (2011). Personal best: Top athletes and singers have coaches. Should you? *The New Yorker*, 87(30).

Granstra, K. (2015). Nurse against nurse: Horizontal bullying in the nursing profession. *Journal of Healthcare Management*, 60(4), 249–257.

Grant, A. M., Passmore, J., Cavanagh, M., et al. (2010). The state of play in coaching. *International Review of Industrial and Organizational Psychology*, 25, 125–168.

Hargreaves, J., & Lane, D. (2001). Delya's story: From expert to novice, a critique of Benner's concept of context in the development of expert nursing practice. *International Journal of Nursing Studies*, 38, 389–394.

Hattie, J., & Timperley, H. (2007). The power of feedback. *Review of Educational Research*, 77, 81–112.

Hattie, J. A., Biggs, J., & Purdie, N. (1996). Effects of learning skills intervention on student learning: A meta-analysis. *Review of Research in Education*, 66, 99–136.

Hattie, J., & Timperley, H. (2007). The power of feedback. *Review of Educational Research*, 77, 81–112.

Homer (2014). *The odyssey* B. B. Powell, trans. New York: Oxford University Press.

International Coach Federation. (2017a). *How does ICF define coaching?* Retrieved from <www.coachfederation.org/about/landing.cfm?ItemNumber=844&navItemNumber=617> (Accessed 16 June 2017).

International Coach Federation (2017b). *Core competencies*. Retrieved from <www.coachfederation.org/credential/landing.cfm?ItemNumber=2206&navItemNumber=576> (Accessed 16 June 2017).

Johnson, C. E., Keating, J. L., Boud, D. J., et al. (2016). Identifying educator behaviours for high quality verbal feedback in health professions education: literature review and expert refinement. *BMC Medical Education*, 16, 96. doi:10.1186/s12909-016-0613-5.

Jowett, S., Yang, X., & Lorimer, R. (2012). The role of personality, empathy, and satisfaction with instruction within the context of the coach–athlete relationship. *International Journal of Coaching Science*, 6(2), 3–20.

Kilminster, S., Cottrell, D., Grant, J., et al. (2007). Effective educational and clinical supervision. AMEE Guide No. 27. *Medical Teacher*, 29, 2–19.

Kilminster, S. M., & Jolly, B. C. (2000). Effective supervision in clinical practice settings: A literature review. *Medical Education*, 34(10), 827–840.

Kluger, A. N., & DeNisi, A. (1996). The effects of feedback interventions on performance: A historical review, a meta-analysis, and a preliminary feedback intervention theory. *Psychological Bulletin*, 119(2), 254–284.

Kolb, D. A. (1984). *Experiential learning: Experience as the source of learning and development*. Englewood Cliffs, NJ: Prentice Hall.

Kruger, J., & Dunning, D. (1999). Unskilled and unaware of it: How difficulties in recognizing one's own incompetence lead to inflated self-assessments. *Journal of Personality and Social Psychology*, 77, 1121–1134.

LaDonna, K. A., Hatala, R., Lingard, L., et al. (2017). Staging a performance: Learners' perceptions about direct observation during residency. *Medical Education*, 51(5), 498–510. doi:10.1111/medu.13232.

Lamberth, B. (2015). Workplace bullying in healthcare: Part 1. *Radiology Management*, 37(1), 12–16.

Lewin, K. (1946). Action research and minority problems. *Journal of Social Issues*, 2, 34–46.

Ling, M., Young, C., Shepherd, H., et al. (2016). Workplace bullying in surgery. *World Journal of Surgery*, 40(11), 2560–2566.

Mann, K. V., van der Vleuten, C., Eva, K., et al. (2011). Tensions in informed self-assessment: How the desire for feedback and reticence to collect and use it can conflict. *Academic Medicine*, 86, 1120–1127.

Min, H., Morales, D. R., Orgill, D., et al. (2015). Systematic review of coaching to enhance surgeons' operative performance. *Surgery*, 158(5), 1168–1191.

Passmore, J., & Gibbes, C. (2007). The state of executive coaching research: What does the current literature tell us and what's next for coaching research? *International Coaching Psychology Review*, 2(2), 116–128.

Patterson, R. (1999). Fear and loathing in residency. *Canadian Medical Association Journal*, 161(4), 419.

Peña, A. (2010). The Dreyfus model of clinical problem-solving skills acquisition: A critical perspective. *Medical Education Online*, 15, doi:10.3402/meo.v15i0.4846.

Pendleton, D., Scofield, T., Tate, P., et al. (1984). *The consultation: an approach to learning and teaching*. Oxford: Oxford University Press.

Perrella, A. (2017). Room for improvement: Palliating the ego in feedback-resistant medical students. *Medical Teacher*, 39(5), 555–557.

Rassbach, C. E., & Blankenburg, R. (2017). A novel pediatric residency coaching program: outcomes after one year. *Academic Medicine*, July, 11. doi:10.1097/ACM.0000000000001825.

Salter, T. (2014). Mentor and coach: Disciplinary, interdisciplinary and multidisciplinary approaches. *International Journal of Evidence Based Coaching and Mentoring*, Special Issue 8, 1–8.

Shannon, S. E. (2015). Ebola, team communication and shame: But shame on whom? *American Journal of Bioethics*, 15(4), 20–25.

Silverman, J. D., Kurtz, S. M., & Draper, J. (1996). The Calgary-Cambridge approach to communication skills teaching: Agenda-led, outcome-based analysis of the consultation. *Education in General Practice*, 7, 288–299.

Subramaniam, A., Silong, A. D., Uli, J., et al. (2015). Effects of coaching supervision, mentoring supervision and abusive supervision on talent development among trainee doctors in public hospitals: Moderating role of clinical learning environment. *BMC Medical Education*, *15*, 129. doi:10.1186/s12909-015-0407-1.

Tingle, J. (2013). What NHS staff think of the NHS: 2012 survey results. *British Journal of Nursing, 22*(6), 348–349.

Venkatesh, B., Corke, C., Raper, R., et al. (2016). Prevalence of bullying, discrimination and sexual harassment among trainees and Fellows of the College of Intensive Care Medicine of Australia and New Zealand. *Critical Care and Resuscitation, 18*(4), 230–234.

Watling, C., Driessen, E., van der Vleuten, C. P. M., et al. (2014). Learning culture and feedback: An international study of medical athletes and musicians. *Medical Education, 48*(7), 713–723.

11

Translating expert practice for clinical learning

Clare Delany and David Beckett

Introduction

In 2002, Grant Gillett described/discovered the 'land of clinicum'. Gillett (2002) suggested that when people enter this land (of healthcare institutions), they become patients and are required to fit in with 'clinicum's' routines and customs (e.g. attention to cleanliness; constant health monitoring and testing; roving teams of clinicians who visit the bedside early in the morning; rotating clinicians and 'chiefs' who determine when a patient can leave clinicum). In this chapter we extend Gillett's metaphor about the experience of entering the land of clinicum, by expanding its population to include novice clinicians, trainees or students, all of whom are required to learn its customs, and pass assessments to become accepted into a particular tribe within this clinical land. We think that a novice learner's experience when they first enter clinical placements as novice students, or when they transition from one placement to another, aligns with the bewilderment a patient feels when they first enter the 'land of clinicum'.

Although students and trainees enter clinicum armed with vast amounts of clinical knowledge, they often struggle to absorb the customs and to grasp the expertise required to integrate and contribute as a member. Clinical educators are one group of inhabitants of clinicum, and they are responsible for guiding these students and trainees. However, as the chapters in this book have highlighted, they, too, find it challenging to explain and translate the type of knowledge and skills required or the 'know-how' of clinicum's clinician inhabitants. For students, attaining expertise in a given clinical disciplinary area is perceived by them as an individual endeavour. Students are awarded individual marks for written and oral examinations and for their performance of procedural skills. Yet the notion of 'professional expertise' is increasingly understood through its manifestation in relationships. There are three kinds of foundational concepts that, taken together, construct expertise. First, even in an individual practitioner (such as a nurse), the expertise is *extended* beyond cognitive knowledge, to include the affective (feelings, for example), and both these contribute to the nurse's professional judgments (Menary & Kirchhoff, 2014). Second, expertise is apparent in how the nurse's workplace functions; that is, it is *distributed* across the learner, the teacher, the learning and practice environment (Williamson & Cox, 2014), and within the explicit and implicit cognitive patterns of practice (Roepstorff, Niewöhner, & Beck, 2010). Third, for everyone in a practice environment, such as a ward or a theatre in a hospital, expertise is *embodied* — arising from technical skills, perceptions, understandings, prior experiences and reactions to people and working situations (Dreyfus & Dreyfus, 2005). These three kinds of concepts and relationships between people and between knowledge, emotions and learning environments, are exemplified in common clinical experiences such as antenatal and maternity wards, where groups of professionals engage new parents; in surgery, where medical teams cluster around the operating table; and in aged care facilities, where chronic health conditions need to be case-managed often for years on end, by evolving small groups of clinical experts.

Accordingly, locating and translating expertise within *webs of relationships* has profound implications for clinical educators in their role of guiding students to learn and practise their health professional work within multidisciplinary teams and dynamic and complex clinical contexts.

In this chapter, we first present excerpts of published and unpublished data from a project examining the experiences of working within a large paediatric public hospital — which can be regarded as a form of clinicum. The data illuminates the types of cognitive, procedural and relational capacities (Winch, 2014) required to negotiate and contribute within a multidisciplinary healthcare context. We then use these insights into professional expertise 'in action', to highlight the task for clinical educators of translating this knowledge and expert know-how so that novices can gain access to and move — in Lave and Wenger's (1991) terms — from the periphery of practice towards more meaningful participation and membership of the clinical community within clinicum.

The underpinning premise of this chapter is that developing practical expertise and know-how in a health professional disciplinary domain is more complex — but more fruitful — than attaining mere competence in procedural skills and in disciplinary-specific clinical reasoning. As our examples above suggest, developing expertise for clinical practice is a rich and highly relational notion that requires a learner not only to think and act independently, and to self-regulate and monitor the impact of their practice on others, but also to move beyond these individual cognitive-based learning processes into building relationships and collaborating with colleagues from different disciplines. In short, one's own sense of agency becomes, ideally, a *collaborative sense of agency*. Winch (2014) describes these notions of practice as a type of occupational capacity, requiring similar holistic agency to project management:

> *Project management becomes more of a unified form of agency to the extent that the project is complex, has a relatively defined and recognised goal, encompasses a wide range of operations and involves freedom from direct managerial control. When the latter two conditions are present, the ability to manage a project becomes a central component of occupational capacity.*

Importantly, if practice novices are required to learn these complex and multidimensional facets of expertise for fully professional work, then educators must also develop an understanding of how they can guide learners on this pathway. This includes assisting them to see the journey towards such an 'occupational capacity' (or what we can call experts' know-how) as an ongoing commitment over the course of their careers. Accordingly, we suggest that the critical pedagogical task of the clinical educator is one of *translation* (Chen, 2016), but not via a technical or mechanical explanation, or the mere transfer of knowledge about skills and techniques. Rather, following Chen (2016), we see translation as creatively opening up spaces for practice-based dialogue and exploration. Starting with close and explicit attention to cases and situations that arise in the daily 'doing' of practice on the ward, in surgery, and in the aged care facility can invite novice practitioners to develop a critical awareness and understanding of their agency (the skills, behaviours and relationships) that contributes to professional practices for all they collaborate with, in the workplace they share. This is not esoteric activity. Talking through what needs to be done, why it should be done, what would be better to do and how a different outcome could be achieved (next time) are simple and sensible conversations in any workplace amongst colleagues. This is, we claim, how expertise is constructed. It is, in this book, how clinical learning and, eventually, professional identity, is established.

The clinical teaching methods which flow from this pedagogical basis should lead a novice to test and discover for themselves how well they can plan, coordinate, work with others and manage the 'project' of what has been termed *sustained professional learning* (Boud & Falchikov, 2006). These conceptions of clinical learning and teaching approaches align more broadly with ideals of higher education, where the role of the educator is to provide the educational space in which dispositions of critical thinking can flourish (Barnett, 2015).

In this chapter, we will illuminate practice-based approaches to facilitating learning to achieve these goals, by addressing four main questions:

1. What are some typical examples of situations where complex professional expertise is required but is hard for students to access? *(case study 11.1)*
2. How does professional expertise manifest in clinical workplaces? *(empirical data from the land of clinicum)*
3. What pedagogical concepts support the development of this type of expertise? *(a section about theory)*
4. What clinically-based teaching approaches flow from this pedagogy of health professional expertise? *(a return to case study 11.1)*

Case study 11.1: Carl and two supervisors

Carl is in the first week of his first-year intern placement in the emergency department.

One supervisor takes a sequential teaching approach, and limits Carl's involvement to first interviewing patients only, and then consulting him as to what should be the next step ... Carl feels frustrated and useless, and worries that if he had to suddenly step up he wouldn't know what to do. He watches and listens to other doctors to try to pick up some key elements.

In the second week, Carl has a new supervisor who gives him a patient list and expects him to manage the whole load. Carl is overwhelmed with this responsibility, and feels under-prepared and worries he might miss something.

How does professional expertise manifest in clinical workplaces?

To illustrate how clinical expertise manifests in everyday clinical practice, we present a series of quotations derived from semi-structured interviews examining allied health practitioners' experiences of working within a public hospital environment (Breckenridge et al., 2012). We have claimed in this chapter from the outset that health professional expertise requires more than atomistic and disciplinary-bounded knowledge. Framed as a type of project management activity, health practice requires a broader set of capacities and dispositions, shaped by ordinary and often messy experiences, where personalities, hierarchies and established work patterns are at play. It is substantial relational work — *extended, distributed and embodied* — as we set out in the introduction to this chapter.

The examples presented below, drill down to the everyday relational work of allied health practice in the context of a large tertiary paediatric teaching hospital in Melbourne, Australia. The original goal of the project was to document the ethical dimensions of the everyday experiences of rehabilitation professionals working in a paediatric setting, in both rehabilitation and acute clinical contexts. In paediatric health settings, there has been comparatively little research into the concerns and experiences of members of the paediatric rehabilitation team, particularly about how individual professionals negotiate their role within broader health teams (Clark et al., 2007; Irvine et al., 2002), and how the interprofessional team as a whole make decisions about the best interests and management plan for a child within their family context (Kenny & Adamson, 1992). The focus on the daily ethical challenges encountered by rehabilitation professionals working in multidisciplinary teams in paediatric practice was purposefully chosen for this study, as a counter to the large body of bioethical literature in paediatric healthcare that has analysed doctors' experiences and challenges of high-stakes decision-making, such as withdrawal of care (Burns et al., 2001; Durall et al., 2012). Ethics approval for this project was provided in 2009 by the hospital human research ethics committee (Ref. no. 29082 D). Findings from the research have been separately published in four papers (Delany & Conwell, 2012; Delany & Galvin, 2014; Delany et al., 2010; Delany et al., 2017).

In the following quotations, consider the significance of the conversations reported by the individual clinical practitioners to the construction of expertise. We claim that these show how extended, distributed and embodied 'expertise' really is — that is, beyond the expertise that already resides in the individual clinician —and that the individual clinician is better, because of this!

In quotation (1), an educational play therapist describes how she negotiates her practice to distract a child undergoing medical resonance imaging. Her description of working closely with other clinicians in the room, and monitoring exactly when she is needed, is a good example of a team (all of whom bring different skills), working synchronously and harmoniously with the shared goal of supporting the child:

(1) *In medical imaging, I know when to step in because they'll look at me and give me a nod of 'we need you now', or I know by their actions that they don't need me at all, they're handling the situation really well, so I just step back. It's about that 'give and take', that you don't own what you do as a play therapist. You want to be able to give those skills across to other colleagues so that when you're not there, they're utilising it, and I think you need to respect it enough that if something is going well, you don't need to jump in. (play therapist) (Delany & Conwell, 2012, p 143)*

In quotation (2), a social worker distinguishes between her focus on the social dimensions of care and the clinician's focus on the clinical aspects. The comment also illustrates her awareness of the impact of authority and hierarchy within the peer relationship, and she expresses some caution about attempting to change the clinical mindset of the doctor:

(2) *It's the [physicians'] assessment in the end, it's whether I guess we can influence them in trying to balance up social and medical … So yeah, we have social workers listening to them [families] about the way things are, but I don't feel confident pushing a [physician] to do something they don't feel completely happy about … (social worker, oncology) (Delany et al., 2017, pp 507–508).*

In quotations (3) and (4), below, two different social workers move from a pragmatic acknowledgment of the limits of knowledge and influence apparent in quote (2), to a recognition of the need to push for a different explanation from the doctor (quote 3); and the need to deepen and add background context to a nurse's understanding about a family (quote 4).

(3) *I remember a doctor suggesting to the mother that, 'I think your baby needs a nasogastric tube because he's not gaining weight'. But from my experience, like I know you need to give a basic explanation and I know you can't predict how long it is, but actually it's far more invasive and involved in the long term than what [the doctor] was suggesting, and this makes me feel uncomfortable that I have this knowledge that the parent doesn't have, so I try to, again, talk to the doctor and sort of change their thinking, or get them to see that this is actually quite a big deal for the family and they might need more explanation. (general medicine) (Delany et al., 2017, p 507)*

(4) *The social work role is to sometimes to give context. I remember a nurse said 'oh this mum, she never feeds her baby', and I said 'well, she actually had quite a traumatic birth of the child … she's not confident, she really worried he's going to choke. So she's not feeding him. She's too scared … Once I give that context, [the nurse seemed to understand more]. (Delany et al., 2017, p 508)*

In the following series of previously unpublished quotes from the same study, physiotherapist participants describe their experiences of working within interprofessional teams. In quote (5), the therapist expresses frustration that her skills are sometimes not recognised or used as effectively as they could be within the team. In quote (6), the therapist exemplifies our main claim of 'relational expertise', when she highlights the importance of developing relationships (*extended* and *distributed*) with colleagues, and, in quote (7), the importance of being physically present (*embodied*) within the team is emphasised.

(5) *We don't have the autonomy to make that decision at the bedside. A lot of that would be dependent on the nurse [who] is looking after the child. […] It happens in other areas, but to some degree we don't know what's not referred. We only find out further down the track when you finally get referred the kid and think I would have been of real help had I known about this kid earlier on. Or you get the opposite, where people refer patients to you [who] really don't need physiotherapy. (Int 8)*

(6) *I think definitely some teams have more of a respect in your opinion than others, and it depends on those relationships I suppose that you build, but then, other times … I find doctors to be very strong personalities. (Int 6)*

(7) *(We would have a weekly meeting), then as a team we would be able to make the decision as to what the plan would be, and I found that incredibly useful and supportive to guide my treatment, and how hard I should be pushing, because you just don't know. (Int 1)*

A recurring theme from the physiotherapy interviews was the need to be included and be present when team meetings occur, because it was in the formal and informal meetings where the real decisions and discussions occurred. The formal systems of documentation may not reveal what is actually going on or being considered (quotes 8 and 9). In quote (10), the therapist also emphasises the importance of developing a strong sense of one's disciplinary role and expertise to effectively join and be accepted within these multidisciplinary teams:

(8) *When I started the job I was like 'Oh, I'm not getting any referrals' and stuff like that. They told me it's all about referral systems, so I'd then have to go up and scan the list. They refer some things, but then I'd scan the list for what I think we can help with. So it's also making sure that we don't miss anything in relation to that. (Int 6)*

(9) *It would never be documented, and I think that's why team meetings are really important and you get to know who's who. In a ward environment you are often running in and out of a patient's room, and the doctor wouldn't know me from a bar of soap a lot of the time. … I think our area is one that's really fragmented. (Int 8)*

(10) *Yes (you need to have a strong sense of your own role) and everyone else's and perspective, which can be hard, because communication and doctors, you can read through their notes and have no idea what's happening with a patient. I had a patient like that semi-recently, and in the notes you could tell things were changing and they were trying different treatments, but there wasn't anything documented. But really, what had happened in the space of a couple of weeks was that she had been made palliative, but it wasn't actually documented anywhere. So you really have to go to the meetings and listen, and if you don't go to the meetings you actually don't know what is happening. (Int 4)*

These quotes show how physiotherapy practitioners move between, on the one hand, describing and justifying their own individual professional expertise, and on the other, recognising the need to integrate their knowledge and practice with other colleagues and to strategically position themselves within the team processes. At several points, the data shows how richer their practices became when they were able to work collaboratively with others, and at other points, the data suggests they struggled to contribute when they were not included within team processes and decisions. The quotes also highlight that teams of clinicians working together represent a type of complex system where the impact of each person's input cannot be linearly combined (Lancaster, 2012). Instead, the goals and outcomes emerge from the relationships between members of the group.

This is not particular to medical and allied health professionals. Right across the spectrum of adults' workplaces, the momentum for improving practice is not merely individualistic, but increasingly collaborative. Groups of between 2 and about 12 practitioners who share a single workplace can be regarded as a site of expertise. Moreover, such a site can readily *grow* expertise. People learn powerfully amongst each other, where there are strong local emotional and social bonds, and where there is a joint commitment to a shared outcome. This was particularly apparent in quotation (1). Project management is one common form of this type of work (as Winch has pointed out), with banking, schooling, governments, and even families providing familiar and ubiquitous examples of the ways small groups form and re-form to get important work done well.

Note that what we may call 'co-present' groups (Hager & Beckett, in press; Lancaster, 2012) are glued together not by disciplinary knowledge (such as typically provided by medical and allied health degrees), but instead by shared processes and goals and by relationships within the group.

From a pedagogical perspective, and recognising that the opportunity to work with others represents a point of entry to professional formation, we suggest that the trajectory from novice to expert occurs best when students are given some guidance about how to integrate their individual professional knowledge with the combined work of the interprofessional group. To use Winch's term, there is an *occupational capacity*, which flourishes when collaboration is apparent. We have claimed from the outset of this chapter that expertise is relational in three interwoven ways, and that understanding this aspect of expertise should be a key purpose of relevant professional pedagogies. In the next section we dicuss how educators might orient their practice towards facilitating learning to achieve this educational goal.

Pedagogical concepts for professional expertise

Based on notions of professional expertise emerging from collaborative relationships in the workplace, two key questions arise for clinical educators:

1. What is the essential translation work for educators to introduce students to 'co-present' groups within their organisations and institutions?
2. How can educators explicitly draw from the interactional component of co-present groups (i.e. groups of clinicians) working within clinical settings?

Chen (2016) suggests that educators should consider moving beyond the traditional conveyor belt of introducing students to specific and procedurally-based skills, and instead move to thinking about teaching as a process of facilitating learning to open up a space for identifying and moving between disciplinary boundaries. This changes to the role of the educator from presenting what needs to be known to guiding the learner to better understand the enterprise of learning and practice through signposting and illuminating expertise as a form of interprofessional collaboration. In short, we advocate a pedagogy for *translating expert practice for clinical learning*. Our pedagogy is based on the nature of learning and practice being grounded in collaborations between people and co-present groups, and the consequent need to provide signposts, information and space for translation work to occur. Educational theories relevant for these pedagogical purposes are:

- *Situated learning* (Lave & Wenger, 1991), where learners are actively supported to move into the centre of system-related knowledge and practice where interprofessional team work occurs.

- *Translational learning and teaching* (Chen, 2016), where educators signpost and open up spaces for noticing and discussing key features of the workplace, including the interests, values, intentions, emotions and understandings of individual colleagues and of groups or teams of practitioners.

- *Critical reflection* (Schön, 1987), where students are encouraged to reflect and make sense of their own contribtuions so that they can recognise the whole 'project' (Winch, 2014) of professional expertise.

Teaching concepts which flow from this pedagogical understanding mean understanding expertise as an emergent phenomenon that is constructed between people who share working together (see McGivern, 2014, pp 693–695); expecting clinical practice to be affectively and constructively melded by disciplinary and interdisciplinary relations, and seeing professional independence and agency as partly attributable to and dependant on the collaborative understandings and actions of groups.

These concepts give rise to specific types of practical and translational roles of the clinical educator:

- to create a space and environment that allows the novice or newcomer to draw on their own experiences and knowledge, not only to promote their individual professional agency but to identify how their perspective and understanding might influence and be influenced by others in the workplace;

- to focus beyond the learning of individual procedures to situating disciplinary-based learning within the collaborative project of disciplinary practice.

Clinical education methods for professional expertise

In case study 11.1, Carl's experiences with his supervisors represent two commonly used approaches for supporting a student to access practice knowledge. The first approach focuses on what might be termed a 'shallow-end' or 'sequential supervisory' approach, where students are given incremental learning tasks to gradually introduce them to the practice tasks.

Shallow-end or sequential learning is based on conceptions of:

- the significance of *cognition* as the primary focus of learning (which may suit the acquisition of theory, but does little to engage the messiness of practice);

- *linearity* as the trajectory from novice to expert (which may suit the acquisition of behavioural and procedural skills, but does little to develop higher-order capacities, such as insight into the dynamics of team processes and decision-making);

- the *sole practitioner* as the source of professional agency (which may suit some clinical decisions, but does little to engage the collaborative agency now a part of most workplaces).

Sequential learning is a very common approach to facilitating learning, and it has its place, in particular, for learning specific procedural skills, and it allows the educator to control the learner's engagement with the patient. The disadvantages are that it is a fragmented approach, and it separates cognition about a task from the doing of a task — splits the thinking from the action. This is a disadvantage, because it diminishes the agency of the learner — it means they rely on the teacher to set tasks. They don't have to plan, coordinate or work in with others.

The second approach can be construed, in contrast, as a 'deep-end' approach, which (in the context of learning to swim) involves an immersive, whole-body experience where 'jumping in' dramatically heightens the sensation of being within and surrounded by water, and which has the effect of forcing the learner to work out how to stay afloat. Facilitating learning from a deep-end perspective requires learning to be provoked through collaborative experience, and the onus is shifted to the learner to self-regulate their response and adjust (in this case for survival). By contrast, the shallow-end approach involves gradual immersion, where the essential skills for staying afloat are developed in a sequential way. The shallow-end learner is somewhat more dependent on the teacher to set the skills agenda, and their agency to prepare, plan and coordinate is restricted to their individual performance.

For the deep-end approach to be effective rather than frightening or unsafe, it requires prior planning and supports to be in place, and ideally the novice swimmer is provided with information and preparation about the goals of the experience and the supports available.

Both the deep- and shallow-end approaches represented by Carl's contrasting supervisory experiences, and his reactions to the supervisor responses, highlight the need to better understand and incorporate collaborative and co-present groups within clinical education.

We therefore argue for a more supported version of the deep-end approach, where explicit attention is given to translating the collaborative and relational work of clinical practice. Teaching approaches that focus on translating practice will focus on explaining the meaning of work within its context. The aim becomes one of illuminating everyday work contexts and professional tasks, which can appear to be opaque and inaccessible to newcomers or novices, by opening up space for conversations which not only provide information but intentionally privileges the novice's values, previous experiences and understanding, and which supports them to recognise the gap or zone between their knowledge and understanding and the more nuanced or complex understanding required to contribute to professional practice.

An example of this teaching as a 'translation of meaning' approach can be found in a the context of supporting international medical graduates (IMGs), who usually begin their clinical practice while very unfamiliar with the new country's health context. The program of teaching as a form of facilitating learning, which was developed to guide these doctors (Harris & Delany, 2013), involved forming critical reflection groups that came together in a program of monthly lunchtime discussion sessions. Although the context was an informal lunchtime meeting, a specific order of discussion was purposefully designed. The first step was to identify and acknowledge the expertise IMG doctors already bring from their previous country of work. The second involved orienting the doctors to the features of their particular land of 'clinicum' enabling them to 'see' — understand and notice particular and salient features of the workplace dynamic (relationships, context, the way things are done). In the IMG program this was done by inviting in a specialist or expert clinician to highlight how things are done in the particular hospital setting, and who was responsible for delivery of their specialised tasks (e.g. a pharmacist, a person from the medical records department, an allied health professional from the rehabilitation unit). The third step was to provide time for the IMG doctors to discuss differences between their prior understanding and experience and what they now see is required to function within the particular hospital context. The specific and practical steps of the lunchtime tutorial for IMGs were:

1. Begin by asking doctors/trainees/students to describe their experiences of, and understanding of, a particular aspect of a 'new' or 'unfamiliar' clinical practice or clinical knowledge area.
2. Discuss how this aspect of clinical practice is undertaken in the specific hospital, or invite a clinician/staff member to discuss how the procedure is done or how the system/team works.
3. Invite the doctors/trainees/students to identify key features of the 'new system' and how it differs from their previous work/knowledge, and discuss, and then problem-solve for themselves what they will need to do, or who they will need to talk with, to adjust their practice.

These steps are examples of the translational work of designing learning and teaching sessions to assist students to zoom in on their own understanding and experience of a particular area of practice, and then, via the information about how that type of clinical practice operates within the team and the systems of the local workplace, to zoom out to see the bigger picture — context, relationships, communication patterns and systems of work (Kanter, 2011).

PRACTICAL TIPS

The steps outlined above can be used in a variety of learning events within clinical placements. They comprise:

1. focusing on what a student knows and/or is unsure of;
2. orientating the student to the environment, relationships, expectations and the 'way things are done' in the particular clinical context;
3. providing opportunities for the student to identify what they need to do to bridge their gap between their current knowledge and understanding, and their capacity to work with others in the specific placement.

Conclusion

Earlier in this chapter, we highlighted three fundamental concepts and relationships that, taken together, construct professional expertise. First, the idea of expertise being a type of *extended* 'know-how' beyond cognitive knowledge, to include the affective; second, that expertise is both *distributed* across the learner, the teacher, and the learning and practice environment, and is *implicit* within cognitive patterns of practice; and third, that expertise is *embodied* — it arises from technical skills, perceptions, understandings, prior experiences and reactions to people and working situations. These relationships and patterns of practice represent the structure of the 'real' clinical curriculum. They pave the way for a new education research agenda that not only seeks to use theory to frame and explain how clinical learning occurs, influenced by contexts, specific workplace affordances and embedded within communities of practice, but also seeks to describe and understand practice-based decisions, judgments, relationships and teamwork, to directly inform approaches to learning and teaching and curricula content.

This chapter has highlighted the need for educators to consider disciplinary cognition, understanding and reasoning as situated and embodied in the project of professional practice (Winch, 2014). We have suggested that assisting students to access and contribute within clinical workplaces requires a type of translational work. Chen (2016) describes this as exposing knowledge, communication and relationships that contribute to the meaning and practice of work. We see this wider notion of translation as assisting novices to make sense of the 'micropolitics' of workplaces (Bleakley, 2006). We also suggest that explicit, creative translation work is essentially the new work of educators in medical and allied health.

Practitioners learn from their 'doing', that much we know; but their *expert* learning arises from the translation of their increasingly collaborative practices, such as around the operating table, during surgery — and also afterwards, in the debriefing and professional development sessions — and even from routine team meetings. This is indeed practice in the deep end of the pool of professionalism. We think a deep-end immersive approach to professional education is highly relevant and transferrable to health professional learning for clinical situations, including placements. The opportunity to develop the necessary 'occupational capacities' is key to what Nguyen and Walker (2016) call 'sustainable learning' where learners recognise they mainly need each other to engage and overcome particular professional problems and obstacles, and to address the messiness of practice, and the complexity and diversity within most workplaces including 'clinicum'.

References

Barnett, R. (2015). A curriculum for critical being. In M. Davies & R. Barnett (Eds.), *The Palgrave handbook of critical thinking in higher education* (pp. 63–76). New York: Palgrave MacMillan.

Bleakley, A. (2006). A common body of care: The ethics and politics of teamwork in the operating theater are inseparable. *Journal of Medicine and Philosophy: A Forum for Bioethics and Philosophy of Medicine, 31*(3), 305–322. doi:10.1080/03605310600732826.

Boud, D., & Falchikov, N. (2006). Aligning assessment with long-term learning. *Assessment and Evaluation in Higher Education, 31*(4), 399–413.

Breckenridge, J., Jones, D., Elliott, I., et al. (2012). Choosing a methodological path: Reflections on the constructivist turn. *Grounded Theory Review, 11*(1), 64–71.

Burns, J. P., Mitchell, C., Griffith, J. L., et al. (2001). End-of-life care in the pediatric intensive care unit: Attitudes and practices of pediatric critical care physicians and nurses. *Critical Care Medicine, 29*(3), 658–664.

Chen, Y.-S. (2016). Translation, the knowledge economy, and crossing boundaries in contemporary education. *Educational Philosophy and Theory, 48*(12), 1284–1297.

Clark, P. G., Cott, C., & Drinka, T. J. (2007). Theory and practice in interprofessional ethics: A framework for understanding ethical issues in health care teams. *Journal of Interprofessional Care, 21*(6), 591–603. doi:10.1080/13561820701653227.

Delany, C., & Conwell, M. (2012). Ethics and teamwork for pediatric medical imaging procedures: Insights from educational play therapy. *Pediatric Radiology, 42*(2), 139–146.

Delany, C., & Galvin, J. (2014). Ethics and shared decision-making in paediatric occupational therapy practice. *Developmental Neurorehabiliation, 17*(5), 347–354.

Delany, C., Richards, A., Stewart, H., et al. (2017). Five challenges to ethical communication for interprofessional paediatric practice: A social work perspective. *Journal of Interprofessional Care, 31*(4), 1–7. Reprinted by permission of the publisher (Taylor & Francis Ltd, http://www.tandfonline.com).

Delany, C., Spriggs, M., Fry, C. L., et al. (2010). The unique nature of clinical ethics in allied health pediatrics: implications for ethics education. *Cambridge Quarterly of Healthcare Ethics, 19*(4), 471–480. doi:10.1017/S0963180110000368.

Dreyfus, H. L., & Dreyfus, S. E. (2005). Peripheral vision: Expertise in real world contexts. *Organization Studies, 26*(5), 779–792.

Durall, A., Zurakowski, D., & Wolfe, J. (2012). Barriers to conducting advance care discussions for children with life-threatening conditions. *Pediatrics, 129*(4), e975e982.

Gillett, G. (2002). *Getting over informed consent.* Paper presented at the Informed Consent in Australia — the 10th Anniversary of Rogers v Whitaker, ACT Canberra.

Hager, P., & Beckett, D. (in press). *The emergence of social complexity.* Dordrecht: Springer.

Harris, A., & Delany, C. (2013). International medical graduates in transition. *The Clinical Teacher, 10*(5), 328–332. doi:10.1111/tct.12021.

Irvine, R., Kerridge, I., McPhee, J., et al. (2002). Interprofessionalism and ethics: Consensus or clash of cultures? *Journal of Interprofessional Care, 16*(3), 199–210.

Kanter, K. R. (2011). Zoom in, zoom out. *Harvard Business Review, 89*(3), 112–116.

Kenny, D., & Adamson, B. (1992). Medicine and the health professions: Issues of dominance, autonomy and authority. *Australian Health Review, 15*(3), 319–334.

Lancaster, J. (2012). The complex systems of practice. In P. Hager, A. Lee, & A. Reich (Eds.), *Practice, learning and change: Practice-theory perspectives on professional learning* (pp. 119–131). Dordrecht: Springer Netherlands.

Lave, J., & Wenger, E. (1991). *Situated learning: Legitimate peripheral participation.* Cambridge: Cambridge University Press.

McGivern, P. (2014). Emergent expertise? *Educational Philosophy and Theory, 46*(6), 692–708. doi:10.108 0/00131857.2013.779217.

Menary, R., & Kirchhoff, M. (2014). Cognitive transformations and extended expertise. *Educational Philosophy and Theory, 46*(6), 610–623. doi:10.108 0/00131857.2013.779209.

Nguyen, T. T., & Walker, M. (2016). Sustainable assessment for lifelong learning. *Assessment and Evaluation in Higher Education, 41*(1), 97–111.

Roepstorff, A., Niewöhner, J., & Beck, S. (2010). Enculturing brains through patterned practices. *Neural Networks, 23*(8), 1051–1059.

Schön, D. (1987). *Educating the Reflective Practitioner.* San Francisco: Jossey-Bass.

Williamson, K., & Cox, R. (2014). Distributed cognition in sports teams: Explaining successful and expert performance. *Educational Philosophy and Theory, 46*(6), 640–654. doi:10.1080/00131857.2013.779215.

Winch, C. (2014). Education and broad concepts of agency. *Educational Philosophy and Theory, 46*(6), 569–583. doi:10.1080/00131857.2013.779211.

12

Peer learning in clinical placements

Joanna Tai, Samantha Sevenhuysen and Phillip Dawson

Introduction

Peer learning has existed in one format or another for hundreds, if not thousands, of years; however, its formalisation as a pedagogy has only recently occurred. Within clinical settings, there are many situations that might be considered peer learning: students aiding each other in their learning, trainees discussing best practice for a situation, even consultant surgeons asking each other for their opinion on a difficult case. These situations are likely to arise of their own accord. In clinical education, educators may also wish to develop, engineer or otherwise make room for opportunities that explicitly utilise peer learning.

This chapter aims to provide practical support for clinician educators who wish to implement peer learning in their setting. First, we provide an overview of what peer learning is and its benefits and potential pitfalls. We then introduce a case study for clinician educators. We examine educational theory which supports peer learning, alongside practical examples and tools, and the case study is then resolved. Together, these three elements provide a solid basis for readers to adapt and develop peer learning activities for their own setting and context. Some directions for future educational research are also provided to highlight current gaps in the literature, and we conclude with practical advice from experts on peer learning and its implementation.

What is peer learning?

Peer learning as we consider it today draws on the work of Keith Topping, who published seminal works on the potential for peer learning within higher education and schools simultaneously (Topping, 1996, 1998). His now ubiquitous definition of peer-assisted learning is 'people from similar social groupings who

TABLE 12.1: Types and examples of peer learning in clinical education

Peer learning term	Example within clinical education
Peer teaching	Learners have a weekly session where pairs prepare and deliver a 20-minute presentation on an allocated topic of relevance to the placement
Peer tutoring	Two learners meet regularly; each week one helps the other with a topic they are having difficulty with
Peer discussion and reflection	Learners on surgical placements meet regularly in a group of 6–8 to talk about their experiences of medical ethics throughout the placement
Role-play with peers	Learners take turns to be the health professional and the patient; they role-play a history-taking or explanation situation
Practising clinical skills with peers	Learners practise application of bandages and slings on each other
Peer observation	A pair of learners go to see a patient; one learner performs the history-taking while the other observes
Peer modelling	One learner observes a peer in practice without the intent to assess or provide feedback
Peer feedback	One learner provides feedback on an observed performance to the other — this occurs after role-play, practising clinical skills or observing a peer with a patient
Peer assessment	One learner grades/marks another learner on some aspect of performance — clinical skills, communication skills and professionalism are common topics

are not professional teachers helping each other to learn and learning themselves by teaching' (Topping, 1996, p 322). You will note that we have chosen the less wordy 'peer learning' over 'peer-assisted learning'. This is partially pragmatic, but we believe there is also value in semantics. By including 'assisted', there is an implied reduction of the utility of peer learning — it suggests that peer learning can only be an assistant or helpmeet to the actual learning (likely from experts), rather than being a valuable source of learning in and of itself. This is not to say that we do not believe in the value of expertise, but that peer learning can provide opportunities which a traditional master–apprentice/expert–novice configuration cannot.

Under the broad umbrella of 'peer learning', there are many activities that may be considered a type of peer learning. Peer learning can occur both in formal settings, where it is part of a curriculum and structured for specific learning outcomes, and more informally. Informal peer learning is usually initiated by students and while also aiming to achieve learning outcomes, is not part of a formal or stated curriculum. Table 12.1 provides some terms with clinical education examples. You will note there is some overlap — peer teaching and tutoring could be very similar. Peer feedback is only likely to occur after observation, role-play or practising a technique or skill. The key element in the included examples is that the learner is interacting with their peers in some way, and with the exception of peer feedback, all other types could occur as standalone activities.

When discussing peer learning, standardised formats for reporting have been proposed. While some focus largely on peer assessment (Gielen et al., 2011; van Gennip et al., 2009), Topping (2005) recommends considering 12 organisational variables for peer learning in general:

1. Context: what facilitators and barriers are there within your local situation?
2. Objectives: what are the desired learning outcomes from the peer learning activity?
3. Curriculum area: this is likely to be linked to the objectives, but if the objectives are about a transcendent skill (e.g. communication), what topic will you ground the content in?
4. Participants: who will be involved? Where will they be drawn from? Do they have similar or complementary (e.g. in the case of interprofessional peer learning) previous ability? Are their roles static or rotational? Will you be matching up learners, or will they form their own groups? What size groups will be used?

5. Helping technique — or learning methods: what activity will they participate in? Is it something they have done before/that exists within the literature or will you design a new activity? How does this activity fit within their learning placement?
6. Contact: what is the location (including online), frequency and duration of meetings?
7. Materials: will you need any special equipment for the activity, including checklists, worksheets and recording devices?
8. Training: what training is required for the learners involved, but also for the educators facilitating the process?
9. Process monitoring: how will you ensure that learners are experiencing quality learning?
10. Assessment: will learners be assessed on the process of peer learning, or the product? Is peer assessment a suitable means?
11. Evaluation: how will you know whether the peer learning worked?
12. Feedback: what feedback will be provided for participants either during or after the activity, for how they might improve in future peer learning activities?

These considerations provide a detailed guide for designing and implementing a formal peer learning activity, ensuring that all important elements are contemplated. Informal peer learning, on the other hand, occurs more spontaneously, and it is likely that the learners involved will have little regard for these considerations, especially points 8–12.

Why same-level peer learning?

Peer learning group configurations can consist of same-level peers or near-peers. Near-peers are learners who are not at the same point in their studies, with there being one or more years' difference between those involved. Learning activities in these situations are usually more unidirectional in their interactions, and senior learners are more likely to be educator substitutes rather than relative equals in an interaction. We choose to focus on same-level peer learning because:

- This can be the more difficult form of peer learning to implement due to both learner and educator perceptions of such activities being less worthwhile (due to a lack of 'expertise' in this configuration).

- It can be the most realistic and practical form of peer learning to implement, due to the logistics of clinical placements, and the likelihood of learners at the same level being on clinical placements at the same time, and for the same duration.

- Both learners and educators are very likely to be familiar with a model of learning within an expert–novice dyad, and less familiar with how to optimise outcomes within a novice–novice dyad, so the need for strategies and tools for implementation is much greater within the space of same-level peer learning.

There may also be cases where near-peer learners do have similar levels of previous exposure to a topic or skill. In these cases, despite otherwise being in different year levels of a course, this would still be considered a form of same-level peer learning.

Benefits and pitfalls of same-level peer learning

There are both practical and educational benefits to peer learning in clinical education. While the practical benefits have frequently driven the implementation of peer learning, the pedagogical benefits are commonly now the rationale for using peer learning as a form of 'active' learning which engages students more deeply than other formats of learning (Topping, 2005).

The educational benefits of peer learning are multiple (Burgess et al., 2014; Santee & Garavalia, 2006; Secomb, 2008; Tai, Molloy et al., 2016; Yu et al., 2011). Peer learning is compatible with adult learning theory, which requires an active learning environment. In almost all cases, when assessed, students demonstrate comparable knowledge of skill gain in the area on which they undertook peer learning. Tai, Molloy and colleagues (2016) identified more detailed benefits to students, including the ability to reflect, increased confidence (and reduced anxiety), motivation to participate in learning, problem-solving skills, evaluative judgment, feedback skills, the sense that they are learning in a supportive environment, and developing a responsibility to their peers. These benefits also potentially extended to patients in the form of students' improved communication, procedural and education skills, with increased empathy and ability to develop rapport. Finally, clinical educators also benefited from the introduction of peer learning, as they found it enjoyable, it allowed them to develop a wider repertoire of education skills and it frequently provided them with additional information on student performance when peer assessment was included. Those acting as peer tutors may experience additional benefits, including a deeper level of understanding than those they have been tutoring (Burgess et al., 2014; Yu et al., 2011), though in these reviews, learners who were peer tutors were near-peers rather than same-level peers.

Peer learning has previously been promoted as a time-saving measure for clinical supervisors responsible for more than one student at a time. However, some studies have demonstrated that the time commitment has remained constant, regardless of placement model (Ladyshewsky, 1995; Ladyshewsky et al., 1998; Sevenhuysen et al., 2014). Logistically, using a peer learning model may also allow for an increase in the number of students placed at a site or with a service, as it can provide a framework for educators to supervise multiple students concurrently.

The most commonly cited pitfall is a concern from educators that learners will not find the peer learning activity useful for their learning, since peers are not experts — what could possibly be learned from them? As indicated above, peer learning has been shown to be effective, so the pitfall is that others involved in the educational endeavour may have negative perceptions of peer learning, and especially peer assessment. Papers frequently cite learner concerns that they are not qualified to provide feedback on or mark their peers' work (Tai, Haines et al., 2014; Tai, Molloy et al., 2016). However, the selection of the peer learning activity, the orientation of learners to the task and appropriate training for both educators and learners are likely to remedy this. It is only through practising those skills that students are able to develop better judgment of work, whether it be their own or others (Tai, Canny et al., 2016). Tai, Canny and colleagues (2016) recommend that learners making credibility judgments about the capacity of the feedback source is an important lifelong skill. For example, part of the strength of peer learning as an educational strategy is that students need to identify and declare the boundaries of their knowledge and skill, and therefore the aspects of work they feel adequately qualified to comment upon. For example, an observing peer in year two of a medical course may declare that they can provide feedback on their fellow peer's communication skills in a physical examination of a patient, but that they do not feel comfortable in commenting on the quality of the neurological examination technique.

Overall, the additional benefits of peer learning usually outweigh any potential pitfalls, which can usually be reduced through careful attention to the design of the peer learning activity. Case study 12.1 introduces both educator and student experiences with peer learning.

Case study 12.1: Ben and Corinne

Ben (clinical educator)

Ben is a physiotherapist relatively new to a senior role. He works in a rehabilitation ward within a hospital which has acute, subacute and mental health units. He has previously assisted with the supervision of students as a junior clinician and acted as lead supervisor for three students. There is one other senior physiotherapist, Michelle, who is part-time and works on the acute wards in the hospital.

The hospital that Ben and Michelle work for partners with a local university to provide clinical education placements for physiotherapy students. The university has recently implemented a peer learning student allocation model, where students are allocated to clinical educators in pairs for each placement. Educators are able to structure the placement according to the clinical environment and workflow; the few formal requirements include basic attendance records and a placement assessment form. Students are accustomed to working in pairs and groups from their prior university studies but have no formal peer learning activities mandated by the university while on clinical placement. Ben and Michelle have attended a one-hour briefing at the university relating to supervising two students simultaneously.

Interview with Ben

'Michelle and I each have two third-year (of a four-year undergraduate degree) students allocated to us for one of their core clinical placements next month. I've only ever supervised one student at a time previously and I'm a bit anxious about supervising two students. When Michelle and I have both had a student each in the past, we have sometimes asked them to work together with a patient. It's worked well, so I know we can use some of these strategies, but having full responsibility for two students is quite different. I feel like it will be twice the work, having two sets of paperwork to complete and two lots of feedback to give every time. At the briefing the facilitator said we should encourage peer learning between the students, but won't it be the "blind leading the blind"?'

Corinne (student)

Corinne is a third-year physiotherapy student preparing for her second clinical placement, which will be supervised by Ben. She was paired with another student on her last placement and enjoyed having someone to debrief with. Corinne was anxious about her first placement and it really helped to have someone to talk to. She also found it useful to brainstorm treatment ideas with her peer and practise patient assessment procedures on one another.

In the pre-clinical years, physiotherapy students at this university participate in a broad range of learning activities. Many of these involve types of collaborative or peer learning, such as case-based learning (where a patient case scenario is presented and small groups of students share tasks to devise an assessment and treatment plan), procedural skills labs (where students practise procedural skills on one another) and peer-assisted study sessions (where students meet informally to revise and discuss relevant topics).

Interview with Corinne

'In my last placement, I was paired with Mary, who is pretty similar to me. It was great to have someone with you during the first placement. I'm really looking forward to being able to do a few more things independently in my second placement, now that I am more confident seeing patients. I hope that I won't have to do everything with my peer as I really want to show my supervisor what I can do. After all, that's the point of placement, to learn how to manage patients on your own. The student who I'm placed with this time, Maxine, has struggled a bit in tutes, so I'm a bit worried about how that's going to go. I want to make sure that the educator judges me on my performance and gives me enough individual feedback. I mean, I know there's things you can learn from your peer, but at the end of the day the educator is the expert and the one assessing you, so that's who you really want to hear from.'

Educational theories relating to peer learning

Several educational theory perspectives could shed light on Ben and Corinne's experiences. We have selected three from the social psychology literature that are used to explain the learning, motivational and relational aspects of peer learning. These are: social constructivism, particularly its notion of the zone of proximal development, which helps understand how people learn through working with more capable peers; self-determination theory, which explains motivation to engage in peer learning through a desire to meet fundamental human needs; and social exchange theory, which covers reciprocity in peer learning. While there are also sociocultural theories that help explain the formation of peer learning groups, such as Lave and Wenger's (1991) 'communities of practice' and the associated concept of 'legitimate peripheral practice', these apply more to situations where practitioners of various skill levels are working and learning together, rather than same-level peers learning together, which is the focus of this chapter.

Social constructivism

The theoretical perspective of social constructivism is strongly associated with Vygotsky's work (Vygotsky, 1978). Social constructivism begins from the premise that knowledge is not absolute, rather it is constructed within learners' minds, and through social interactions. Taking the two students in the case, each already possesses certain capabilities. There are some things Corinne can do that Maxine can't do, and vice versa. Social constructivism argues that effective learning should take place when Corinne and Maxine are extending each other by operating within their 'zone of proximal development' (ZPD). The ZPD is the set of things a learner cannot do on their own, but can do with the assistance of a more capable other (Vygotsky, 1978).

From a ZPD perspective, peer learning (both formal and informal) works by learners engaging in activities that are beyond their individual capabilities but within their collective capability. In a peer learning context, educators need to manage the activities that students undertake in order to ensure they spend maximum time in their collective ZPD (Topping, 2005). The ZPD concept also implies that learners in a peer learning context should not be asked to undertake activities that are beyond their collective competence. Ben could operationalise the ZPD through helping Corinne and Maxine to identify their own capabilities, and encouraging them to collaborate where their collective competence is greater than their individual competence.

While Maxine may learn much from Corinne through working in her ZPD, it sounds like the relationship may be somewhat one-sided, with Corinne learning less from Maxine. If Ben wishes to leverage the ZPD, he may want to consider spending more time extending Corinne. This may run counter to his instincts as an educator; we often want to help students of lower ability first. But Maxine's ZPD is already rather large with Corinne's support, while Corinne's ZPD is small with only Maxine's help.

Self-determination theory

Given the rather small ZPD for Corinne from peer learning, what does she really have to gain? Rather a lot, if we consider the perspective of self-determination theory (Deci & Ryan, 1985). This perspective builds on empirical work that identified basic human needs: a sense of competence; a sense of autonomy; and a sense of relatedness. When these needs are fulfilled, learners feel more intrinsically motivated; conversely, when these needs are not fulfilled, educators may find themselves using extrinsic motivators (e.g. grades or praise) as primary motivators, which can harm learners' intrinsic motivation (Deci & Ryan, 1985).

Development of a sense of competence is both a fundamental human need and a powerful intrinsic motivator for learning (Deci & Ryan, 1985). Although Corinne is worried about being paired with a less capable student, this may give her more opportunities to develop her sense of competence. Peer learning is particularly useful in developing learners' sense of competence as it offers more opportunities for learning through doing. However, for Corinne to fully meet her need for a sense of competence, Ben needs to remain engaged with her, evaluating her work and providing feedback.

Corinne expressed that she feels more motivated because she thinks she will be more independent in this placement, and this is supported by self-determination theory (Deci & Ryan, 1985). The more self-directed nature of peer-led approaches in contrast to teacher-led approaches may support Corinne and Maxine in developing their sense of autonomy even further. Ben can support them in developing their sense of autonomy even further by providing them with opportunities to set the agenda, and guide their learning towards their self-identified needs.

The fundamental human need for a sense of relatedness — a sense of belonging and being connected to others (Deci & Ryan, 1985) — may be particularly powerful in the placement setting; as Corinne notes, it's important to have someone with you. Ben can help support the peer relationship between Maxine and Corinne by encouraging them to spend time together, even if it's not always on-task.

Social exchange theory

However, there is a chance that Corinne will weigh the potential benefits of peer learning against all the effort it requires and decide that it's not worth it. This sort of decision is the core of social exchange theory, which argues that people enter into and maintain relationships based on an analysis of the costs, benefits and likelihood of those costs and benefits (Emerson, 1976). Pairing Corinne with someone less capable, like Maxine, may tilt Corinne's unconscious cost–benefit analyses in such a way that she decides not to invest in peer learning.

What can Ben do to support Corinne to engage meaningfully in peer learning? He may wish to clarify what the benefits of peer learning are for more capable students. A core benefit is that by demonstrating how to do particular activities, Corinne will learn them more. Ben may also wish to directly address Corinne's needs for competence, relatedness and autonomy, and explain how peer learning can support those. However, peer learning is not a panacea, and it is subject to the social exchange theory concept of 'diminishing returns', which functions similarly to its namesake in economics: the more someone receives a particular sort of benefit (such as the nice feelings one gets from helping a peer), the less rewarding any additional amount of that benefit is (Emerson, 1976). Ben must be wary not to rely too much on any particular benefit as convincing Corinne, and he should watch out for peer learning burnout for Corinne if she is relied upon too heavily to 'teach' Maxine.

Case study 12.1 (continued): Ben and Corinne

Ben (clinical educator)

Ben is looking forward to the end of the student placement block. He didn't think there had been *more* work during this block, but he'd found his educator role was different from previous blocks and he'd had to change the way he normally operated. Ben had participated in a workshop about peer learning previously as part of his clinical education training and learned about how others had implemented it in their placements (Currens & Bithell, 2003; Ladyshewsky et al., 1998; Lekkas et al., 2007; Sevenhuysen et al., 2014). Ben and Michelle used the information they had learned in the workshop and further reading to work together and develop a program of activities that they thought would maximise the value of peer learning for their four students collectively. They focused on the use of self-determination theory, reasoning that students on their second placement were looking to develop their autonomy on clinical placements. Regular activities for students included peer observation and feedback (using a template that was modelled from the placement assessment form), assessing and/or treating patients together, and asking them to reflect and discuss their key learning and challenges, at the end of the day, to form a summary for Ben and Michelle. Ben also ensured that there were allocated sessions for him to work with Corinne and Maxine separately, to fulfil his assessment responsibilities.

Interview with Ben

'The main thing I've taken out of this placement is that it isn't twice the work, but it's not less work either — it's just different. You really need to "let go" of your traditional views of 1:1 clinical education and be prepared to work differently. I can see that how I set up the placement and the learning activities is crucial to getting students to work constructively with each other. You can't just throw the students in and say "treat this patient together and let me know what you think".

In the beginning I think I needed to talk more about what we were doing and why, what was in it for them. I did that along the way in the last placement, but next time I want to spend more time on it at the beginning. The students also told me that it would've been better if they'd seen me in practice a bit more, so they could see what they were aiming for. Then they would have something to compare to when they observe and give feedback to each other. So that's something else I will add in next time: observation of the clinical educator. I think they could watch me and how I go about clinical practice, but also how I have feedback discussions as well. When the sessions were set up well, it was actually really surprising what the students came up with. Then it just became habit and the students initiated the set-up themselves, so I could begin to step away. It was sometimes difficult to balance their independence with safety and patient care — we used tools like the SNAPPS (Summarise history and findings; Narrow the differential; Analyse the differential; Probe preceptor about uncertainties; Plan management; Select case-related issues for self-study) (Wolpaw et al. 2009) so they could quickly run me through their clinical reasoning and I could be confident in the direction they were heading. By the end they had developed a great routine and had really helped each other progress, so it wasn't the blind leading the blind after all.'

Corinne (student)

Corinne arrived at this placement not knowing exactly what to expect. She was happy to discover her educator, and the other educator at the hospital, had developed a structure for the placement, with a range of activities she and Maxine could do together. That meant that Maxine also had to contribute, rather than Corinne doing everything as she'd done in the past with group assignments on campus with other students. It also meant that Corinne never had to fish around for ideas on what to do with Maxine — there was always a list to go back to, even if they weren't required to do them all. Ben seemed to be entrusting a fair bit of the patient load to them, though of course they had to discuss all their findings and decisions before they could proceed with treatment. Again, having a peer on the placement meant she was less anxious about seeing patients — having Maxine there meant that she had moral support.

Interview with Corinne

'It turns out Maxine struggled in tutes because she was trying to understand things very deeply and got caught up on points while the rest of the class had moved on. Going through this detail actually helps me to understand the theory better, and at the same time I can help Maxine come to grips with the practical side of management in a clinical setting. I thought I would be better on placement with someone who was similar to me, but us having different approaches to learning has actually worked quite well. I do learn by working with Maxine, and Ben has given me positive feedback on it and how it contributes to my own performance. He has made sure that we both receive individual feedback and learning activities targeted at our own level. We've worked together but we've also worked separately — Ben has balanced that really well and involved us in the discussion and allocation of tasks on our timetable. Maxine's feedback is not as in-depth as Ben's, but it gives me another perspective. It might be "little things" like closing the curtains around the patient's bed or making eye contact when I am taking a subjective assessment, but Ben is not always available and it all makes a difference. Sometimes the peer feedback and discussion covers off on a lot of the queries and thoughts I have, so that with Ben we can hone in on the clinical reasoning and more sophisticated understanding.'

Strategies for implementing peer learning
Formal and informal peer learning activities

We are careful to include both formal and informal peer learning activities as strategies, because both can be facilitated by clinical educators. Formal peer learning activities are not only structured, but also facilitated by educators and implemented as part of the required learning for a placement — whether this be in the setting of a tutorial, a patient bedside consultation, or an activity which learners perform independently. Informal activities are therefore those excluding the formal activities — tasks that students might organise themselves, or that are outside the formal curriculum. Educators can still have a role in providing structure, activities and recommendations for learners on what to do or who to see, what the learning outcomes from those situations might be and generally establishing and promoting an environment where collaboration is expected.

We return to Table 12.1, which is now expanded and includes specific examples of tasks and the associated evidence for them in Table 12.2.

TABLE 12.2: Peer learning activities for clinical placements

Type of peer learning	Description	References in the literature
Peer teaching	Learners have regular sessions where they prepare and deliver a presentation on an allocated topic of relevance to the placement. Learners may be allocated topics individually or in groups, depending on the number of students and topics.	Learners who participated in teaching sessions (5-minute presentations, no slides) performed better on an exam than those who just received traditional lectures (Wirth et al., 2015).
Peer tutoring	Learners meet regularly; configurations can vary from 1:1 to several students in a group taking turns to act as a 'tutor'. Compared with peer teaching this may not be as facilitated and structured by clinical educators. Learners usually choose a particular topic to concentrate on.	Zaidi et al. (2012) implemented a model where students who demonstrated 'positive deviance' in their approach to clinical learning coached small groups of their peers. Students reported that the additional motivation aided them in achieving their learning goals.
Peer discussion and reflection	Learners on similar or the same placement meet regularly in a group of 6–8 to talk about their experiences throughout the placement. Topics might include diagnosis and management of conditions, ethical considerations, or more generally a debriefing and support group for students.	Learners meet in person (Chou et al., 2011; Liu et al., 2016) or online (Duke et al., 2014; Ladyshewsky & Gardner, 2008), and this can be supported through requiring preparation of a written piece, which may or may not be shared.

Continued

TABLE 12.2: Peer learning activities for clinical placements — cont'd

Type of peer learning	Description	References in the literature
Role-play with peers	This may occur more formally in a structured skills session (or OSCE practice), where students take it in turns to be the patient. Alternatively, this may be an informal activity for learners to do in pairs in their own time to practise and revise particular areas in preparation for seeing patients.	Communication skills in paediatrics have been a focus for this, with learners playing the role of a parent in a consultation session (Bosse et al., 2010; Bosse et al., 2015).
Practising clinical skills with peers	Learners practise application of bandages and slings on each other.	Areas of practice have extended to include ophthalmoscopy (Milani et al., 2013) and giving injections (Chunharas et al., 2013).
Peer collaboration	Peers perform a patient assessment or intervention together.	Tools such as the SNAPPS (Wolpaw et al., 2009) can be completed by the students together and presented back to the clinical educator as a summary.
Peer cooperation	Student A takes the patient's history, while student B performs the physical examination. Putting their information together, both students develop a management plan.	Establishing a climate of cooperation and consideration of 'reward structures' (Ladyshewsky, 2006) is important for these kinds of tasks.
Peer observation	A pair of learners see a patient; one performs the history-taking while the other observes.	Providing a rubric or longitudinal assessment form (if used) could help frame the notes taken during an observation (Stegmann et al., 2012).
Peer feedback	One learner provides feedback on an observed performance to the other — this occurs after role-play, practising clinical skills or observing a peer with a patient.	Peers can be extremely helpful in providing alternative perspectives and pick up on concerns that learners may have (Ladyshewsky, 2013). In one study (Ladyshewsky, 2002) students performed better when reciprocal peer coaching was used. Easy-to-learn feedback models (such as Pendleton et al., 2003) should be introduced early to enable learners to do best practice.
Peer assessment	One learner grades or marks another learner on some aspect of performance: clinical skills, communication skills and professionalism are common topics.	Assessment by peers is more fruitful if learners have had a prior learning relationship (Chou et al., 2013).

Developing a culture of peer learning

In addition to individual favourable experiences of peer learning (e.g. a successful pilot program), promoting a general culture or attitude that expects peer learning is likely to facilitate both students and educators being more willing to adopt peer learning methods (Tai et al., 2017). In case study 12.1, Corinne had ample exposure to peer learning activities prior to arriving in clinical placement. Thus, she had already experienced several peer learning types, and knew some of the benefits and pitfalls, but was overall willing to participate in it. Conversely, clinical educators Ben and Michelle were less familiar with peer learning and so more hesitant on how it would work. By normalising the expectations that peers will be a source of good learning — priming them for the social exchange — the challenge remains only in the logistics of doing it well, rather than winning individuals over to peer learning as an educational method.

Depending on your position as a clinical educator, it may or may not be your role to be involved in changing educational culture. As an individual, setting baseline expectations that peer learning occurs on placement could reinforce learners' previous experiences and prepare them for future learning. It is unlikely that learners will cease to learn once they graduate and become qualified in their discipline; they will acquire new knowledge, skills and attitudes over the course of their working life. Since work is not an individual pursuit, especially within the health professions, it is likely that the people one learns from in work environments will be peers of a sort, and so to practise peer learning from the start is a useful strategy, as part of learning to be a professional.

Directions for evaluation and research

We are aware that clinical educators have many competing demands on their time, and so research and evaluation of educational interventions may not be a high priority. However, by including some direction here, we hope that it may spark interest and indicate the limitations and boundaries of the evidence provided in this chapter.

General evaluation principles apply. First, clear goals are necessary for a peer learning intervention to be valuable: if the program intends to promote learning of skills, then this implies that evaluation should focus on how well those skills have been learned. Peer learning interventions are frequently implemented with learning goals, but evaluated in terms of how much students like them. Second, evaluation should not be post-hoc, but should be planned and begin with evaluation of the peer learning design, and even the rationale for using peer learning. Using realist methods may assist in untangling the complexities and variances in clinical education (Wong et al., 2012) and may also support theory-building to illuminate the contexts, mechanisms and outcomes of effective peer learning.

Robust data collected through well-designed trials are often lacking in clinical education research. There are many challenges, including logistical and ethical considerations in creating and randomising cohorts of learners among the myriad of other requirements when arranging clinical placements. The 'crossover' and 'stepped-wedge' (Brown & Lilford, 2006) designs have been used in clinical education research (Sevenhuysen et al., 2014; Sevenhuysen et al., 2017) and may be useful in addressing the ethical concerns of ensuring that students are equally exposed to interventions which may be beneficial for their learning. Both designs allow all participants to receive the intervention. The order in which they receive the intervention can be determined at random, meaning the designs can meet the gold standard 'randomised controlled trial'.

There are many potential directions for research in peer learning in clinical education. Demonstrating superior learning outcomes is still a goal, and cost-effectiveness of alternative education methods is an emerging key interest. We would particularly draw attention to the concept of evaluative judgment, the capability to make informed decisions about the quality of work of self and others. This is an essential component of becoming an independent practitioner, in knowing the limits of one's own and others' abilities, and knowing when additional assistance is required. Peer learning has been suggested to play a large role in the development of evaluative judgment, providing opportunities to interact with tacit or explicit standards of practice, and practise judgment making (Tai, Canny et al., 2016). Further research in this area could examine more carefully which forms of peer learning, under which conditions, contribute best to developing learners' evaluative judgment.

PRACTICAL TIPS

Advice from Melanie, an experienced clinical educator (personal communication):

'It's really important to set the scene in the beginning. Often students come to clinical placements with the expectation that it will be very different from their previous learning experiences, so they don't always think about how the skills they've developed can be translated into the workplace setting. Some students expect that clinical placements will be all about getting "hands on" and learning from experts, so they might think that learning from peers is not as valuable, or even that having to "share" their learning experiences with peers will get in the way of them performing tasks themselves or demonstrating independence. So right up front you need to talk to them about how peer learning will feature in the placement and what the benefits are for them. I often talk to them about how much I utilise my own colleagues to discuss cases, how we work with junior staff, assistants and other health professionals, so these collaborative skills are really important not just for learning but also for being a good practitioner. The students should be involved and active in this discussion — they can talk about what peer learning activities they've been involved in previously, what types of learning approaches work for them, what their strengths and weaknesses are and if they have any reservations about peer learning.

I really like to use a timetable, especially in the beginning, to plan tasks and activities. That way I can set the expectation around how peer learning will work and what tasks I expect, but also I can demonstrate clearly that there will be a balance between peer learning and individual activities and that the allocation of tasks is equitable between the students. The timetable doesn't have to be full; often the students will fill in the gaps and that way we can be responsive to the demands of the workload that day. Over time the peer learning activities change — in the beginning the students might do a lot together and gradually they will be more independent, but still work together when something more complex comes up or maybe one gets to see an unusual diagnosis. Often they will brainstorm with one another or even just debrief at the end of the day. I usually find if I set it up well in the beginning, they get into a good rhythm and just keep going with the peer learning tasks themselves.

One of the benefits for me as an educator is that the students utilise one another as a resource and it saves me having to be that resource for them all the time. They can come to me when they can't solve the problem themselves, or for something more complex. I feel more confident when they head off to treat a patient when they are together, so my feeling is that it promotes independence rather than hinders it. When the students have the right structure and expectations, I have found that they can provide each other with some very constructive feedback. They will often provide a good base level of feedback, and I can just come in with suggestions related to clinical reasoning or other more complex issues. In the past I've found that students can never get enough feedback; no matter how much you give them, they always want more. But since I've been using peer learning models, with the students giving each other feedback, they seem more satisfied and it takes the pressure off me to provide feedback all the time.'

Conclusion

Though peer learning has been occurring for a long time, only recently have we amassed evidence evaluating the impact and demonstrating the benefits of peer learning. Peer learning can act as an adjunct and enhancement to traditional conceptions of clinical placement learning. Expertise in the facilitation and implementation of peer learning is required, though many peer learning interventions have simply originated from a need to host more learners on a clinical placement. Developing appropriate attitudes and a culture of peer learning, scaffolding learning activities and having a sound understanding of educational theory applicable to peer learning are all important for success.

References

Bosse, H. M., Nickel, M., Huwendiek, S., et al. (2010). Peer role-play and standardised patients in communication training: A comparative study on the student perspective on acceptability, realism, and perceived effect. *BMC Medical Education, 10*, 27. doi.org/10.1186/1472-6920-10-27.

Bosse, H. M., Nickel, M., Huwendiek, S., et al. (2015). Cost-effectiveness of peer role play and standardized patients in undergraduate communication training. *BMC Medical Education, 15*(1), 183. doi.org/10.1186/s12909-015-0468-1.

Brown, C. A., & Lilford, R. J. (2006). The stepped wedge trial design: A systematic review. *BMC Medical Research Methodology, 6*(1), 54. doi.org/10.1186/1471-2288-6-54.

Burgess, A., McGregor, D., & Mellis, C. (2014). Medical students as peer tutors: A systematic review. *BMC Medical Education, 14*(1), 115. doi.org/10.1186/1472-6920-14-115.

Chou, C. L., Johnston, C. B., Singh, B., et al. (2011). A 'safe space' for learning and reflection: One school's design for continuity with a peer group across clinical clerkships. *Academic Medicine*, 86(12), 1560–1565. doi.org/10.1097/ACM.0b013e31823595fd.

Chou, C. L., Masters, D. E., Chang, A., et al. (2013). Effects of longitudinal small-group learning on delivery and receipt of communication skills feedback. *Medical Education*, 47(11), 1073–1079. doi.org/10.1111/medu.12246.

Chunharas, A., Hetrakul, P., Boonyobol, R., et al. (2013). Medical students themselves as surrogate patients increased satisfaction, confidence, and performance in practicing injection skill. *Medical Teacher*, 35(4), 308–313. doi.org/10.3109/0142159X.2012.746453.

Currens, J. B., & Bithell, C. P. (2003). The 2:1 clinical placement model. *Physiotherapy*, 89(4), 204–218. doi.org/10.1016/S0031-9406(05)60152-6.

Deci, E., & Ryan, R. (1985). *Intrinsic motivation and self-determination in human behavior*. New York: Plenum.

Duke, P., Grosseman, S., Novack, D. H., et al. (2014). Preserving third year medical students' empathy and enhancing self-reflection using small group 'virtual hangout' technology. *Medical Teacher*, (January), 1–6. doi.org/10.3109/0142159X.2014.956057.

Emerson, R. M. (1976). Social exchange theory. *Annual Review of Sociology*, 2, 335–362.

Gielen, S., Dochy, F., & Onghena, P. (2011). An inventory of peer assessment diversity. *Assessment & Evaluation in Higher Education*, 36(2), 137–155. doi.org/10.1080/02602930903221444.

Ladyshewsky, R. K. (1995). Enhancing service productivity in acute care inpatient settings using a collaborative clinical education model. *Physical Therapy*, 75(6), 503–510. http://www.ncbi.nlm.nih.gov/pubmed/7770496.

Ladyshewsky, R. K. (2002). A quasi-experimental study of the differences in performance and clinical reasoning using individual learning versus reciprocal peer coaching. *Physiotherapy Theory and Practice*, 18(1), 17–31. doi.org/10.1080/095939802753570666.

Ladyshewsky, R. K. (2006). Building cooperation in peer coaching relationships: Understanding the relationships between reward structure, learner preparedness, coaching skill and learner engagement. *Physiotherapy*, 92(1), 4–10. doi.org/10.1016/j.physio.2005.11.005.

Ladyshewsky, R. K. (2013). The role of peers in feedback processes. In D. Boud & E. K. Molloy (Eds.), *Feedback in higher and professional education: Understanding and doing it well* (pp. 174–189). Abingdon, Oxon: Routledge.

Ladyshewsky, R. K., Barrie, S. C., & Drake, V. M. (1998). A comparison of productivity and learning outcome in individual and cooperative physical therapy clinical education models. *Physical Therapy*, 78(12), 1288–1298, 1299–1301. http://www.ncbi.nlm.nih.gov/pubmed/9859948.

Ladyshewsky, R. K., & Gardner, P. (2008). Peer assisted learning and blogging: A strategy to promote reflective practice during clinical fieldwork. *Australasian Journal of Educational Technology*, 24(3), 241–257. doi.org/10.14742/ajet.1207.

Lave, J., & Wenger, E. (1991). *Situated practice: Legitimate peripheral participation*. Cambridge, UK: Cambridge University Press.

Lekkas, P., Larsen, T., Kumar, S., et al. (2007). No model of clinical education for physiotherapy students is superior to another: A systematic review. *The Australian Journal of Physiotherapy*, 53(1), 19–28. http://www.ncbi.nlm.nih.gov/pubmed/17326735.

Liu, G. Z., Jawitz, O. K., Zheng, D., et al. (2016). Reflective writing for medical students on the surgical clerkship: Oxymoron or antidote? *Journal of Surgical Education*, 73(2), 296–304. doi.org/10.1016/j.jsurg.2015.11.002.

Milani, B. Y., Majdi, M., Green, W., et al. (2013). The use of peer optic nerve photographs for teaching direct ophthalmoscopy. *Ophthalmology*, 120(4), 761–765. doi.org/10.1016/j.ophtha.2012.09.020.

Pendleton, D., Schofield, T., Tate, P., et al. (2003). Learning and teaching about the consultation. In T. Schofield, P. Tate, & P. Havelock (Eds.), *The new consultation: Developing doctor–patient communication* (Vol. 1968, pp. 64–84). Oxford: Oxford University Press.

Santee, J., & Garavalia, L. (2006). Peer tutoring programs in health professions schools. *American Journal of Pharmaceutical Education*, 70(3), Article 70.

Secomb, J. (2008). A systematic review of peer teaching and learning in clinical education. *Journal of Clinical Nursing*, 17(6), 703–716. doi.org/10.1111/j.1365-2702.2007.01954.x.

Sevenhuysen, S., Skinner, E. H., Farlie, M. K., et al. (2014). Educators and students prefer traditional clinical education to a peer-assisted learning model, despite similar student performance outcomes: A randomised trial. *Journal of Physiotherapy*, 60(4), 209–216. doi.org/10.1016/j.jphys.2014.09.004.

Sevenhuysen, S., Thorpe, J., Molloy, E., et al. (2017). Peer-assisted learning in education of allied health professional students in the clinical setting: A systematic review. *Journal of Allied Health*, 46(1), 26–35. http://www.ncbi.nlm.nih.gov/pubmed/28255594.

Stegmann, K., Pilz, F., Siebeck, M., et al. (2012). Vicarious learning during simulations: Is it more effective than hands-on training? *Medical Education*, 46(10), 1001–1008. doi.org/10.1111/j.1365-2923.2012.04344.x.

Tai, J., Canny, B. J., Haines, T. P., et al. (2016). The role of peer-assisted learning in building evaluative judgement: Opportunities in clinical medical education. *Advances in Health Sciences Education*, 21(3), 659. doi.org/10.1007/s10459-015-9659-0.

Tai, J., Canny, B. J., Haines, T. P., et al. (2017). Implementing peer learning in clinical education: A framework to address challenges in the 'real world'. *Teaching and Learning in Medicine*, 29(2), 162–172. doi.org/10.1080/10401334.2016.1247000.

Tai, J., Haines, T. P., Canny, B. J., et al. (2014). A study of medical students' peer learning on clinical placements: What they have taught themselves to do. *Journal of Peer Learning*, 7, 57–80.

Tai, J., Molloy, E., Haines, T., et al. (2016). Same-level peer-assisted learning in medical clinical placements: A narrative systematic review. *Medical Education*, 50(4), 469–484. doi.org/10.1111/medu.12898.

Topping, K. J. (1996). The effectiveness of peer tutoring in further and higher education: A typology and review of the literature. *Higher Education, 32*, 321–345. http://www.springerlink.com/index/n724l17269g79xkj.pdf.

Topping, K. J. (1998). Peer assessment between students in colleges and universities. *Review of Educational Research, 68*(3), 249–276. doi.org/10.3102/00346543068003249.

Topping, K. J. (2005). Trends in peer learning. *Educational Psychology, 25*(6), 631–645. doi.org/10.1080/01443410500345172.

van Gennip, N. A. E., Segers, M. S. R., & Tillema, H. H. (2009). Peer assessment for learning from a social perspective: The influence of interpersonal variables and structural features. *Educational Research Review, 4*(1), 41–54. doi.org/10.1016/j.edurev.2008.11.002.

Vygotsky, L. S. (1978). M. Cole, V. John-Steiner, S. Scribner, et al. (Eds.), *Mind in society*. Cambridge, MA: Harvard University Press.

Wirth, K., Malone, B., Turner, C., et al. (2015). A structured teaching curriculum for medical students improves their performance on the National Board of Medical Examiners shelf examination in surgery. *American Journal of Surgery, 209*(4), 765–770. doi.org/10.1016/j.amjsurg.2014.09.036.

Wolpaw, T., Papp, K., & Bordage, G. (2009). Using SNAPPS to facilitate the expression of clinical reasoning and uncertainties: A randomized comparison group trial. *Academic Medicine, 84*(4), 517–524.

Wong, G., Greenhalgh, T., Westhorp, G., et al. (2012). Realist methods in medical education research: What are they and what can they contribute? *Medical Education, 46*(1), 89–96. doi.org/10.1111/j.1365-2923.2011.04045.x.

Yu, T., Wilson, N., & Singh, P. (2011). Medical students-as-teachers: A systematic review of peer-assisted teaching during medical school. *Advances in Medical Education and Practice, 2*, 157–172. http://www.ncbi.nlm.nih.gov/pmc/articles/PMC3661256/.

Zaidi, Z., Jaffery, T., Shahid, A., et al. (2012). Change in action: Using positive deviance to improve student clinical performance. *Advances in Health Sciences Education, 17*(1), 95–105. doi.org/10.1007/s10459-011-9301-8.

13

Educating for professional practice through simulation

Debra Nestel and Suzanne Gough

Introduction

Although simulation-based education (SBE) has a very long history, it has surfaced as an important learning method in contemporary health professions education. In this chapter, we orientate readers to definitions, key concepts and theoretical underpinnings of SBE and introduce two frameworks to enhance SBE practice. Given that this book is about learning and teaching in clinical contexts, it is important to make connections between simulation and clinical settings. It is far too easy for SBE to become disconnected from the very service it is designed to support, to seem so very specialised that it risks exclusivity. There are many educational alliances between teaching and learning in simulated and clinical settings. We highlight some of these while focusing on the features of simulation.

We provide an overview of two simulation frameworks that can be used to facilitate robust design, delivery and evaluation of SBE for professional practice. The first is the integrated simulation and technology enhanced learning (ISTEL) framework, which highlights interlinking components that underpin the simulation design, delivery and evaluation of a short course, curriculum or in situ simulation. The second, from a national training program in Australia (NHET-Sim), provides a systematic approach to SBE and focuses on a single simulation event. We apply these frameworks in two case studies. In case study 13.1, we illustrate how the ISTEL framework is used to support the design of a scenario to develop effective teamwork in a computerised human patient (manikin)–based simulation. In case study 13.2, we explore how the NHET-Sim framework has been used to support the development of patient-centred communication skills and clinical judgment of medical students in a simulated patient (SP)–based scenario. These case studies show how carefully designed and executed SBE can offer a safe learning environment to enable learners to explore routine, evolving and complex clinical situations, leading to safer professional practice.

Definitions and contemporary context of simulation-based education

Simulation is commonly described as a 'technique — not a technology — to replace or amplify real experiences with guided experiences that evoke or replicate substantial aspects of the real world in a fully interactive manner' (Gaba, 2004, p i2). In healthcare, this has resulted in the development of a multimillion dollar industry that manufactures simulators (e.g. task trainers, manikins, virtual reality and other screen-based simulators), simulated environments (e.g. replica specialist clinical environments) (Kneebone et al., 2010; Staropoli et al., 2017), purpose-designed audio-visual recording and replay systems and other data management tools. Alongside these developments there has been certification of specialist simulation educators and technicians (or operation specialists) and accreditation of simulation-based programs and facilities (Nestel et al., 2017).

Simulation is now widely used in health professions education in the preparation for entry to practice, during specialty training and in continuing professional development. In 2009, Sir Liam Donaldson, then Chief Medical Officer in the United Kingdom, reported that 'simulation in all its forms will be a vital part of building a safer healthcare system' (Donaldson, 2009). In the United States, Hayden and colleagues (2014) reported the findings of a major study in nursing education where conventional nursing curricula substituted clinical placement with 10%, 25% or 50% simulation-based activities — no statistically significant differences were found in the practice of 666 student nurses six months after graduation (Hayden et al., 2014). Similar but smaller scale studies in Australia in professional physiotherapy education identified similar outcomes for physiotherapy graduates (Watson et al., 2012; Blackstock et al., 2013).

In 2010, a critical review in the context of medical education summarised the 12 best features and practices for SBE as follows: curriculum integration, outcome measures, simulation fidelity, skill acquisition and maintenance, team training, feedback, deliberate practice, mastery learning, transfer to practice, high-stakes testing, instructor training, and educational and professional context (McGaghie et al., 2010). Although many of these features are part of the current discourse in healthcare simulation educational practice and research, some remain highly contested (e.g. fidelity), others have gathered high-level evidence (e.g. mastery learning), while others continue to be investigated (e.g. feedback, instructor training). We explore some of these ideas in this chapter.

Any educational practices must be ethical and in simulation this has even greater importance since SBE has the potential for harm, despite somewhat ironically the safety it often espouses. SBE is safe for patients (since they are not directly involved) but it may be unsafe for learners as tasks, environments and outcomes can be manipulated, learners can be pushed beyond their competence and debriefing can place learners at risk, at times threatening their identity. Emmerich and colleagues (2018) explored the role of virtue ethics in SBE while, Sanko Nestel and colleagues (2018) have raised the importance of humanism in SBE, especially with reference to simulated participants.

SBE has many features that may be harder to foster in clinical contexts, including:

- being truly learner-centred since no real patients are present;
- orienting learners to clinical environments;
- designing learning opportunities to acquire specific elements of clinical practice;
- breaking clinical activities into components so that competence in each can be achieved before moving to the next;
- individualising learning activities;
- standardising learning opportunities;
- slowing down or speeding up clinical activities to a pace that supports teaching and learning;
- providing repetitive practice with feedback to achieve competence prior to clinical practice;
- increasing progressively the level of complexity of clinical activities;
- providing learners with the opportunity to work at the edges of their competence;
- ensuring that learners have exposure to infrequently occurring clinical events;
- video-assisted debriefing, since there are no real patients;
- providing linked learning activities following learning through simulation, such as reflective writing, case discussions, workshops and sequential scenarios.

SBE is often characterised by briefing (intentional preparation for learning activity) and debriefing (focused discussions on what was done, how, why and what next) activities, although these features have relevance for learning and teaching in the workplace.

An exciting area of development is conducting simulation in clinical settings, often referred to as in situ simulation, although this language has recently been contested (Posner et al., 2017). Kneebone and colleagues (2004) described the benefits of enabling learners to move between simulated and real clinical settings as their expertise develops (Kneebone et al., 2004). Locating simulation facilities near to clinical ones has many benefits since this movement between settings is enabled.

There is almost nothing that cannot be simulated, at least in part! What is important is making sensible decisions about what is optimally and feasibly taught and learned using simulation.

Theories, principles and concepts that inform simulation-based education

In any educational practice, theories, principles and concepts play an important role. For contemporary SBE this includes theories from the traditions of behaviourism, cognitivism and constructivism. Battista and Nestel (in press) describe key theories linked to these traditions that are often cited in SBE literature. They include theories, principles and concepts such as mastery learning, deliberate practice, instructional design, cognitive load, scaffolding, zone of proximal development, participatory learning and reflective practice. They also note the emerging discussion of complexity theory in SBE. As it is beyond the scope of this chapter to discuss these in depth, we direct readers to other chapters in this book and the references at the end of this chapter. However, we make an exception for mastery learning and the interrelated concepts of instructional design and deliberate practice, as well as those relating to complexity theory that fall under the banner of sociomateriality.

Mastery learning draws on the concepts of *instructional design* and *deliberate practice*. It is characterised by a focus on individual rather than time-based milestones, on baseline and progressive testing, on the clear description of learning objectives, on the development of sequenced skills and on opportunities for repetitive practice with feedback (McGaghie, 2015a). Instructional design draws on cognitive load theory that considers the mental effort to manage a task and points to specific types of 'load'. Reedy (2015) describes the role of cognitive load for SBE. Deliberate practice is a particular approach to the development of expertise in which a highly motivated individual has opportunities to repetitively practise and receive feedback on their performance (Ericsson, 2015). Additionally, the learner sets goals incrementally beyond their current stage of development. It is easy to see how simulation works so well with this approach. It has particular relevance to the development of clinical examination and procedural skills with simulation modalities such as task trainers, manikins and simulated patients.

Sociomaterial theories (e.g. complexity theory, cultural historical activity theory and actor-network theory) focus on the recognition of the collective dynamics of learners and influences that materials have on their thoughts, attitudes, behaviours and interactions with others (Ericsson, 2015). Complexity theory lends itself to the development of SBE scenarios and debriefing in terms of exploring simple, complicated or complex interactions, the linear or non-linear processes of a skill/task, and the rapidly changing or unpredictable nature of clinical practice. Key principles of complexity theory that may be incorporated into the design of clinical scenarios include emergence (acknowledging diverse ways of thinking, acting and responding to change), materiality (equipment and environmental considerations), attunement (to what is unfolding during a scenario), disturbance (promoting/amplifying disturbances or routine practice) and experimentation (through provision of diverse learning and feedback/debriefing opportunities) (Fenwick & Dahlgren, 2015).

Simulation frameworks

The use of a framework to design SBE promotes and strengthens learning (Fenwick & Dahlgren, 2015). An additional benefit includes enhancing the quality of reporting SBE research. Cheng and colleagues (2016) identify the following items as essential for reporting in SBE research: participants' orientation, simulator type, simulation environment, simulation event/scenario, instructional design, and feedback or debriefing approach. These items should probably fit within any SBE framework. Several approaches to designing SBE have been presented in the literature. Examples include frameworks for nursing education

(Alexander et al., 2015), interprofessional manikin-based simulation (Dieckmann, 2009), and instructional design and media selection (Chiniara et al., 2013).

In the following sections we discuss two frameworks that have widespread application and relevance for different learner populations, learning focus, simulation modality and setting.

- The ISTEL framework was developed from a literature review, methodological design and findings from a doctoral study on the SBE in physiotherapy. The development of this framework is presented elsewhere (Gough et al., 2016).

- The NHET-Sim framework is used in a national faculty development program in Australia and offers a systematic approach to the design of any simulation-based learning activity (The NHET-Sim Monash Team, 2012). It draws on theories that inform broader educational practice.

The ISTEL framework

The ISTEL framework provides a structured approach to the design, implementation and evaluation of SBE. It integrates three interlinking components — preparation, intervention and evaluation/research — which are divided into eight elements: 1) learner, 2) facilitator, 3) theories and educational practices, 4) learning design characteristics, 5) pre-brief and debrief, 6) linked learning activities, 7) outcomes, and 8) economic evaluation (see Fig. 13.1). It is acknowledged that these elements will be subject to differing factors, which may include staffing, equipment and logistical (e.g. accessibility/timetabling) considerations, as well as financial constraints. These factors should be accounted for when designing SBE interventions to promote

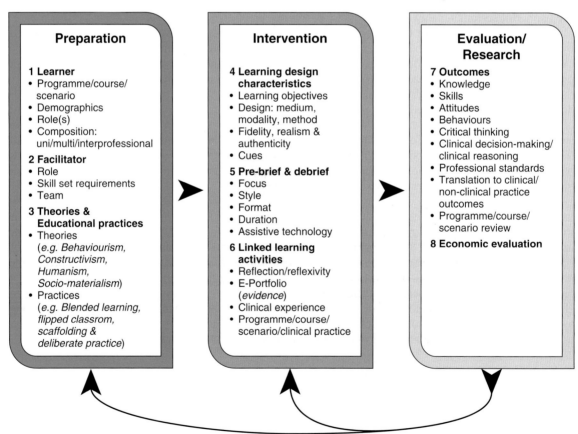

Figure 13.1: Integrated simulation and technology enhanced learning (ISTEL) framework (version 2)

Source: Copyright Manchester Metropolitan University, 2016. Authored by Suzanne Gough.

equitable learning experiences that are scalable and sustainable within an organisation. To illustrate, we provide an example of a manikin-based scenario to enhance effective teamwork and explore unconscious bias (see case study 13.1 later in the chapter) within a cardiorespiratory module at a university or for student physiotherapists on clinical placement. The costs of designing, piloting and delivering this simulation scenario are presented in Table 13.1 later in the chapter.

The preparation component

The first component is preparation, which features three elements: learner, facilitator and identification of relevant theories and educational practices. It is valuable to use or develop a scenario design template to document the components. This permits consistency of design and documentation of scenarios and standardisation of delivery between staff (facilitators, technicians and simulated patients).

Learner In this context, learners are defined as participants who engage in the SBE intervention with the purpose of developing knowledge, skills, attitudes and behaviours relevant to professional practice. The overall number of learners will influence design considerations relating to the roles that the learners will be required to play during the intervention (simulation activity). The allocation of learners to clearly defined observer roles and scenario participants permits greater numbers to be actively involved in the intervention, while promoting vicarious learning (O'Regan et al., 2016). This is illustrated in case study 13.1. There are a number of factors that may affect the decision to include learners from the same and/or different professional groups, such as the overall number of learners, the logistics of timetabling, access to simulation facilities/clinical areas or equipment and the availability of facilitators.

Facilitator Considerations include defining the roles and number of facilitators required to provide equitable, scalable and sustainable learning experiences. Further detailed considerations of the essential facilitator skills set requirements are comprehensively detailed elsewhere (Department of Health, 2011; INACSL, 2016a). The number of facilitators will probably depend on local need and availability. A document published by the Department of Health in the United Kingdom (UK) (2011) recommends the identification of a strategic lead facilitator, who should ensure that staff and learners have access to relevant simulation and technology to appropriately meet clearly defined curricula/patient/service needs.

Theories and educational practices Consideration of appropriate learning theories and educational practices will influence the design of the intervention (learning design characteristics, pre-briefing and debriefing, linked learning activities) and evaluation or research components. Several theories, concepts and educational practices have already been outlined. Educational practices such as the flipped classroom approach (Roehl et al., 2013) may be desirable in some circumstances, to ensure that all learners have the desired prerequisite knowledge prior to participating in a scenario. However, it is not always possible to provide preparatory learning or pre-simulation exercises. The need to provide additional opportunities for deliberate practice (Ericsson, 2015) to achieve mastery (McGaghie, 2015a) of professional competencies or capabilities will also influence the design of the intervention (simulation activity).

The intervention component

The intervention component focuses on three elements: learning design characteristics, pre-brief and debrief, and linked learning activities.

Learning design characteristics Considerations relate to the identification of learning objectives, the creation of a safe learning environment through effective instructional design (medium, modality and methods) of the simulation activity, pre-briefing and debriefing requirements, and the development of linked learning activities. All of these activities should be clearly documented, ideally on a scenario design template. In addition, role profile templates can be used to provide clear information for participants involved in the simulation activity such as facilitators and/or simulated patients (SPs). The development of learning objectives has been reported as an important aspect of developing SBE resources (McGaghie, 2015b; INACSL, 2016a). Learning objectives should address all domains of learning, be correlated to the learner's level and experience, correspond to the overall course or curriculum outcomes, feature evidence-based practice and be achievable within a realistic timeframe (INACSL, 2016b). For example, using a behaviourist approach, the development of learning activities starts with the objectives, such as desired achievement of changes in the cognitive (knowledge), psychomotor (skills) and affective (attitude) domains, which are often written in SMART format: specific, measurable, achievable, relevant and timed (Gould, 2009). A cognitive approach focuses on the learning process, rather than content, and places more emphasis on understanding in the learning objectives (Gould, 2009), whereas in a humanistic approach learning is considered to be both learner-centred and learner-driven (Gould, 2009).

Instructional design principles may be used to facilitate the design of SBE (Schaefer et al., 2011; Chiniara et al., 2013). It is important that the most appropriate simulation modality is selected to enable learners to achieve the learning objectives (Department of Health, 2011; Chiniara et al., 2013). The Department of Health (2011) recommends that the simulation design should be reviewed regularly to ensure that its application continues to meet the needs of learners and provides value for money. The instructional design medium refers to the mode of delivery (e.g. textbook learning, lectures, e-learning or simulation), modality is the characteristics that affect the learning experience (e.g. computer-based, simulated patient, procedural simulation or simulated clinical immersion) and method is either self-directed or facilitator-led learning (Chiniara et al., 2013). Chiniara's 'zone of simulation matrix' may be used to help identify learning activities that are most suited to SBE (Chiniara et al., 2013). Additional factors influencing simulation design considerations may include the accessibility and availability of specialist equipment and environments, timetabling and staffing constraints, and financial costs.

Once the learning outcomes and most appropriate/optimal simulation design have been selected, the focus is directed towards consideration of fidelity, realism and authenticity requirements. There is currently no universally adopted definition of fidelity in healthcare. The INACSL standards define fidelity as believability or 'the degree to which a simulated experience approaches reality; as fidelity increases realism increases' (INACSL, 2016c). Fidelity can also be defined according to several dimensions including physical (environmental and equipment factors), psychological (emotions, beliefs and learner self-awareness) and conceptual (realistic relationship of elements within the scenario, e.g. the vital sign parameters accurately reflect the diagnosis) (INACSL, 2016c; Lopreiato, 2016). While fidelity is sometimes used synonymously with realism and authenticity (INACSL, 2016c), Bland and colleagues (2014) differentiate between fidelity and authenticity and their contribution to learning. They define simulation fidelity as the close as possible reproduction of object reality, while authenticity is considered to be a subjective interpretation or response in relation to a constructed interactional situation between learners, facilitators and varying degrees of technology fidelity. Thus, as the interpretation of authenticity can be highly variable, increasing fidelity and realism does not necessarily increase authenticity.

Intricate cues can be incorporated into scenarios to guide the learners to achieve the overall learning objectives. Careful consideration of the learners' demographics is required to ensure optimal cognitive load (Reedy, 2015) to enable achievement of the learning objectives. Specific design considerations relating to antecedent cures (e.g. temporal, interpersonal and covert cues) are provided elsewhere (Burton et al., 1996; INACSL, 2016c). The incorporation of conceptual and reality cues to enhance the conceptual dimension of fidelity/realism and aid achievement of the learning objectives is also detailed by others (Ahmed et al., 2012). In addition, verbal and/or written cues can be provided by facilitators/simulated patients to enable learners to discriminate conditions for behaving in a way that returns the desired consequence in a scenario (e.g. normalisation of physiological responses to a given intervention).

Pre-brief and debrief Both of these phases have common design and implementation considerations relating to the focus, style, format, duration and use of assistive technology. It is important to outline the specific format of the pre-brief within the scenario design template, including specification of the role of facilitators, technicians (where required/available) and learners during the simulation activity and debrief. This may be provided to the learners in advance or immediately before they participate in the simulation activity. Separate briefings may be offered to simulated patients (Nestel & Gough, 2018) so as not to reveal pertinent information ahead of time to the learners.

The style of pre-brief/debrief refers to face-to-face or digital resource considerations (e.g. incorporation of an orientation video of the simulation and debrief facilities, which can be particularly useful to learners prior to their first exposure to the equipment and/or environment). The provision of pre-brief information for learners also includes clarification of the use of assisted technology and may include: 1) providing video podcasts to provide an orientation to the facilities or simulated patient introduction to set the scene during the pre-brief; 2) establishing consent for video recording or live streaming; and 3) specifying whether video recordings will be used during the debrief or made available for linked learning activities. Establishing the duration of the pre-brief is advisable, particularly when this is to be factored into a timetabled teaching session. Pre-briefing or briefing immediately prior to the simulation activity provide an important opportunity to establish the similarities and differences between the scenario and reality (Nestel & Gough, 2018).

The scenario design template should clearly outline the focus, style, format, duration and use of assisted technology during the debrief. While there is currently no gold standard approach to debriefing, key considerations to optimise debriefing practices have been published (Sawyer et al., 2016; INACSL, 2016d). Typically, debriefing occurs within-event or post-event (Sawyer et al., 2016; Nestel & Gough, 2018) and may be described as facilitator-guided or self-guided. Multiple debriefing structures have been published — examples include debriefing with good judgment (Rudolph et al., 2006), TeamGAINS (Kolbe et al., 2013), promoting excellence and reflective learning (PEARLS) (Eppich & Cheng, 2015) and the diamond debrief (Jaye et al., 2015). Sawyer and colleagues (2016) provide a critical review of different simulation debriefing methods. Optimal timing, duration, format and use of video within debriefing have yet to be defined (Grant et al., 2010; Ahmed et al., 2012; Krogh et al., 2016; Nestel & Gough, 2018). Guidelines for the use of debriefing and video-assisted debriefing have been published (Krogh et al., 2015; Nestel & Gough, 2018; INACSL, 2016d), but evidence of the optimal use remains unclear. Krogh and colleagues (2015) identified that the value of the role of the debriefer is often underestimated, and a new model (the practice development triangle) has been proposed to provide insight into how organisations may seek to develop expert debriefers (Krogh et al., 2016).

Linked learning activities Considerations include the development of post-debrief activities. Examples may include further post-simulation reflection, provision of additional study tasks focusing on key learning objectives and formalisation of links action plans arising from the debrief or identification of related learning opportunities (e.g. a more complex scenario later in the debrief/course/clinical placement). The provision of digital resources (e.g. small video excerpts/vodcasts) arising from simulation-based activities has the potential to enhance the learner's educational experiences and facilitate repetitive post-event reflection (Gough, 2018). These may be incorporated into e-portfolios or web folios by learners as evidence of personal and professional development. Such linked learning activities may be voluntary or mandatory, depending on the reason for the simulation activity being developed (e.g. inclusion of part of course, academic module, clinical placement or informal learning opportunity in practice).

The evaluation/research component

The final component has two elements that focus on designing and undertaking meaningful evaluation of the outcomes of simulation-based learning activities and identification of the associated economic costs.

Outcomes Evaluation and research of SBE require careful consideration to ensure that they are meaningful and representational, in order to drive changes in simulation preparation and intervention and ultimately impact on healthcare practice. Evaluation considerations may focus on observation, measurement and/or exploration of knowledge, skills (performance/retention), attitudes, behaviours (e.g. non-technical skills), critical thinking, clinical decision-making, clinical reasoning, professional standards, translation to clinical/non-clinical practice outcomes, and program course or scenario review. It is essential that an evaluation of the simulation preparation and intervention is undertaken to evaluate the effectiveness and/or assess the achievement of the desired outcomes and value for money (Department of Health, 2011; TRAC Development Group, 2015; INACSL, 2016b). There is no universally accepted approach to evaluation, due to the tensions derived from the diversity of instructional design and application of SBE in healthcare (Inventures, 2010; Maloney & Haines, 2016; Lin et al., 2018). Additionally, it is important to establish key timeframes for evaluation and in research that are appropriate and will generate meaningful information. The actual timing of such evaluation/research data collection may be determined by the timetabling of teaching and assessment activities, clinical placement timing or optimal timeframes within a research study (e.g. repeated measures over a period of time).

Economic evaluation It is widely acknowledged that SBE in healthcare education and practice can be costly. However, publication of SBE costs and return on investment is scarce (Black & Marcoux, 2002). Black and Marcoux (2002) reported delivery costs of US$1760.60 for 19 physiotherapy students completing a 90-minute SP-based physiotherapy scenario and Shoemaker and colleagues (2011) identified a cost of US$500 for 64 physiotherapy and occupational therapy students participating in a 4-hour exercise featuring three complex SP-based scenarios. However, the true cost of designing and implementing this intervention was under-reported, as the authors acknowledged their figure did not account for actual staff time for the design and implementation.

The UK Department of Health has stated that the facilitation lead should be able to evidence the appropriate integration of SBE, value for money, equity of access and evaluation of provisions to ensure that simulation interventions meet the needs of the learners and organisation (Department of Health, 2011). There are many ways to conduct economic evaluations in healthcare including cost description analysis, cost minimisation analysis, cost effectiveness analysis, cost utility analysis, cost benefit analysis and cost consequence analysis. Guidance on undertaking economic evaluations is provided elsewhere (Kernick, 2003; Maloney & Haines, 2016; Lin et al., 2018; Nestel, Brazil et al., 2018).

TABLE 13.1: Detailed example of total costs for designing and delivery of the physiotherapy case study

TRAC component	Description (requirements for 16 learners: 4 groups, 3-hour session)	Total ($)
Pay costs	1 facilitator: scenario design, pilot scenario, 3-hour session delivery including debrief (6 hours) 1 technician: pilot session, set up and clear away, session delivery including debrief and uploading videos (5 hours)	618
Indirect costs	Estates and facilities costs for specialist teaching space	303
Non-pay costs	Sleeping bag, acute illness management consumables kit, authentic odour creation (alcohol, cigarette smoke, urine and aftershave) and charity shop clothes	75
Total		996
Ongoing delivery costs for 16 learners: 4 groups, 3-hour session		
Pay costs	1 facilitator: session delivery including debrief (3 hours) 1 technician: set up and clear away, session delivery including debrief and uploading videos (4 hours)	371
Indirect costs	Estates and facilities costs for specialist teaching space	168
Non-pay costs	Acute illness management consumables kit, authentic odour creation (alcohol, cigarette smoke, urine and aftershave), and laundering of clothes and sleeping bag	36
Total		575
TRAC component	Description (requirements for 4 learners: 1 group, 1 hour session)	Total ($)
Pay costs	1 facilitator: scenario design, pilot scenario, 1-hour session delivery including debrief (3 hours) 1 technician: pilot session, set up and clear away, session delivery including debrief and uploading videos (3 hours)	395
Indirect costs	Estates and facilities costs for specialist teaching space	225
Non-pay costs	Sleeping bag, acute illness management consumables kit, authentic odour creation (alcohol, cigarette smoke, urine and aftershave) and charity shop clothes	75
Total		695
Ongoing delivery costs for 4 learners: 1 group, 3-hour session		
Pay costs	1 facilitator: session delivery including debrief (1 hour) 1 technician: pilot session, set up and clear away, session delivery including debrief and uploading videos (3 hours)	150
Indirect costs	Estates and facilities costs for specialist teaching space	56
Non-pay costs	Acute illness management consumables kit, authentic odour creation (alcohol, cigarette smoke, urine and aftershave) and laundering of clothes and sleeping bag	36
Total		242

Source: Copyright Manchester Metropolitan University, 2017. Authored by Suzanne Gough.

In Table 13.1, we provide a cost description for case study 13.1, which was undertaken using the transparent approach to costing (TRAC) method (TRAC Development Group, 2015). The total cost is calculated by adding individual staff pay costs, indirect costs and non-pay costs for the design, pilot and delivery of the SBE intervention. As the resources for utilising SBE are finite, it is important to identify the optimal delivery methods to maximise the achievement of learning objectives (Maloney & Haines, 2016). Economic evaluations can also be used to determine the optimal use of SBE resources and inform decision-making for scarce resource allocation within education and clinical practice (Maloney & Haines, 2016; Lin et al., 2018; Nestel, Brazil et al., 2018). Additionally, economic evaluation can be used to determine the value, scalability and sustainability of SBE.

The NHET-Sim framework

The NHET-Sim framework has been described elsewhere (The NHET-Sim Monash Team, 2012) and is summarised here. The six phases represent a cycle of educational design: preparing, briefing, simulation activity, feedback and/or debriefing, reflecting and evaluating (see Fig. 13.2). To illustrate the framework, we provide an example of a simulated patient-based scenario designed to support the development of patient-centred communication skills and clinical judgment — see case study 13.2 later in the chapter.

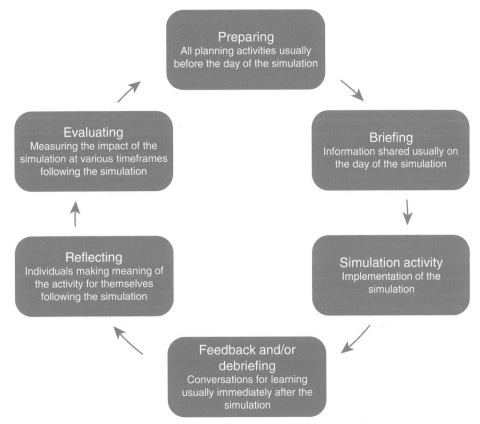

Figure 13.2: NHET-Sim program framework: phases in simulation design
Source: Copyright 2016, Manchester Metropolitan University, Authored by Suzanne Gough

The **preparing** phase includes all planning activities that occur usually before the day of the simulation. This includes: identifying learners' needs, articulating learning objectives, and locating or aligning them with a curriculum (if there is one) or with other clinical activities; consulting with learners, subject matter experts, patients or others as deemed appropriate; developing the learning activity; and identifying the most suitable simulator, setting, medical equipment, props etc. Logistics need to be considered and will depend on local simulation facilities. It is often important to rehearse simulation activities to ensure that they are feasible within the timeframe and will provide the learning opportunity that is intended.

On the day of the simulation, learners and others involved in the simulation activity are briefed. The importance of the **briefing** phase sometimes goes unrecognised but it is essential for optimal learning. Although often briefed separately, faculty and learners (and anyone else involved in the simulation) will probably need information on the learning objectives; the learners' characteristics; logistics such as timeframes, starting, pausing and ending the simulation activity; simulator programing; technical support; communication with the control room (if there is one); audio-visual capability; debriefing and feedback processes; reflective exercises; evaluation forms etc. (Nestel & Gough, 2018). It is also important for learners to consider their own objectives within the parameters of the simulation activity. Learners must be oriented to the simulation, the simulator and the setting in which it occurs. Observing students can be given active roles (O'Regan et al., 2016), the outcomes of which can be shared during the debriefing/feedback. Because in simulation the learning environment can be manipulated, it can be stressful for participants as they are usually being observed with judgments being made about their performance. The way that these judgments are invited and how they are later shared is crucially important. Establishing a trusting relationship with learners is important. Before the simulation commences, it is helpful to ask whether there are any further questions.

The **simulation activity** phase hopefully plays out as planned. For example, learners working with task trainers to develop psychomotor skills for a procedural skill may receive concurrent (during) feedback from peers and/or experts, or the feedback may be generated by the simulator. In scenario-based simulations, there may be a pause and discuss option in which a 'time out' is called and discussion occurs about what has happened so far, what the next best steps are and how they might be achieved. Although unexpected events sometimes occur, if the briefing has been successful and trust has been established, valuable learning may still occur. Observers should be enabled to undertake their tasks. If audio-visual recording is occurring, it should be started and notations made for use during the next phase.

Immediately after the simulation, the **feedback and/or debriefing** phase occurs. There are many published approaches to feedback/debriefing that are theory-based (Rudolph et al., 2006), empirically based (Arora et al., 2012; Ahmed et al., 2013), experience-based (Pendleton et al., 1998; Phrampus & O'Donnell, 2013; Jaye et al., 2015) or a combination of all (Sawyer et al., 2016). Several of these were shared above for the ISTEL framework. Some debriefing/feedback approaches have developed from teaching and learning in real clinical settings and have been applied to SBE while others have emanated from SBE. There is no single 'best' way to debrief/feedback. As above, after task-trainer simulations, feedback may be described as terminal (referring to timing) and may be offered by peers and/or experts or be simulator-generated. Following scenario-based simulations, facilitators usually explore learners' feelings and experiences of the simulation, address learning objectives, explore unplanned issues, summarise learning, affirm positive behaviours and establish new goals.

Although one goal of debriefing/feedback is to promote **reflection**, in the NHET-Sim program reflection is considered as important as debriefing/feedback and so it has its own phase. It is during reflection that individuals make meaning of the simulation activity for themselves, relative to their past, current and future practice. This phase also includes setting goals and so encompasses the notion of feeding forward, making plans to maintain or develop future practice. Of course, there is overlap between these phases and reflecting can occur during briefing, the simulation activity and debriefing.

Evaluating refers mainly to the extent to which the simulation activity supported the learner in meeting the objectives. Nestel and Gough (2018) describe how this phase benefits from the involvement of all stakeholders, although practically it often involves only learners, faculty and simulated participants. Complex learning interventions may require equally complex evaluations, using qualitative and quantitative methods, drawing on multiple sources, and triangulating data alongside different levels of impact and in different timeframes (Nestel & Gough, 2018).

Having described these phases, it may seem that SBE is extraordinarily complex with so many considerations. However, simulations can also occur almost spontaneously and could still be represented by this framework. For example, a medical student on a clinical placement in the emergency department is required to close a patient's wound. The medical student has previously learned suturing in a clinical skills lab but she has little experience in a clinical setting. The patient is ready, the wound has been cleansed, local anaesthesia administered and consent obtained for the student to complete the task. Immediately prior to closing the wound under supervision, the student quickly refreshes her skill by first using a suture pad to rehearse the technique. *Preparing* involves ensuring access to appropriate simulators and kit, the student identifies her strengths and areas for development before starting, she is observed and given *feedback*, immediately *reflects* on her performance before attending to the patient. The whole event from preparation to reflection takes minutes. After closing the wound, the student and faculty may *evaluate* the simulation activity in preparing her for the task.

Case study 13.1: A scenario designed using the ISTEL framework to enhance effective teamwork and explore unconscious bias

The following information provides details of the design, implementation and evaluation considerations of a scenario to replicate the hospital ward environment within a university. In clinical practice this scenario could be undertaken in a clinical ward area. The learners are required to participate in pairs in a 20-minute scenario. Two learners adopt the role of student physiotherapists who are asked to undertake the assessment and provide initial physiotherapy management for a deteriorating patient who has recently been admitted to hospital.

The preparation component

Learners

The learners are final-year pre-registration physiotherapy students. Physiotherapy class sizes vary between 16 and 30 students. This simulation activity was designed for a group of 16 physiotherapy students and timetabled for a 3-hour session within a cardiorespiratory module. Options for delivery with groups of four students (e.g. on clinical placement) are also provided.

Facilitator

The implementation of this scenario required two facilitators, with experience of facilitation skills, operating a computerised patient manikin (simulator) and video-assisted debriefing. The facilitator/technician operating the simulator is also responsible for the audio-visual equipment used to livestream and record the scenario. At least one facilitator should have experience and skills in both facilitation and debriefing, to provide continuity for the learners of the transition between the simulation activity and debrief.

Theories and educational practices

The scenario design was influenced by social constructivism and sociomaterial (complexity) theoretical perspectives (Ericsson, 2015; Fenwick & Dahlgren, 2015). The scenario aims to simulate the complexity of physiotherapy practice when managing an acutely deteriorating patient within a hospital ward setting. The complexity of the scenario promotes the learners to use their prior knowledge and clinical skills, coupled with critical thinking and clinical decision-making skills to provide optimal patient management without unconscious bias. Learning is thus socially situated and knowledge is constructed through interaction with others during the scenario and debrief.

The scenario builds on prior cardiorespiratory physiotherapy and acute illness management knowledge and skills, which have been embedded throughout the pre-registration physiotherapy curriculum. Relevant prior learning resources including lectures, study tasks and skills videos are provided via the virtual learning environment (e.g. Moodle platform). This flipped classroom approach provides learners with access to resources in order to develop prerequisite knowledge and skills (McGaghie, 2015b). Scaffolding is provided by the facilitator during the scenario and debrief by offering varying levels of support to help the learners reach higher levels of comprehension and skill acquisition that they may not be able to achieve without assistance. Vicarious learning is promoted by providing learners with specific tasks to undertake as an observer (O'Regan et al., 2016).

The intervention component

Learning design characteristics

The scenario is designed to support the learners (student physiotherapists) in:

- demonstrating safe and effective assessment and management of an acutely deteriorating medical in-patient;
- demonstrating clinical reasoning and problem-solving skills to select, plan, justify and evaluate the assessment and treatment of patients with uncomplicated, predictable cardiorespiratory pathology;
- critically discussing unconscious biases that may arise during the management of patients.

This scenario is designed to augment but not replace clinical practice.

Design, fidelity, realism, authenticity and cues

The instructional medium includes high-fidelity (equipment, environmental and psychological) simulation, featuring a computerised patient simulator (manikin) situated on a hospital bed in a simulated side room. An immersive clinical simulation (modality) is used to replicate two acutely deteriorating medical in-patients (Mr Tony Johnson or Mr John Flemming). The instructional method includes facilitator-guided learning during the scenario and debrief. A high degree of realism is achieved through the use of authentic artefacts (equipment and environment) and scenario design to replicate the complexities of the clinical situation.

Cues are pre-programed onto the manikin software package to provide realistic physiological timing of responses to interventions. Interpersonal cues (verbal prompts) are outlined in the scenario design template and patient role profiles. Verbal, visual patient monitor display and written cues are provided to enable the learners to discriminate between conditions and prompt the desired consequence to actions as they unfold during the scenario (e.g. normalisation of physiological status in response to appropriate physiotherapy intervention). Differences in the room odour and cleanliness of the manikins and the application of tattoo sleeves to Mr Johnson are intended to stimulate potential unconscious biases during the scenario.

Scenario design template

The scenario design template contains details of the specific requirements including equipment list, pictures of the environmental setup, operational requirements, information as to how the scenario will progress, manikin programing information and debriefing requirements. A patient role profile is also developed featuring specific information/cues that are to be provided to the learners during the scenario.

Pre-brief and debrief

Pre-brief

The facilitator is required to work with all 16 learners in groups of four during this 3-hour session. Each group of students participates in one of the two scenarios (Mr Johnson or Mr Flemming). Group members are required to allocate roles: two observers (one person to draw a concept map of the scenario and one to complete the checklist of observations relating to clinical and non-technical skills) and two active participants in the scenario (student physiotherapists). The facilitator provides the pre-brief information to all groups at the start of the session (10 minutes). The simulation activity (scenario) rotation takes approximately 20 minutes per group and all learners then participate in a 1-hour facilitator-guided post-event group debrief.

Note: If the session is to be undertaken with one group of four students (e.g. on clinical placement) the timings can be modified as follows: 5–10 minute briefing, 20–minute simulation activity and 20–minute debrief.

Pre-brief synopsis

- Mr Tony Johnson: Nurse Foster has referred Mr Johnson for a respiratory physiotherapy assessment, as she is concerned that he has developed a chest infection. There is very limited history available. Over the past few days he has become tired, increasingly short of breath with a cough productive of dark-green sputum. In the early hours of this morning he suddenly became worse and admitted himself to the emergency department. On admission, he was in possession of an open can of alcohol and was moderately intoxicated. His possessions include a sleeping bag and small rucksack of clothing, which is heavily soiled and smells of urine, nicotine and alcohol.
- Mr John Flemming: Nurse Foster has referred Mr Fleming for a respiratory physiotherapy assessment, as she is concerned that he has developed a chest infection. There is very limited history available. The patient is not able to give a history and the information has been provided by his daughter on admission. Mr Fleming is a 69-year-old man with chronic obstructive pulmonary disease (COPD). Over the past few days he has become tired, increasingly short of breath with a cough productive of dark-green sputum. In the early hours of this morning he suddenly became worse and was admitted to the emergency department from home.

Simulation activity

Two simulation rooms are set up to simulate the equipment and environment of a single-bedded hospital side room. An acute illness management consumables kit is provided in the room on a trolley. The manikin in each room is dressed according to the patient role profile information:

- Mr Johnson is lying in the bed dressed in soiled clothing with a tattoo sleeve on each arm. A bag of clothes is placed at the bedside along with a sleeping bag. All items of Mr Johnson's clothing should be nicotine-stained and smell of urine and alcohol.
- Mr Flemming is dressed in clean clothing and the room smells of men's aftershave.

Although the patient role profiles have different personal information, the presenting physiological signs and symptoms are identical.

A facilitator is required to offer support/assistance and cues throughout the scenario. The other facilitator/technician should be positioned in the control room to operate the manikin software, provide verbal responses to learners through the voice of the manikin and operate the audio-visual equipment

The observers in each group complete the observations and concept maps. This can be undertaken from within the simulated environment via an observation window or by watching a livestream of the scenario.

Debrief

A 1-hour facilitator-guided debrief is scheduled immediately after the last group has completed its scenario. The facilitator incorporates feedback from the active participants and observers (including completed checklist information and concept maps) to explore achievement of the learning objectives. The SHARP debriefing tool is used to provide a structured debrief (Ahmed et al., 2013). The concept map information can be used to illustrate any differences and similarities in the assessment and management of the two patients (Mr Flemming and Mr Johnson). An action plan is agreed relating to future modifications to improve clinical practice (and specific to this scenario, to minimise the influence of potential unconscious biases).

Linked learning activities

Specific linked learning activities are provided to enhance and consolidate the scenario and overall module learning outcomes. These include:

- written activities to direct the learners to develop problem lists and evidence-based management plans;
- workshop activities to consolidate core cardiorespiratory physiotherapy skills pertinent in readiness of forthcoming clinical placements;
- unconscious bias resources to supplement the debrief discussions.

When a video recording of the simulation activity is generated, this permits copies to be made available to the groups via the virtual learning environment. This provides opportunities for further post-event reflection, which can be embedded by learners into their e-portfolio or web folio.

Note: These activities can similarly be provided if the simulation activity is undertaken on clinical placement.

The evaluation/research component

Outcomes

The overall module learning outcomes are assessed via a 40-minute oral clinical reasoning and practical examination at the end of the term. The learners are required to demonstrate three aspects of physiotherapy practice related to a patient case study, followed by an oral clinical reasoning discussion based on the physiotherapy management provided. The module assessment design allows the learners to:

- demonstrate their ability to relate the structure and function of the cardiorespiratory system to the pathology and clinical features of selected complex cardiorespiratory pathologies;
- plan, critically discuss and explain assessment, treatment and rehabilitation approaches for patients with selected complex cardiorespiratory pathologies;

- safely and accurately demonstrate physiotherapy assessment and management techniques for the selected pathologies;
- practise within the rules of professional conduct and communicate clearly and coherently using appropriate terminology.

Economic evaluation

The design, pilot and delivery costs for this 3-hour session have been calculated using the TRAC method and a detailed example is provided in Table 13.1.

Source: Copyright Manchester Metropolitan University, 2017. Authored by Suzanne Gough.

Case study 13.2: An example of an SP-based scenario to promote patient-centred communication skills and clinical judgment using the NHET-Sim framework

The patient has come into the emergency department in severe pain. The medical student is required to assess the patient and make a differential diagnosis. The patient has renal stone disease. The scenario is designed to support the medical student in:

- communicating effectively with a patient experiencing pain;
- obtaining relevant medical information from the patient;
- practising clinical decision-making.

Preparing

Tutor

- Ensure that the topic content aligns with the current stage of the curriculum (patient-centred communication and clinical judgment).
- Develop the scenario including the student task and SP role.
- Prepare student priming material and send to the students.
- Identify or develop an *observation* guide for observing students.
- Ensure room bookings and suitable facilities for video-assisted debriefing.
- Identify plan for feedback/debriefing.
- Prepare student reflection activities.
- Prepare evaluation forms for tutors, students and SPs.
- Ensure SP is booked and trained for role portrayal and feedback.
- Rehearse SP role with SP if it is a new one — check level of complexity for learners.

Students

- Complete written priming task.
  - How do you feel about your interview with the SP?
  - What skills do you want to focus on in your patient-centred interview? (List three.)
  - Is there anything specific you would like the tutor to observe and give you feedback on? Briefly outline.
  - Is there anything specific you would like the SP to observe and give you feedback on? Briefly outline.
- Review patient-centred interviewing skills.
- Review assessment questions for a patient experiencing pain.

Simulated patient

- Read the SP role and attend training and rehearsal for role portrayal and feedback.
  - You are Leon Walsh, a 54-year-old man who is married with three children and who works as a courier driver. Today you have had the most severe pain you have ever experienced. You were perfectly well until 6 hours ago when you developed an excruciating pain in your left loin which has moved to your groin. At one point you were rolling around the floor in pain. Nothing seemed to help. The pain was so bad you actually called out. It took about half an hour to settle. After it had passed, you felt totally drained. During the pain, you passed urine, which was a rose colour. You had no clots, no stinging, no adjustment to stream. After another 2 hours, the pain slowly came back

and you had the same experience all over again. That settled an hour ago during which time you came to hospital. You are very concerned that this is cancer. You have always worried about getting cancer. You have no real other clue about what else could cause this pain. You have no other symptoms. You have had no problems with your urine in the past. Actually, you have always kept very good health. You have never had pain like this before. If asked, the pain was 10/10! You are expecting that you will be examined in the emergency department and that tests will be done. You are relieved to speak with the medical student and look forward to the assessment by a doctor.

- Review responsibilities as an SP in formative assessments.

Briefing

Faculty/tutor

- The tutor will work with four students in the session, each of whom will interview a different patient in this 3-hour session.
- The rotation will take approximately 30 minutes: 10 minutes for briefing, 10 minutes in the simulation activity and 10 minutes in the debriefing/feedback.
- Meet the SP to make sure they are clear about their role.
- Ensure that the tutor can operate the audio-visual capture and replay.
- Inform the tutor of their role in briefing the students.

Students

- The tutor welcomes students. The tutor shares the learning objectives; reviews the interviewing student's priming activities; asks about prior experiences of simulation, assessing patients in pain and patient-centred communication skills; shares observation guide; offers time out; orientates to reflective activity; and checks for questions.
- Task: Mr Leon Walsh (54 years old) has come to the emergency department and is describing severe abdominal pain. Please assess him and consider a differential diagnosis.

Simulated patient

- Check that the SP knows this role in portrayal and feedback.
- Check that the SP knows logistics plan outlined above.
- The tutor shares student's goals with SP if different to learning objectives.
- Check whether any further questions.

Simulation activity

- SP is seated in the consultation room.
- Observers are seated appropriately.
- Audio-recording is started.
- Timing is noted.

Feedback and/or debriefing

- The tutor uses the following protocol but is also flexible to be responsive to the students and the SP.
  - *To interviewing student:* Can you briefly state how you felt during the interview? [Students should be encouraged to simply name the emotion/s they experienced and not the rationale or thoughts for those feelings. The purpose of this question is to raise the student's awareness of the link between feelings and behaviour.] Can you describe two aspects of the patient-centred interview that worked well? And of your pain assessment?
  - *To the SP:* Can you identify two communication skills that the student used that were effective?
  - *To the observer students*: Based on the observation guide, can you identify two communication skills that the student used that were effective?
  - The tutor provides specific feedback on skills that they observed that worked well.
  - The entire process is repeated, this time focusing on what could be improved.
  - One of the students summarises everything that has been discussed and the reflective activity is flagged.

- Video-assisted debriefing to facilitate the debriefing process.
  - Select two or three short clips of 30–45 seconds illustrative of achievement of the learning objectives and of areas for development; use to promote discussion.

Reflecting

- Students complete a written reflection based on their experience.
  - What did you learn during the simulation and debriefing about your patient-centred communication skills and clinical judgment?
  - What was similar to your prior experience? What was different?
  - How will you maintain the skills you were good at?
  - What knowledge do you need to better manage a situation like this?
  - What skills do you need to develop to better manage a situation like this?
  - How will you gain the knowledge and develop the skills?

Evaluating

- Students, faculty and tutors complete an evaluation form evaluating the extent to which the learning objectives were met, and the role of each simulation phase in achieving the objectives.

Source: Copyright 2016, Manchester Metropolitan University, Authored by Suzanne Gough

PRACTICAL TIPS

We offer the following practical tips for simulation practice. However, deeper reflection of values about learning and teaching are also important.

- Careful planning/preparation can be key to optimal learning outcomes.
- Actively build trust with learners, especially during the (pre-) briefing.
- Create safety for learners — do not assume it. This mainly occurs during the briefing and is then enacted during the simulation and the feedback/debriefing.
- Be clear about the learning objectives.
- Design the simulation activity with the objectives in mind, avoiding distractions — unless that is one of the objectives!
- Align SBE content with others types of learning activities.
- Choose a simulation modality that is fit for purpose; that is, the simulator that can best support the learner in meeting the learning objectives.
- Choose the simulation setting that optimises learning (e.g. in a clinical setting) balanced with convenience and clinical service needs.
- Use a simulation framework to avoid omissions.
- For scenario-based simulations, at a minimum do a run-through before using the scenario for the first time.
- Provide opportunities for learners to repeat the learning activity (or a related learning activity) in simulation and where possible in clinical practice too.
- Ensure that learners receive feedback on their performance.
- Encourage learners to reflect on their experiences and plan how they might use the learning in their practice.
- Build evaluation strategies into all SBE to create a process of quality improvement — it can be quite simple.
- Review standards for simulation practices and consult with simulation educators.

Conclusion

Simulation is an exciting educational method with tremendous relevance in health professional education. There are many facets of simulation practice that resonate with learning and teaching in clinical contexts. A key difference between the settings is that in simulation, learning can be truly learner-centred. However, in clinical settings, patients must always be at the centre of the care process and so being truly learner-centred is compromised. In simulation, there is an opportunity to adjust the learning activity to meet the needs of the learner, which is harder to achieve in clinical settings. The frameworks offered in this chapter provide a basis for bringing learning and teaching in both simulated and real settings together. Features of simulation, especially key practices during the briefing, observer roles during the simulation activity, feedback/debriefing and reflecting, all have relevance for supporting learning in clinical contexts too. The role of conversation for learning in SBE can have a profound impact on learners. Many of its principles are likely to be equally powerful in clinical contexts.

References

Ahmed, M., et al. (2012). Identifying best practice guidelines for debriefing in surgery: A tri-continental study. *The American Journal of Surgery, 203*, 523–529.

Ahmed, M., et al. (2013). Operation debrief: A SHARP improvement in performance feedback in the operating room. *Annals of Surgery, 258*(6), 958–963.

Alexander, M., et al. (2015). NCSBN simulation guidelines for prelicensure nursing programs. *Journal of Nursing Regulation, 6*(3), 39–42.

Arora, S., et al. (2012). Objective structured assessment of debriefing (OSAD): Bringing science to the art of debriefing in surgery. *Annals of Surgery, 256*(6), 982–988.

Battista, A., & Nestel, D. (in press). Simulation in medical education. In T. Swanwick (Ed.), *Understanding medical education*. Brisbane: Wiley.

Black, B., & Marcoux, B. (2002). Feasibility of using standardized patients in a physical therapist education program: A pilot study. *Journal of Physical Therapy, 16*(2), 49–56.

Blackstock, F. C., et al. (2013). Simulation can contribute part of a cardiorespiratory physiotherapy clinical education. *Simulation in Healthcare, 8*, 32–42.

Bland, A., Topping, A., & Torbell, J. (2014). Time to unravel the conceptual confusion of authenticity and fidelity and their contribution to learning within simulation-based nurse education. A discussion paper. *Nurse Education Today, 34*(7), 1112–1118.

Burton, J. K., Moore, D. M., & Magliaro, S. G. (1996). Behaviorism and instructional technology. In D. H. Jonassen (Ed.), *Handbook of research for educational communications and technology*. New York: Macmillan.

Cheng, A., et al. (2016). Reporting guidelines for health care simulation research: Extensions to the CONSORT and STROBE statements. *Advances in Simulation, 11*(1), 238–248.

Chiniara, G., et al. (2013). Simulation in healthcare: A taxonomy and a conceptual framework for instructional design and media selection. *Medical Teacher, 35*(8), 1380–1395.

Department of Health UK (2011). *A framework for technology enhanced learning*. London: Department of Health.

Dieckmann, P. (Ed.), (2009). *Using simulations for education, training and research*. Lengerich, MI: PABST.

Donaldson, L. (2009). *150 years of the chief medical officer's annual report 2008*. London: Department of Health.

Emmerich, N., Gormley, G., & McCullough, M. (2018). Ethics of healthcare simulation. In D. Nestel, et al. (Eds.), *Healthcare simulation education: Evidence, theory and practice* (pp. 121–126). Chichester, West Sussex: John Wiley & Sons.

Eppich, W., & Cheng, A. (2015). Promoting excellence and reflective learning in simulation (PEARLS): Development and rationale for a blended approach to health care simulation debriefing. *Simulation in Healthcare, 10*(2).

Ericsson, K. A. (2015). Acquisition and maintenance of medical expertise: A perspective from the expert-performance approach with deliberate practice. *Academic Medicine, 90*(11), 1471–1486.

Fenwick, T., & Dahlgren, M. A. (2015). Towards socio-material approaches in simulation-based education: Lessons from complexity theory. *Medical Education, 49*(4), 359–367.

Gaba, D. M. (2004). The future vision of simulation in health care. *Quality & Safety in Health Care, 13*(Suppl. 1), i2–i10.

Gough, S. (2018). Optimizing learning in simulation-based education using video reflexivity. In D. Nestel, et al. (Eds.), *Healthcare simulation education: Evidence, theory and practice* (pp. 171–180). Chichester, West Sussex: John Wiley & Sons.

Gough, S., Yohannes, A. M., & Murray, J. (2016). Using video-reflexive ethnography and simulation-based education to explore patient management and error recognition by pre-registration physiotherapists. *Advances in Simulation, 1*(1), 1–16.

Gould, J. (2009). *Learning theory ad classroom practice in lifelong learning sector*. Tavistock: Learning Matters.

Grant, J. S., et al. (2010). Using video-facilitated feedback to improve student performance following high-fidelity simulation. *Clinical Simulation in Nursing, 6*(5), e177–e184.

Hayden, J., et al. (2014). The NCSBN national simulation study: A longitudinal, randomized, controlled study replacing clinical hours with simulation in prelicensure. *Nursing Education, 5*(Suppl. 2), S1–S64.

INACSL. (2016a). Standards of Best Practice: SimulationSM facilitation. *Clinical Simulation in Nursing, 12*, S16–S20.

INACSL. (2016b). Standards of Best Practice: SimulationSM outcomes and objectives. *Clinical Simulation in Nursing, 12*, S13–S15.

INACSL. (2016c). Standards of Best Practice: SimulationSM simulation glossary. *Clinical Simulation in Nursing, 12*, S39–S47.

INACSL. (2016d). Standards of Best Practice: SimulationSM debriefing. *Clinical Simulation in Nursing, 12*, S21–S25.

Inventures (2010). *NHS simulation provision and use study summary report*. (Version 23). London: Department of Health.

Jaye, P., Thomas, L., & Reedy, G. (2015). 'The diamond': a structure for simulation debrief. *The Clinical Teacher, 12*, 171–175.

Kernick, D. P. (2003). Introduction to health economics for the medical practitioner. *Postgraduate Medical Journal, 79*(92), 147–150.

Kneebone, R., et al. (2010). Distributed simulation – accessible immersive training. *Medical Teacher, 32*(1), 65–70.

Kneebone, R. L., et al. (2004). Simulation and clinical practice: Strengthening the relationship. *Medical Education*, 38(10), 1095–1102.

Kolbe, M., et al. (2013). TeamGAINS: A tool for structured debriefings for simulation-based team trainings. *BMJ Quality & Safety*, 22(7), 541.

Krogh, K., Bearman, M., & Nestel, D. (2015). Expert practice of video-assisted debriefing: An Australian qualitative study. *Clinical Simulation in Nursing*, 11(3), 180–187.

Krogh, K., Bearman, M., & Nestel, D. (2016). 'Thinking on your feet'—a qualitative study of debriefing practice. *Advances in Simulation*, 1(12), doi:10.1186/s41077-016-0011-4.

Lin, Y., Cheng, A., Hecker, K., et al. (2018). Implementing economic evaluation in simulation-based medical education: Challenges and opportunities. *Medical Education*, 52(2), 150–160.

Lopreiato, J. O. (2016). *Healthcare simulation dictionary*. AHRQ Publication No. 16(17)-0043. Rockville, MD: Agency for Healthcare Research and Quality.

Maloney, S., & Haines, T. (2016). Issues of cost-benefit and cost-effectiveness for simulation in health professions education. *Advances in Simulation*, 1(13).

McGaghie, W. C. (2015a). Mastery learning: It is time for medical education to join the 21st century. *Academic Medicine*, 90(11), 1438–1441.

McGaghie, W. C. (2015b). When I say … mastery learning. *Medical Education*, 49(6), 558–559.

McGaghie, W. C., et al. (2010). A critical review of simulation-based medical education research: 2003–2009. *Medical Education*, 44(1), 50–63.

Nestel, D., Brazil, V., & Hay, M. (2018). You can't put a value on that … Or can you? Economic evaluation in simulation-based medical education. *Medical Education*, 52(2), 139–147.

Nestel, D., & Gough, S. (2018). Designing simulation-based learning activities. In D. Nestel, et al. (Eds.), *Healthcare simulation education: Evidence, theory and practice* (pp. 135–142). Chichester, West Sussex: John Wiley & Sons.

Nestel, D., Roche, J., & Battista, A. (2017). Creating a quality improvement culture in standardized/simulated patient methodology: The role of professional societies. *Advances in Simulation*, 2(18).

Nestel, D., Sanko, J., & McNaughton, N. (2018). Simulated participant methodologies: maintaining humanism in practice. In D. Nestel, et al. (Eds.), *Healthcare simulation education: Evidence, theory and practice* (pp. 45–53). Chichester, West Sussex: John Wiley & Sons.

O'Regan, S., et al. (2016). Observer roles that optimise learning in healthcare simulation education: A systematic review. *Advances in Simulation*, 1(1), 4.

Pendleton, D., et al. (1998). *The consultation: An approach to learning and teaching*. New York: Oxford University Press.

Phrampus, P., & O'Donnell, J. M. (2013). Debriefing using a structured and supported approach. In A. Levine, et al. (Eds.), *The comprehensive textbook of healthcare simulation* (pp. 73–84). New York: Springer Science & Business Media.

Posner, G., Clark, M. D., & Grant, V. (2017). Simulation in the clinical setting: Towards a standard lexicon. *Advances in Simulation*, 2(15).

Reedy, G. (2015). Using cognitive load theory to inform simulation design and practice. *Clinical Simulation in Nursing*, 11, 350–360.

Roehl, A., Reddy, S. L., & Shannon, G. J. (2013). The flipped classroom: An opportunity to engage millennial students through active learning strategies. *Journal of Family and Consumer Sciences*, 105.

Rudolph, J. W., et al. (2006). There's no such thing as 'nonjudgmental' debriefing: A theory and method for debriefing with good judgment. *Simulation in Healthcare*, 1(1), 49–55.

Sawyer, T., et al. (2016). More than one way to debrief: A critical review of healthcare simulation debriefing methods. *Simulation in Healthcare*, 11(3), 209–216.

Schaefer, J. J., et al. (2011). Literature review: Instructional design and pedagogy science in healthcare simulation. *Simulation in Healthcare*, 6(Suppl.), 30–41.

Shoemaker, J. C., Beasley, M., Perkins, R., et al. (2011). A method for providing high-volume interprofessional simulation encounters in physical and occupational therapy education programs. *Journal of Allied Health*, 40(1), 15–21.

Staropoli, P. C., Gregori, N. Z., Junk, A. K., et al. (2017). Surgical simulation training reduces intraoperative cataract surgery complications among residents. *Simulation in Healthcare*, 13(1), 11–15.

The NHET-Sim Monash Team. (2012). *The National Health Education and Training: Simulation (NHET-Sim) Program*. www.monash.edu/medicine/nhet-sim. (Accessed 21 September 2017).

TRAC Development Group. (2015). *TRAC: a guide for senior managers and governing body members*. www.hefce.ac.uk/media/TRAC%20A%20guide%20for%20Senior%20Managers%20and%20Governing%20Body%20members.pdf.

Watson, K., et al. (2012). Can simulation replace part of clinical time? Two parallel randomised controlled trials. *Medical Education*, 46(7), 657–667.

14

Interprofessional learning opportunities for pre-registration students in clinical workplaces

Fiona Kent and Gillian Nisbet

Introduction

Contemporary models of healthcare frequently involve teams of professionals, rather than individuals working in isolation. Collaborative rather than profession-specific practice is required to deliver safe, efficient and integrated care within and across clinical teams (Frenk et al., 2010). However, healthcare teams and systems are complex, and learners require skills in interprofessional practice to navigate this complexity (Kuipers et al., 2014).

Education in the health professions has traditionally been delivered in profession-specific silos. A shift in health professional education has been advocated for, to ensure education includes preparation for working with teams and in complex systems, to better align with both the requirements of health systems and the population they serve (Frenk et al., 2010). In Australia, accreditation bodies are progressing the interprofessional agenda by the inclusion of interprofessional learning criteria in course requirements (Australian Medical Council, 2012; Australian Nursing and Midwifery Accreditation Council, 2012; Physiotherapy Board of Australia & Physiotherapy Board of New Zealand, 2015). Simultaneously, patients are increasingly expecting a collaborative approach from their healthcare team, and make the assumption that their health professionals *are* communicating with one another in order to deliver safe, efficient and effective care. Furthermore, changing patient attitudes, including the growing interest in accessing health information on the internet, demand that health professions develop skills in integrating multiple perspectives and priorities (Cutilli, 2010). Clinical placement settings provide many opportunities for pre-registration students to develop skills in collaborative practice, and increasingly attempts are being made to facilitate educational interventions to maximise interprofessional learning opportunities.

Interprofessional learning in the workplace offers real-world authenticity and complexity to engage pre-registration students. Utilising the workplace for interprofessional learning, where professions are co-located, is also a logical strategy to counter the challenges of bringing together large cohorts of students from different professions and often disparate campuses in the pre-clinical years. A wealth of interprofessional patient engagement opportunities may be utilised, with the potential for students to be prompted to consider the patient's perspective within the complexity of current healthcare models of care (Spencer et al., 2000). Importantly, where the patient's voice is able to be integrated into educational initiatives, students can be exposed to the reason for striving for collaborative practice (Kent et al., 2017).

Interprofessional learning is discussed in this chapter within the context of work-integrated learning (Billett, 2001). Although somewhat contested within the literature (Billett, 2004), we find it useful to conceptualise interprofessional learning opportunities in the workplace in terms of formal and informal learning. We see a role for both formal and informal approaches to interprofessional learning for pre-registration students. We consider formal approaches to interprofessional learning to include those that are pre-designed and scheduled, with set learning outcomes and structured activities for a target group of students. Formal programs might include dedicated interprofessional training wards, student-led clinics, simulation activities and interprofessional student workshops. By contrast, informal learning refers to the unstructured, experiential and non-institutional learning that occurs as part of everyday work practice (Marsick & Volpe, 1999; Regehr & Mylopoulos, 2008).

For healthcare students on placement, we extend the definition of informal learning to encompass the learning that occurs through engaging with other professions as part of a student's everyday workplace practice while on placement. For example, a physiotherapy student may be liaising with an occupational therapy student to safely discharge a patient home from hospital, and later reflect on the importance of communication within the healthcare team. A medical student may observe the interactions within a team meeting and take note of the range of professions contributing to a patient case. A speech pathology student may listen to a conversation between a nurse and a patient, observing how questions are asked to elicit particular information. In each of these interactions, learning may or may not be recognised by the student, as the interaction forms part of everyday work practice (Eraut, 2004).

The approach to informal interprofessional learning presented in this chapter is modelled on a typology of informal learning presented by Eraut (2000) and described in detail for health professionals engaging in informal workplace learning (Nisbet et al., 2013). Eraut (2000) categorises informal learning into:

1. *implicit, unintended learning:* where there is no awareness of learning at the time it takes place;
2. *reactive learning:* where learning is explicit, but it takes place almost spontaneously in response to an event — no time is specifically set aside for it;
3. *deliberative learning:* time is set aside for acquiring new knowledge — earning is deliberately built into work activity.

Table 14.1 provides examples of interprofessional learning scenarios for each category. In this model, there is a continuum of intentionality of informal learning from the implicit unplanned chance learning, akin to the serendipitous interprofessional learning described by Freeth and colleagues (Freeth et al., 2005), to the more deliberate explicit focus on interprofessional learning in workplace interactions. Learning therefore becomes more intentional as we move from implicit to more explicit. However, informal opportunities may not be fully utilised, hence methods to enhance the educational value require exploration.

The goals of this chapter are to: 1) provide an overview of the learning outcomes underpinning collaborative practice for pre-registration students; 2) describe formal models of interprofessional education for pre-registration students in the workplace, and the mechanisms underpinning effective programs as determined by realist methods; and 3) describe strategies for the facilitation of informal learning opportunities in the workplace, and the theory that may underpin this learning. We make a clear distinction between a teacher-centred approach to student learning and our preferred approach: *facilitation* of interprofessional learning.

A case study is used to explore the challenges faced by clinicians in the workplace, seeking methods by which to promote interprofessional learning. After describing the case, and presenting the background and theory, we describe explicit strategies that can be adopted to a range of clinical settings.

TABLE 14.1: Interprofessional learning examples of Eraut categories

Implicit, unintended learning	Reactive learning	Deliberate learning
No awareness of interprofessional learning at the time it takes place	Interprofessional learning is explicit, but takes place almost spontaneously in response to an event. Some degree of individual reflection, but time is not specifically set aside for planning or debriefing	Time is set aside for acquiring new knowledge, skills and insights. Interprofessional learning is deliberately built into work activity. Reflection is key to learning
Examples		
A speech pathology student listening in to a phone conversation between a patient and an occupational therapist	Discussion occurring between team members after a 'near-miss' event on a hospital ward	Shadowing another profession in usual practice. The clinician may also provide explanations of tasks and encourage student participation in activities
Corridor conversation between a student nurse and a physiotherapy student about a patient	An individual's reaction to observing inappropriate communication between staff and patient	A joint patient consultation with another student professional. Includes prior planning, and debriefing afterwards
Pharmacy student raises a drug interaction with a doctor. The doctor thanks the pharmacist and makes the necessary changes to his patient's medications	Participating in a team meeting where an adverse drug reaction is discussed. The pharmacist explains to the team the likely reasons this occurred, proposes an alternative medication, and makes a recommendation to reduce the same reaction occurring in the future	Conducting an audit of drug near-misses in a specific ward or clinical environment

Case study 14.1

Jackie is a physiotherapist in a subacute rehabilitation centre. She enjoys clinical teaching and supervises physiotherapy students through most of the year. Her colleagues from medicine, nursing, occupational therapy and social work also frequently ask whether their students can spend some time watching her in the gym to increase their students' understanding of what a physiotherapist does. Jackie is keen for others to understand the role of physiotherapy, so obliges the multiple requests.

Interview with Jackie: 'I tend to set the observation students up to sit to the side of the gym so they can watch a few of us at work. If a student seems particularly interested, and asks me questions about what I'm doing or why, I'll engage in a conversation with them, but generally the students just stay for an hour or so, then return to their dedicated educator. I've noticed that when students are in pairs, they tend to chat away to one another throughout their time in the gym, but I'm not convinced the discussion has anything to do with what they are observing. I could get more involved with their learning and explain what I am doing, but I spend so much time teaching already, and I'm not sure that it's worth the effort if they are not interested. I've been thinking lately whether there is anything else I could do to make better use of these observation sessions, without increasing the demands on my time.'

Background: definitions, frameworks and theory

Definitions

A range of terms have been used to describe activities combining learners from different professions in education or practice. In this chapter, we have used the following definitions as previously described (Freeth et al., 2005; Reeves et al., 2010).

Interprofessional learning is 'learning arising from interaction between members (or students) of two or more professions. This may be a product of interprofessional education or happening spontaneously in the workplace or in education settings.' (Freeth et al., 2005)

Interprofessional education describes 'those occasions when two or more professions learn with, from and about each other to improve collaboration and the quality of care'. (Freeth et al., 2005)

'Interprofessional teamwork is a type of work which involves different health and/or social professions who share a team identity and work closely together in an integrated and interdependent manner to solve problems and deliver services.' (Reeves et al., 2010)

For this chapter, we propose a range of interprofessional learning opportunities for students within the workplace, a subset of which are formal interprofessional education activities. We acknowledge the variability in the interprofessional practice that students may be exposed to across different settings, and intentionally present a diverse range of approaches.

Frameworks

Education activities benefit from clear learning outcomes (Biggs, 2011), and established interprofessional competency frameworks can be a useful starting point for educators such as Jackie. Multiple broad interprofessional competency frameworks have been both described and compared over the past decade (Canadian Interprofessional Health Collaborative, 2010; Interprofessional Education Collaborative, 2016; The Interprofessional Curriculum Renewal Consortium, 2014). A literature review has identified key interprofessional learning outcomes as communication, roles and responsibilities, teamwork, ethics/attitudes, the patient and learning/reflection (Thistlethwaite & Moran, 2010), and an analysis of the multiple frameworks has generated a list of potential graduate attributes (O'Keefe et al., 2017).

Although competency frameworks provide overarching guidance, contextual considerations will inform local interprofessional learning outcomes. For example, an overarching competency framework may aspire for learners to understand their own role and the role of others, and a learning target that Jackie may identify for her setting is for students to be able to describe the role of a physiotherapist in stroke rehabilitation, and determine when a person suffering a stroke may benefit from referral to physiotherapy. There is the potential for interprofessional learning to be integrated into clinical placements wherever there is a requirement for collaborative practice. A wide range of clinical contexts have structured interprofessional workplace activities, including orthopaedic wards (Jakobsen, 2016), paediatrics (Stewart et al., 2010), disability (Anderson et al., 2010), medication safety (Nagelkerk et al., 2014), mental health (Kinnair, 2012), rehabilitation (Fougner & Horntvedt, 2011) and aged care (Kent et al., 2016b). Informal learning contexts are less frequently described in the literature, and are a focus for our existing research.

Assessment of interprofessional learning is arguably the least developed area of curriculum design. Yet clinical assessment is now considered critical for both assessing *and* improving learning (Imanipour & Jalili, 2016; Norcini et al., 2011; Schuwirth & van der Vleuten, 2011). Failure to have interprofessional learning activities 'count' towards assessment in the clinical setting, and/or unauthentic assessment tasks, discourages student engagement (Thistlethwaite, 2015; Zhao et al., 2015). An international consensus statement on the assessment of interprofessional learning outcomes (Rogers et al., 2017) provides a useful selection of assessment approaches suitable for the clinical setting; for example, peer assessment, team-based projects, an interprofessional portfolio, reflective journalling and clinical observation. We suggest that profession-specific clinical assessment tools could also be better utilised to assess interprofessional competence. For example, many of these tools already contain elements to assess teamwork and a patient-centred approach to care. An *interprofessional* perspective could be incorporated when assessing students on these elements.

Theory

Theory can be useful to inform how and why learning occurs. A broad range of learning and psychological theories have been cited as underpinning formal interprofessional education activities (Barr, 2013; Clark, 2006), notably adult learning theory, experiential learning and reflective practice (Kent et al., 2017). While these theories are important foundations for work-integrated learning generally, we suggest that they alone are not enough to explain the complexities of interprofessional learning within clinical settings. In an investigation of workplace learning within postgraduate learners, Nisbet and colleagues (2013) identified learning theories that help explain interprofessional learning from an *individual* perspective, as well as theories that help explain how new understanding is *socially created* through interaction with others. These theories are briefly described below, and contextualised to interprofessional learning in the workplace.

Social cognitive theory (Bandura, 1986) recognises the influence on student actions and behaviour of individual learner factors (e.g. knowledge of other professions, attitude towards learning from others, and motivations to work collaboratively), *and* environmental factors (e.g. support from profession educators to participate in interprofessional learning activities). Role-modelling is a good example of how social cognitive theory applies to interprofessional learning: students observe other health professionals and how they may or may not interact collaboratively with each other, make meaning out of these observations, and enact similar behaviours. For example, a student who hears her educator constantly criticising other professions for inappropriate referrals may begin to take on similar behaviours when faced with a similar situation. Both negative and positive role-modelling may impact on learning.

Transformative learning challenges learners to revisit and critically examine previously held beliefs, and through discourse and reflection shift their perspective (Mezirow, 2000). Significant shifts in perspective may initially require a new or even disorientating experience. Within the complexity of the workplace, which typically involves multiple professions, teams and systems, the potential to disorientate is high. Through facilitated reflection, there is an opportunity to shift learners from viewing situations through a profession-specific lens towards the recognition of the need for the broader healthcare team. This ultimate shift toward 'interprofessionality' and more cohesive practice may better align with the patient's needs, as a desired target of interprofessional education (D'Amour & Oandasan, 2005).

Constructivism (McInerney & McInerney, 2002) recognises learning as the gradual process of meaning-making. Less emphasis is placed on instructing students, but rather learning approaches are scaffolded and students are encouraged to engage by drawing on past experiences to develop new understanding and apply it to future situations (Hager & Smith, 2004). Social constructivism (McInerney & McInerney, 2002) builds in the social element to learning; that is, learning through interaction with others. Examples where interprofessional facilitators draw on constructivism include asking students to reflect on their past patient care experiences, share their profession-specific knowledge with others in the group, and/or reflect on an encounter with another profession.

While the above theories are useful to theorise the learning process for individuals, sociocultural learning theories assist us in understanding the social connectivity that underpins interprofessional learning. Sociocultural learning theories view learning as participatory, social and contextual (Hager, 2008; Kaufman & Mann, 2010; Morris & Blaney, 2013). Learning occurs through interactions with others, and through interactions with the environment and its culture (Garavan & McCarthy, 2008). Within the complexity of the clinical workplace, it is important for clinical educators to be aware of the systems, procedures and tools that promote and detract from interprofessional learning opportunities (Kent et al., 2016a).

We are not advocating one particular learning theory to explain workplace interprofessional learning. Rather, it is likely that a combination of individual and collective learning theories will contribute to our understanding of the learning process. The theories described above should inform the choice of learning activities and their delivery approach. In particular, they align with our focus on interprofessional *facilitation* rather than teacher-driven approaches to enhance learning, as discussed later.

Formal interprofessional opportunities

Multiple formal interprofessional education models have been implemented for pre-registration students. Interprofessional training wards have operated in Sweden for over 20 years, and longitudinal studies suggest positive and sustained outcomes for student learning (Hylin et al., 2007; Jakobsen, 2016). Training wards typically involve a two-week orthopaedic ward placement, combining medical, nursing, physiotherapy and occupational therapy students, although aged care and emergency department training ward models have also been described (Jakobsen, 2016). The training ward model aims to explicitly bring together students from different professions to provide clinical care on a delegated ward for an extended period. A strength of the model is the opportunity for learning through participation in real patient care while supporting the development of professional identity. A limitation of the model is the ability to deliver training ward interprofessional opportunities at scale, when catering for large student cohorts across multiple professions.

Student-led clinics have been strategically established to facilitate the combination of service delivery in areas of community need and student education (both profession-specific and interprofessional) (Schutte et al., 2015). Informed patient consent for student-led care in clinics allows students the autonomy to engage in clinical consultations to the level of their ability with clinician oversight. Student and educator perceptions of participation in such programs are positive (Kent et al., 2014; Schutte et al., 2015). The scope of student practice from each participating profession, and therefore the supervision required, requires careful consideration in the design of the clinic operations. Strengths of the model are positive patient outcomes related to preventative healthcare (Kent et al., 2016c; Schutte et al., 2015) and the potential for identifying new health issues and medication modifications (Lai et al., 2015). A limitation of student clinics has been the dependency on volunteer students (Kent & Keating, 2015), and financial sustainability, due to the difficulty of student clinics to generate sufficient income through student consultations to cover the costs of operation (Haines et al., 2014).

Case studies and workshops have been delivered in the workplace to opportunistically bring students together during clinical placements. The context for interprofessional cases can be aligned to workplace priorities. The Australian National Standards (Australian Commission on Safety and Quality in Health Care, 2012) represent areas of clinical complexity ideal for interprofessional learning such as 'partnering with consumers', 'medication safety', 'clinical handover' and 'preventing falls and harms from falls'. Occasions of clinical error involving team practice can also provide an engaging base for the development of case studies for student learning (Anderson et al., 2009). An example of an interprofessional workshop that we have found successful for pre-registration students is based on a falls incident, which reveals multiple contributing factors and the need for input from multiple professions. A benefit of case studies and workshops is logistics: they can be completed in only a few hours when placement schedules overlap.

It is useful for educators to understand the mechanisms underpinning the success of formal interprofessional education programs in the workplace. Realist methods seek to analyse what works for whom, under what circumstances, and why, through an analysis of context, mechanism and outcome (Pawson et al., 2005). In a realist review of formal interprofessional education in the workplace, meaningful interprofessional student discussion and reflection were the *mechanisms* aligned with students gaining increased knowledge of the roles of others and of teamwork skills (Kent et al., 2017). Interprofessional education initiatives that involved student teams interacting with a real patient, in addition to discussion and reflection, resulted in the students increasing their awareness of the patient perspective in health, as well as learning about the roles of others and teamwork skills. We argue that regardless of the education format selected, prioritising meaningful interprofessional discussion and reflection should be an aim for clinical educators.

Informal interprofessional opportunities

Informal interprofessional learning has the potential to overcome many of the barriers described within formal programs. First, it does not rely on students being timetabled in the same location. Rather, it takes advantage of students who happen to be on placement together at the same time. Alternatively, students may interact with *staff* from other professions, increasing their exposure to other professions. Secondly, informal learning utilises existing workplace structures; for example, ward rounds and team meetings ensuring authentic and experiential student learning. Thirdly, interprofessional learning can be integrated within existing placement curricula rather than be seen as an 'add-on'. Finally, fourthly, informal learning is arguably less resource-intensive compared with more formal interprofessional learning programs, as it utilises existing placement staff resources (Lait et al., 2011).

However, informal interprofessional learning opportunities may not be recognised or utilised where students are not invited or guided to access the opportunities (Billett, 2014). A lack of encouragement by clinical educators for students to seek interprofessional learning opportunities (Pollard, 2009; Zhao et al., 2015), reduced educator confidence and skill in facilitating interprofessional learning (Pollard, 2008), and poor role-modelling of interprofessional practice (Murray-Davis et al., 2014; Pollard, 2008) may all contribute to reduced uptake. A lack of student awareness of the opportunities for interprofessional learning while on placement, and reduced student confidence to actively seek interprofessional experiences while on placement (Pollard, 2009), also contribute to missed opportunities. Moreover, when an assessment of learning is missing, student engagement may be reduced (Morison et al., 2003).

The above issues have guided the development of a suite of stakeholder-informed interprofessional learning activities for use by educators and healthcare students when on placement. Based on an initial scan of existing resources (see the 'Online resources' section at the end of this chapter) and interviews with potential end-users, the resource package introduces a practical and sustainable approach to promoting interprofessional learning by *integrating* individual activities into students' usual profession-specific placements. The interprofessional activities are linked with already existing placement learning outcomes, and are completed through interaction with other students who happen to be on placement at the same time, observation and interaction with staff from other professions, and through self-directed activities. The resources are accessible on Health Education and Training (HETI) and the University of Sydney's public websites (see 'Online resources'), and include worksheets to prompt reflection after observation of another profession at work, a team meeting or a joint patient consultation.

Informal approaches to interprofessional learning capitalise on existing workplace structures, processes and interactions. However, rather than leave learning to chance, learning using the aforementioned resources is scaffolded by providing worksheet instructions and reflective prompts to guide students through the activity. Students are encouraged to initiate their own learning opportunities by engaging with other students, thus developing their informal social networks, which in turn promotes learning (Garavan & McCarthy, 2008). Debriefing is explicitly included to encourage reflection and promote deeper learning. As with formal interprofessional programs, the *mechanism* of learning through interaction, discussion and reflection is sought.

Facilitation of interprofessional learning

Although a range of terms are used within the literature, we use the term *interprofessional facilitation* to include any or all of the following tasks undertaken in the placement setting: facilitating interprofessional learning activities; mentoring students from other professions; providing feedback to individual students or groups of students from other professions; and assessing students from other professions in relation to providing safe, appropriate and high-quality collaborative patient care. The interprofessional facilitation role may take on a supervisory role in either formal placements (such as student-led clinics) or the more informal interprofessional learning opportunities that occur on placement.

We also deliberately use the term *facilitator*, to shift the focus from the educator as being the profession expert and there to *teach* the students, to one whereby the educator is an enabler of the learning process, working *with* the students (Oandasan & Reeves, 2005). However, this approach may be a paradigm shift for some educators who prefer a more teacher-centred rather than learner-centred approach to student learning. For the *interprofessional* facilitator, the role also includes a focus on the collaborative nature of interprofessional practice. This is apparent in the facilitator role outlined by Freeman and colleagues (Freeman et al., 2010). Although a campus-based program, the role described is pertinent to the clinical setting, which is to: 1) promote the benefits of interprofessional learning for teamwork and patient care; 2) provide direction and focus towards the learning objectives without making decisions for the group; 3) encourage interaction and collaboration; 4) foster the knowledge and skills necessary for good interprofessional teamworking, such as mutual respect and flexibility; and 5) provide encouragement and support (Freeman et al., 2010). Pre-planning is essential to ensure these roles are achievable (Nisbet et al., 2016). This includes session planning, considering any sensitive or contentious issues that may arise, and ensuring support from key stakeholders.

While health practitioners may be involved in the clinical education of students from their own profession, it cannot be assumed that this expertise translates to the skill and confidence required for interprofessional facilitation. The literature reports educators feeling challenged and under-prepared for this new role (Bray, 2008; Egan-Lee et al., 2011; Reeves & Freeth, 2002). Concerns relate to the educator's ability to mentor other professions due to a lack of profession-specific clinical knowledge (Marshall & Gordon, 2010), being able to manage the group dynamics of interprofessional student groups (Anderson et al., 2011), and the ability to identify and capitalise on 'teachable' interprofessional moments (Egan-Lee et al., 2011). Students soon become aware of differences in facilitation approaches; for example, differences in the level of support offered, and the ability to be inclusive of all participating professions (Yang & McAllister, 2017). This can affect the functioning of the student team and student satisfaction (Reeves et al., 2002), and from our own observations can negatively impact on student learning and on students' views on interprofessional practice. Our experience from workshops with potential interprofessional learning facilitators also raises additional concerns from educators about patient safety when supervising students outside one's own profession and the ability to assess students from other professions.

Educator competencies for facilitating interprofessional learning

Published interprofessional competencies exist, outlining the knowledge and skills required of an interprofessional facilitator (Freeman et al., 2010; Freeth et al., 2005; Howkins & Bray, 2008). While many of the included competencies reflect generic small-group facilitation skills — for example, reflecting on and responding to feedback, managing conflict and group dynamics, active listening, and being flexible — the interprofessional context adds an additional dimension and nuance. In particular, Howkins and Bray (Howkins & Bray, 2008) acknowledge the potential power dimensions and hierarchies that may be present across professions and institutions. Similarly Reeves and colleagues (2012) argue:

> a core skill of an interprofessional facilitator then becomes the ability to make explicit for participants, learning moments which can surface the traditional power hierarchies amongst the professions and then move participants to common ground, which is most often an integrated plan for patient care. (p 236)

Recognition of one's own professional identity and personal biases, and the influence these have on interprofessional facilitation is also important (Howkins & Bray, 2008). We would also add an awareness of one's own supervisory style, and whether this style is congruent with interprofessional practice. For example, a supervisory style that values peer learning and encourages students to work through solutions together, rather than being told the answer by the facilitator, encourages collaborative learning as well as independence from the facilitator (Nicol & Forman, 2014). Students learn to seek information *from each other*, in the process learning to trust and respect the knowledge and capabilities of their interprofessional peers. Moreover, allowing students to explain their clinical reasoning to and answer questions from other professions strengthens students' professional-specific knowledge and capabilities (Chipchase et al., 2012). Students need to be clear in their own mind of the concept they are explaining, consider the knowledge level of the recipient(s) of the information, then formulate an explanation to ensure that it is relevant, pitched at an appropriate level, free of discipline-specific jargon and conveys the message intended. We suggest that this is an iterative process that develops the more students are exposed to this process. From our experience, explaining one's thinking and responding to questions not only helps students appreciate their own unique professional expertise, but validates that they do have something useful to contribute to the other professionals' understanding.

Interprofessional facilitators require experience working in an interprofessional setting (Nicol & Forman, 2014; Reeves et al., 2007) and a commitment to its value (Freeth et al., 2005). They also need to role-model interprofessional behaviours, such as respect for other professions, resolving interprofessional conflict, and the ability to work with others in providing patient care (Freeth et al., 2005; Oandasan & Reeves, 2005), as negative role-modelling has been found to be detrimental to successful interprofessional learning initiatives (Nisbet et al., 2008). Likewise, interprofessional facilitators need an understanding of the various professional roles and how they contribute to the care team (Chipchase et al., 2012). However, this does not mean that facilitators need an *in-depth* knowledge of other professions. Rather, interprofessional facilitation requires knowing what services and skillsets other professions can offer, when it might be appropriate to involve another profession, and how the various professions' expertise combine in providing integrated patient care.

Case study 14.1 (continued): Resolution

Jackie and her clinical team have been directed to the multiple existing resources that may be utilised to facilitate active student involvement in interprofessional activities. A team approach to student observations of others at work has been established. When convenient and relevant to all parties, physiotherapy students under Jackie's supervision are able to observe other professions at work, and Jackie has students from other professions observe her. The patient under observation is ideally known to the student, and patient consent is obtained. The process involves the following:

- Clear learning outcomes may be provided to the students by their usual clinical educator to direct the focus of the observation session.
- Prior to the observation, students may be provided with a worksheet with prompt questions, such as: 'What did the physiotherapist do with the patient?'; 'How may this observation assist you in providing patient care?'; 'What did you find out through this observation that you were not previously aware of?'

- When more than one profession is observing a consultation, interaction is encouraged among the students: while they may not be discussing what is directly being observed, the socialisation process that occurs through these more informal interactions assists with breaking down professional barriers.
- Questions to the treating professional are encouraged and invited at the completion of the observation activity. Jackie might ask: 'What did you understand we were trying to achieve in that physiotherapy session?'; 'Why do you think my focus was on ...'
- Questions to the patient are encouraged at the completion of the observational activity. Jackie might ask: 'Is there anything you would like to ask the patient about this session?'
- Finally, the clinical educator who facilitated their students' attendance at the session should follow up each observation session by facilitating a reflection on the experience based on the learning outcomes of interest. A return to the original prompt questions, aligned to the learning outcomes, is useful.

PRACTICAL TIPS

Based on the existing interprofessional learning facilitation literature and our own experiences, we provide a set of practical tips to assist educators when tasked with facilitating interprofessional learning within the placement setting (see Table 14.2). We have deliberately focused on the points of difference from facilitating single-profession groups of students. Our tips are influenced by the work of Carlson and colleagues, who report on their experiences of facilitation within a Swedish hospital training ward (Carlson et al., 2011), and the learnings from the PIPE project (Promoting Interprofessional Education) as detailed by Howkins and Bray in their book on preparing for interprofessional teaching (Howkins & Bray, 2008). Several useful resources have also been developed to assist the interprofessional facilitator, such as *Facilitating interprofessional clinical learning* from the University of Toronto (see the 'Online resources' section at the end of this chapter), *Interprofessional collaboration in practice: A guide for strengthening student learning experiences* from Dalhousie University (Godden-Webster & Murphy, 2014) and *Interprofessional mentoring guide for supervisors, staff and students* from Alberta Health Services (see 'Online resources').

TABLE 14.2: Practical tips for facilitating interprofessional learning

Component of interprofessional learning facilitation	Interprofessional learning points of difference
Initial preparation	Know the professional backgrounds of your students and their prior IPL experience (Howkins & Bray, 2008)
Creating a safe learning environment	Establish ground rules around respect and valuing others' professional opinions (Lie et al., 2016)
	Encourage engagement by all professions — be aware that particular professions may have more of a role to play at certain times, and that some students may be naturally quieter than others
	Welcome differences of opinion — encourage respectful debate. Challenge the view expressed, not the person (or profession) expressing that view (Howkins & Bray, 2008)
	Avoid using professional jargon — where used, ensure terms are explained if necessary (Howkins & Bray, 2008)
	Support all students, not just those in your own profession (Carlson et al., 2011)

Continued

TABLE 14.2: Practical tips for facilitating interprofessional learning — cont'd

Component of interprofessional learning facilitation	Interprofessional learning points of difference
Professional hierarchical barriers	Focus on the needs of patients to guide decisions (Carlson et al., 2011; Orchard et al., 2017)
	Make domains of knowledge and skill expertise from each profession visible (Carlson et al., 2011)
	Discuss areas of overlap between professional roles and scope of practice
	Rotate the leadership in case management (Lie et al., 2016)
	Explore stereotypical perceptions of other professional groups (Egan-Lee et al., 2011)
Self-awareness as an interprofessional learning facilitator	Be professionally neutral — keep your own professional biases at bay (Freeman et al., 2010)
	Keep an open mind — avoid making assumptions about individuals, groups or particular professions (Howkins & Bray, 2008)
	Acknowledge and use other professionals' experience (not just using your own experience) (Howkins & Bray, 2008; Orchard et al., 2017)
	Reflect on and evaluate your interprofessional facilitation skills — for example, complete the 'Interprofessional Facilitation Scale' (Carlson et al., 2011; Sargeant et al., 2010)
Interactive and reflective learning	Include peer learning — this may be unfamiliar to some professions, but part of routine placement for others (Carlson et al., 2011)
	Ask open and probing questions (e.g. 'What are Mrs Jones's main concerns? How best can we address these concerns?'; 'Who is best placed to lead the team?')
	Ask provocative questions to stimulate discussion (e.g. 'You indicated the nurse and doctor do most of the talking in the meeting. Is this appropriate? Why/why not?'; 'Who is leading this team meeting?')
	Recognise that you don't have to be a content expert — draw on the student expertise within the group
	Co-facilitate to role-model collaboration (and assist novice facilitators) (Anderson et al., 2011; Egan-Lee et al., 2011. Lie et al., 2016)
	Include a team reflection — both on the content of the interprofessional session, and on the interprofessional team process (Lie et al., 2016)

Directions, evaluation and research

A key area for more research lies in the development of empirically informed theories that inform what interprofessional learning occurs in the workplace. The *mechanisms* of interprofessional discussion and reflection appear to be important for students to acquire a knowledge of others' roles and some teamwork skills; however, the process required to shift a student from a profession-specific lens to embrace interprofessionality (D'Amour & Oandasan, 2005) requires further investigation. In our experience, this paradigm shift may not be achieved by the point of registration.

Formal interprofessional workplace models have been evaluated discretely, informal less so. Multiple evaluation instruments targeted at the learner, team or organisation have been developed and synthesised by the National Center for Interprofessional Practice and Education (2013). Despite broad uptake of self-rating tools, the ability of these tools to assess student learning has been questioned (Colthart et al., 2008). The Readiness for Interprofessional Learning Scale, which measures attitudes towards shared learning

(Parsell & Bligh, 1999), is perhaps the most commonly cited evaluation tool. However, in addition to the limitations of self-assessment, it is unlikely to be as relevant today as it was 10 years ago, due to a greater acceptance by students of the need for interprofessional learning, with high scores reported at baseline (McFadyen et al., 2010). There is also a need to shift from the attitudinal evaluations and self-rating of competence, to more objective measures of knowledge, skills and behavior, such as the recently developed iTOFT tool (The iTOFT Consortium, 2015), which was designed for students to receive feedback on their teamwork performance. Monitoring of changes over time could be used as a guage of student learning.

Further research is needed to better understand the learning outcomes from informal interactions. Unfortunately, our recent research has demonstrated that interactions between some professional groups (e.g. medical students and occupational therapy or physiotherapy students) on clinical placement may actually be minimal when not facilitated (Rees et al., in press). Pollard (2008) explored students' experiences of interprofessional learning, and raised concerns that some students could not differentiate between appropriate and inappropriate interprofessional behaviour observed in the workplace. Others have reported variability in the depth of learning, with speech pathology students reporting increased knowledge and skills through informal interprofessional interactions (Zhao et al., 2015). To date, only shadowing suggests positive effects on informal learning (Fougner & Horntvedt, 2011; Jain et al., 2012; Wright et al., 2012). However, evaluations of interprofessional learning within the clinical setting need to go beyond evaluation of student learning to also evaluate the impact of student interprofessional activity on service delivery and on patient care. For example, is a student-led interprofessional respiratory clinic enabling more patients to be seen in a timely manner? Are individual patient goals being met more so than when adopting a uni-professional approach to care? How is patient satisfaction impacted? Evaluations that address these and similar questions are required to demonstrate the broader impact of interprofessional learning in the workplace. Such evaluations would enable much-needed cost–benefit evaluations to be undertaken, to justify the inclusion of often labour-intensive and relatively costly interprofessional activity in health professional programs (Haines et al., 2014).

Although multiple models of interprofessional learning have been implemented and evaluated discretely, the variability across workplaces reflects the lack of consensus on the most effective and efficient approaches. Furthermore, despite the need to meet accreditation requirements, until the education research is able to establish a clear link between pre-registration interprofessional learning and the development of a collaborative workforce, the incentive for a broad uptake of such activities in the workplace is low. Whole-of-curriculum and longitudinal approaches to evaluation of interprofessional programs are now required.

Conclusion

University and clinical educators are working to reform education to meet the current needs of patients and systems. This reform requires inclusion of interprofessional learning opportunities for students to interact with health professionals beyond their own profession in the workplace. However, reform is at times a slow process, and until best-practice models can be established there is a role for both formal and informal interprofessional learning opportunities. The challenge remains for educators to ensure that, by the time of their graduation, all students have an awareness of their clinical teams, recognise the roles of others, communicate effectively across teams, and collaborate effectively. Both clinicians and students have the potential to initiate relevant interprofessional interactions within clinical placements, once directed to the multiple possibilities. Formal and informal learning opportunities are dependent on the commitment and skills of clinicians to facilitate these opportunities.

Online resources

Alberta Health Services. Interprofessional mentoring guide for supervisors, staff and students: www.albertahealthservices.ca.
Health Education and Training Institute (HETI). Interprofessional learning resource for placement settings — Literature review: www.heti.nsw.gov.au/Resources-Library/Interprofessional-Learning-Resource-for-Placement-Settings/.
The University of Sydney. Interprofessional learning resources for placements: health-ipl.sydney.edu.au/.
The University of Toronto. Facilitating interprofessional clinical learning: www.ipe.utoronto.ca/tools-resources/tools-toolkits.

References

Anderson, E., Smith, R., & Thorpe, L. (2010). Learning from lives together: Medical and social work students' experiences of learning from people with disabilities in the community. *Health and Social Care in the Community*, *18*(3), 229–240.

Anderson, E. S., Thorpe, L. N., & Hammick, M. (2011). Interprofessional staff development: Changing attitudes and winning hearts and minds. *Journal of Interprofessional Care*, *25*(1), 11–17.

Anderson, E., Thorpe, L., Heney, D., et al. (2009). Medical students benefit from learning about patient safety in an interprofessional team. *Medical Education*, *43*(6), 542–552.

Australian Commission on Safety and Quality in Health Care (2012). *National safety and quality health service standards*. Sydney: Commonwealth of Australia.

Australian Medical Council (2012). *Standards for assessment and accreditation of primary medical programs by the Australian Medical Council 2012*. Canberra: Australian Medical Council.

Australian Nursing and Midwifery Accreditation Council (ANMAC) (2012). *Registered nurse accreditation standards*. Canberra: ANMAC.

Bandura, A. (1986). *Social foundations of thought and action. A social cognitive theory*. Englewood Cliffs, NJ: Prentice-Hall.

Barr, H. (2013). Toward a theoretical framework for interprofessional education. *Journal of Interprofessional Care*, *27*(1), 4–9.

Biggs, J. B. (2011). *Teaching for quality learning at university: What the student does*. Maidenhead: McGraw-Hill Education.

Billett, S. (2001). Learning through work: Workplace affordances and individual engagement, *Journal of Workplace Learning*, *13*(5–6), 209–214.

Billett, S. (2004). Workplace participatory practices: Conceptualising workplaces as learning environments. *Journal of Workplace Learning*, *16*(6), 312–324.

Billett, S. R. (2014). Securing intersubjectivity through interprofessional workplace learning experiences. *Journal of Interprofessional Care*, *28*(3), 206–211.

Bray, J. M. (2008). Interprofessional facilitation skills and knowledge: Evidence from Delphi research surveys. In E. Howkins & J. Bray (Eds.), *Preparing for interprofessional teaching* (pp. 27–39). Oxford: Radcliffe.

Canadian Interprofessional Health Collaborative (CIHC) (2010). *A national interprofessional competency framework*. Vancouver: CIHC.

Carlson, E., Pilhammar, E., & Wann-Hansson, C. (2011). The team builder: The role of nurses facilitating interprofessional student teams at a Swedish clinical training ward. *Nurse Education in Practice*, *11*(5), 309–313.

Chipchase, L., Allen, S., Eley, D., et al. (2012). Interprofessional supervision in an intercultural context: A qualitative study. *Journal of Interprofessional Care*, *26*(6), 465–471.

Clark, P. (2006). What would a theory of interprofessional education look like? Some suggestions for developing a theoretical framework for teamwork training. *Journal of Interprofessional Care*, *20*(6), 577–589.

Colthart, I., Bagnall, G., Evans, A., et al. (2008). The effectiveness of self-assessment on the identification of learner needs, learner activity, and impact on clinical practice. BEME Guide No. 10. *Medical Teacher*, *30*(2), 124–145.

Cutilli, C. C. (2010). Seeking health information: What sources do your patients use? *Orthopaedic Nursing*, *29*(3), 214–219.

D'Amour, D., & Oandasan, I. (2005). Interprofessionality as the field of interprofessional practice and interprofessional education: An emerging concept. *Journal of Interprofessional Care*, *19*(Suppl. 1), 8–20.

Egan-Lee, E., Baker, L., Tobin, S., et al. (2011). Neophyte facilitator experiences of interprofessional education: implications for faculty development. *Journal of Interprofessional Care*, *25*(5), 333–338.

Eraut, M. (2000). Non-formal learning and tacit knowledge in professional work. *British Journal of Educational Psychology*, *70*(1), 113–136.

Eraut, M. (2004). Informal learning in the workplace. *Studies in Continuing Education*, *26*(2), 247–273.

Fougner, M., & Horntvedt, T. (2011). Students' reflections on shadowing interprofessional teamwork: A Norwegian case study. *Journal of Interprofessional Care*, *25*(1), 33–38.

Freeman, S., Wright, A., & Lindqvist, S. (2010). Facilitator training for educators involved in interprofessional learning. *Journal of Interprofessional Care*, *24*(4), 375–385.

Freeth, D., Hammick, M., Reeves, S., et al. (2005). *Effective interprofessional education, development, delivery and evaluation*. Oxford: Blackwell/CAIPE.

Frenk, J., Chen, L., Bhutta, Z. A., et al. (2010). Health professionals for a new century: Transforming education to strengthen health systems in an interdependent world. *The Lancet*, *376*(9756), 1923–1958. doi:10.1016/S0140-6736(10)61854-5.

Garavan, T. N., & McCarthy, A. (2008). Collective learning processes and human resource development. *Advances in Developing Human Resources*, *10*(4), 451–471.

Godden-Webster, A., & Murphy, G. (2014). *Interprofessional collaboration in practice: A guide for strengthening student learning experiences*. Halifax: Dalhousie University, Faculty of Health Professions.

Hager, P. (2008). Learning and metaphors. *Medical Teacher*, *30*, 679–686.

Hager, P., & Smith, E. (2004). The inescapability of significant contextual learning in work performance. *London Review of Education*, *2*(1), 33–46.

Haines, T., Kent, F., & Keating, J. (2014). Interprofessional student clinics: An economic evaluation of collaborative clinical placement education. *Journal of Interprofessional Care*, *28*(4), 292–298.

Howkins, E., & Bray, J. (2008). *Preparing for interprofessional teaching: Theory and practice*. Oxford: Radcliffe Publishing.

Hylin, U., Nyholm, H., Mattiasson, A-C., et al. (2007). Interprofessional training in clinical practice on a training ward for healthcare students: A two-year follow-up. *Journal of Interprofessional Care*, *21*(3), 277–288.

Imanipour, M., & Jalili, M. (2016). Development of a comprehensive clinical performance assessment system for nursing students: A programmatic approach. *Japan Journal of Nursing Science*, *13*, 46–54.

Interprofessional Education Collaborative (IPEC) (2016). *Core competencies for interprofessional collaborative practice: 2016 update*. Washington DC: IPEC.

Jain, A., Luo, E., Yang, J., et al. (2012). Implementing a nurse-shadowing program for first-year medical students to improve interprofessional collaborations on health care teams. *Academic Medicine*, 87(9), 1292–1295.

Jakobsen, F. (2016). An overview of pedagogy and organisation in clinical interprofessional training units in Sweden and Denmark. *Journal of Interprofessional Care*, 30(2), 156–164.

Kaufman, D. M., & Mann, K. V. *Teaching and learning in medical education: How theory can inform practice*. In T. Swanwick (Ed.), *Understanding medical education: Evidence, theory and practice*. Chichester: Wiley-Blackwell.

Kent, F., Drysdale, P., Martin, N., et al. (2014). The mixed discipline aged care student clinic: An authentic interprofessional learning initiative. *Journal of Allied Health*, 43(1), 51–56.

Kent, F., Francis-Cracknell, A., McDonald, R., et al. (2016a). How do interprofessional student teams interact in a primary care clinic? A qualitative analysis using activity theory. *Advances in Health Sciences Education: Theory and Practice*, 21(4), 749–760. doi:10.1007/s10459-015-9663-4.

Kent, F., Hayes, J., Glass, S., et al. (2017). Pre-registration interprofessional clinical education in the workplace: A realist review. *Medical Education*, 51(9), 903–917.

Kent, F., & Keating, J. (2015). Interprofessional education in primary health care for entry level students — a systematic literature review. *Nurse Education Today*, 35(12), 1221–1231.

Kent, F., Lai, F., Beowich, B., et al. (2016b). Interprofessional student teams augmenting service provision in residential aged care. *Australasian Journal on Ageing*, 35(3), 204–209.

Kent, F., Martin, N., & Keating, J. (2016c). Interprofessional student led clinics – an innovative approach to the support of older people in the community. *Journal of Interprofessional Care*, 30(1), 123–128.

Kinnair, D. J., Anderson, E. S., & Thorpe, L. N. (2012). Development of interprofessional education in mental health practice: Adapting the Leicester Model. *Journal of Interprofessional Care*, 26(3), 189–197. doi:10.3109/13561820.2011.647994.

Kuipers, P., Ehrlich, C., & Brownie, S. (2014). Responding to health care complexity: Suggestions for integrated and interprofessional workplace learning. *Journal of Interprofessional Care*, 28(3), 246–248.

Lai, F., Kent, F., & Dodic, M. (2015). Student-led interprofessional clinics may improve health management in patients with chronic disease. *Medical Journal of Australia*, 203(10), 402.

Lait, J., Suter, E., Arthur, N., et al. (2011). Interprofessional mentoring: Enhancing students' clinical learning. *Nurse Education in Practice*, 11(3), 211–215. doi:10.1016/j.nepr.2010.10.005.

Lie, D. A., Forest, C. P., Kysh, L., et al. (2016). Interprofessional education and practice guide no. 5: interprofessional teaching for prequalification students in clinical settings. *Journal of Interprofessional Care*, 30(3), 324–330.

McFadyen, A. K., Webster, V. S., Maclaren, W. M., et al. (2010). Interprofessional attitudes and perceptions: Results from a longitudinal controlled trial of pre-registration health and social care students in Scotland. *Journal of Interprofessional Care*, 24(5), 549–564.

McInerney, D. M., & McInerney, V. (2002). *Educational psychology: Constructing learning* (3rd ed.). Sydney: Prentice Hall.

Marshall, M., & Gordon, F. (2010). Exploring the role of the interprofessional mentor. *Journal of Interprofessional Care*, 24(4), 362–374.

Marsick, V. J., & Volpe, M. (1999). The nature and need for informal learning. *Advances in Developing Human Resources*, 1(1), 1–9.

Mezirow, J. (2000). *Learning as transformation: Critical perspectives on a theory in progress*. San Francisco: Jossey-Bass.

Morison, S., Boohan, M., Jenkins, J., et al. (2003). Facilitating undergraduate interprofessional learning in healthcare: Comparing classroom and clinical learning for nursing and medical students. *Learning in Health and Social Care*, 2(2), 92–104.

Morris, C., & Blaney, D. (2013). Work-based learning. In T. Swanwick (Ed.), *Understanding medical education: Evidence, theory and practice*. Chichester: Wiley-Blackwell.

Murray-Davis, B., Marshall, M., & Gordon, F. (2014). Becoming an interprofessional practitioner: Factors promoting the application of pre-qualification learning to professional practice in maternity care. *Journal of Interprofessional Care*, 28(1), 8–14.

Nagelkerk, J., Peterson, T., Pawl, B. L., et al. (2014). Patient safety culture transformation in a children's hospital: An interprofessional approach. *Journal of Interprofessional Care*, 28(4), 358–364. doi:10.3109/13561820.885935.

National Center for Interprofessional Practice and Education (2013). *Measurement instruments Minnesota 2013*. Minneapolis, MN: National Center for Interprofessional Practice and Education. https://nexusipe.org/advancing/assessment-evaluation-start.

Nicol, P., & Forman, D. (2014). Attributes of effective interprofessional placement facilitation. *Journal of Research in Interprofessional Practice and Education*, 4(2).

Nisbet, G., Hendry, G. D., Rolls, G., et al. (2008). Interprofessional learning for pre-qualification health care students: An outcomes-based evaluation. *Journal of Interprofessional Care*, 22(1), 57–68.

Nisbet, G., Lincoln, M., & Dunn, S. (2013). Informal interprofessional learning: An untapped opportunity for learning and change within the workplace. *Journal of Interprofessional Care*, 27(6), 469–475.

Nisbet, G., O'Keefe, M., & Henderson, A. (2016). Twelve tips for structuring student placements to achieve interprofessional learning outcomes. *MedEdPublish*, 5(3), 1–10. doi.org:10.15694/mep.2016.000109.

Norcini, J., Anderson, B., Bollela, V., et al. (2011). Criteria for good assessment: Consensus statement and recommendations from the Ottawa 2010 Conference. *Medical Teacher*, 33(3), 206–214.

Oandasan, I., & Reeves, S. (2005). Key elements for interprofessional education. Part 1: The learner, the educator and the learning context. *Journal of Interprofessional Care*, 19(Suppl. 1), 21–38.

O'Keefe, M., Henderson, A., & Chick, R. (2017). Defining a set of common interprofessional learning competencies for health profession students. *Medical Teacher*, 39(5), 463–468.

Orchard, C., Pederson, L. L., Allen, D., et al. (2017). Can preparation of clinical teachers in IPC concepts and competencies impact their approach to teaching students in clinical practice? A promising approach. *International Journal of Practice-based Learning in Health and Social Care*, 5(1), 98–115.

Parsell, G., & Bligh, J. (1999). The development of a questionnaire to assess the readiness of health care students for interprofessional learning (RIPLS). *Medical Education*, 33(2), 95–100.

Pawson, R., Greenhalgh, T., & Harvey, G. (2005). Realist review — a new method of systematic review designed for complex policy interventions. *Journal of Health Services Research and Policy*, 10(Suppl. 1), 21–34.

Physiotherapy Board of Australia, & Physiotherapy Board of New Zealand. (2015). *Physiotherapy practice thresholds in Australia and Aotearoa New Zealand*. Melbourne/Wellington:Physiotherapy Board of Australia/Physiotherapy Board of New Zealand.

Pollard, K. (2009). Student engagement in interprofessional working in practice placement settings. *Journal of Clinical Nursing*, 18(20), 2846–2856. doi:10.1111/j.1365-2702.2008.02608.x.

Pollard, K. C. (2008). Non-formal learning and interprofessional collaboration in health and social care: The influence of the quality of staff interaction on student learning about collaborative behaviour in practice placements. *Learning in Health and Social Care*, 7(1), 12–26.

Rees, C. E., Crampton, P., Brown, T., et al. (2018). Understanding students' and clinicians' experiences of informal interprofessional workplace learning: an Australian qualitative study. *BMJ Open*, (in press).

Reeves, S., & Freeth, D. (2002). The London training ward: An innovative interprofessional learning initiative. *Journal of Interprofessional Care*, 16(1), 41–52.

Reeves, S., Freeth, D., McCrorie, P., et al. (2002). 'It teaches you what to expect in future …': Interprofessional learning on a training ward for medical, nursing, occupational therapy and physiotherapy students. *Medical Education*, 36(4), 337–344

Reeves, S., Goldman, J., & Oandasan, I. (2007). Key factors in planning and implementing interprofessional education in health care settings. *Journal of Allied Health*, 36(4), 231–235.

Reeves, S., Lewin, S., Espin, S., et al. (2010). *Interprofessional teamwork for health and social care*. Oxford: Wiley-Blackwell/CAIPE.

Reeves, S., Tassone, M., Parker, K., et al. (2012). Interprofessional education: An overview of key developments in the past three decades. *Work (Reading, Mass.)*, 41(3), 233–245.

Regehr, G., & Mylopoulos, M. (2008). Maintaining competence in the field: Learning about practice, through practice, in practice. *Journal of Continuing Education in the Health Professsions*, 28(Suppl. 1), S19–S23.

Rogers, G. D., Thistlethwaite, J. E., Anderson, E. S., et al. (2017). International consensus statement on the assessment of interprofessional learning outcomes. *Medical Teacher*, 39(4), 347–359.

Sargeant, J., Hill, T., & Breau, L. (2010). Development and testing of a scale to assess interprofessional education (IPE) facilitation skills. *Journal of Continuing Education in the Health Professions*, 30(2), 126–131.

Schutte, T., Tichelaar, J., Dekker, R. S., et al. (2015). Learning in student-run clinics: A systematic review. *Medical Education*, 49(3), 249–263.

Schuwirth, L. W. T., & van der Vleuten, C. P. (2011). Programmatic assessment: From assessment of learning to assessment for learning. *Medical Teacher*, 33(6), 478–485. doi: 0.3109/0142159X.2011.565828.

Spencer, J., Blackmore, D., Heard, S., et al. (2000). Patient-oriented learning: A review of the role of the patient in the education of medical students. *Medical Education*, 34(10), 851–857.

Stewart, M., Purdy, J., Kennedy, N., et al. (2010). An interprofessional approach to improving paediatric medication safety. *BMC Medical Education*, 10(1), 19.

The Interprofessional Curriculum Renewal Consortium (2014). *Curriculum renewal for interprofessional education in health*. Canberra: Commonwealth of Australia, Office for Learning and Teaching.

The iTOFT Consortium (2015). *Work-based assessment of teamwork: An interprofessional approach*. Canberra: Australian Government, Office for Learning and Teaching.

Thistlethwaite, J., & Moran, M. (2010). Learning outcomes for interprofessional education (IPE): Literature review and synthesis. *Journal of Interprofessional Care*, 24(5), 503–513.

Thistlethwaite, J. E. (2015). Assessment of interprofessional teamwork – an international perspective. In D. Forman, M. Jones, & J. E. Thistlethwaite (Eds.), *Leadership and collaboration* (pp. 35–152). Basingstoke: Palgrave.

Wright, A., Hawkes, G., Baker, B., et al. (2012). Reflections and unprompted observations by healthcare students of an interprofessional shadowing visit. *Journal of Interprofessional Care*, 26(4), 305–311.

Yang, K., Nisbet, G., & McAllister, L. (2017). Students' experiences and perceptions of interprofessional supervision on placement. *International Journal of Practice-based Learning in Health and Social Care*, 5(2), 1–18.

Zhao, D., Nagarajan, S., & Nisbet, G. (2015). Informal learning opportunities matter: The interprofessional learning experiences of undergraduate speech pathology students. *International Journal of Practice-based Learning in Health and Social Care*, 3(2), 17–31.

15

Pedagogically-rich activities in hospital work
Handovers, ward rounds and team meetings

Stephen Billett, Christy Noble and
Linda Sweet

Introduction

This chapter discusses healthcare activities held to be pedagogically rich, their qualities, and how their educational worth can be realised in clinical settings. Beyond identifying and elaborating the pedagogical qualities of these activities, the aim here is to propose how their potential can be optimised, not only through what they offer in terms of learning-related tasks and interactions, but also through students' and practitioners' engagement with them. The chapter commences by discussing the importance of these learning experiences, and then outlines some of their pedagogical qualities from earlier research into learning through workplaces. These pedagogical qualities are illustrated by examining the practices of handovers, ward rounds and team meetings. Strategies for optimising them to promote effective learning are then advanced. These considerations include how these activities might be used to promote: 1) students' or novice practitioners' learning; 2) the ongoing development of healthcare practitioners across and within their working lives; and 3) effective interprofessional working and learning. In sum, sets of principles and practices used to promote the efficacy of these experiences are identified, presented and illustrated as a means to assist with promoting effective learning in clinical settings.

Pedagogically-rich work activities

Everyday work activities and interactions in healthcare ordinarily offer a range of opportunities for the initial and ongoing learning of the occupational knowledge required for patient care (Cooke et al., 2010; Dornan, 2012; Teunissen & Wilkinson, 2010). Practice-based experiences are central to the initial development and ongoing learning of healthcare professionals (Billett, 2016; Eppich et al., 2016). Yet some work activities and interactions offer learning experiences that are particularly pedagogically-rich. Usng the examples of handovers, ward rounds and team meetings, we demonstrate how they: 1) provide practitioners access to healthcare knowledge through others' insights and practices; 2) permit comparisons and appraisals with what these practitioners know, can do and value; and 3) offer interactions and access to that knowledge, which might not otherwise be available. More than assisting the refinement and reinforcement of what individuals know, these work activities have the potential to extend and transform healthcare practitioners' knowledge in ways that might not otherwise occur. These activities require practitioners to consider clinical cases and their management, and articulate, discuss and evaluate them with others, and are directed towards healthcare practice. All of these occur in complex clinical contexts with high work demands and finite resources.

Effective provision of clinical care is dependent on healthcare professional capabilities, such as an in-depth understandings of disease states and treatments, along with effective communication skills and clinical reasoning, while valuing the compassionate and attentive delivery of care (Cleland et al., 2014). By engaging in clinical tasks, practitioners can develop many of these kinds of capabilities, including strategic procedural knowledge (Collins et al., 1989; Ericsson & Lehmann, 1996), deep conceptual outcomes (Groen & Patel, 1988), critical appraisal abilities, and the exercising of individuals' dispositions (e.g. values). Moreover, practitioners' engagement in particular work activities, such as handovers, ward rounds and team meetings, can extend and augment what healthcare workers know, can do and value in specific ways, because these activities have an inherently rich pedagogical potential. While all workplace activities and interactions can be generative of professional capabilities, some have qualities that make them pedagogically-rich learning experiences, and can be accessed as part of daily healthcare work activities.

A primary pedagogical advantage of workplace activities and interactions such as handovers, ward rounds and team meetings (e.g. mortality and morbidity meetings) is that they are part of everyday healthcare practice, and thus provide accessible and authentic learning experiences. This accessibility and authenticity is in contrast to experiences intentionally designed and enacted for similar purposes, such as simulations and virtual reality, which are substitutes and not as readily accessible, and require extensive planning, resources and support to replicate authentic workplace experiences.

Moreover, the range of pedagogically-rich work activities are unlikely to be found and accessed elsewhere (O'Keefe et al., 2011). Even the most sophisticated simulations and virtual realities may not capture the quality of authentic activities. For the learning potential of these workplace experiences to be optimised, they need to be effectively enacted and effortfully engaged in by practitioners and students. For practitioners and educators to realise these benefits, the key qualities of these pedagogically-rich activities (PRAs) need to be identified, and strategies for optimising professional learning outcomes need to be elaborated.

We commence by presenting an illustrative example in the form of a vignette of nurses' handovers. Then, drawing on literature and recent empirical work, the concept of PRAs is examined, their key qualities identified, and how these activities might be engaged with and be optimised in the healthcare sector is advanced. The theoretical propositions underpinning such claims are advanced by discussing how people have learnt through practice across human history; that is, from personally mediated processes, rather than being taught or directly guided (Billett, 2014a; Byrne & Russon, 1998; Donald, 1991). We propose that while workplace experiences such as handovers, ward rounds and team meetings are not intentionally established for educational purposes, they offer potentially rich learning experiences to those who participate in them (e.g. practitioners and students). Hopefully, this contribution will also assist in opening up discussions on what constitutes worthwhile and legitimate learning experiences, both for the initial and ongoing development of healthcare practitioners' abilities to provide patients with safe and effective care.

Case study 15.1: Field observation of nurses' handovers

It was a normal, busy day at the Moncrieff Medical Centre in the east of a large Australian metropolitan city. The day shift of the nursing staff in the general ward was coming to a close. The incoming late shift of nurses entered the staffroom individually or in pairs, sipping on hot drinks, some of them finishing snacks as they completed the preparation of their uniforms, and assembling their notepads, keys and other accoutrements. Some of these nurses were of mature age, but most seemed quite young. Among them were final-year student nurses working on the ward, but they looked no different to the other nursing staff. They were all chatting among themselves when the nurse unit manager from the day shift entered the room. There were perfunctory greetings, followed by a handing around of sheets of paper about the patients currently on the ward.

Also, entering were two first-year nursing students, who were quite distinct, not so much by their age, although they seemed a bit younger than the other nurses, but by their uniform and prominent badge indicating the university where they were studying. This appeared a routine activity for the students, as they were not given, nor appeared to require an introduction, or be consciously drawn into the handover proceedings. They also did not look particularly engaged. Then the nurse unit manager left the room, and individual nurses from the day shift came in and discussed their patients in turn. There was a set procedure for this discussion, comprising details about: 1) the patient; 2) their condition(s); 3) their treatment(s); 4) their progression; and 5) their prognosis.

The handover commenced with a discussion about the patient, which comprised age (gender was usually apparent), some family considerations (e.g. whether the patient had relatives visiting, making enquiries, raising concerns; or the patient's domestic circumstances). Then the patient's condition and the treatments being provided were mentioned, usually together. Sometimes one of the incoming-shift nurses would raise a question about the treatment, its stage or appropriateness. At this point, there was discussion, which was not restricted to the nurse who raised the question, or to the day-shift nurse who was reporting and responding to the question, but included others in the room. Then the discussion moved on to how the patient was progressing and what the prognosis was for the future; for instance, in terms of when they might be discharged, or any additional treatments or therapies (e.g. strategies for addressing access to the patient's apartment) that might be required. These topics tended to generate a degree of interaction and discussion, usually initiated by the incoming-shift nurses, particularly those who would be caring for the specific patient. However, other nurses, including graduate-year nurses, would engage in discussion and offer suggestions, opinions, concerns and commentary.

All of this progressed in a fairly perfunctory way as the day-shift nurses rotated through the room. Occasionally, there was a slight halt in the proceedings while the next nurse came in for the handover. During these breaks, the incoming shift of nurses often chatted, sometimes about the cases, but not always. During one such break, one of the two student nurses leant across to the other and said 'Let's go', and they both left the room midway through the handover. When the final handover case had been discussed, the incoming shift of nurses briefly chatted among themselves, some of which was about arrangements for patient care or prioritising activities, and then the nurses left the handover room and went into the ward to commence their nursing care.

Elements of pedagogically-rich activities from the case study

There are a range of pedagogical elements evident in this vignette. First, the focus was on real patients, who had a medical condition or conditions, and the particular levels and types of support they had outside of the hospital, as well as the individuals who might need to be consulted or advised about their progress. Secondly, there were also opportunities for the articulation and discussion of patient conditions, treatments and progress. Thirdly, as some of the nurses had roles associated with the care of these patients, they had reason to engage intentionally and in directed ways. This activity provided an opportunity for the nurses' occupational concepts, procedures and values to be utilised, appraised and, potentially, extended.

The nurses had an occupational knowledge base from which to form judgments about this complex of interrelated factors. By drawing on this knowledge, through listening or responding to the discussions in the handovers, they were applying and appraising what they know, can do, and value about nursing. It was not necessary for all of them to verbally articulate their understandings, preferences for procedures or values for it to be a rich learning experience. They could conduct an appraisal without verbal articulation. Those expressing their views, importantly, provided bases for others to make judgments about their own knowledge (e.g. what they understood or did not know about, would have done, or would have prioritised). So, while articulation is helpful for the learning process, it is not necessary for all participants to engage verbally (Manias & Street, 2000). Fourthly, the quality of engagement here is important, because each healthcare practitioner will have particular kinds of understandings based on their prior experience, and will construe the case being discussed (Meißner et al., 2007) in person-particular ways.

In these ways, the handover experience provided: 1) goal-directed activities, within an authentic context; 2) a structure through which patient care can be understood and appraised; and 3) opportunities for cases to be discussed, and perspectives entertained and appraised. Such processes and outcomes are supportive of learning, as well as of patient care. These processes are generative of learning, albeit not often referred to as such, nor always recognised by educators, whose focus is often on the provision of teaching-led activities, and practitioners, whose focus is patient care.

The likely richness of learning outcome is, however, contingent on the degree of effort individuals exercise in comparing and contrasting what is being discussed with what they know, the current or proposed treatments with what they would do, and the overall regimen of care with what they value as nurses (Ericsson, 2006; Ericsson & Lehmann, 1996; and see Chapter 12 of this book). It is difficult, of course, to gauge the level of participation during these handovers. It is likely that the nurses caring for particular patients follow their cases more closely, because they will be responsible for their care. Others might engage in the discussion if they have contributions to make; for example, a preference for particular kinds of treatments, knowledge of the patient or previous experiences with this health-related issue. In this way, the quality of learning arising for each nurse is likely to be contingent upon the quality of what they know and also how they elect to engage in this activity.

For these nurses, there were tangible reasons for engaging in this activity, as they would be soon caring for these patients, and perhaps assisting their colleagues with others on the shift. Hence, the potential richness of this everyday learning activity is premised not only on what it afforded them in terms of activities and interactions, and even guidance by teachers and clinicians, but also how the nurses come to engage with them — the duality of what is afforded and how individuals participate and learn (Billett, 2001a).

The centrality of learner engagement was demonstrated in the actions of the two student nurses who left midway through the handover session. As these students were intentionally engaged in learning about nursing, one would assume that they would be engaging effortfully in this event. It might have been presumed that they would follow each case with interest and seek to listen to the propositional statements, and attempt to make causal links and associations about the patients' health and treatments, as the more experienced nurses discussed them. However, none of this appeared to be the case. These students did not have assigned patients to care for, and were not involved in the next shift. They also did not appear to understand or appreciate the potential richness of the handover as an opportunity to learn. This session, it seemed, was something they were obliged to attend, but they did not seem to be aware of the value of their participation. In this instance, it was enacted as an obligation to be fulfilled with the least effort possible, rather than something from which they could learn much about nursing.

Had the students been required to lead the commentary on one of the cases, or to personally evaluate or reiterate any one of them, they would have likely been far more involved in the discussions, and the outcomes might have been more generative of learning. In this example, the students' participation not only lacked effortful engagement, it was not purposefully directed. Hence, their readiness to engage in and learn through these experiences was not just a product of their nascent knowledge base. It also was a product of a lack of affordances, such as the intentional use of, and response to, patients' cases using the five-point handover rubric to participate and learn effectively. This issue will be taken up later in the chapter.

Background theory related to PRAs

This section presents the background theory and empirical evidence informing PRAs, and, based on these propositions, the key qualities of PRAs are presented. To begin, the four key theoretical perspectives informing this chapter include:

1. learning occurs without teaching;
2. learning outcomes are influenced by the degree of practitioner engagement;
3. effective practitioner engagement in practice contributes to learning, and the remaking or transformation of practice;
4. learning is influenced by the workplace's invitational qualities — that is, affordances.

Firstly, learning is not dependent on teaching. There is a tendency to consider learning and teaching as inseparable and irreducible concepts. This is not surprising given that we all live in societies where schooling is compulsory and education ubiquitous. However, quite the opposite is the case. Indeed, there is no separation between participation in everyday activities, such as work, and the processes of engaging human cognition and the change arising from that engagement, referred to as learning (Billett et al., 2017; Rogoff & Lave,

1984; Scribner, 1984). As we participate in everyday thinking and acting, we draw on what we know, can do and value, and in doing so we bring about change within ourselves (i.e. learning). That is, legacies arise, in the form of extensions of what we know, can do and value, through engaging with them in our everyday activities (Anderson, 1982).

Engagement in work activities in healthcare is no exception here. Indeed, the daily processes of using our knowledge, evaluating its utility, and monitoring patients' progress with treatment, leads to the elaboration and transformation of understandings about, and procedures associated with, healthcare. This is how much of the higher-order forms of knowledge required for complex problem-solving required in healthcare is generated (Groen & Patel, 1988). Whether referring to the honing of specific- or the development of strategic-procedural capacities (i.e. how we effectively achieve goals) (Anderson, 1993), the development of propositions through the building of causal links (Goldman, 2003) that comprise deep understanding, or the nuancing of the dispositions (i.e. values) associated with occupations (Tobias, 1994) — all of these arise through practice (Billett, 2001b).

Secondly, while there are roles for teaching and direct guidance by more experienced practitioners, ultimately, the processes of an individual's learning are shaped by how they come to engage what they know, can do and value, when participating in the workplace and interacting with others. This is how we have learnt occupations across human history. For the vast majority of humans, prior to modern schooled societies, access to intentional educational experiences and teaching was not available (Billett, 2014b). It was reserved for a tiny minority of privileged individuals (Roodhouse, 2007). Even then, the processes that we would recognise in an era of mass education as comprising teaching were notably absent. Teaching, as in classroom instruction, as we have come to know it, and how educational institutions have been organised in contemporary schooled societies, is a relatively recent phenomenon (Jordan, 1989), and commenced with the advent of modern nation states and mass education. While education and teaching contribute to learning, most learning across human history, and across individuals' lives, arises through personally mediated learning processes, not teaching (Billett, 2014b).

Moreover, even though much learning is personally mediated, this does not mean that the knowledge required for an occupation is a product of individual discovery. Occupational knowledge is a product of history, culture and situation. The evolving knowledge of the occupations arises through societal institutions, such as research centres, hospitals and universities, but also has manifestations in particular situations. What might constitute effective healthcare practice in one community may be quite inappropriate in another. Moreover, the kinds of health-related issues which might plague one community might be totally absent in another. The key point is that the knowledge required for healthcare occupations has to be accessed and engaged with between individuals and the social world (Billett, 2006). This process requires individuals to access this socially derived knowledge on the one hand, and engage with it on the other; that is, construe and construct it in applicable ways. It follows then that learning such knowledge is dependent on: 1) the kinds of interactions and activities available to or afforded individuals; and 2) how individuals elect to engage with those affordances. That is, learning is shaped by the provision of 'experiences' and the processes of 'experiencing' them.

Thirdly, when individuals engage in work activities, another kind of change arises: the active remaking of occupational practice. As healthcare practitioners engage in their work activities at a particular point in time and place, and in response to specific patients' needs, they are actively engaging in the process of remaking their occupational practice. As our knowledge of healthcare evolves, it is healthcare practitioners who often innovate and implement those changes in their practice. Whether it is about reducing antimicrobial prescribing, being confronted by increasing numbers of young people with depressive conditions, or dealing with the increased frequency of older patients with delirium and dementia, it is healthcare practitioners who remake their occupational practice in their healthcare settings, as they confront these occupational requirements.

Therefore, as practitioners, such as the nurses in case study 15.1, engage in their work they are both learning about and remaking healthcare practice. The specific focus here is that particular experiences provide the bases for both their learning, and the effective remaking of that practice. The latter is important, because, if the practice is remade in inappropriate or perilous ways, there can be detrimental consequences for patients, as has been experienced recently in hospital systems in the United Kingdom (Francis, 2013) and Australia (Garling, 2008).

Fourthly, workplaces afford significant opportunities for diverse learning experiences — but not all experiences are considered equal, with some resulting in detrimental outcomes. It is important to identify the qualities of clinical activities and interactions that are particularly educationally- or pedagogically-rich. It is well understood that everyday activities and interactions in clinical workplaces support the development of practitioners' knowledge (Cooke et al., 2010). Repeating activities that have already been learnt and practised assists in honing and refining their enactment, and understanding the breadth of their applicability (Billett, 2001a). Workplace activities and interactions that are novel or new to practitioners can assist them in developing new understandings, practices and values. Both routine and new activities arising through everyday work activities contribute to healthcare practitioners' learning and development (Dornan, 2012).

Yet some activities and interactions have particular potency in terms of their potential to promote learning, and learning of specific kinds. That is, they have particular qualities that make knowledge accessible in ways that might not otherwise occur through educational actvities. Workplace activities that provide opportunities to discuss, compare, contrast and evaluate what has occurred or is occurring are particularly valuable. These kinds of experiences extend to opportunities to subsequently observe, monitor progress and evaluate what is being achieved. Hence, these processes can lead to learning associated with clinical understandings, procedures and values. These contributions are now elaborated in terms of what is afforded by PRAs.

Qualities of pedagogically rich activities

This section discusses the key qualities of PRAs, and delineates and elaborates their particular educational worth in terms of their potential for developing adaptable knowledge (e.g. principled understandings, strategic procedures and nuanced dispositions) (Goldman, 2003; Vosniadou et al., 2002). These qualities, and how they lead to the optimisation of learning through everyday activities and interactions in healthcare settings, are then advanced. This includes how healthcare practitioners and students might come to most effectively engage with those experiences. Optimising the potential of these learning experiences is premised on the duality of what is afforded by practitioners in terms of the quality of these activities and interactions, on the one hand, and how healthcare practitioners and students take up and engage with what is afforded them, on the other (Billett, 2006). Informed by the theoretical and empirical literature presented earlier in this chapter, it is proposed that the key qualities of PRAs are five-fold (see Box 15.1).

Box 15.1: Key qualities of pedagogically-rich activities

1. Engage learners in authentic, goal-directed work activities.
2. Have complex practice-based scenarios.
3. Offer opportunities for verbalisation of occupational knowledge by experts.
4. Involve narratives and discussions supporting recall and appraisal.
5. Are set within authentic work experiences.

Beginning with the first PRA quality, authentic experiences press individuals into goal-directed activities that require them to generate responses to healthcare tasks based on what they know and can do, and what they value (Anderson, 1993). It is these kinds of situations that are generative of purposive learning about the occupational practice (Scribner, 1984). Through authentic, goal-directed experiences, individuals are required to generate potential responses, evaluate options and priorities, and appraise them in relation to specific patient care regimens and outcome goals (Mayer, 1992; Scribner, 1992). In this way, they are engaging and extending their knowledge of what they know, can do and value against those of others.

Secondly, PRAs are usually context-rich, complex, practice-based scenarios. They constitute individual cases involving patients who have names, families, particular conditions and variabilities. These individually and collectively constitute context-rich scenarios that generate and support indexing (i.e. how we organise and order knowledge in memory) (Anderson, 1982; Ericsson & Simon, 1980), and recall of knowledge (Royer et al., 2005; Sweller, 1990), and offer what Barsalou (2009) refers to as *simulations* (i.e. multimodal ways in which we construe and organise what we know, can do and value). Rather than human cognition being founded on single sensory processes, it seems that multimodal and sensory processes shape human thinking and acting. Hence, these rich scenarios provide the means by which human cognitive, sensory and even neural processes come to engage with what they are experiencing, and generate cognitive structures, forms and ordering of that knowledge, often known as *illness scripts* or *mnemonics*.

Thirdly, the verbalisation of knowledge provides declarative or statable forms of knowledge that permit concepts and propositions to be understood, and causal links and associations to be formed and developed further

(Goldman, 2003). In particular, verbalisation by more experienced practitioners allows novices or less-experienced workers to have access to propositional bases and procedural considerations of those practitioners in ways which might not otherwise be accessible (Vosniadou et al., 2002). This verbalisation permits all participants to consider and appraise what these practitioners are proposing (Goldman, 2003). Even if individuals do not express either assent or disagreement with what is being verbalised, they can still compare and contrast what they know, can do and value against what others are stating. This permits the ability to evaluate these procedures and procedural responses without having to experience them directly themselves.

Fourthly, the process of discussing authentic, practice-based cases generates narratives which can further act as mnemonics to assist recall, and bases for the appraising of individuals' knowledge. These narratives have significant mnemonic value, as they assist not just based recall, but also provide the details of circumstances to be engaged with. Mnemonics are used extensively to assist recall within healthcare and to remember complex cases (Rice, 2010; Sinclair, 1997).

Fifthly, PRAs provide access to sets of activities and interactions which, while being highly authentic, are unlikely to be generated through other means (Barsalou, 2008). These kinds of experiences are those that educational technology seeks to generate so that they can be readily accessed by learners. Yet they are accessible as part of particular kinds of workplace activities. It is on these bases that these activities be potentially pedagogically rich.

What has been proposed here is that these qualities, in sum or in part, are those that can make work activities inherently pedagogically rich.

Bases of engagement by learners

The realisation of the potential of workplace PRAs is as much in the engagement by learners as what is afforded them. The quality of engagement is likely to be shaped by: 1) individuals' readiness to engage effectively in these experiences as premised on what they know, can do and value; and 2) the degree by which they elect to engage in them (Billett & Sweet, 2015). (See Box 15.2.)

Box 15.2: Factors influencing learner engagement

1. Learner readiness
   - what they know
   - what they can do
   - what they value.
2. Degree learners elect to engage.

For instance, the two student nurses in case study 15.1 may not have the readiness to be able to engage in making a prognosis about the outcomes for the patients. That is, their level of knowledge may have been insufficient to engage productively in that process. Yet their readiness might have put them in a position to understand the patient's condition and the kinds of treatments they were undertaking. That is, they might have been able to make links between what they have learnt in the university setting (i.e. in lectures, tutorials or practical skills sessions) to what is being discussed in the handover. As they were on placement, it could have been assumed they were ready to engage in that kind of activity. In the case study, the graduate nurses actively engaged in discussions about the patient treatment and outcomes, both in terms of responses and prognoses. This demonstrates that their range and extent of experiences provided them the readiness to engage in that kind of discussion.

The second factor is the degree by which the learners engage effortfully or with agency in these activities (Bhaskar, 1998), or in their mediational means (Wertsch, 1991). That is, how individuals exercise their engagement as learners, and the effort they use to engage what they know, can do and value (Valsiner, 1998), will influence learning. In the case study, it was suggested that the agency of individual nurses might be most exercised by those providing the care to the patients. For the less-experienced nurses, this focus might be pre-eminent; however, for more experienced nurses, both individual cases and overall considerations of cases on the ward might be the basis by which they come to engage. Certainly, the nurse unit manager would have a different set of bases for engagement than individual nurses.

When making use of PRAs, it is important to consider both their affordance, and the ways individuals come to engage with these activities and learn through them. This includes the challenges that might be faced by experienced practitioners when they must change their practices. For instance, healthcare workers who have previously prescribed antimicrobials in non-judicious ways need to change their antimicrobial prescribing practice to address over-prescribing and subsequent antimicrobial resistance. This change requires practitioners to identify alternative treatments to address patients' symptoms, while engaging in, sometimes, complex communications with patients to temper their concerns. The worth of these experiences needs to be made explicit in an era where reforms, such as telehealth, can limit their dialogic qualities and bases for engagement. So there is a need to acknowledge and augment their pedagogical worth.

Bringing pedagogy to practice

PRAs are embedded in practice. The key pedagogical concerns are about access to, participation, and potentially some guidance, when engaging in PRAs. That is, firstly providing access to these kinds of activities as learning experiences, and then finding ways of encouraging effortful engagement with them. Such engagement is likely to be of a progressive kind. Novice practitioners, new staff members, or students might not initially play an explicit role in the discussions, but rather participate through observation, following through the narratives, comparing and contrasting, critically appraising, and attempting to predict what might next occur. The process of actively appraising what is occurring, and predicting what might happen next, or considering the likely outcomes, are well-established bases for improving learning outcomes from these kinds of experiences. For example, first-year medical students might begin by attending ward rounds to understand there structure, processes and intentions; while final-year students might present cases, describe their thinking, or conduct patient examinations. Indeed, this process, also referred to as *reciprocal teaching and learning* (Palinscar & Brown, 1984) in education, is a key instructional process whereby teachers explicitly state their thinking processes. This provides a model for students to understand the processes they need to learn, and, through observation and hearing what the teacher has modelled, students are then invited to engage in similar kinds of thinking processes, such as think-aloud techniques or making thinking visible (Ritchhart et al., 2011).

This strategy can be adopted within PRAs. First, those positioned as learners (e.g. students, junior staff, novice practitioners) would seek to follow through what senior clinicians or practitioners talk about, in terms of the cases, and begin to identify the processes through which patient history and information about their health are discussed. Secondly, the learners might be encouraged to participate in ways commensurate with their level of understanding and confidence. For instance, they might introduce a case or lead a handover of the patient. Third, as with the graduate nurses in the case study handover, progressively they might be invited to discuss features of the patient's health, or illness conditions and their treatments. Throughout, they might be reminded of the importance of positioning themselves in the 'driver's seat', so to speak. That is, to position themselves as if they were the decision-makers, and to consider how they would progress the conversation, and identify what kinds of information they need, and how they draw that information together when making judgments about patient health and outcomes. This can be achieved through careful facilitation and focused questioning.

In Table 15.1, the five characteristics of PRAs are set out in the left column, strategies for augmenting learning in the middle column, and then examples are provided in the right column about how these activities can be structured to enable effective learning and be more pedagogically potent. Much of what is in the table demonstrates the ways in which individuals are provided with access to PRAs, and how they can be encouraged to participate in these activities, to enhance learning outcomes. Also, in Table 15.1, considerations are given of how these PRAs, including handovers, ward rounds and team meetings, might be used to promote learning for: 1) different learner capabilities (i.e. novice through to expert practitioner); and 2) different types of learning goals (e.g. augment effective interprofessional working and learning) (see Chapter 14 for further details on student engagement in interprofessional learning). These considerations are important, because firstly the degree of learner readiness influences engagement, and secondly, different learning goals are likely to require different strategies when engaging in and affording PRAs. For example, if the goal is to augment interprofessional working and learning while on a ward round, then considerations might be given to ensuring that all of the professional groups are engaged by inviting them to verbalise their clinical reasoning and appraise others' reasoning.

TABLE 15.1: Strategies and examples

Key qualities	Strategies for augmenting learning	Practical examples
1. Engage learners in authentic goal directed work activities	Preparatory work to enhance readiness before engaging in goal-directed activities (e.g. background readings or discussions with a clinical educator) Identify and articulate roles for novice learners to play when engaging in goal-directed activities Consider the level of guidance required to facilitate learner engagement	**Novice:** Invite learners to read up on a patient's condition (e.g. claudication) before handover, to augment their conceptual knowledge. Learners are allocated roles (Walton & Steinert, 2010) (e.g. present a few cases during handover or be responsible for tasks on ward rounds) **Mid-career:** Invite practitioners to read an article that challenges current practices (e.g. ward rounds), and in collaboration with the supervisor identify new ways of practicing and enact these practices **Senior:** Self-evaluate, and invite others to evaluate their role in work activities **Interprofessional learning focus:** Develop meeting structures, guidelines and templates to supporting professional groups engagement and limit hierarchial structures
2. Have complex practice-based scenarios	Use authentic cases, as in handovers, mortality and morbidity meetings, ward rounds Invite learners to consider perspectives of healthcare disciplines other than their own Support understanding through observation and appraisal of what is occurring by providing explanation Construct progressive learning opportunities to facilitate understanding of practice complexities	**Novice:** Invite learners to lead the case presentation, and later a discussion about cases in these meetings. Provide clear frameworks or overviews of the meeting, handover or ward round structures, to support understanding of processes. Invite learners to follow patients' journeys (e.g. from admission to discharge) to understand the purpose and intentions of the different activities (e.g. handover; ward round) **Experts:** Revise and generate structures and processes to agument learner engagement; invite critique from peers
3. Offer opportunities for the verbalisation of occupational knowledge by experienced others	Experts use 'think-aloud' techniques (Pinnock et al., 2015) or 'making thinking visible' (Delany & Golding, 2014) to articulate clinical reasoning Consider the influence of hierarchy, and ensure that all of the professions involved have 'a voice'	**Novices:** During ward rounds, have trainees present a case and senior clinicans 'think aloud' to provide additional insights. Encourage learners to seek explanation of decision-making and clincial reasoning when working with more experienced practitionrs. Learners' voices can be fostered by using tools such as SNAPPS to promote learner-centred case presentations (Wolpaw et al., 2003) **Experts:** Make thinking explicit, invite peers and juniors to critique their 'think-aloud' and debate approaches to practice, and/or have experts self-evaluate aloud and role-model to juniors **Interprofessionl learning focus:** Encourage all professions to engage in discussion during ward rounds, handover and team meetings

Continued

TABLE 15.1: Strategies and examples — cont'd

Key qualities	Strategies for augmenting learning	Practical examples
4. Involve narratives and discussions supporting recall and appraisal	Participation in meetings to follow through the description and discussion, and predicting treatments, progress and prognoses. Create opportunities for recall and appraisal (Warmington & McColl 2017). Share both professional and patient stories during handover, ward rounds and team meetings (Gray, 2009)	**Novice:** Following the meetings' conversations, discussions and conclusions by developing illness scripts to enhance clinical reasoning, and debriefing after ward rounds or meetings (Warmington & McColl, 2017) **Experts**: Consider the types of stories they are sharing, and how these are likely to influence learners' understanding. Invite peers to challenge their reasoning.
5. Set learning within authentic work experiences	Systematically examine the practice setting to identify learning opportunities not likely to be generated through other means. Support/sensitise the clinical team to recognise PRAs. Press participants to appraise their clinical decision-making processes, and about how they decide to proceed with them	**Novices:** Effortfully attend and progressively engage in the processes of handover, ward round and team meetings. Engage in the actual care of cases discussed to consolidate learning. Question and clarify areas of confusion or poor understanding **Experts:** Maximise clinical presentations for learning. Identify useful examples to meet the learning needs of all team members

Potential directions for evaluation and research

The PRAs discussed in this chapter are increasingly being recognised as learning opportunities (Benassi et al., 2017; Nisbet et al., 2015); however, strategies for optimising learning from them require further investigation. While there has been a focus on supporting the development and learning of novices, further investigation into how these activities contribute to expert practitioners is likely to be worthwhile.

In terms of evaluation, the learning outcomes from engaging in these activities will not always be explicit, measurable or easy to identify, and may resist effective measurement. This situation is, in part, likely due to the challenges associated with capturing learning processes. However, we know that the kinds of human performances that are most measurable are those that are of relatively low importance. Capturing the capacities that underpin human performance, such as possessed by expertise, requires evaluation processes that are sensitive to articulation, justification and tolerance to variations and complexity. Indeed, events such as PRAs are circumstances where such performance can likely be evaluated through the actions, utterances and procedures adopted by those leading the discussions. Further research is required to ensure informed contributions to the benefits (or not) of these experiences are illuminated.

Tips for augmenting learning

Case study 15.2: Back to the nursing handover

Having observed the nursing students leave the handover early, Jo, one of the senior nurses, considers some of the factors likely to have caused the students to leave early, and makes the following suggestions to her team to improve student engagement. First, she suggests that a nurse meets with the students five minutes before handover to describe what is going to occur, and prepares them for the patients and the conditions likely to be discussed. Secondly, the students are given particular roles during handover, such as taking note of anything they have not heard of, so they can look it up later (e.g. claudication). Thirdly, Jo suggests that the students are allocated roles and tasks to follow up after the handover, such as interview a patient with a condition discussed, or follow up on a discharge plan (e.g. the occupational therapist home visit).

Case study 15.3: Maximising workplace learning through PRAs

Sarah has been a health professional for 15 years. Despite busy work schedules where she needs to balance outpatient and ward commitments, she has been recognised as an excellent clinical educator. The team, interprofessional colleagues and students all note that when working with Sarah on ward rounds, in handover or team meetings, they consistently learn from her guidance and the learning opportunities she fosters for them.

You ask Sarah about her tips for augmenting learning:

You have been a clinician and facilitating clinical learning for 15 years, and, despite your extremely busy schedule, those working with you are impressed by your ability to support their learning. What strategies do you use to ensure that rich learning is enabled through activities such as handover, ward rounds or team meetings?

Sarah responds:

The key idea underpinning my approach is to think about each of these experiences as opportunities to learn, and I consider the potential learning opportunities and how I can best encourage people to engage. Next I consider who is going to be involved and what is their learning level (i.e. readiness) — that is, what do they know, what can they do and what do they value? — as well as considering what level of guidance they are likely to require.

To explain further, let us consider each activity in turn.

PRACTICAL TIPS

Handovers: I appreciate that engaging in handover [*complex practice-based scenario*] can be overwhelming for junior clinicans; however, given its importance for ensuring patient safety, it is essential that they are supported in their engagement. Because our juniors often have not had much in the way of handover training, I started to consider ways in which I could enhance juniors' learning through practice. Firstly, to *support narratives and discussions*, we base our handover structure on patient reporting systems such as I-PASS (or ISBAR). The menominc I-PASS refers to:

- **I**llness severity (e.g. whether the patients is stable, 'watcher' or unstable).
- **P**atient summary, including a summary statement, the events leading up to admission, and an overview of the patient's course in hospital and the plan.
- **A**ction list, including a to-do list, and a timeline and ownership.
- **S**ituation awareness and contingency; that is, knowing what's going on and planning for what might happen.
- **S**ynthesis by receiver, which is achieved by inviting the receiver to summarise what was heard, ask questions and restate key action and 'to-do' items (Starmer et al., 2012).

This mnemonic, along with ensuring a consistent approach to handover, supports the juniors' understanding of handover discussions along with being able to appraise them. This means that the purpose of handover is clear and we are sharing how we work here with the team members. This approach also highlights the role of the juniors, by ensuring the action list items are allocated to a team member. Finally, with new and junior team members, the senior members, by leading the handover discussions using the I-PASS, will be role-modelling practices and verbalising their knowledge, while increasingly engaging the junior members. For the development of experienced practitioners, we invite peers to observe and critique the effectiveness of the handover structure and approach. For final-year students, I might ask them to present a case, using I-PASS, during handover; whereas first-year students might be asked to attend several handovers so that they can understand the structure, process and importance of sharing knowledge.

Ward rounds: We have really struggled with effectively enhancing interprofessional engagement on our ward rounds. We acknowledge the importance of effective interprofessional working for patient safety. To address this challenge, we have revised our practices and use the model called structured interdisciplinary rounds (SIDR) (O'Leary et al., 2010; O'Leary et al., 2011). A key consideration was ensuring that there were opportunities for all of the professional groups to engage in the interdisciplinary ward rounds [*engagement in goal-directed activities*]. To ensure this, we worked together to identify a suitable time for all practitioners. Again, we use a structured communication tool (see O'Leary et al., 2010), and ensure that there is a shared understanding of the purpose of the ward round. Also, the team member roles have been agreed (e.g. the pharmacist presents the medication history; the medical students each present one patient; the occupational therapist presents the discharge planning), and this approach has ensured that decisions are shared and everyone is engaged in the round. The ward round is co-led by nursing and medical staff, to attempt to address hierarchy challenges, and all of the professions are invited to articulate their clinical reasoning. However, we are aware of the importance of engaging patients in ward rounds, and so are reviewing our structures and considering strategies for enhancing the patient voice.

Team meetings: One of our team meetings — the morbidity and mortality meeting — has been an area of practice which we acknowledge as a key learning opportunity for all pracitioners of all levels of experience. Our goal has been to establish a meeting environment where it is safe for all to contribute. However, fostering this has been challenging, as there is a long tradition of using a somewhat hierarchical approach. To begin the process of change, we made simple changes, such as rearranging the seating to promote discussion by using circular seating arrangements, and encouraging the senior practitioners to sit in the outer circle and the juniors in the inner circle. Already we are seeing an increased engagement of the junior practitioners. All of the professional groups are invited to the meeting, and the meeting chair has also been primed to ensure interprofessional participation and collaborative case discussion (Benassi et al., 2017). Again, we use a standardised meeting format, including a structured approach to root cause analysis, and ensure that the meeting concludes with a clear action list for improvement.

Conclusion

This chapter has sought to identify and promote the learning potential of particular healthcare activities held to be pedagogically rich. Beyond identifying and elaborating the particular pedagogical qualities of these activities, we have proposed how their potential can be optimised through their affordance and through practitioners' engagement with them. It commenced by discussing the importance of these learning experiences, and then outlined some of their pedagogical qualities by drawing on earlier research into learning through workplaces, including clinical settings. These qualities are illustrated by making reference to what occurs within handovers, ward rounds and team meetings. Following this elaboration of the qualities of these activities, the means by which they might be optimised to promote effective learning were then advanced. These considerations include how these activities might be used to promote: 1) novices', students' or new workplace entrants' learning (e.g. junior or student doctors, nurses, midwives); 2) the ongoing development of healthcare practitioners across and within their working lives; and 3) effective interprofessional working and learning. In sum, the sets of principles and practices used to promote the efficacy of these experiences have been identified, presented and illustrated, as a means to assist with promoting effective learning in clinical settings.

References

Anderson, J. R. (1982). Acquisition of cognitive skill. *Psychological Review, 89*(4), 369–406.

Anderson, J. R. (1993). Problem solving and learning. *American Psychologist, 48*(1), 3544.

Barsalou, L. W. (2008). Grounded cognition. *Annual Review of Psychology, 59,* 617–645.

Barsalou, L. W. (2009). Simulation, situated conceptualisation, and prediction. *Philosophical Transcactions of the Royal Society of London. Series B, Biological Sciences, 364,* 1281–1289.

Benassi, P., MacGillivray, L., Silver, I., et al. (2017). The role of morbidity and mortality rounds in medical education: A scoping review. *Medical Education, 51*(5), 469–479. doi:10.1111/medu.13234.

Bhaskar, R. (1998). *The possibility of naturalism.* London: Routledge.

Billett, S. (2001a). *Learning in the workplace: Strategies for effective practice.* Crow's Nest, NSW: Allen and Unwin.

Billett, S. (2001b). Learning through work: Workplace affordances and individual engagement. *The Journal of Workplace Learning, 13*(5/6), 209–214.

Billett, S. (2006). Relational interdependence between social and individual agency in work and working life. *Mind, Culture, and Activity, 13*(1), 53–69. doi:10.1207/s15327884mca1301_5.

Billett, S. (2014a). *Mimetic learning at work: Learning in the circumstances of practice.* Dordrecht, The Netherlands: Springer.

Billett, S. (2014b). Mimesis: Learning through everyday activities and interactions at work. *Human Resource Development Review, 13*(4), 462–482.

Billett, S. (2016). Learning through healthcare work: Premises, contributions and practices. *Medical Education, 50*(1), 124–131.

Billett, S., Harteis, C., & Gruber, H. (2017). Developing occupational expertise through everyday work activities and interactions. In K. A. Ericsson, R. R. Hoffman, & A. Kozbelt (Eds.), *Cambridge handbook of expertise and expert performance* (2nd ed.). New York: Cambridge University Press.

Billett, S., & Sweet, L. (2015). Understanding and appraising healthcare students' learning through workplace experiences: Participatory practices at work. In J. Cleland & S. Durning (Eds.), *Researching medical education*. Oxford: Wiley.

Byrne, R. W., & Russon, A. (1998). Learning by imitation: A hierarchical approach. *The Behavioral and Brain Science, 21*(5), 667–721.

Cleland, J., Leaman, J., & Billett, S. (2014). Developing medical capacities and dispositions through practice-based experiences. In C. Harteis, A. Rausch, & J. Seifried (Eds.), *Discourses on professional learning: On the boundary between learning and working* (pp. 211–219). Dordrecht: Springer.

Collins, A., Brown, J. S., & Newman, S. E. (1989). Cognitive apprenticeship: Teaching the crafts of reading, writing and mathematics. In L. B. Resnick (Ed.), *Knowing, learning and instruction: Essays in honour of Robert Glaser* (pp. 453–494). Hillsdale, NJ: Erlbaum & Associates.

Cooke, M., Irby, D., & O'Brien, B. C. (2010). *Educating physicians: A call for reform of medical school and residency*. San Francisco: Jossey-Bass.

Delany, C., & Golding, C. (2014). Teaching clinical reasoning by making thinking visible: An action research project with allied health clinical educators. *BMC Medical Education, 14*(1), 20. doi:10.1186/1472-6920-14-20.

Donald, M. (1991). *Origins of the modern mind: Three stages in the evolution of culture and cognition*. Cambridge, MA: Harvard University Press.

Dornan, T. (2012). Workplace learning. *Perspectives on Medical Education, 1*(1), 15–23.

Eppich, W., Rethans, J. J., Tueunissen, P. W., et al. (2016). Learning to work together through talk: Continuing professional development in medicine. In S. Billett, D. Dymock, & S. Choy (Eds.), *Supporting learning across working life: Models, processes and practices* (pp. 47–73). Dordrecht: Springer.

Ericsson, K. A. (2006). The influence of experience and deliberate practice on the development of superior expert performance. In K. A. Ericsson, N. Charness, P. J. Feltowich, et al. (Eds.), *The Cambridge handbook of expertise and expert performance* (pp. 685–705). Cambridge: Cambridge University Press.

Ericsson, K. A., & Lehmann, A. C. (1996). Expert and exceptional performance: Evidence of maximal adaptation to task constraints. *Annual Review of Psychology, 47*, 273–305.

Ericsson, K. A., & Simon, H. A. (1980). Verbal reports as data. *Psychological Review, 87*(3), 215–251.

Francis, R. (2013). *Report of the Mid Staffordshire NHS Foundation Trust Public Inquiry*. London: The Stationery Office.

Garling, P. (2008). *Final Report of the Special Commission of Inquiry Acute Care Services in NSW Public Hospitals*. Sydney: Special Commission of Inquiry: Acute Care Services in New South Wales Public Hospitals, State of New South Wales.

Goldman, S. R. (2003). Learning in complex domains: When and why do multiple representations help? *Learning and Instruction, 13*, 239–244.

Gray, J. B. (2009). The power of storytelling: Using narrative in the healthcare context. *Journal of Communication in Healthcare, 2*(3), 258–273. doi:10.1179/cih.2009.2.3.258.

Groen, G. J., & Patel, P. (1988). The relationship between comprehension and reasoning in medical expertise. In M. T. H. Chi, R. Glaser, & R. Farr (Eds.), *The nature of expertise* (pp. 287–310). New York: Erlbaum.

Jordan, B. (1989). Cosmopolitical obstetrics: Some insights from the training of traditional midwives. *Social Science and Medicine, 28*(9), 925–944.

Manias, E., & Street, A. (2000). The handover: Uncovering the hidden practices of nurses. *Intensive and Critical Care Nursing, 16*(6), 373–383.

Mayer, R. E. (1992). *Thinking, problem solving, cognition* (2nd ed.). *A series of books in psychology*. New York, NY: W H Freeman/Times Books/ Henry Holt & Co.

Meißner, A., Hasselhorn, H. M., Estryn-Behar, M., et al. (2007). Nurses' perception of shift handovers in Europe — results from the European Nurses' Early Exit Study. *Journal of Advanced Nursing, 57*(5), 535–542.

Nisbet, G., Dunn, S., & Lincoln, M. (2015). Interprofessional team meetings: Opportunities for informal interprofessional learning. *Journal of Interprofessional Care, 29*(5), 426–432. doi:doi:10.3109/13561820.2015.1016602.

O'Keefe, M., McAllister, S., & Stupans, I. (2011). Health service organisation, clinical team composition and student learning. In S. Billett & A. Henderson (Eds.), *Developing learning professionals: Integrating experiences in university and practice settings* (pp. 187–200). Dordreht, Netherlands: Springer.

O'Leary, K. J., Buck, R., Fligiel, H. M., et al. (2011). Structured interdisciplinary rounds in a medical teaching unit: Improving patient safety. *Archives of Internal Medicine, 171*(7), 678–684.

O'Leary, K. J., Wayne, D. B., Haviley, C., et al. (2010). Improving teamwork: Impact of structured interdisciplinary rounds on a medical teaching unit. *Journal of General Internal Medicine, 25*(8), 826–832. doi:10.1007/s11606-010-1345-6.

Palinscar, A. S., & Brown, A. L. (1984). Reciprocal teaching of comprehension-fostering and comprehension-monitoring activities. *Cognition and Instruction, 1*(2), 117–175.

Pinnock, R., Young, L., Spence, F., et al. (2015). Can think aloud be used to teach and assess clinical reasoning in graduate medical education? *Journal of Graduate Medical Education, 7*(3), 334–337. doi:10.4300/jgme-d-14-00601.1.

Rice, T. (2010). Learning to listen: Auscultation and the transmission of auditory knowledge. *Journal of the Royal Anthropological Institute (NS), 16*, S41–S61.

Ritchhart, R., Church, M., & Morrison, K. (2011). *Making thinking visible: How to promote engagement, understanding, and independence for all learners.* Chichester: John Wiley & Sons.

Rogoff, B., & Lave, J. (Eds.), (1984). *Everyday cognition: Its development in social context.* Cambridge, MA: Harvard University Press.

Roodhouse, S. (2007). Special issue introduction. *Education + Training, 49*(3), 161–169.

Royer, J. M., Mestre, J. P., & Dufresne, R. J. (2005). Introduction: Framing the transfer problem. In J. P. Mestre (Ed.), *Transfer of learning from a modern multi-disciplinary perspective* (pp. vii–xiv). Washington: Information Age Publishing.

Scribner, S. (1984). Studying working intelligence. In B. Rogoff & J. Lave (Eds.), *Everyday cognition: Its development in social context* (pp. 9–40). Cambridge, MA: Harvard University Press.

Scribner, S. (1992). Mind in action: A functional approach to thinking. *Quarterly Newsletter of the Laboratory of Comparative Human Cognition, 14*(4), 103–110 (Reprint of 1983 lecture).

Sinclair, S. (1997). *Making doctors: An institutional apprenticeship.* Oxford: Berg.

Starmer, A. J., Spector, N. D., Srivastava, R., et al. (2012). I-pass, a mnemonic to standardize verbal handoffs. *Pediatrics, 129*(2), 201–204.

Sweller, J. (1990). Cognitive processes and instructional procedures. *Australian Journal of Education, 34*(2), 125–130.

Teunissen, P. W., & Wilkinson, T. J. (2010). Learning and teaching in workplaces. In T. Dornan, K. Mann, A. Scherpbier, et al. (Eds.), *Medical education: Theory and practice* (pp. 199–203). Edinburgh: Churchill Livingstone.

Tobias, S. (1994). Interest, prior knowledge, and learning. *Review of Educational Research, 64*(1), 37–54.

Valsiner, J. (1998). *The guided mind: A sociogenetic approach to personality.* Cambridge, MA: Harvard University Press.

Vosniadou, S., Ioannides, C., Dimitrakopoulou, A., et al. (2002). Designing learning environments to promote conceptual change in science. *Learning and Instruction, 11*(4–5), 381–419.

Walton, J. M., & Steinert, Y. (2010). Patterns of interaction during rounds: Implications for work-based learning. *Medical Education, 44*(6), 550–558. doi:10.1111/j.1365-2923.2010.03626.x.

Warmington, S., & McColl, G. (2017). Medical student stories of participation in patient care-related activities: The construction of relational identity. *Advances in Health Sciences Education, 22*(1), 147–163. doi:10.1007/s10459-016-9689-2.

Wertsch, J. W. (1991). A sociocultural approach to socially shared cognition. In L. B. Resnick, J. M. Levine, & S. D. Teasley (Eds.), *Perspectives on socially shared cognition* (pp. 85–100). Washington, DC: American Psychological Association.

Wolpaw, T. M. M. D., Wolpaw, D. R. M. D., & Papp, K. K. P. (2003). SNAPPS: A learner-centered model for outpatient education. *Academic Medicine, 78*(9), 893–898.

16

Learning in community-based contexts

Jennifer Johnston, Nigel Hart and
Gerard Gormley

Introduction

Whether it is seeking advice about a persistent cough, having a cut forehead cleaned and dressed, or seeking contraceptive advice, many of us will have experienced community healthcare. Throughout this chapter, we use this term to mean *primary care*, delivered in the places where we live and work through the collaborative efforts of multi-professional teams. Primary care is consonant with clinical generalism, with longitudinal healthcare across a lifetime and above all with a deep appreciation of the patient as a whole person within their own context.

Considering these affordances, education within primary care offers unique opportunities for learning. Embedded within their local communities, primary care nurses, doctors and other health professionals work within a distinct clinical paradigm, quite separate from the life and culture of hospital-based care. Primary care clinicians value continuity while embracing complexity and uncertainty, and rarely restrict their focus to a purely biomedical model of health and illness.

In this chapter, we situate learning and teaching within the two paradigms of primary and secondary care, and introduce the principles of primary care pedagogy, drawn from social theories of learning, in practical ways. With a major focus on the importance of context and the relationships between people, these concepts can be used to help clinicians to share their discipline with learners right across the educational continuum. We then illustrate some of these principles by unpacking two very different case studies from general practice (family medicine) education: one deals with undergraduate teaching in our own UK institution; the other looks at how new technologies can bring people together, blurring paradigm differences to create new communities of practice while still maintaining the primacy of the patient. Next, we consider some of the global political contexts in which primary care currently exists, and think about education as a means of addressing marginalisation and bringing about positive social change. Finally, we finish with some practical suggestions for those who are working within primary care contexts who want to either get started in education or deepen their pedagogical practice.

The primary care paradigm

If you were to enter a primary healthcare facility for the first time, one of the most striking aspects would probably be the diversity of the staff. Healthcare delivery in the community, as in hospital settings, depends on a functional relationship between different professional groups. The average multidisciplinary team might include doctors, nurses, receptionists and management staff, and possibly pharmacists, occupational therapists and social workers. Within each of these groups, there will be further subgroups that reflect different professional interests and areas of expertise.

Thinking about all these professionals as belonging to one paradigm — primary care — helps us to understand the ties that bind such diverse teams together (Bhatia & Rifkin, 2013). In science, paradigms define the sorts of questions that can be asked and the answers that can be found, thus dictating the rules of engagement (Kuhn, 1962). A paradigm is simply a particular way of looking at the world. The primary care paradigm offers a particular perspective and a way of approaching healthcare, and it is this distinctive affordance that makes learning in this setting so valuable. Not everyone who rotates through primary care as part of their training will end up working there. All healthcare professionals, however, must understand what happens to patients once they leave secondary care to resume their normal lives. Illness is a sometimes devastating biographical disruption (Bury, 1982), which may be emphasised by inpatient and outpatient contacts with secondary care. Primary care sits closer to home, to work, to family and offers familiarity in its longitudinal aspect.

As a concept, primary care education is substantially different from learning in other healthcare arenas. Primary care has a distinctive *ontology* and *epistemology* which are socially, culturally and historically defined. Things that are quite unobservable, or seemingly unproven, are an accepted part of practice (Ghosh, 2004; French, 2002). Depression, fibromyalgia and pain, for example, are quite as 'real' as less ephemeral infection, cancer or hypertension. 'Hard' scientific evidence, such as that from randomised controlled trials, certainly occupies an important position, but is mediated by the complementary expertise of the patient and the clinician (Wilson, 2000; Greenhalgh et al., 2014; Fulford, 2008). Understanding that this way of working constitutes an alternative understanding, and not an inferior one, goes a long way to addressing the traditional perceived difference in the status of hospital and community medicine (Norredam & Album, 2007). The underpinning philosophy of primary care, and its place within the wider healthcare world, is one of the most important tasks for educators introducing neophyte learners to their world.

More practically, learners are also likely to find that clinical encounters differ significantly in scope and function from those in secondary care. Primary healthcare practitioners welcome all those in need, whether the presenting complaint is a devastating illness or an ingrowing toenail. Because it is situated in the community, primary care sits closer to the real-life contexts of patients; it is centred on an understanding of health and illness as they are experienced by people. Longitudinal clinical relationships offer the opportunity to work with families across births, deaths and major life events (Sturmberg, 2000; White et al., 2016). This aspect is often cited as one of the most satisfying aspects of community medicine, with the clinician in a highly trusted position (RCGP, 2017a). Longitudinal primary care follows the contours of the patient's life journey, tiding them over some of life's most challenging times. Even a short glimpse of this way of working can be profound for learners accustomed to a more anonymous or short-lived relationship with patients.

One further aspect of importance is that learners begin to understand the breadth and depth of conditions seen (Kringos et al., 2010). Complexity and uncertainty are cornerstones of practice (Evans & Trotter, 2009; Gerrity et al., 1992; World Association of Family Doctors, 2015). Since primary care is often patients' first port of call, primary care clinicians must be equipped to recognise and manage undifferentiated illness (Henry, 2006). In our own pedagogy, we often use the analogy of 'horses and zebras' to teach this concept: which is the more likely to appear in any given situation? For example, a 15-year-old with a cough is probably more likely to have an upper respiratory tract infection than a non-small-cell lung cancer. A 15-year-old immigrant from a developing country, living in crowded housing, may however turn out to have tuberculosis. Context is everything, and the breadth of the work means that every clinician will occasionally encounter a zebra disguised as a horse (Evans & Rafi, 2016). Risk management involves the development of a finely tuned clinical instinct, in conjunction with a type of evidence-based decision tree (Gabbay & le May, 2004). These are sophisticated skills, honed over a lifetime. For undergraduate learners or those 'passing through', the educator's job is to make familiar the nuances of this form of practice (Bird, 2011; Howe, 2001). For trainees who have chosen primary care as their life's work, it is about helping them to take their first few steps on this rich and rewarding, if challenging, pathway.

Primary care pedagogy

Moving to primary care from secondary care contexts, particularly technology-rich environments such as cardiology or anaesthetics, can represent a significant paradigm shift for learners. Primary care pedagogy draws on the contexts outlined above to focus on the importance of relationships and environment. A few important concepts drawn from social learning theory can help illuminate the primary care paradigm's educational possibilities.

Dialogue

In our experience, primary care clinicians tend to do a lot of talking! In fact, for GPs like ourselves, the consultation is an essential part of our practice and, consequently, our shared identity (Stott & Davis, 1979). The therapeutic value of simple relational care is taken for granted (Balint, 1957). Learning to consult in primary care involves learning to understand people in all their diversity, and is a central way by which practitioners come to understand themselves and their place within the world of healthcare. Both patients and the primary care context play a role in the co-construction of clinical encounters (May et al., 1996). Indeed, primary care consultations can be seen as an *epistemological act* (Johnston, 2015). In simple terms, they come to define how we know and understand the world of medicine.

Clearly, this sophisticated form of consulting relies heavily on communication. Primarily this takes the form of spoken (and written) language, but it also includes other subtle forms of communication such as body language, dress, manner and either overt or 'hidden' cues (Friedman, 1979). These are all culturally defined, as with other aspects of medical practice (Horne et al., 2004). Subtle differences in non-verbal communication between a doctor and a patient of different cultural backgrounds, for example, are fertile grounds for the development of misunderstanding. A patient who has been subject to abuse in the past may have difficulty in articulating their concerns or their needs directly. Consultations with those seeking asylum often involve complex physical and emotional presentations which must be mediated by a third-party interpreter (Robb & Greenhalgh, 2006). Particular care must be taken in all such circumstances to avoid dysfunctional consulting, which may interfere with the quality of information given or received, and hence impede diagnosis, investigation or management (Neighbour, 1987). Within healthcare too, care must be taken in managing the dynamics of communication between different members of the multidisciplinary team and the primary–secondary care interface. Excellent communication here includes written mediums such as referral letters, prescriptions and team protocols.

Dialogue is the lifeblood of the consultation, as well as interdisciplinary cooperation. Engaging in dialogue is how we make sense and meaning from the world around us, so it is a very important concept in educational theory terms. The theorist who expounded the idea of dialogue, and who is most deeply associated with it, is Bakhtin. He drew a lot of his thinking from literary texts, and saw dialogue everywhere: between ourselves and others, the world around us, our own past selves and even the people we might become in future. Each of these conversations contribute to the way we understand the world and find meaning in it (Bakhtin, 1981).

Since all this dialogue involves numerous different 'voices' potentially talking at once, it is no wonder that some will be harmonious and some a bit more discordant. Bakhtin called this chorus *polyphony* or *multi-voicedness* (Bakhtin, 1981). Polyphony is a second important concept for learning and teaching in primary care, because it allows us to think about the perspectives of other people and groups. It is helpful in facilitating learners to understand the diversity of patients' backgrounds and experience, something we return to at the end of the chapter, and encourages the development of an empathic understanding of illness experience.

Dialogue is an essential aspect of primary care, exemplified by the co-constructed primary care consultation referred to earlier. The clinician can, by developing a dialogic consultation style, be of considerable therapeutic value simply through their engagement with their patients (Balint, 1957). Realising what may be achieved in terms of 'hard' clinical outcomes, through the simple means of communication and relationship building, can be a revelation for learners. This is valuable for those who will work in secondary care, since they may not encounter such an emphasis on consultation skills in other specialties. For those destined to work in primary care, meanwhile, engaging in such dialogue allows them to begin to develop an identity within their chosen field. In doing so, they become part of a larger community of clinical practice (Endsley et al., 2005).

Relational learning

One specific type of dialogue is particularly useful in primary care pedagogy, and that is the relationship that develops between the clinical educator and the learner. Just as the clinician may have a therapeutic impact in clinical encounters, so too can they have a positive impact on learners (Boendermaker et al., 2000). We explore this in detail later, in case study 16.1. Taking place in ambulatory settings, primary care teaching is of course often physically different from that which takes place in hospitals. As people are usually seen in primary care clinics, or sometimes in their own homes, there is no traditional bedside teaching with ad hoc clinical educators. The setup of primary care instead often affords a privileged opportunity for valuable one-on-one or small-group teaching (Gordon, 2003), as well as for a degree of longitudinal engagement, with tutor and learner often able to form a meaningful relationship over a longer term.

This relationship can be a powerful driver for learning, as a safe shared space is developed between learner and mentor. In the technical language of social theory, we call this safe shared space the *zone of proximal development (ZPD)* or *zoped* (Vygotsky, 1978). This idea was developed in the early 20th century by Vygotsky and has been hugely influential in education and psychology. The zoped represents the extra distance that learners can manage to travel through a supportive relationship with a mentor or educator, relative to what might be possible if they were working on their own. Relational learning, in other words, expands the horizons of learning. From this perspective education is a very social endeavour, and one that is embedded in cultural surroundings. It is more than an individual undertaking. In practical terms, constructing a zoped with learners may be facilitated by welcoming learners into the fabric of the unit's work, and developing a supportive and honest, but non-judgmental, teaching style (Anderson et al., 2017). Positive feedback based on clear evidence, and an openness to discussion and questioning on the part of the clinical teacher, go a long way in building learner confidence (Cantillon & Easton, 2015). Role modelling, too, such as watching an experienced clinician consult, is a powerful teaching tool which, with appropriate debriefing, can be used in the same vein (Cruess et al., 2008).

One further affordance of this type of relational learning is that a zoped does not always have to be constructed between a clinical mentor and a learner. People also learn from relationships with patients (for clinicians, this is a lifelong dialogue), and from other multidisciplinary team members, as well as from the broader community. Learning is not just about content knowledge, but about clinical and consultation skills, and the process knowledge needed to function within any given environment (Billett, 2001). For example, a GP trainee or community nursing learner will quickly assimilate contextual local knowledge.

We are based in Belfast, Northern Ireland, a city where aspects of the civil conflict known as 'The Troubles' still form part of general practice consultations (Ferry et al., 2008). Certain legacies have been left in terms of deprivation, physical and mental illness, and manifest in ways that clinicians embedded here understand and work with. Any learner situated within this context will need to learn to manage home visits, for example, which might involve 'interface' areas of the city. These are neighbourhoods in which social deprivation and periodic political unrest are a lingering reminder of old conflicts. Clinicians must understand how to conduct themselves, to use the correct language, even simply to navigate the streets where signs were once removed as an act of civil resistance. Thus, this contextual knowledge forms a critical part of workplace learning, without which it would be impossible to practise competently. As clinicians of long standing in this context, there are few surprises here for us, but there may be many for learners coming from more sheltered backgrounds, or from other countries. One of the privileges of being a clinician educator, indeed, is the ability to look around with the fresh eyes of the learner, and thus learn something new about your own practice. The zoped in this sense can work in both directions: the tutor–learner relationship offers profound opportunities for dialogue and development.

Case study 16.1: Undergraduate general practice education in Northern Ireland: the patients, professionals and processes

Fionnuala is a 22-year-old medical learner at a UK-based medical school. She is about to embark on her general practice placement. Prior to this the majority of her learning has been in the secondary care setting. This often involves being part of a small group of learners sitting in an outpatient clinic passively observing a senior doctor interact with a patient in a defined speciality area, or interviewing patients on a medical ward after they have been assessed by medical staff. Her sense of general practice has largely been shaped by her own limited personal experience of primary care, and by the views of healthcare professionals on general practice. Not all views have been positive towards general practice. For the first time she will experience a one-to-one learning relationship with a clinical educator.

Clinical placement in general practice

Northern Ireland is a region of the UK with a population of approximately 1.8 million people (NISRA, 2012). Community-based (primary) healthcare is provided here by just over 1100 GPs, under the auspices of the UK National Health Service (NHS) (Health and Social Care, 2017). Undergraduate medical education is currently delivered by Queen's University Belfast (QUB), which admits both undergraduate and graduate entrants to a five-year integrated curriculum. As with many other medical schools in the UK, the majority of clinical teaching at the university is currently hosted in hospital settings. There is, however, an increasing presence of community-based education across the five years of training.

In the fourth year of studies at QUB, medical learners experience their first formal clinical placement in the discipline of general practice. The ethos of this module is to provide learners with a grounding in how healthcare is provided in a community setting. Learners are introduced to the professionals, processes and, most importantly, patients that make up this important clinical learning environment. They are provided with the opportunity to embrace the richness and diversity of this unique learning environment, under the supervision of experienced and enthusiastic GP tutors. Of the 343 general practices in Northern Ireland, just over 140 host medical learner clinical placements. These teaching practices range from single-handed to large-group practices, and from rural to inner-city practices, serving patients and populations from all social classes.

In the first week, medical learners are oriented and sensitised to the concept and realities of general practice through lectures and small-group work, delivered by clinicians and clinical academics. Rather than being confronted with an array of disease-oriented learning outcomes, learners cover broad-based primary care–oriented topics such as: chronic disease; women's, men's and children's health; common conditions; primary care emergencies; prescribing; consultation skills; health promotion; and clinical ethics. This introductory week uses a constructivist learning approach with an emphasis on participation, and thus engages learners early on in the dialogue which, as we outlined earlier, is such a feature of both learning and clinical practice in this context. The theoretical element prepares learners for their immersion into the vibrant learning environment of general practice.

Nurturing and supporting safe learning

GP tutors who host learners in their practices are encouraged to build supportive learning relationships. Most of these relationships are with one or two learners at a time. Coming from busy hospital placements of multiple students, feedback from learners is that they are consistently delighted to discover that they will be a significant part of the practice team during their placement. Staff often already know their name before they arrive.

Following an initial learning needs assessment with their tutor, learners embark on their planned learning activities. A structured logbook, including appropriate workplace-based assessment, helps guide their learning and ensure that minimal standards and experiences are achieved. Though learners have a designated GP placement tutor, they are assigned to the *practice* and not to a single GP. This promotes a more inclusive experience for learners and makes them feel an integral part of the practice, as well as allowing access to a range of clinical interests and consultation styles.

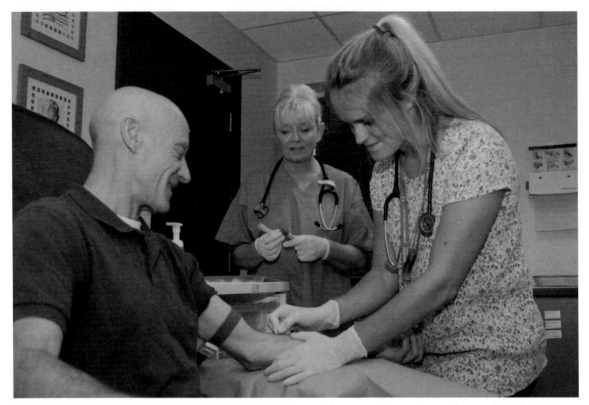

Figure 16.1: A medical learner gaining experience with a practice nurse, illustrating the relationship learning between learner and mentor — such a safe and shared space (zone of proximal development) can be a powerful driver for learning and learner development

Being part of the team

While the majority of time is spent seeing and consulting with patients under the supervision of a GP, learners also typically spend time with the community nursing team, other healthcare professionals such as the practice pharmacist, community midwife or health visitor, as well as the practice manager and reception team (see Fig. 16.1).

This enables learners to develop an understanding of the cogwheels of primary care and its inherent multidisciplinary and cooperative nature. Such experiences are not just a process of passive observation. Instead, learners explore the various roles of the healthcare team through dialogue and interaction, appreciating the contribution of each to patient care. This deeper understanding of each team member's role provides them with situated experience of the primary healthcare team. Such dialogue promotes relational learning and allows the creation of a safe space for both learner and educator development (i.e. zoped) (Vygotsky, 1978).

Advancing consultation skills

Developing learners' consultation skills is an important learning objective for their time in general practice. The consultation carries enormous weight in general practice, being the central tool of the trade. After being taught the theoretical aspects of consultation skills during preparatory lectures and role-play, learners translate theory into practice with real patients. This is an invaluable opportunity for consultation development beyond simulation, under the tutelage of an experienced clinician teacher.

In our context, learners observe GPs as they go about their usual consultations with patients. These clinics are interspersed with conversations and unpacking of the complexities of the interactions. Observation then progresses to a more active phase, where GPs actively involve learners in the consultation. This may involve taking a history or examining under direct supervision, or suggesting a possible management plan. Finally, learners progress to indirect supervision, 'swapping seats' with their GP tutor to take the lead in the consultation (see Fig. 16.2).

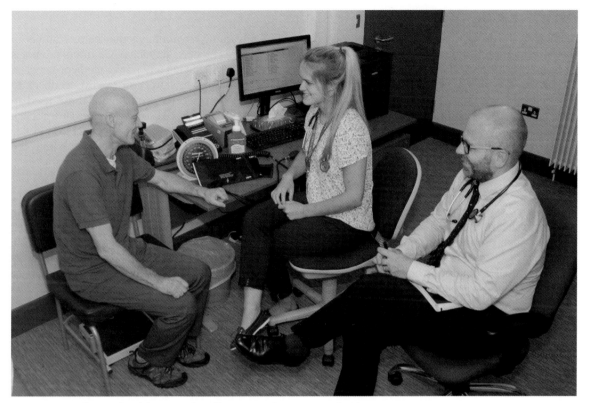

Figure 16.2: A medical learner leading a patient consultation

During this phase, learners may interview patients first, with their consent, then present their findings. As learners develop, practices organise a mini-surgery, where a small number of real patients have booked to see the learner primarily. In this case, the GP will follow up by conducting their own consultation (van der Zwet, 2011). This stepwise teaching approach aims to improve learner confidence by providing them with a sense of empowerment and responsibility with actual patients, but in a safe and supportive environment. Dialogue is an important mediator in such learner development.

Lastly, all learners in our program have the opportunity to undertake a video surgery. This footage is used to help learners explore the components of what makes a good consultation, and provide indictors of how to improve their consultation skills in the future. The use of video in this manner is commonplace in postgraduate medical education and a major feature of the Royal College of General Practitioners' licensing exam. Its use in an undergraduate setting thus aligns with the aims, objectives and methods used in postgraduate GP training in the UK and elsewhere.

People and patients

One thing that general practice is not short of is the opportunity for interaction with patients and their families. The relative autonomy and responsibility presented to learners within this role is a significant privilege and educationally very powerful. The chance for learners to accompany GPs on home visits, where GPs consult with frail elderly patients or others unable to attend surgery in the patient's own home, opens up further learning experiences for learners. Visiting a patient's home adds further important contextual and situational aspects of patienthood. For example, an elderly patient with multiple co-morbidities may be struggling to carry out their activities of daily living (e.g. washing, dressing, shopping, feeding). Such insights can place the patient and their illnesses in context, and help the learner, in conjunction with their GP tutor, to formulate an individual patient-centred management plan.

An envelope of feedback

At the core of the placement is the intention of providing a learning environment that helps learners in their development as future doctors. Feedback is fundamental to this process. Training of GP tutors promotes good practice in providing learner feedback. Emphasis is placed on reducing any power gradient between the learner and the GP tutor, and on building a learning relationship that allows constructive feedback to flow in both directions. Formative workplace-based assessment tools are used, mirroring those used in postgraduate training (e.g. MiniCEXs and case-based discussions) (RCGP, 2017b), but informal feedback is considered equally valuable and is signposted throughout the placement. This often occurs over coffee and is highly valued educational dialogue for both parties. Additionally, learners receive feedback from the other members of staff as well as patients after they have consulted with them.

Taking stock and feeding forward

On the last day of the module, small-group feedback is facilitated at the university by GP tutors, facilitating learners in sharing their learning experiences. In coming together, they build a shared dialogue about general practice which supports the community of practice. Furthermore, this exercise provides a 'snapshot' of life in general practice across Northern Ireland as seen through the eyes of our learners. This final day serves to consolidate learning over the course of the placement and to underline the key message about primary care that we hope learners will take with them back into secondary care. Prior to moving onto their next hospital-based module, we help learners to articulate how best they can interact with general practice in their future careers.

No two learners will have the same experience, hence the importance of sharing a range of experiences to build a conceptual framework of the diversity of general practice. Patients vary, their conditions vary, doctors vary and communities vary: in short, clinical variation is very much part of the fabric of real clinical practice. Such insights aim to promote learners' ability to embrace diversity in the future.

Case study 16.2: Building new communities of practice

James is a 28-year-old doctor in training for general practice. Following four years working in various hospital departments, James has started his first community placement in primary care. His experience to date has been largely ward-based with secondary care populations. He is at the beginning of learning to manage the complexity and uncertainty of working in a primary care setting. While James has an experienced GP trainer, he is worried about how, in the short training program, he will achieve sufficient experience in managing a range of conditions common to the primary care setting. He enrols to become a participant in a Project ECHO program on common dermatology problems in primary care. This connects James with his GP trainee peers in distant locations, helping him to develop his clinical knowledge and also his fledgling sense of identity as a GP.

New technologies and GP training

Contemporary primary care-based general practice situated in the UK context is varied and challenging, involving the diagnosis and management of a wide range of undifferentiated illnesses and the management of long-term conditions within community settings. In the UK, postgraduate GP trainees follow a well-defined, broad-based training curriculum including competencies across numerous clinical specialties (RCGP, 2017c).

This vocational training scheme is completed within a relatively short three-year time period. The majority of learning for general practice takes place in clinical attachments in the workplace. Commonly, this involves beginning with placements in hospital settings (18 months) and subsequently in general practice itself (18 months). A key element of GP training requires trainees to reflect actively on their experiences (Kolb, 1984) and, under the supervision of their trainers, to incorporate their learning into their daily work with their patients. For the clinical attachments in the GP setting, trainees are normally placed on a 'one trainee per trainer' basis. There is usually only one trainee in each general practice at a given time. As with undergraduate teaching, GP trainees are widely scattered geographically, which makes formal instruction for a cohort across a region challenging. Given the intensity of workload, there is relatively limited opportunity for formal teaching outside the workplace. New technologies and a novel approach to building communities of practice have the potential to blur the boundaries.

The ECHO model

Project ECHO (Extension for Community Healthcare Outcomes) (Project ECHO, 2017) is a new technology supporting community healthcare education. The model (originally developed in New Mexico) is designed to support and train primary healthcare providers in rural and underserved areas so that they can better manage patients with complex health needs, and to improve access to what is considered to be specialised (usually synonymous with secondary) care. The ECHO model does this by creating an opportunity for healthcare professionals from various backgrounds to participate in a community of learners in conjunction with specialist mentors. As such, it has particular relevance to primary healthcare in bridging the primary–secondary care interface and thus allowing new communities of practice to develop.

Using webcams and videoconferencing technology, Project ECHO enables healthcare professionals to link in from 'spokes' to a central 'hub' for case-based discussions. This overcomes the problems of geographical dispersion. The ECHO session starts with a short 15-minute didactic presentation on a topic relevant to the clinical area of that particular session. Following this presentation, participants present and discuss the background history, clinical presentation, examination findings, investigation and management of actual clinical cases they have encountered.

Evidence is growing that the use of this innovative approach to learning has significant potential. A systematic review of the impact of Project ECHO on patient and provider outcomes identified 39 studies across 17 distinct disease groups (Zhou et al., 2016). For example, participation in Project ECHO led to changes in primary care providers' behaviour, improvements in primary care providers' knowledge and confidence, and improvements in patient outcomes for people affected by dementia, diabetes and hepatitis C (Project ECHO NI, 2016).

Exploring the contributions of new technologies to community-based learning

Embracing new approaches such as Project ECHO can greatly enhance primary care education. ECHO brings together a community of learners who are at the same time situated in their place of work and who use technology to support a social learning space (Socolovsky et al., 2013). Socolovsky and colleagues suggest that the success of Project ECHO for community-based learning can be explained by situated learning and community of practice theories (Lave & Wenger, 1991) and by social cognitive theory (Bandura, 2001). The participants in Project ECHO are situated within the community-based context for which they are seeking to acquire knowledge, insights and skills and they come together to learn as a community, albeit aided by technology-enhanced remote access. Lave and Wenger's work, with which many medical educators will already be familiar, explains that a community of practice (CoP) is a group of people undertaking shared activities and interests. The CoP normally has a domain, a community and a practice, and practitioners who develop a shared repertoire of resources. The CoP is seen as a conduit to promote innovation, develop social capital and facilitate the spread of tacit knowledge within the group. The community develops its practice through the finding, sharing and transferring of knowledge. This is a major advantage of using the ECHO model to bridge the primary–secondary care interface (see Fig. 16.3).

An example of meeting challenges for curriculum coverage with ECHO

An example of a curricular area for UK GP training, and a useful heuristic for the use of Project ECHO in primary care education, is 'care of people with skin problems'. This is one of the core competencies of the national licensing exam of the Royal College of General Practitioners (MRCGP) (RCGP, 2017c). It is also a key area for the development of new GPs since around 24% of the population consult their GP with a skin problem in any 12-month period (RCGP Birmingham Research Unit, 2006) and approximately 14% of all GP consultations are in relation to disorders or concerns about the skin (Kerr et al., 2007). Thus, establishing and maintaining competence in this area is essential for any GP trainee. Undergraduate training in dermatology is, however, variable and often limited, and only a few will gain deeper experience in the management of skin problems through clinical attachments in the hospital setting. This can lead to gaps in confidence and competence at the postgraduate level (Davies & Burge, 2009; Chiange et al., 2008). Ensuring adequate

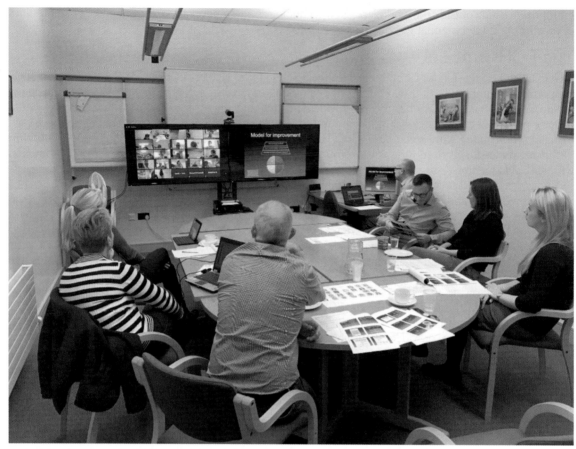

Figure 16.3: Example of an ECHO session

opportunity to increase knowledge of and competence in this important clinical area has the potential to have a career-long impact for future cohorts of GPs and the communities they serve.

We note from personal experience the encouraging outcomes of an evaluation of a pilot ECHO project for dermatology among GP trainees (Project ECHO NI, 2016). In the context of this case study we can reflect on the opportunity for experiential learning (Kolb, 1984) while at the same reflecting on learning that has been facilitated through the establishment of a socially active 'situated' learning community (Lave & Wenger, 1991; Bandura, 2001). Unusually and encouragingly, this is a community that crosses interdisciplinary boundaries and, crucially, links primary and secondary care paradigms for the benefit of patients.

Reflecting on the case studies: community education in action

Contrasting these two case studies demonstrates that learners have different needs at different stages of training. The educational aim of time spent in the community will vary depending on the stage of development and the learner's career intention. Case study 16.1 deals with an undergraduate medical learner. At a stage of training where learners are relatively undifferentiated, the focus is on a basic grounding in the principles and practice of primary care. In case study 16.2, the learner is a postgraduate medical trainee who has entered primary care medicine after time spent rotating around hospital posts. Having made a firm commitment to working within this paradigm, he is now firmly committed to primary care and clinical generalism. His learning needs are different from those of his specialist, hospital-based peers.

There are, however, many commonalities in the education of both of these groups. Relational learning through authentic clinical encounters is central to primary care education. In the primary care setting, learners are often highly visible and keen to engage. In our experience, one of the joys of community teaching is the manner in which learners or trainees strive to reach a level that may have been previously beyond them. They experience graded exposure with consulting under first direct and then remote supervision, and finally consulting in the room next door with the tutor coming in at the end.

As ever, feedback is essential in helping learners and trainees to move forward. In practice, however, feedback inevitably exists outside formal processes; coming from mentor, patient or team member, it is often conveyed more subtly by a nuanced tone or look in the course of normal conversation. Debriefing is often necessary, where a consultation or a clinic can be dissected post hoc within a safe space. Given the autonomous nature of primary care consultations compared with the teamwork of, say, a ward round, debriefing is a useful safety net, a means of conveying feedback, of managing challenging emotions that may arise from the proximity of patient experience, and of consolidation. Assessments, both formative and summative, should always have a strong orientation to primary care. Patient satisfaction questionnaires and multi-source feedback can be an important source of feedback for learners at all stages (RCGP, 2017d).

Linking across healthcare paradigms

Relational learning is the hallmark of primary care education, but can extend beyond interpersonal connections. Learners also develop an educational relationship with whole cultures and paradigms, broadening their understanding of medicine, patients and their own place within healthcare.

Universal experience in both primary and secondary care can potentially ameliorate misunderstanding between different types of healthcare, for the benefit of patients. Time spent in primary care also has a second benefit of addressing longstanding assumptions about the nature of the work. Historically, our own field of general practice has been perceived within medicine as being of lower status than hospital practice (Giles, 2007; Petchey et al., 1997). The inequality is based on multiple assumptions about clinical generalism and the perceived lack of technical 'difficulty' of general practice. Hospital specialties, even now, can be seen as more scientific, more challenging and more appropriate for a talented young doctor to choose (Lambert et al., 2012). Yet although many primary care doctors will have trained in hospital settings, the same is not always true of secondary care doctors. Experience of learning within primary care settings may help to prevent negative stereotypes of primary care work and help to attract young clinicians to make their career in primary care (Alberti et al., 2017).

Spending time embedded within primary care units also has a direct benefit to patients in terms of clinical safety. The primary–secondary care interface is a well-known pinch-point for healthcare, but is routinely traversed by patients as they move from community to hospital and back to community. Common issues encountered at this interface include problems with discharge letters, reconciling medication and referral pathways. Experiencing both sides of the interface is an important way of improving patient safety (Werrett et al., 2001). One practical example of education across clinical paradigms is the increasing use of longitudinal integrated clerkships (LICs) (Walters et al., 2012). Rather than dividing training into specialty-based silos, learners follow the healthcare journeys of patients as they navigate a route between the two. Not only does a curriculum including LICs promote teamwork and paradigm harmony, but it is also highly patient-centred. Skills learned in primary care are easily portable into secondary care, and vice versa, meaning that links between the two are more easily made. LICs are one potential route for health professional education in the future that may overcome many of the issues we have discussed above.

Global and political contexts

Naturally, local context influences on-the-ground practice. There is enormous variation in the delivery of primary healthcare, and therefore its education, across the world. Commercialisation is, of course, an abiding concern in North America (Oberlander, 2012); at the time of writing, the socialised healthcare initiative Obamacare had just survived another attempt at repeal (Pear & Caplan, 2017). In developing countries, meanwhile, primary care may face entirely different problems, with gross pathology, infectious disease and infant mortality serious challenges. Here, primary care may have a more visceral nature, developed and delivered in conjunction with non-governmental organisations and perhaps even military forces. Health inequalities are written large (WHO, 1978). Vaccination, maternal and child health, and patient education programs are essential here, but not straightforward. The Ebola outbreak in West Africa in 2016 is a key example (WHO Ebola Response Team, 2016). Civil unrest contributes to lack of availability of reliable primary care funding and delivery, and places the developing world at ongoing risk from further epidemics.

We are GPs within the UK NHS and our perspective is embedded within this context. Here, the role of clinical generalists is inseparable from the structure of the NHS, a public healthcare system founded on socialist principles in 1948. NHS family doctors have long prided themselves on providing patient-centred cradle-to-grave care (Simon et al., 2014) but this model is currently under considerable strain. Given its overt ideological position as a socialised healthcare system, the NHS sits uncomfortably within the political context of modern neoliberalism (Brookes & Harvey, 2016; Pownall, 2013). Meanwhile, primary care in other countries takes place within the broader contexts of healthcare.

In short, politicisation is inevitable in primary care systems. The 'inverse care law' states that those most in need of good medical care are the least likely to be able to access it, and that this relationship is only exacerbated in the presence of significant market forces (Hart, 1971). Finally, then, primary care education has an innate responsibility to introduce learners to the politics of patient advocacy and change. Advocacy is deeply embedded within primary care medicine and, indeed, has long been one of the World Organization of Family Doctors' (WONCA's) stated roles of the family doctor (Leuwenhorst Group, 1974). Primary care's patient-centredness, sheer breadth and close associations open a window on marginalisation, stigma and issues of social justice, which can at times be uncomfortable for practitioners, and even more potentially uncomfortable for learners introduced to this aspect of care for the first time. As with all challenging experiences in healthcare education, debriefing, feedback and support for learners in the form of role modelling are essential. It may help learners from all stages and backgrounds to consider that patient advocacy can have very real positive consequences. One successful group in Scotland has, with the support of Glasgow University and the RCGP, made significant advances in improving health inequalities in that area, as well as providing crucial peer support for GPs working in difficult circumstances (Deep End GP Group, 2009).

For primary care doctors, patient advocacy occupies a privileged position. When considered in this light, political and geographical variations in primary care are crucial considerations for educators. As clinical generalists engaged in longitudinal relationships with patients, one of our most important roles is that of smoothing out the wrinkles and complexities of modern healthcare. Often this includes navigating the primary–secondary care interface, multiple agencies and the politically determined local availability of resources. Understanding, and indeed participating in, this central role of the generalist can represent profound social learning.

Research and scholarship

Research and scholarship into primary care education may take a number of forms, drawing on the underpinning primary care epistemology (Hutchison & Becker, 2004). Medical education research typically uses a variety of frames, from the sociological to the psychological, and primary care offers a key context for scholarship. There is also an important overlap with clinical and health services research; educationalists have much to offer in expanding this sort of work beyond traditional positivist boundaries. In general, 'how' or 'why' questions lend themselves to qualitative methods, but there are also interesting questions that can be addressed using statistics. Suggestions for primary care research projects might include:

- research into the consultation;
- research into prescribing practices;
- research into identity development;
- how clinicians work within primary care teams;
- how clinicians navigate the structures of healthcare;
- how patients navigate the structures of healthcare.

For clinical educators, teaching rather than research is often the main focus of their involvement. Educational scholarship for this group can often deepen teaching practice and encourage self-reflexivity, as well as innovation. Suggestions for areas of scholarship might include:

- reflective practice;
- what educators can learn from engagement with learners;
- what works in specific contexts;

- evaluation of new ways of teaching;
- innovative teaching methods;
- working with patients.

PRACTICAL TIPS

It is worth reflecting on the fact that many medical education professionals are already teaching and mentoring as part of their everyday practice. For those who take part in annual appraisal, formally expressing a wish to become more involved in education can open doors. Even simply reading, reflecting and developing as a practitioner is an important foundation for any educator.

Often, some of the first things are to decide how much time to devote, whether undergraduate, postgraduate or both, and where you would like to see learners — within university contexts or embedded within your own clinical workplace? If the latter, some work is required to set up the appropriate supporting infrastructure, such as physical space and equipment, timetables and supervision.

Linking in with a local academic primary care or postgraduate training organisation will often allow access to other educators and resources for continuing professional development. Courses in medical education, targeted at clinician educators, are now widely available for those who want to take the next step.

As with any area of the healthcare professions, role models and mentors are important in helping you to find and develop your identity as a primary care educator. Support networks, too, will help you to either link in with an existing community of practice, or start developing a new one (Bartle & Thistlethwaite, 2014).

Conclusion

We hope that reading this chapter has helped to open up your own vocation for primary care education and to inspire you in your own educational contexts. We have drawn on a primary care perspective on community education. In future, of course, the lines of healthcare may be redrawn, with a greater proportion of secondary care situated in communities and a blurring of paradigm boundaries. It will be clear that we write from a particular vantage point: our own position is unequivocally and passionately as GPs and as educationalists. This chapter is imbued with our own experience and that of our learners. Ultimately, we teach for the benefit of our patients, and we have never regretted the choice to share our passion and experience with a new generation. We hope you will have a similarly transformative experience of primary care education.

References

Alberti, H., Randles, H. L., Harding, A., et al. (2017). Exposure of undergraduates to authentic GP teaching and subsequent entry to GP training: a quantitative study of UK medical schools. *British Journal of General Practice*, 67(657), e248–e252.

Anderson, C., Lee, K., Wakeling, J., et al. (2017). An enhanced induction programme for general practice specialty training: a qualitative study of trainee perceptions and experience. *Education for Primary Care*, 28(2), 102–110.

Bakhtin, M. M. (1981). *The dialogic imagination: four essays.* Austin, TX: University of Texas Press.

Balint, M. (1957). *The doctor, his patient and the illness.* London: Churchill Livingstone.

Bandura, A. (2001). Social cognitive theory of mass communication. *Media Psychology*, 3(3), 265–299.

Bartle, E., & Thistlethwaite, J. (2014). Becoming a medical educator: motivation, socialisation and navigation. *BMC Medical Education*, 14, 110.

Bhatia, M., & Rifkin, S. B. (2013). Primary health care, now and forever? A case study of a paradigm change. *International Journal of Health Services: Planning, Administration, Evaluation*, 43(3), 459–471.

Billett, S. (2001). Learning through work: workplace affordances and individual engagement. *Journal of Workplace Learning*, 13(5), 209.

Bird, D. (2011). General practice and the Foundation Programme. *British Journal of General Practice*, 61(591), 633.

Boendermaker, P. M., Schuling, J., Meyboom-de Jong, B., et al. (2000). What are the characteristics of the competent general practitioner trainer? *Family Practice*, 17(6), 547–553.

Brookes, G., & Harvey, K. (2016). Opening up the NHS to market: using multimodal critical discourse analysis to examine the ongoing commercialisation of health care. *Journal of Language and Politics*, 15(3), 288–302.

Bury, M. (1982). Chronic illness as biographical disruption. *Sociology of Health and Illness*, 4(2), 167–182.

Cantillon, P., & Easton, G. (2015). A new series on current thinking in education for the busy primary care educator. *Education for Primary Care*, 26, 1.

Chiange, Y., et al. (2008). Undergraduate dermatology education: a survey of UK medical students. *British Journal of Dermatology*, 159(Suppl. 1).

Cruess, S. R., Cruess, R. L., & Steinert, Y. (2008). Role modelling—making the most of a powerful teaching strategy. *British Medical Journal*, 336(7646), 718–721.

Davies, E., & Burge, S. (2009). Audit of dermatological content of UK undergraduate curricula. *British Journal of Dermatology*, 160, 999–1005.

Deep End GP Group. (2009). *General practitioners at the Deep End*. www.gla.ac.uk/media/media_430491_en.pdf. (Accessed 28 July 2017).

Endsley, S., Kirkegaard, M., & Linares, A. (2005). Working together: communities of practice in family medicine. *Family Practice Management*, 12(1), 28–32.

Evans, L., & Trotter, D. R. M. (2009). Epistemology and uncertainty in primary care: an exploratory study. *Family Medicine*, 41(5), 319–325.

Evans, W. R. H., & Rafi, I. (2016). Rare diseases in general practice: recognising the zebras among the horses. *British Journal of General Practice*, 66(652), 550–551.

Ferry, F., Bolton, D., Bunting, B., et al. (2008). *Trauma, health and conflict in Northern Ireland: a study of the epidemiology of trauma related disorders and investigation of the impact of trauma on the individual*. Psychology Research Institute: University of Ulster.

French, P. (2002). What is the evidence on evidence-based nursing? An epistemological concern. *Journal of Advanced Nursing*, 37(3), 250–257.

Friedman, H. S. (1979). Nonverbal communication between patients and medical practitioners. *Journal of Social Issues*, 35, 82–99.

Fulford, K. W. M. (2008). Values-based practice: a new partner to evidence-based practice and a first for psychiatry? *Mens Sana Monographs*, 6(1), 10–21.

Gabbay, J., & le May, A. (2004). Evidence based guidelines or collectively constructed 'mindlines?' Ethnographic study of knowledge management in primary care. *British Medical Journal*, 329, 1013.

Gerrity, M. S., Earp, J. A. L., DeVellis, R. F., et al. (1992). Uncertainty and professional work: perceptions of physicians in clinical practice. *American Journal of Sociology*, 97(4), 1022–1051.

Ghosh, A. K. (2004). On the challenges of using evidence-based information: the role of clinical uncertainty. *Journal of Laboratory and Clinical Medicine*, 144, 60–64.

Giles, S. (2007). Just family. *Canadian Family Physician*, 53(7), 1212.

Gordon, J. (2003). One to one teaching and feedback. *British Medical Journal*, 326(7388), 543–545.

Greenhalgh, T., Howick, J., & Maskrey, N. (2014). Evidence based medicine: a movement in crisis? *British Medical Journal*, 348, g3725.

Hart, J. T. (1971). The inverse care law. *The Lancet*, 297(7696), 405–412.

Health and Social Care, Business Services Organisation. (2017). *Northern Ireland GP/practice lists for professionals*. www.hscbusiness.hscni.net/services/1816.htm. (Accessed 30 July 2017).

Henry, M. S. (2006). Uncertainty, responsibility, and the evolution of the physician/patient relationship. *Journal of Medical Ethics*, 32, 321–323.

Horne, R., Graupner, L., Frost, S., et al. (2004). Medicine in a multi-cultural society: the effect of cultural background on beliefs about medications. *Social Science & Medicine*, 59(6), 1307–1313.

Howe, A. (2001). Patient-centred medicine through learner-centred teaching: a learner perspective on the key impacts of community-based learning in undergraduate medical education. *Medical Education*, 35, 666–672.

Hutchinson, A., & Becker, L. A. (2004). How the philosophies, styles, and methods of family medicine affect the research agenda. *Annals of Family Medicine*, 2(Suppl. 2), s41–s44.

Johnston, J. L. (2015). *The road to general practice: constructing identity in GP training*. PhD thesis. Belfast: Queen's University.

Kerr, O. C., Benton, E. C., Walker, J. J., et al. (2007). Dermatological workload: primary versus secondary care. *British Journal of Dermatology*, 157(Suppl. 1).

Kolb, D. (1984). *Experiential learning*. Englewood Cliffs, NJ: Prentice-Hall.

Kringos, D. S., Wienke, D. W. B., Hutchinson, A., et al. (2010). The breadth of primary care: a systematic literature review of its core dimensions. *BMC Health Services Research*, 10, 65.

Kuhn, T. S. (1962). *The structure of scientific revolutions*. Chicago: University of Chicago Press.

Lambert, T., Goldacre, R., Smith, F., et al. (2012). Reasons why doctors choose or reject careers in general practice: national surveys. *British Journal of General Practice*, 62(605), e851–e858.

Lave, J., & Wenger, E. (1991). *Situated learning: legitimate peripheral participation*. Cambridge: Cambridge University Press.

Leuwenhorst Group (1974). *The general practitioner in Europe: a standard by the working party appointed by the European Conference on the teaching in general practice*. Leeuwenhorst: The New Leuwenhorst Group.

May, C., Dowrick, C., & Richardson, M. (1996). The confidential patient: the social construction of therapeutic relationships in general medical practice. *The Sociological Review*, 44, 187–203.

Neighbour, R. (1987). *The inner consultation*. Lancaster: MTP Press.

Norredam, M., & Album, D. (2007). Prestige and its significance for medical specialties and diseases. *Scandinavian Journal of Public Health*, 35, 655–661.

Northern Ireland Statistics and Research Agency (NISRA). (2012). *Census 2011: key statistics for Northern Ireland*.

www.nisra.gov.uk/sites/nisra.gov.uk/files/publications/2011-census-results-key-statistics-northern-ireland-report-11-december-2012.pdf. (Accessed 28 July 2017).

Oberlander, J. (2012). The future of Obamacare. *New England Journal of Medicine, 367*, 2165–2167.

Pear, R., & Caplan, T. (2017). *Senate rejects slimmed-down Obamacare repeal as McCain votes No. New York Times.* www.nytimes.com/2017/07/27/us/politics/obamacare-partial-repeal-senate-republicans-revolt.html. (Accessed 28 July 2017).

Petchey, R., Williams, J., & Baker, M. (1997). 'Ending up a GP': a qualitative study of junior doctors' perceptions of general practice as a career. *Family Practice, 14*(3), 194–198.

Pownall, H. (2013). Neoliberalism, austerity and the Health and Social Care Act 2012: the coalition government's programme for the NHS and its implications for the public sector workforce. *Industrial Law Journal, 42*(4), 422–433.

Project ECHO. (2017). *Project ECHO: a revolution in medical education and care delivery.* University of New Mexico. echo.unm.edu/. (Accessed 28 July 2017).

Project ECHO NI (2016). *Evaluation of Project ECHO (Extension for Community Healthcare Outcomes) Northern Ireland programme 2015–16. HSC NI.* echonorthernireland.co.uk/wordpress/wp-content/uploads/2016/05/ECHO-NI-Evaluation-Report-2015-2016.pdf. (Accessed 28 July 2017).

Robb, N., & Greenhalgh, T. (2006). 'You have to cover up the words of the doctor': the mediation of trust in interpreted consultations in primary care. *Journal of Health Organisation and Management, 20*(5), 434–455.

Royal College of General Practitioners. (2017a). *Continuity of care. RCGP.* www.rcgp.org.uk/policy/rcgp-policy-areas/continuity-of-care.aspx. (Accessed 28 July 2017).

Royal College of General Practitioners. (2017b). *MRCGP workplace based assessment (WPBA). RCGP.* www.rcgp.org.uk/training-exams/mrcgp-workplace-based-assessment-wpba.aspx. (Accessed 28 July 2017).

Royal College of General Practitioners. (2017c). *Welcome to the online curriculum. RCGP.* www.rcgp.org.uk/training-exams/gp-curriculum-overview/online-curriculum.aspx. (Accessed 28 July 2017).

Royal College of General Practitioners. (2017d). *The multi-source feedback (MSF).* www.rcgp.org.uk/training-exams/training/mrcgp-workplace-based-assessment-wpba/msf-for-workplace-based-assessment.aspx. (Accessed 28 July 2017).

Royal College of General Practitioners Birmingham Research Unit. (2006). *Weekly returns service annual report 2006.* www.rcgp.org.uk/clinical-and-research/our-programmes/research-and-surveillance-centre.aspx. (Accessed 28 July 2017).

Simon, C., Everitt, H., van Dorp, F., et al. (2014). *Oxford handbook of general practice.* Oxford, UK: Oxford University Press.

Socolovsky, C., Masi, C., Hamlish, T., et al. (2013). Evaluating the role of key learning theories in ECHO: a telehealth educational program for primary care providers. *Progress in Community Health Partnerships: Research, Education, and Action, 7*(4), 361–368.

Stott, N. C. H., & Davis, R. H. (1979). The exceptional potential in each primary care consultation. *Journal of the Royal College of General Practitioners, 29*(201), 201–205.

Sturmberg, J. P. (2000). Continuity of care: towards a definition based on experiences of practising GPs. *Family Practice, 17*(1), 16–20.

van der Zwet, J., Zwietering, P. J., Teunissen, P. W., et al. (2011). Workplace learning from a socio-cultural perspective: creating developmental space during the general practice clerkship. *Advances in Health Sciences Education, 16*(3), 359–373.

Vygotsky, L. S. (1978). *Mind in society: the development of higher psychological processes.* Cambridge, MA: Harvard University Press.

Walters, L., Greenhill, J., Richards, J., et al. (2012). Outcomes of longitudinal integrated clinical placements for learners, clinicians and society. *Medical Education, 46,* 1028–1041.

Werrett, J. A., Helm, R. H., & Carnwell, R. J. (2001). The primary and secondary care interface: the educational needs of nursing staff for the provision of seamless care. *Advanced Nursing, 34*(5), 629–638.

White, E. S., Pereira Gray, D., Langley, P., et al. (2016). Fifty years of longitudinal continuity in general practice: a retrospective observational study. *Family Practice, 33*(2), 148–153.

Wilson, H. J. (2000). The myth of objectivity: is medicine moving towards a social constructivist medical paradigm? *Family Practice, 17*(2), 203–209.

World Association of Family Doctors. (2015). *The world book of family medicine.* WONCA Europe. www.woncaeurope.org/sites/default/files/009%20%E2%80%93%20Complexity%20and%20Primary%20Care.pdf. (Accessed 28 July 2017).

World Health Organization. (1978). *Declaration of Alma-Ata.* www.who.int/publications/almaata_declaration_en.pdf. (Accessed 28 July 2017).

World Health Organization Ebola Response Team. (2016). After Ebola in West Africa — unpredictable risks, preventable epidemics. *New England Journal of Medicine, 375,* 587–596.

Zhou, C., Crawford, A., Serhal, E., et al. (2016). The impact of project ECHO on participant and patient outcomes: a systematic review. *Academic Medicine, 91,* 1439–1461.

17

Identifying and working with underperformance

Margaret Bearman, Damian Castanelli and Charlotte Denniston

Introduction

Underperformance in clinical education is a significant challenge. Underperformance is more than the routine mistakes and errors associated with learning. It is persistant, and concerns those learners who do not work at the expected level of competency for an extended period of time. These learners are at risk of failing clinical placements.

Much of the published literature overlooks the phase where students are at risk, instead focusing on the point of failure and beyond. The 'remediation' literature (Cleland et al., 2013) considers ways to address gaps in knowledge skills and attitudes, generally *after* learners actually fail. It often takes place outside of the immediate clinical education environment. Equally, an extensive body of work explores the moment of failure, particularly when clinical educators 'fail to fail' learners whom they know do not meet the required competency criteria. However, decisions to fail and remediation generally come at the end of the placement or after. By this time, it is too late for the learner to learn from the opportunities within that particular placement environment.

This chapter takes an alternative view. It offers strategies for working with underperformance within the clinical placement. The focus is on the educational processes that assist both the learner and the clinical supervisor to make the best out of the situation at hand. It asks the question: How can learners who underperform be assisted to build their capacities?

The challenge of underperformance for clinical educators

Learners who are at risk of failing clinical placements have enormous impact on clinical educators' workload and stress levels, irrespective of profession (Health Workforce Australia, 2010). This may be because clinical educators report *failing* students as extremely challenging, with a high negative emotional impact. In many instances, clinical educators feel as though they themselves are insufficient (Salm et al., 2016). For instance, a nurse preceptor describes emotions after failing a student: 'I felt like I killed somebody. I killed somebody's career' (Hrobsky & Kersbergen, 2002, p 552). Qualitative studies note the complexity of emotion that clinical educators can experience while assisting students who underperform (Luhanga et al., 2008; Salm et al., 2016). At an extreme, clinical supervisors may also have concerns about legal action or bullying accusations. These emotions reflect the tensions of the clinical education environment.

Clinical education requires the supervisor to take on many roles with competing responsibilities, such as teaching, assessment and patient care (Bearman et al., 2012). The tensions between these roles are exacerbated when students underperform. Often, educators are stretched to provide appropriate patient care while simultaneously allocating meaningful tasks to students who have not yet reached an expected level of competency. Likewise, it may be difficult to provide mentorship to students, while simultaneously assessing them as being below expectations. Underperformance also increases the many bureaucratic requirements of liaising with academic institutions, complying with the competency standards of the profession, and ensuring that the safety measures of the workplace are met. All of this must be managed in a busy work environment, where time and other resources are often very scarce. Moreover, clinical supervisors are frequently placed in this challenging supervisory situation with limited professional development in educational skills (Bearman et al., 2017).

In a study of physiotherapy clinical supervisors, Bearman and colleagues (2012) noted that the supervisors had limited strategies for managing underperformance and coined the term 'more more more' to describe their general approach. The clinical supervisors gave *more* of the same feedback, *more* of the same activities, and *more* oversight to learners who were underperforming. It is noteworthy that, for the most part, they didn't do anything *differently*. This is common across different professional contexts: Cleland and colleagues' (2013) systematic review of remediation in health professional education suggests that remediation is likewise 'more of the same' generally focused on 'getting' the learner over the line. They critique remediations as 'tailored to improve performance to the standard required to pass a re-sit or re-take rather than to support the development of effective lifelong learning skills' (Cleland et al., 2013, p 247). This underpins the point: clinical educators lack *educational* strategies to develop learners; they are concerned with how the learner can pass, rather than *educating* the learner on how they can succeed in the future. This chapter seeks to address this gap.

This chapter provides practical strategies for working with underperformance, grounded in educational theory. First, we discuss how clinical educators can identify underperformance. This is strongly grounded in the clinical educator's perspective. Next, we explore two specific theories that provide means of understanding the learners' perspectives in underperformance. Throughout this chapter, we suggest that appreciating the learner's perspective is essential to supporting the learner to develop the necessary skills both to pass the placement and to manage their own future learning. Finally, we draw from both theory and practice to outline strategies for working with underperformance, which focus on developing the learner and supporting the supervisor.

In order to explore these ideas, we use two case studies. The first is set in a postgraduate specialist medical training environment. The second concerns undergraduate occupational therapy. From a clinical education perspective, the set-up of the placement *from commencement* is significant in how underperformance is identified and managed. For this reason, we start our case studies, before the underperformance becomes apparent.

Case study 17.1: Anaesthetic training — introducing Kate and Antoine

Kate is supervisor of training in anaesthesia in a tertiary hospital. She is responsible for the junior anaesthetic trainees in her hospital, who face significant challenges as their prior training has been in suburban and country hospitals, and this is their first placement in a tertiary hospital. Although some of the operations are familiar, the patients have more co-morbidities and are frailer. The trainees will be getting their first exposure to anaesthesia for some subspecialties, such as neurosurgery, and oesophageal and cardiac surgery. Many of the patients are having operations and procedures that make it complex and challenging to provide anaesthetic care.

Soon after the trainees arrive, Kate organises to meet with them individually to set their learning priorities and help them adjust to their new workplace.

Antoine is an anaesthetic registrar who is six years post medical school graduation. He recently commenced the third year of his anaesthetic training. Antoine has moved between hospitals frequently, so is used to establishing new working relationships. However, this hospital is significantly larger than his previous placement, and there are many more supervisors and co-workers. As is the case in many areas of healthcare, individual anaesthetists have their own rules and preferences when caring for patients, and Antoine must discern these as he negotiates an appropriate level of independence to facilitate his learning.

Antoine prepares for this initial meeting with Kate by completing a learning plan. He details what he hopes to achieve, based on the curriculum requirements and his understanding of the learning opportunities the placement would provide. With Kate's help, he modifies this, and Kate also emphasises how the level of performance expectation has now increased as he has completed basic training and is now an advanced trainee.

Case study 17.2: Occupational therapy — introducing Ethan and Sarah

Ethan, a junior occupational therapist, is the primary supervisor of two third-year occupational therapy students. Ethan has limited experience supervising students, but in a busy department the student load has been shifted to some of the junior occupational therapy staff. Sarah and Chloe are in Ethan's department for three months spending a six-week placement with him in a general medicine stream and then another six-week placement with his colleague in paediatrics. Ethan is keen to make this placement worthwhile for Sarah and Chloe, so he puts in effort to develop a timetable and provide a detailed orientation handout for them. Ethan has also blocked out weekly supervision sessions. Although he knows these sessions are important, Ethan is struggling to manage his time between Sarah and Chloe, as well as his own patient caseload and the 'quality project' he is completing for the department.

At the end of the first week, Ethan sits down to reflect on the performance of Sarah and Chloe. Ethan can see that, although there are some areas that need improvement, Chloe is demonstrating the expected level of competence and has in fact identified some learning goals herself during their first supervision session. Ethan realises that he hasn't spent as much time observing Sarah as he has with Chloe, and finds it hard to think about what specific feedback to give Sarah about her performance. She reports that 'everything is going well' and she has 'no concerns'. Ethan thinks she's 'pretty confident', and he makes a concerted effort to observe Sarah more in the second week so they both can make the most of their supervision time.

Identifying underperformance

Identifying underperformance is a different task to helping learners *overcome* underperformance, although clinical educators often do both simultaneously. While based on interactions with the learner, identifying underperformance is primarily the work of the clinical educator. This is in contrast to underperformance, where the strategies need to be more learner-centred so that the work belongs mostly to the learner, with the clinical educator in support.

In *identifying* underperformance, Steinert (2013) suggests that there are three areas of performance that are worth interrogating: knowledge, skills and attitudes. She also notes: 'teachers often assume that it is the learner who has the problem' (Steinert, 2013, p e1037). As a first step, Steinert suggests identifying whose 'problem' is prompting concerns: does the problem belong to the learner, the teacher or the system? Contemplating this type of question can be beneficial when grappling with a situation that is ambiguous and potentially challenging. For example, in case study 17.2 Ethan hasn't spent sufficient time observing Sarah. This is a 'teacher problem'. Another 'teacher problem' can result from clinical educators finding it easier to work with people they identify with; for example, sharing the same cultural background, class, gender and so on. It's important to be aware of the potential for these unconscious preferences. In clinical education, 'system problems' often relate to a lack of opportunity for practice. Another common system issue is a challenging or toxic practice environment, in which all learners will struggle. It's worth noting that, while asking 'who's problem?' is a valuable first question, it's not always easy to answer. This is partially because systems problems and teacher problems are exacerbated when a learner persistently underperforms.

So how can clinical educators know whether underperformance is more significant than just the normal errors and challenges of progression? Paice and Orton (2004) suggest looking for 'flags' that indicate a trainee is having difficulties. These 'flags' are signs of a potential problem that is more significant than usual, and include:

- *poor clinical performance*, including inadequate note-taking, difficulty in recognising urgency associated with a particular clinical situation, and so on;
- *unexplained absences*, which may be particularly related to broader issues, including bullying or depression;
- *rigidity*, including self-righteousness and an inability to accept responsibility for actions;
- *outbursts*, which may be strongly associated with stress;
- *failure to gain the trust of others*, which may also be related to systems issues, such as bullying of the trainee.

Both Steinert (2013) and Paice and Orton (2004) suggest identifying *situations* that are of concern, rather than focusing on the trainee as a 'problem'. This is a valuable approach, because, as Hodges and Lingard (2012) note, competency is not a fixed notion nor a fixed quantity. A person is not inherently incompetent or competent. Indeed, we all progress from mostly incompetent to mostly competent as we move from novice to expert. As future professionals who will take responsibility for their future conduct and learning throughout their career, learners should understand that competency (or incompetency) is not a stable personality trait, and that individuals can learn to develop. Thus, we also emphasise that the focus on the situation, not the learner, is appropriate. As a corollary, it is worth being careful about how underperformance labels are articulated and applied. We suggest shifting from the terms 'underperformers', 'struggling students', 'poorly performing learners' and 'problem students', and instead referring to 'students or trainees who underperform'. This acknowledges the problematic situation without providing a sense that it is permanent or personal.

Identifying underperformance is the easier part of the equation. Helping the learner to improve their performance is a knottier problem for most clinical educators, particularly when it is not a matter of more practice or more knowledge. Steinert (2013) notes that clinical educators often find attitudinal difficulties particularly difficult to manage. This is where educational theory can assist.

Case study 17.1 (continued): Anaesthesia training — identifying underperformance

Almost four weeks into the placement, Kate is pulled aside in the corridor by the anaesthetic charge nurse. He tells her that his staff are worried about Antoine. They have told him that they think he is indecisive, lacks confidence, that he is slow in preparing for cases after-hours, and doesn't clearly tell them what he wants from them before or during cases. A few of them have started to notify the other registrar who is on overnight with other duties when Antoine is doing a case, so they are around, 'just in case'.

Kate thanks her colleague, and tells him that she will monitor the situation. She knows that not every issue that is flagged to her will turn out to be significant. Sometimes, a trainee might not get along with one or two people, or have had a 'bad day', as anyone's performance can fluctuate.

Later that afternoon, Kate sees a colleague, Paul, who worked with Antoine the previous week. She asks Paul how he has found working with Antoine. Paul says that Antoine was not as 'sharp' as he expected the new trainees to be. He seemed unsure of himself and unprepared for the cases.

Kate checks the roster and sees that Antoine is working with Kim today. As it is now nearing the end of the day, she calls Kim to ask how Antoine's performance has been. Kim says she thinks Antoine has had a bad day. Even though the cases were ones he would have seen before, the patients have all had significant co-morbidities and have been challenging. Antoine was slow to react when the patients' condition required intervention, and she had been surprised that she had needed to step in a number of times. He also took a very long time and wasn't ready for the afternoon list, even though she let him out of the morning list early.

Kate decides she will need to investigate Antoine's performance more systematically. She doesn't want to miss the early signs of underperformance, because she knows remediation takes time, and that issues only get harder to deal with if they persist. Kate runs into Antoine in the department and asks how he is finding the new placement. Antoine reassures her, saying he is 'finding his feet'. Kate says that is good, and asks to catch up next week to discuss matters in more detail.

Case study 17.2 (continued): Occupational therapy — identifying underperformance

On Monday afternoon, Ethan observes Sarah with Mrs Peirce, an 86-year-old lady who was admitted over the weekend after a fall at home. This is Mrs Peirce's initial assessment and first contact with anyone from the allied health team since she arrived. The cause of her fall is still under investigation, with notes from the general medicine team stating 'IMP: ?AF for Cardiol r/v.' After reading the notes, Sarah enters Mrs Peirce's room to find her attached to an electrocardiogram (ECG), oxygen therapy, and pulse oximeter. Sarah introduces herself and proceeds to gather a detailed history from Mrs Peirce. Ethan is pleasantly surprised with Sarah's performance, and feels comfortable leaving Sarah to complete the rest of the assessment while he answers a page from the physiotherapist.

Some minutes pass. While on the phone, Ethan witnesses Sarah and Mrs Peirce walking with no walking aids or attachments towards the corridor. Sarah is striding half a metre in front of Mrs Peirce, leading her to the bathroom to assess her self-care performance. Ethan notices Mrs Peirce slow down, reach for the wall and (luckily) find a seat on a wheelchair that has been left in the corridor. Sarah takes a little while to realise what has happened, and inquires as to what is wrong. Mrs Peirce states she is 'feeling a bit dizzy and would like to return to bed'. Ethan steps in to check Mrs Peirce's vital signs by applying the portable pulse oximeter. Her oxygen is at 89%; however, the probe is struggling to find a trace. Mrs Peirce is still dizzy as Ethan wheels her back to her bed, where her ECG and oxygen are reattached. Ethan immediately alerts the nursing staff to take over providing essential care to Mrs Peirce, and takes Sarah aside. As it is nearing the end of the day, Ethan suggests that Sarah write in Mrs Peirce's notes, and that they meet in the morning to have a chat about what happened.

Theories which inform working with underperformance

We propose exploring underperformance through the lens of two very different but complementary theories: 'communities of practice' and 'self-determination theory'. Neither of these are explicitly about underperformance, but we have chosen these theories to encourage educators to think deeply about the underperformance situations they encounter from different perspectives. The aim is to shift how clinical educators conceptualise and manage underperformance. These theories draw from very different traditions. One focuses on the broader social environment of the learner; the other focuses on individual internal processes.

Learning as social participation: communities of practice

Conceptualising learning as a social act may help explain why underperformance presents so many challenges. One of the best-known theories of social learning is 'communities of practice' (Lave & Wenger, 1991). This grew from Lave and Wenger's study of apprenticeship, and how apprentices moved from the 'periphery' of a practice to being an 'old-timer' at the centre of activity. Wenger (1998) suggests that there are three necessary elements to a community of practice:

- mutual engagement;
- joint enterprise;
- shared repertoire.

Mutual engagement

Workers interact with each other, and these social interactions are central to the community of practice itself. The community is formed by participation. In this way, the novice healthcare worker learns not just through observing, but also through interaction and joint tasks, buttressed by social interactions. This may explain why clinical supervisors can find disinterested learner attitudes so challenging: if they refuse to participate, they cannot learn.

Joint enterprise

The workers must have shared purposeful activities. In the case of clinical education, this is the general work of the department, unit or practice. The enterprise is constantly emerging through 'negotiation', which forms evolving practices rather than static rules. This evolution is constantly 'negotiated' by the members of the community, and necessarily entails 'mutual accountability'. This underlines how useful it is to make the tacit 'ways things are done around here' as explicit as possible for novices.

Shared repertoire

There is a set of common tools for a community of practice. These include the language of the clinical environment, as well as the daily practices: a ward round, conducting 'obs' (observations), taking a history. A novice often lacks the shared repertoire, and part of the work of learning in a clinical environment is coming to enact these common tools through participating in the work of the unit. These three aspects — mutual engagement, joint enterprise and shared repertoire — are interlinked, and by their nature cannot be reduced from the sum of their parts. In a nutshell, learning in a community of practice can only occur through experiencing it.

Other implications of communities of practice theory

Communities of practice theory suggests that novices craft an inbound trajectory through the community. They shift from the inexperienced and inexpert periphery into 'identities of participation'. Wenger (1998) distinguishes 'peripherality' of novices from 'marginality', where there is no inbound trajectory to take the individual more deeply into the community.

'Marginality' is an identity of *non-participation*. Considered in this way, performance issues can position an individual on the margins of a community; this is further out than the periphery, because there is no way to work towards 'full' participation. Viewed in the context of clinical education, this marginality is more impactful than the failure of the student who does not do well in an academic exam. Even in the circumstances of exam failure, a learner can still participate in student life: attend lectures, study groups. Clinical underperformance means that learners are frequently not allowed to perform certain tasks, and become marginalised from the practice community. This can be an immediate form of social exclusion, and may arouse strong negative emotions, which can impede learning further. Moreover, the very act of investigating underperformance can amplify the sense of marginality.

While communities of practice does not immediately suggest strategies for working with learners, it raises some key ideas: participation is necessary for learning; tacit rules should be made as clear as possible; and social interaction supports bringing learners into the community. In addition, non-participation leads to learners feeling marginalised from their learning environment. We draw from these ideas later in this chapter.

Critiques of communities of practice theory

One major critique of 'communities of practice' theory is that it does not put enough emphasis on what the *learner* brings to the community (Fuller et al., 2005). Other theorists, such as Stephen Billett, do highlight the role of the learner. Billett (2014, p 5) notes that '... humans are active meaning makers and constructors of knowledge that arises through their experiencing … albeit premised on what they have previously experienced and learnt'. He then suggests that, in workplace learning, the degree of effort undertaken by the learner to engage their past experience with the current circumstance is 'premised on their interest, desire and energy'. In short, education in the workplace is a 'duality' of 'personal and social contributions'. Against this complexity, how is a clinical educator to move forward? If sociocultural theories such as communities of practice theory help clinical supervisors to understand the reasons for the emotional challenges of underperformance, other approaches may help with orienting the individual to improvement.

In underperformance, one of the biggest challenges to supporting individuals is when learners do not acknowledge that they have deficits. This is the 'insight problem'. Often clinical educators find this very difficult to manage, and we spend a moment on this concern before outlining how our next theoretical approach can provide assistance.

The 'insight problem' reconsidered

Clinical educators often describe the 'insight problem' as the biggest problem of all (Steinert, 2013). However, the 'insight problem' is sometimes mis-labelled. It may not be the learner's insight that is in question. The dual roles of the clinical educator as both assessor and teacher mean that learners often do not want to reveal their weaknesses. In other words, they may know that they have problems, but don't want to acknowledge this in front of someone who will be assessing them. At the same time, without learners being prepared to declare weaknesses, it can be very difficult for clinical educators to provide solutions for improvement. As one physiotherapy clinical supervisor noted: 'Some of [the students] just keep up the big, fake bravado, keep the blind down — "I'm not going to let you know anything about me because that might expose some weakness that you might see in me." They're the ones that are really unsuccessful.' (Bearman et al., 2011). An additional layer of complexity is that sometimes learners do genuinely lack insight. From a patient safety perspective, irrespective of what learners think of their own situation, clinical educators must judge learners against the required standards, including hard-to-measure aspects such as professionalism. One way of addressing this dilemma is to move beyond the 'insight problem'. Taking an educational development perspective, we suggest focusing on the learner's motivations.

Self-determination theory

Self-determination theory (SDT) (Ryan & Deci, 2000) looks at the 'interests, desires and energy' of the learner. Drawing from the cognitive theoretical tradition, it describes the necessary conditions for intrinsic motivation. This is the motivation to learn that springs from the learner themselves, rather than from outside interests. Ryan and Deci (2000, p 70) write: 'Perhaps no single phenomenon reflects the positive potential of human nature as much as intrinsic motivation, the inherent tendency to seek out novelty and challenges, to extend and exercise one's capacities, to explore, and to learn.' This helps reframe the 'insight problem'. We suggest it is more valuable to focus on how we enhance the learner's capacity to drive learning than focusing on lack of 'insight', given that the latter may or may not exist.

Ryan and Deci (2000) propose three types of motivational states. The first to be *amotivational*; when a person lacks any motivation. This is rare to find in clinical learning contexts. The second is when motivation is *controlled*; when learners are driven by external conditions, including notions of self-esteem based on others' opinions. Finally, there are *autonomous regulated* motivations. These are when individuals control their own motivational states, either through intrinsically enjoying the task, or because the desired behaviour aligns with their own 'personal goals and identities' (Gagné & Deci, 2005). Underpinning autonomously regulated motivations are feelings of *competence*, *relatedness* and *autonomy*. Autonomy is noted by Gagné and Deci (2005) as particularly important. Any learning environment can provide more or less opportunity for learners to achieve autonomously regulated motivations. In some instances, clinical contexts can have a significantly negative impact, and in other instances be profoundly inspiring.

Underperformance automatically challenges the conditions for autonomously regulated motivation, as the feeling of competence is removed. It is therefore critical that feelings of relatedness and autonomy are maintained, so that the learner has some degree of control over their learning and choices. Often the choices that are made by clinical supervisors — the 'more more more' — are precisely in the opposite direction. In a 2015 study of medical students who had failed final re-sit exams, one participant noted that: 'I did [go to my personal tutor] … but kind of always felt there was always an issue of trust. […] How much of this is a degree of policing rather than true help?' (Patel et al., 2015, p 49). Being told once more that you are doing something poorly or being offered the same activity (which you have already failed) again or being burdened with even more oversight are at odds with building feelings of autonomy, as well as further degrading any feelings of competence.

SDT helps frame the core challenge for clinical supervisors: what educational strategies promote autonomy and relatedness, while at the same time sufficiently scaffolding underperformance and ensuring patient safety? The rest of this chapter investigates this question. There is limited research in this area, so these strategies are drawn from diverse bodies of work, some of which are specific to underperformance and some of which are more general.

Case study 17.1 (continued): Anaesthesia training — initial approach to underperformance

In preparation for the meeting, Kate talks to some more of the consultants who have worked with Antoine. She is not reassured. They tell her that Antoine has difficulty integrating the requirements of complex patients and surgery, that he seems under-prepared and reluctant to start complex cases, lacks vigilance, and is reticent to intervene when required. When they meet, Kate is keen to hear Antoine's side of the story. Antoine says that he has found the placement challenging, and has been working longer and doing extra reading. He remarks there is so much to take into account when deciding what is the right thing to do, but he thinks he is managing okay.

Kate relays the consultants' concerns. Antoine points out that they haven't said anything directly to him, and that he expects them to intervene whenever they think it is appropriate, so he hadn't thought anything was wrong. Kate gives a few specific examples, and explains how each consultant separately had thought his performance might be an exception, but when taken together their reports are consistent and indicate a real issue.

When Kate asks him how he is finding working with the anaesthetic nurses, he says he hasn't given it much thought; they generally seem happy to do what he tells them to do. Kate tells him that the nurses are concerned when they work with him, and that they are getting the other registrar to stand by when he does a case. Antoine is surprised to hear this, and is concerned what his peers will think.

Next, Kate checks on Antoine's health and home life. He doesn't report any issues, and, given she doesn't have any way to check personally, she decides to take this response at face value.

Kate tells Antoine that the situation as reported to her indicates his performance is below that expected, and that they will need to agree a remediation plan. Antoine is reluctant to acknowledge that this is required, but agrees to cooperate.

Antoine's roster is changed so that he works with a smaller, select group of consultants whose judgment she trusts, and whom she can rely on to provide specific and honest feedback to Antoine on his performance. She asks them to complete work-based assessments on cases they perceive are appropriately challenging for Antoine, so he will receive useful feedback and she will have a record of his performance and the feedback discussions that take place.

Kate discusses with Antoine the need to articulate his plans to his anaesthetic nurse prior to each case, and to keep them informed of what he is thinking. Kate says she will be asking the nurses to give feedback to her on how he is performing in this area. She organises for Antoine to attend the local simulation centre to help practise prioritisation in decision-making and teamwork. They agree to meet in two and four weeks to review progress.

Case study 17.2 (continued): Occupational therapy — initial approach to underperformance

Ethan prepares some notes for the feedback meeting, and meets Sarah in the meeting room up on the ward the next morning. Despite his preparation, the conversation with Sarah does not quite go to plan. Sarah and Ethan seem to agree that Sarah's history-taking is a strength of hers. She engaged well with Mrs Peirce and had successfully identified some key occupational performance issues, determined relevant acute occupational therapy goals, and commenced discharge planning. When asked to identify areas that she did not do so well, Sarah answers, 'Well, not much. She [Mrs Peirce] never made it to the bathroom, so I don't know if she is safe to go home.' When Ethan prompts about any other safety issues of concern, and what might have impacted on

Mrs Peirce's performance during the assessment, Sarah answers, 'Well, she has no rails at home in her shower or toilet, so we will need to assess that.'

From Ethan's perspective, Sarah is missing the significant safety issues with her performance with Mrs Peirce. She seems offended when Ethan tells her that 'the way you mobilised Mrs Peirce without checking with the nursing or medical staff was unsafe'. Additionally, even if she had the go-ahead, 'she should have kept her ECG and oxygen attached'. Not to mention Sarah's unsafe manual handling as 'you were not close enough to Mrs Peirce, especially as she was a falls risk'. Sarah says nothing after Ethan finishes reading his prepared notes, and she shrugs off his request to catch up later in the day before he watches her see Mrs Peirce again. Their feedback meeting is quickly wrapped up, as other health professionals begin entering the room for the Tuesday morning multidisciplinary team meeting. Sarah spends the entire meeting looking at the floor.

Practical strategies for working with underperformance

Two types of practical strategies assist with underperformance. Firstly, there are general approaches that are valuable for all forms of clinical learning, but particularly necessary for underperformance. We need to outline these first, as they form the foundational platform to build underperformance specific strategies. Secondly, there are strategies specifically designed for learners who underperform. Different types of strategies and how they are used, both generally and specifically with underperformance, are outlined below. The next sections outline these strategies in more detail.

PRACTICAL TIPS

General and specific strategies for working with underperformance.

Pedagogical approach	General strategies across the spectrum of performance	Specific strategies for working with underperformance
Learning plan	Learning plan drawn up at the beginning of the placement to be revisited at regular points	Returning to the learning plan more frequently, revisiting previously agreed standards
Workplace curriculum	Identifying and sequencing tasks as part of a workplace curriculum. Role-modelling tasks, articulating knowledge, skills and attitudes	Rethink tasks to be at the right level/size to challenge learning. Focused and explicit demonstration
Relationship-building	Building an 'educational alliance'	Educator reflective practice, such as 'pause and think'
Feedback and assessment	Refer to Chapter 20	Feedback and goal-setting on smaller, achievable tasks
Educational administration	High-level documentation, reviewed and agreed by the learner	All documentation reviewed and agreed by the learner. Engage institutional supports

General strategies across the spectrum of performance

Learning plan

The first tool of choice at the commencement of a placement is the joint development of a learning plan. The emphasis here is on the *joint* construction. It is through this upfront investment that ground rules for the placement are set, the engagement of the learner begins, and an educator–learner relationship is established. In case study 17.1 (anaesthesia), Kate has tools from the accreditation body to assist her in developing this learning plan. Ethan, inexperienced and unsupported, does not have the expertise to develop this from the start. Learning plans allow the learner and the educator to develop goals together for the placement. They allow the learner to declare areas of concern, and for educators to flag transitions that the learner finds difficult. Most of all, they allow the explicit and agreed declaration of standards. This serves as a useful benchmark for later conversations about performance. For example, the presence of explicit standards would be very useful in Ethan's conversation with Sarah.

Workplace curriculum

The educator allocates tasks to the learner that constitute a workplace curriculum. In a placement experience that goes according to plan, the general notion is that through work the supervisor guides the learner. This allows the learner to complete increasingly difficult tasks and assume greater independence. From an SDT perspective, the learner's needs for *relatedness*, *competence* and *autonomy* are all met. From a communities of practice perspective, the learner progresses on a *trajectory* into the community.

Like many clinical educators, Kate and Ethan articulate this curriculum more tacitly than explicitly. They may never consciously consider some of the educational tools at the clinical educator's disposal. These are well described by Billett (2001), and include:

- role-modelling of the expected standards;
- sequencing of tasks, from those that are easier to those which are more challenging;
- consideration of tasks that are routine (most for students), to those which are non-routine (more important for post-graduates);
- opportunities to learn outside of the workplace environment; for example, reading for knowledge or using simulation for skills development;
- manipulation of levels of responsibility, so that the learner is always working within their zone of challenge;
- explicit articulation of 'the way things are done around here' — so that the learner can understand some of the tacit approaches;
- explicit links between the particular situation and other situations — to assist the learner in transferring their learnings to other situations.

In both Ethan's and Kate's situations, these tools have not all been employed. Sarah, in particular, would benefit from more exposure to the expectations of practice through role-modelling and articulation 'of the way things are done around here'. Antoine is clearly being provided with opportunities outside of the workplace, but Kate could be reviewing these with him to ensure they are the *right* ones. Antoine could also benefit from explicit *positive* links from his previous rotation to his current one. In these examples, these activities and conversations serve multiple roles. First, they help Sarah and Antoine with the tasks at hand. Secondly, they provide them with the *shared repertoire* of the community of practice. Finally, they allow Ethan and Kate to facilitate feelings of *relatedness* (through the building of the relationship), *competence* (through the exposure of tacit practices) and *autonomy* (through the investment in them as potential colleagues).

Building relatedness: the educational alliance

As can be seen, the role of the educator–learner relationship in devising a workplace curriculum is significant. Most learners, let alone those who may be underperforming, are in a vulnerable place, as they are on the periphery of the *community of practice* and have lower feelings of *competence* due to their novice status. Thinking about the clinical supervision process as an 'educational alliance' may assist. Drawing from the psychotherapy notion of the 'therapeutic alliance' between a therapist and a patient, the notion here is that the learner's perception of the relationship between the clinical supervisor and the learner is central to the value of the feedback. As Telio, Ajjawi and Regehr (2015, p 612) note:

> … the learner is likely to be actively exploring and testing the supervisor's commitment to the learning process from the first moment of their first meeting. Almost immediately, the learner will be asking himself or herself questions such as the following: Does this supervisor care about me as a person? Am I present in this person's mind? Does this supervisor care about my goals in this context? Is he/she trying (and able) to understand where I am starting from and where I want to get to? Does this supervisor have my best

interests at heart? Is this relationship about my becoming the best clinician I can be, or are there other agendas here?

This educational alliance framework suggests that it is important from the commencement of the placement that a clinical supervisor demonstrates a commitment to the learner's progress. The learners can therefore grasp that the clinical educators' efforts are designed to benefit the learner. Both Ethan and Kate have positioned themselves well to form an educational alliance with their learners; they clearly have taken time and effort to observe and work with the learners. However, the communication of their commitment is not necessarily clear, and some of their actions actively undermine this. In particular, Kate letting Antoine know that the nurses will be reporting back on him is closer to surveillance than educational observation.

The educational alliance, like all things relational, is not an easy prescription. They are founded on relationships and, as mentioned earlier, humans tend to more easily connect with those of similar background. As noted in the section on insight, learners don't find it easy to be vulnerable with those who will make decisions about their progress. However, we suggest that learners do find it easier to be vulnerable with those clinical educators who obviously have the learners' best interests at heart.

Feedback and assessment tasks

The educational alliance serves as one model for feedback relationships; there are many others. The significance of feedback associated with formative and summative assessment tasks in clinical education is well covered in other sections of this book. We refer readers to Chapter 20 for in-depth discussions of this important foundation of clinical education practice.

Educational administration: documentation

It is important to document learner progress. This includes records of learning plans, formal meetings and observed performances. If this is routine, then it assists in signalling to the learner that this is part of building their trajectory, not a surveillance that can undermine their motivations.

Specific strategies when managing underperformance

Learners who are underperforming also require particular attention. Here are some specific strategies which we suggest can help with managing these difficult situations. We encourage educators to reflect on how these may work with respect to their situations.

Learning plans: revisiting standards and the workplace curriculum

Revisiting the learning plan is very helpful when managing underperformance. It is important to be clear about what the aims of the activity are. By making learning plans as explicit as possible, the learner can begin to recognise the required standards within the community of practice. That is to say, the learning plan should have explicit markers of progress with expected standards as a series of short-term goals. This learning plan then establishes the learner as part of the community, and provides them with a clear understanding of what is required for progression. This establishes a path for their *trajectory*, as well as a concrete representation of their planned participation. Contrast this with a learner being increasingly excluded from tasks without any explanation or discussion. The shared learning plan reinforces *peripherality* (the natural state of the novice) rather than *marginality*.

SDT provides guidance on how to structure tasks to meet the learning plan. First, consider the learner's feelings of *competence*. It is critical that some tasks be achievable. This may mean giving the learner time to practise skills they are already competent at (possibly out of the placement environment), or to demonstrate skills with a very low level of challenge. The next element to consider is feelings of *relatedness*; coming from an educational alliance perspective may help here. This means that the stance of the clinical supervisor is not about the person, but about the situation. If the underperformance concerns are in the area of dishonesty or other areas where the learner's character is called into question, this becomes much more challenging, but even in this circumstance it is most useful to focus on expected behaviours of the future. It is helpful to refer to evidence, as collected by documentation. It is useful to provide any data to the learner in a sensitive manner, possibly in advance, so that they can start to make sense of what can be very distressing information in their own time. Providing the opportunity to offer suggestions, and genuinely considering these suggestions, promotes feelings of *autonomy*. When the clinical educator and the learner sit down together to form a remediation plan, it is useful to frame this as an exercise in joint problem-solving. If possible, the plan should provide for some independent practice; this may mean giving learners easier tasks to do without oversight that do not impair patient safety.

In case study 17.2 (occupational therapy), Ethan's management of Sarah unintentionally removed much of her *autonomy*. While it is appropriate that she should not be managing patients independently until Ethan is sure that she can do so safely, she can be supported towards a path where she can work safely by herself. While Sarah was told explicitly that what she had done was not right, it may have been difficult for her to have understood what she should have done instead. This is an opportunity for a focused and explicit demonstration of the expected standard. Sometimes things that are very self-evident to experienced clinicians, bewilder novices.

Relationship management: 'pause and think'

As noted, underperformance invokes heavy emotions. This means that a clinical supervisor must be managing their own emotions as much as those of their learner, as they are having to maintain the learner's motivations. We suggest a very simple practical strategy: 'pause and think' at every juncture when the clinical supervisor feels the stress of underperformance. We suggest they ask themselves the following questions before having a feedback conversation or devising a learning plan or considering what to do next:

- How is your current situation and environment affecting what you are thinking and feeling? (For example, are there clinical or administrative or staffing issues? What other stresses do you have?)
- What is the learner's impact on you? (For example, is it 'more more more'? What impact is it having on your feelings of competence, relatedness and autonomy?)
- What is your impact on the learner? (For example, what impact are you having on their feelings of competence, relatedness and autonomy?)

Take stock of all these things; it may be that some feedback exchanges must happen right now, and others can be shelved for later. The learner may need space to come to grips with their own situation. Alternatively, it may be that now is the perfect time for a quick discussion in a quiet place.

Specific feedback strategies

Feedback is very challenging with underperformance. Most feedback models are designed to take account of deficits, as all learners make errors, and feedback exchanges about the gap between performance and standard are generally par for the course. All models, however, are prone to tokenism. For example, the clinical educator may tokenistically use learner-centred phrasing, but the message is clear: the learner has done something wrong, and the clinical educator is telling them what ought to be done to fix it. This is a common type of message. The problem is that it not only reduces a learner's sense of *competence* (a necessary part of coming to grips with underperformance), but also simultaneously impairs the learner's sense of *relatedness* and *autonomy*.

Focusing on building *relatedness* and *autonomy* may give learners the intrinsic motivation (and possibly the 'insight') to work towards improvement. Whichever feedback model is employed, consider how the feedback exchange can maintain the learner's sense of relatedness and autonomy. The former is relatively easy. As mentioned earlier, focusing on situations and behaviours rather than personalities can assist. Body language and tone are also important, as these are critical in terms of building a sense of relatedness. Autonomy is more challenging. This is why feedback models often seek the learner's input into solutions: how can the learner 'own' the situation and the way forward? Goal-oriented feedback may prove helpful. In this model of feedback, either before or after the task the clinical supervisor will ask for the learner to nominate a preferred focus for the feedback exchange. This can assist in giving the learner a sense of control.

It is important to have a discussion of alternative pathways to progression; they can and should be provided as real options. Withdrawal or failure is sometimes necessary, and may be important for the learner's trajectory. Underperformance may be transient and due to external factors; in these circumstances, time away from the clinical environment can be restorative. Kate made attempts to identify whether there are external factors that may have been troubling Antoine, but had no way to confirm his response. We appreciate these conversations can be difficult for both parties; an *educational alliance* may help create an environment in which learners/trainees are willing to share this type of information.

Administration: documentation and referrals

Documentation is even more critical once underperformance is identified. Underperformance is rarely a single person's problem; there is usually a broader system involved. Make sure that documentation is exchanged with that broader system: the accrediting body, university or employer. The learner will need to know this, but they can also be informed that this is a common situation and it is for their own benefit as well. Also make sure that the learner is provided with all the assistance that the broader system offers. In particular, mental health supports, disability supports and mentoring are all great resources that can be underutilised. As clinical educators, it can be difficult to remember that the learner is a member of more than one community of practice, and that these other communities may provide appropriate assistance.

Case study 17.1 (continued): Anaesthesia training — a different approach to underperformance

In spite of the measures Kate and Antoine agree to, Antoine continues to struggle. He does not seem to take in the feedback he receives, is unsure of himself when working without direct supervision, and is reticent in his dealings with the anaesthetic nurses. He has become reluctant to attend meetings with Kate or the other supervisors, and has had many days absent from work.

Kate is worried that all of the extra effort that the department is putting in to help Antoine is not working, so she seeks advice from Richard, a more experienced supervisor who supervised her. Richard asks her what Antoine thinks he needs to do to improve, and she realises she hasn't really asked him — that they have mostly been telling him where he has failed and what they think he needs to do. Richard points out that in the end it is Antoine who has to learn, and that their feedback needs to support his confidence and autonomy. She decides to start again by first asking Antoine what he thinks he should do.

It takes some work to convince him, but she meets with Antoine and asks him whether he thinks the remediation plan is working. He doesn't think so. He feels like he is under a microscope and that whatever he does is wrong, and even though he thinks he knows more about what he is doing and is not overwhelmed anymore, no one seems to notice. He says he's no longer confident even with work he knows how to do. Kate realises that everyone trying to be helpful and telling Antoine where he is going wrong has not had the effect they had hoped for. When Kate asks him what he thinks he should do, he says he would like to 'turn back time' and go back to his previous role, where he was comfortable and competent and felt at home.

Kate organises for Antoine to return to his previous workplace for the next placement, where the staff know him well. Together with the supervisor there, Kate helps Antoine to plan what he can do to regain his confidence and sense of competency through setting tasks to be at right level to challenge his learning within a supportive environment. They also make specific plans that he can practise to better prepare for dealing with the more complex work he will face when he returns. Kate plans in the meantime to try out a new feedback model with her colleagues so that if Antoine does need more help on his return they can do a better job of it.

Case study 17.2 (continued): Occupational therapy — a different approach to underperformance

Over morning tea, Ethan takes time to reflect on the feedback meeting with Sarah. He knows it hasn't gone too well, but is unsure of what other approaches to take. Sarah was unsafe, but telling her about her deficits didn't seem to have the effect Ethan was after. She doesn't seem aware that she had areas to improve on, nor is interested in improving. Short of coaching her step-by-step through her next session with Mrs Peirce, or outlining the patient safety items on her assessment tool, Ethan is not sure how to motivate her to change her practice.

Ethan starts to consider the situation from an alternative perspective. He realises that he could have engaged with Sarah in a different way. What is it that motivates Sarah? Reflecting on the time he has spent with her, Ethan acknowledges that he has yet to explore Sarah's personal goals or what she hopes to achieve at this placement. What are her learning goals? Perhaps Ethan can use yesterday's example with Mrs Peirce to explore what Sarah hopes to achieve, and outline some strategies to move towards achieving the expected level of performance. Ethan also considers the value of Chloe and Sarah working together in a more collaborative learning approach. He can easily schedule some time for Chloe and Sarah to work together. They could present client cases to each other, and discuss the key things they have learnt. Ethan could prompt them to highlight the key safety aspects of each case, with a view to helping Sarah see the importance and the need to check the safety signs of patients, and to be mindful for potential risks that may occur.

Failure and its consequences

Successfully working with a learner who is underperforming does not always mean that the learner passes. In our case studies, Ethan and Kate have reworked their plans to take account of Sarah and Antoine's perspectives, and these changed approaches may well provide them with the opportunity they need to meet the requisite standard. However, there are no guarantees. Failure occurs; learners sometimes do not meet the requirements for a whole host of reasons. Learners may never acknowledge any deficits; there are intractable situations where a learner and a clinical educator's views never converge — these are but two examples. However, it is not the clinical educator's responsibility to make the learner pass. Their responsibility is to create a curriculum and environment where learners have an opportunity to succeed. 'Failure to fail' has many negative impacts, most notably on patient care, but also on the learner themselves. A practitioner who never feels competent may never feel comfortable in their profession.

Potential directions for evaluation and research

The area of underperformance is a very open area for further research. There are many potential avenues that could usefully inform both academic understandings and clinical education. Most notably, it would be very helpful to have qualitative and quantitative data that support particular strategies for working with underperformance. Much of the work in this space is drawn from theory and from expert clinical education practice. It would be useful to know what the various impacts of different approaches have on both learners and clinical educators. One particularly interesting area for investigation is the notion of team rather than individual competence.

Conclusion

Underperformance is a challenging area for clinical educators and learners alike. Failing to meet standards is unpleasant all round. This emotionally negative situation may be compounded by insufficient educational training. This chapter has offered some theoretical insights and practical suggestions. The take-home message can be summarised simply: if you notice yourself saying or doing the same thing over and over again, then it may be time to think differently. Learners need autonomy in order to progress, and the art of clinical education is working out how to give them this in a way that is safe and constructive.

Acknowledgment

The authors would like to acknowledge Alyce Folan (Monash Health) for her contribution to the occupational therapy case study.

References

Bearman, M., Ajjawi, R., Molloy, E. K., et al. (2011). *'They can't see it': Characterising the poorly performing student in the clinical environment*. Paper presented at the Association of Medical Education Europe, 29–31 August 2011, Vienna.

Bearman, M., Molloy, E., Ajjawi, R., et al. (2012). 'Is there a Plan B?': Clinical educators supporting underperforming students in practice settings. *Teaching in Higher Education, 18*(5), 531–544. doi:10.108 0/13562517.2012.752732.

Bearman, M., Tai, J., Kent, F., et al. (2017). What should we teach the teachers? Identifying the learning priorities of clinical supervisors. *Advances in Health Sciences Education*, doi:10.1007/s10459-017-9772-3.

Billett, S. (2001). *Learning in the workplace: Strategies for effective practice*. Sydney: Allen & Unwin.

Billett, S. (2014). Integrating learning experiences across tertiary education and practice settings: A socio-personal account. *Educational Research Review, 12*, 1–13. doi: http://doi.org/10.1016/j.edurev.2014.01.002.

Cleland, J., Leggett, H., Sandars, J., et al. (2013). The remediation challenge: Theoretical and methodological insights from a systematic review. *Medical Education, 47*(3), 242–251. doi:10.1111/medu.12052.

Fuller, A., Hodkinson, H., Hodkinson, P., et al. (2005). Learning as peripheral participation in communities of practice: A reassessment of key concepts in workplace learning. *British Educational Research Journal, 31*(1), 49–68.

Gagné, M., & Deci, E. L. (2005). Self-determination theory and work motivation. *Journal of Organizational Behavior, 26*(4), 331–362. doi:10.1002/job.322.

Health Workforce Australia. (2010). *Clinical Supervisor Support Program Discussion Paper*. [Host website disestablished, but available via online search.]

Hodges, B. D., & Lingard, L. (2012). Introduction. In B. D. Hodges & L. Lingard (Eds.), *The question of competence: Reconsidering medical education in the twenty-first century* (pp. 1–13). Ithaca NY: Cornell University Press.

Hrobsky, P. E., & Kersbergen, A. L. (2002). Preceptor's perceptions of clinical performance failure. *Journal of Nursing Education, 41*(12), 550–553.

Lave, J., & Wenger, E. (1991). *Situated learning: Legitimate peripheral participation*. Cambridge: Cambridge University Press.

Luhanga, F., Yonge, O., & Myrick, F. (2008). Precepting an unsafe student: The role of the faculty. *Nurse Education Today, 28*(2), 227–231.

Paice, E., & Orton, V. (2004). Early signs of the trainee in difficulty. *Hospital Medicine, 65*(4), 238–240.

Patel, R., Tarrant, C., Bonas, S., et al. (2015). The struggling student: A thematic analysis from the self-regulated learning perspective. *Medical Education, 49*(4), 417–426. doi:10.1111/medu.12651.

Ryan, R. M., & Deci, E. L. (2000). Self-determination theory and the facilitation of intrinsic motivation, social development, and well-being. *American Psychologist, 55*(1), 68–78. doi:10.1037/0003-066X.55.1.68.

Salm, T. L., Johner, R., & Luhanga, F. (2016). Determining student competency in field placements: An emerging theoretical model. *Canadian Journal for the Scholarship of Teaching and Learning, 7*(1), 5. http://dx.doi.org/10.5206/cjsotl-rcacea.2016.1.5.

Steinert, Y. (2013). The 'problem' learner: Whose problem is it? AMEE Guide No. 76. *Medical Teacher, 35*(4), e1035–e1045. doi:10.3109/0142159X.2013.774082.

Telio, S., Ajjawi, R., & Regehr, G. (2015). The 'educational alliance' as a framework for reconceptualizing feedback in medical education. *Academic Medicine, 90*(5), 609–614.

Wenger, E. (1998). *Communities of practice: Learning, meaning, and identity*. UK: Cambridge University Press.

Section 3

Assessment for learning in the workplace

18

Workplace-based assessment

James Crossley

Introduction

Assessment is part of learning

Assessment is an essential part of learning. It has the potential to show whether learning has taken place, and to direct the nature and content of learning. Learners make their learning choices paying careful attention to their upcoming assessments. They can also learn from the assessment experience and the assessment outcome. Thus, assessments can be designed to support learning in several ways: to plan learning (assessment *for* learning), to promote learning (assessment *as* learning), or to test learning (assessment *of* learning).

Assessment takes many forms, including: written cognitive tests; observations of skill in controlled situations; and judgments based on real work activity. So what defines assessment? It is distinctive because it aims to measure performance against explicit criteria. It is the approximation to measurement, and the defining of criteria that sets assessment apart from other evaluation activities such as appraisal. Some learning is easy to measure and some is difficult, but assessment always aspires to being systematic, fair and defensible.

Define what you are measuring

With any measurement process, the first step is to define what you are measuring. Even with physical measurements you have to decide what feature you are measuring before you start (volume, melting point, density, etc.).

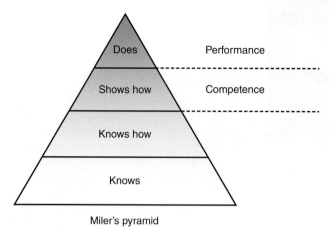

Figure 18.1: A model of cognitive and behavioural levels of learning

Source: Adapted from Miller, G. E. (1990). The assessment of clinical skills/competence/performance. Academic Medicine, 65(9Suppl), S63–S67.

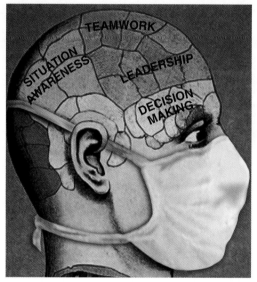

Figure 18.2: A cartoon representation of non-cognitive constructs as anatomically-based traits

Source: Reprinted with permission of Springer Nature. Yule, S., Flin, R., Maran, N., Rowley, D., Youngson, G., & Paterson-Brown, S. (2008). Surgeons' nontechnical skills in the operating room: Reliability testing of the NOTSS behavior rating system. World Journal of Surgery, 32(4), 548–555

Defining what type of learning to measure is much more difficult than defining a physical property. At the very least, we need to identify whether we are interested in what learners know or don't know (cognition), in what they can or can't do (skill), or in their value-driven real-world actions. Learning operates at many levels. Cognition ranges from superficial recall to deep understanding and creativity. Skill ranges from bare competence under predictable conditions, to unconscious mastery and everyday adaptability. Miller's pyramid (see Fig. 18.1) models learning as a progression through four levels, where cognition underpins skill, and skill underpins action. This simple but effective framework helps to focus assessments in healthcare education where both cognitive and behavioural learning are important.

However, this way of defining learning is situation-specific. To give an obvious example: I can read quite well (unconscious mastery), but I can't play the cello at all (don't even know the notes). In some situations — for example, selection — we're more concerned with what a learner *is* than with what they have *learned*. We might describe the learner using traits such as IQ, psychomotor skill, situational awareness, empathy, conscientiousness, etc. (see Fig. 18.2).

Unfortunately, the measurement of traits is elusive. The second half of the chapter will return to this issue.

Define why you are measuring

The second step is to define the purpose (why you are measuring). This is because different methods are suited to different purposes. To return to the physical world analogy, I wouldn't carry around a heavy atomic clock to keep me on time for my next meeting, and I wouldn't use a cheap wristwatch to measure the speed of light. Different measurement methods have different characteristics and are therefore suited to different purposes. So do different assessments:

- Some are more accurate than others and will produce the same results every time. This characteristic is called *reliability*.
- Some reflect the intended learning more faithfully than others (e.g. a true/false multi-choice questionnaire reflects recall well, but doesn't reflect understanding so well). This characteristic is called *validity*.
- Some lend themselves to supporting learning (e.g. an observed performance followed by a debrief), but others do not. This characteristic is designated *educational impact*.
- Some are straightforward to implement, but others are difficult in terms of *cost, feasibility* or *acceptability*. (Who wants to volunteer as the assessment case for a novice surgeon?).

The key point here is that the purpose of the assessment determines the relative importance of the characteristics. For example, assessments that grant a license need to be reliable so that the learners, the institution(s) and the public can be assured that no one who is incompetent enters practice. On the other hand, regular assessments of an evolving procedural skill, such as suturing, might be designed mainly to support learning through the observations of an experienced practitioner who can provide useful feedback. In this situation, it may be less important that individual practitioners' judgments vary and reliability is limited.

The golden rule of assessment

Out of these two principles of measurement flows a simple rule for all assessors: choose or design an assessment process that is likely to measure the learning you're interested in, and has measurement characteristics consistent with the purpose of your assessment.

This may sound a very simple and obvious statement, but many problems with existing assessments stem from a failure to observe this rule.

The aim of the chapter is to apply this golden rule to the specific example of real-world practice. By providing educators with good strategies for measuring the highest levels of learning we can improve the quality and safety of care that patients receive from tomorrow's healthcare professionals. There is still a place for assessing the lower levels of cognitive learning and competence. Early in a learner's progression, both knowledge tests and relatively scripted behavioural assessments in controlled situations are valuable to help plan teaching and learning activites, to support learning, and to measure progress. But here is the important point: once the learners have moved beyond scripted performances and are beginning to participate in the workplace, what we are measuring is a different thing, and no amount of knowledge testing, competence assessment, or trait measurement will substitute for assessing real working practice or 'workplace-based assessment' (WBA).

Case study 18.1: St Mary's International Hospital

The board of St Mary's International Hospital has approached the hospital's multi-professional education team for help. There are not enough doctors to assess and treat the patients coming to the emergency department, and the human resources department can't find an effective way to attract them away from St Joseph's Hospital in the capital city. The university is willing to train experienced nurses, physiotheraptists and pharmacists as 'advanced practitioners' to do the work of a doctor. There are modules on anatomy, biochemistry, physiology, pathology, taking a patient history, undertaking a physical examination, ordering tests, and prescribing medications. Each module is assessed using an extensive knowledge examination and, where appropriate, a skills assessment.

St Paul's Hospital, in the neighbouring district, has started employing the graduates from this program to work alongside the doctors in the emergency department as part of the medical team. However, there is a problem. Patients and other staff don't think that the practitioners are ready for the job they are being asked to do. Some of the practioners themselves agree. Several of them have left their jobs within the first six months.

The board of St Mary's wants to employ advanced practitioners, too. But they're worried the practitioners won't stay if patients lack confidence in them and they feel unprepared for their role. They want the multi-professional assessment team to develop an assessment that will help the practioners to grow into the role, and will reassure other staff and the public that they can assess patients safely.

You are the assessment lead on the team. You have looked at the literature and discussed the problem with colleagues in other hospitals. You have concluded that you should use workplace-based assessment (WBA) to assess the practitioners in practice. This way, what is being assessed is representative of authentic clinical practice (validity), and the process will provide the opportunity for feedback (educational impact). You have been shown the assessment forms that the doctors use when they are assessing postgraduate trainees. There's a MultiSource Feedback form (MSF), a mini-Clinical Evaluation eXercise form (mini-CEX), a Case-Based Discussion form (CBD), and a Directly Observed Procedural Skill form (DOPS).

However, there is a hitch. Your colleague at St Peter's has tried this approach and says that neither the clinical educators nor the practitioners liked using WBA.

- The complexity of the cases and the pressure in the workplace are very variable. Practioners undergoing mini-CEX forms had complained that it was unfair to compare their performance on a difficult case, or under pressure, with their performance on a simple case with plenty of time.
- Practioners also felt that different clinical educators had different standards and different ways of doing things. Consequently, it seemed unfair to compare the judgment of one educator directly with the judgment of another. Perhaps the assessment said more about the educator than the performance.
- Sometimes the forms seemed to miss the point. For example, a practitioner might 'tick all the boxes' on an assessment, but the educator wouldn't want the practitioner to treat a member of their own family. Sometimes the reverse was true, and a good performance wouldn't tick all the boxes.
- Also, because they didn't want to disrupt the working relationship, educators almost always ticked the box that said 'excellent'. For their part, the practitioners found the assessments threatening, so they avoided difficult cases. This didn't help the practioners to develop.

The research you have read doesn't provide many answers to these problems, except to suggest that 20 or so separate observations are needed for each assessment to be reliable. You are caught between two stools. It seems that controlled assessments at the university aren't predicting the practioners' readiness for the workplace, but WBA (which should be the right approach) isn't working in practice. How will you apply the golden rule to help solve this problem?

First, let's look at some of the theory that will inform your decisions. Then we'll apply the principles we have reviewed to the assessment challenge above.

Assessment theory

The case study illustrates some common assessment problems at the interface between formal education and the workplace. It would be reasonable to summarise the problems raised by the case into three main issues, and the chapter will address each in turn:

- the relationship between formal academic assessments and workplace performance;
- the problem of performance variability in the workplace;
- the problems of subjectivity and authenticity in judgment-based assessment.

The relationship between formal academic assessments and workplace performance

> **Problem 1: why the university assessment doesn't work — the wrong kind of learning**
> * Only the right framework can define the right kind of learning.
> * Possessing the learning doesn't guarantee using it in practice.
> * Procedural learning is different from declarative learning.
> * Entrustable professional activities (EPAs) provide a promising synthetic framework for the workplace.

The university identified all of the learning required for the advanced practioners to be able to do the work of a doctor. The modules included both cognitive learning (e.g. physiology) and behavioural learning (e.g. undertaking a physical examination). Each module was carefully assessed using a method that provided a valid indication of the expected learning and gave reliable results. However, practioners who succeeded at university were not necessarily ready for practice. This is not just a problem for advanced practioners. Until recently, many universities have assessed healthcare learners' readiness for practice in exactly the same way, with very similar outcomes. How do we apply the golden rule to understand and solve this problem?

Learning frameworks

The golden rule says that the first step in planning any assessment is to define what learning you are measuring — so how do we do that? The focus here is not on *what learning* to choose, but rather about *how to approach* the problem of defining 'learning'. The kind of learning we choose will depend on the framework we apply. Learning is a complex domain; different frameworks conceive that domain in different ways and thus divide it up differently. Pangaro and ten Cate (2013, e1197) identify three types of frameworks: 'Analytic[al] frameworks deconstruct competence into individual pieces, to evaluate each separately. Synthetic frameworks attempt to view competence holistically, focusing evaluation on the performance of real-world activities. Developmental frameworks focus on stages of, or milestones in, the progression toward competence.' (It's probably worth adding that developmental frameworks are usually synthetic, so the intitial choice is between an analytical or synthetic framework.)

In the context of assessing and treating undifferentiated patients attending the emergency department (see case study 18.1), an analytical framework would attempt to list all of the learning that underpins performance. It might look something like Box 18.1.

By contrast, a synthetic framework views performance as a whole. It acknowledges complexity, but doesn't attempt to reduce it to its component parts. Epstein and Hundert (2002, p 226) capture this when they define competence as: 'the habitual and judicious use of communication, knowledge, technical skills, clinical reasoning, emotions, values, and reflection in daily practice for the benefit of the individuals and communities being served'.

The university has used an analytical framework to define the learning that underpins workplace practice. That framework has determined the structure of the whole curriculum, including the assessment strategy. Have they chosen the wrong type of framework?

The relationship between knowledge and performance

Miller's pyramid is one example of a learning framework. Consequently, it embraces certain assumptions about the nature of learning:
* it integrates the analytical and synthetic views of learning;
* it integrates cognitive and behavioural learning into one whole;
* it suggests that synthesis increases as learning progresses (a narrowing pyramid);
* it suggests that each new level builds on *and adds to* the learning of the level below (a building pyramid).

Miller (1990, p S63) put the last assumption in the following way:

> *… while it may be reasonable to assume that either action or performance implies achievement of the more basic elements of the triangle, measurement of the infrastructure (i.e., knowledge and competence) cannot be assumed to predict fully and with confidence the achievement of the more complex goals.*

Box 18.1: An analytic description of the learning required to assess and treat a patient

Core learning for the task

- Knowledge of, or ideally experience of, a wide range of clinical presentations, and the possible diagnoses, investigations and treatment options relevant to them
- Sufficient understanding of basic biological sciences in heath and disease to extrapolate from first principles where necessary
- The skills to gather clinical data (history-taking and examination), and to communicate with patients, carers and other members of the team
- The 'art' of bringing those elements together in a real and unique situation, using an inductive or deductive reasoning process to formulate and negotiate a diagnosis and a plan of management

Generic learning that is simultaneously employed in the task

- Prioritising time-management decisions
- Deciding how to interact with other team members (e.g. asking for help when appropriate)
- Inferring the personal beliefs and preferences of the patient to individualise the communication and management planning approach
- Weighing risk–benefit ratios, forecasting worst-case-scenario probabilities, and considering potential safety-nets

Reflective self-monitoring relevant to the task (questions the practitioner asks themselves)

- What is my level of uncertainty; is this safe?
- How do I feel about this person/this task? Is that affecting my performance?
- Do I have what it takes to undertake this task? grow into this new professional identity?
- What am I learning from this? Am I good enough? How can I improve?

If Miller is right, then he has identified the problem with the university assessment. Performance is built on knowledge and competence, but it is more than the sum of all of the knowledge and competence. So was Miller right; what does the evidence suggest?

To investigate the relationship between competence and performance, Rethans and colleagues (1991) arranged for 4 covert standardised patients to visit 36 general practitioners during normal surgery hours. The actors depicted four clinical problems and assessed the performance of the doctors they saw. The doctors were then taken to an assessment centre, where they saw the same problems represented and assessed in exactly the same way. The doctors' competence in the assessment centre was completely uncorrelated with their day-to-day practice. Clearly, actual practice depends on more than just competence. Most follow-up studies have shown similar or very low correlations. Cognitive tests are similarly poor at predicting actual performance (Ram et al., 1999).

Bruning and colleagues (1999) highlight a learning distinction made by cognitive psychologists. They describe what a learner knows (and can tell or show) as *declarative knowledge*, and what they do with that learning as *procedural knowledge*. Just like the study above, many experimental studies in cognitive psychology demonstrate that sound declarative learning doesn't necessarily lead to procedural learning.

In summary, knowledge and competence in controlled assessments don't predict real-world performance, even if those assessments test all of the formal learning that is required for the task. The next obvious question is: why not?

Declarative learning versus procedural learning

The occupational competency movement of the 1960s provided a clear critique of formal academic assessments in relation to workplace practice. In his seminal paper, McClelland (1973, p 7) wrote: '… testers have got to get out of their offices where they play endless word and paper-and-pencil games into the field … If you want to test who will be a good policeman, go find out what a policeman does'. McClelland's thesis was that Bloom's (1971) learning silos of knowledge, skills and attitudes did not add up to occupational competence. He went on to offer a reason why. In the workplace, learners must integrate these silos into a whole that is more than the sum of its parts. Furthermore, the integration is orchestrated through more generic traits and values. A 'competency' was an occupation-oriented unit of learning defined by the ability to undertake a real task in the real world. And, in the real world, each task is completely unique.

Donald Schön (1987) highlights the importance of case-uniqueness in professional practice. While, formal education often assumes that there are right and wrong solutions to a problem, real practice is full of situation-specific factors that the learner must 'handle' by making choices about manner, pace, priorities, certainty, safety-netting, etc. Schön (1987, p 6) calls these the: '… indeterminate zones of practice that have uncertainty, uniqueness and values conflicts. These indeterminate zones of practice elude the canons of technical rationality'.

In summary, the analytical framework chosen by the university is simply not the right way of viewing learning for practitioners. An analytical framework defines declarative learning outcomes — the parts. But the procedural learning required for practice is all about synthesis and application — building a case-unique whole that is more than the sum of the parts.

A synthetic framework for the workplace

The preceding sections have shown us why the university assessments don't work. To assess performance in the workplace, we need a synthetic framework, and we need to be in the workplace. So what synthetic frameworks can we draw on to focus our assessments?

Thirty years ago the answer would have been a competency-based framework. A 'competency' was understood to mean the ability to do a real task in the real world. Unfortunately, the value of the term competency has become eroded, because it carries at least four meanings in the education literature:

- competency as a unit of learning:
  - the ability to do a real-world task (see competency movement);
  - a personal trait;
- competency (competence) as a level of learning:
  - satisfactory in controlled representations of practice;
  - satisfactory at the 'minimum safe level'.

Into this confused context, ten Cate (2006) has provided a new term to recapture the essence of the competency movement. He argues that the best integrated measure of workplace learning is 'entrustability'. From this he derives a synthetic work-oriented unit of learning: the entrustable professional activity (EPA), which is defined as 'a unit of essential professional practice … for qualified professionals … that requires the integration of specific knowledge, skills and attitudes gained through training' (Chapter 20).

For example, a diagnostic EPA could be: 'Safely and efficiently assesses a patient presenting with chest pain such that the clinical educator does not need to re-assess the patient.' This represents an integration of many types of learning, around a purposeful and representative professional activity, to a specified level or standard. Chapter 20 provides a detailed description of EPAs, and practical guidance on how they can focus assessments in the workplace.

To summarise the learning from this section:

- The university assessments fail to predict workplace performance because they are built around the wrong framework. An analytical framework that is useful for academic curriculum design and delivery is not the right framework for focusing work-oriented assessments.

- The evidence suggests that knowledge and competence, even when exhaustively defined and tested, do not predict real workplace performance. In the language of cognitive psychology, declarative learning does not predict procedural learning.

- The occupational competency movement provides one of the reasons for this disconnect. In the workplace, a practitioner's main task is to synthesise and apply their learning to build a case-unique whole that is more than the sum of its parts.

- Miller's pyramid encapsulates the same idea. It indicates that some new learning must take place to move from knowledge and competence to actual workplace performance, and that this involves synthesis.

- Consequently, work-oriented assessments are best planned using synthetic frameworks that consider performance as a whole.

The problem of performance variability in the workplace

Problem 2: dealing with workplace variability — sample widely and focus on reflection in action
- Many situational, personal and case-related factors affect performance in the real world.
- Controlled assessment methods don't predict workplace performance, however.
- Therefore, sample challenges widely to assess how learners respond to unplanned factors.
- Focus on reflection-in-action to assess meaningful variations in practice.

In case study 18.1, practioners from St Peter's had complained about the unfairness of comparing assessments on difficult cases seen under pressure with assessments on easy cases seen at leisure. It's easy to understand their concern; all assessments aspire to being systematic, fair and defensible, but case variation doesn't seem fair. This is not just a problem for the case study; it's one of the complaints many clinical educators and learners perceive with WBA. So how do we apply the golden rule to understand and solve this problem?

Factors affecting workplace performance

The Cambridge model (Rethans et al., 2002) shows how performance assessment is different from competence assessment, because performance is affected by a whole range of personal and situational factors (see Fig. 18.3).

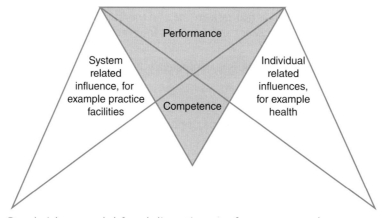

Figure 18.3: The Cambridge model for delineating performance and competence
Source: Rethans, J., Norcini, J. J., et al. (2002), The relationship between competence and performance: implications for assessing practice performance. Medical Education, 36, 901–909. doi:10.1046/j.1365-2923.2002.01316.x

However, in some ways, this understates the variability challenge in WBA. As we learned in the last section on the occupational competency movement, in the real world the learner brings together knowledge, skills, traits and values in a unique way by applying them to a unique situation. From any conventional perspective, this looks like a measurement nightmare!

The assessment literature is therefore full of attempts to control variation in workplace assessments in an attempt to yield more reliabile results. We will review these attempts briefly, and then explain why it is better to exploit variation rather than control it.

Controlled assessment methods and performance

Because workplace performance is affected by so many factors, some educators have wanted to move back down Miller's pyramid. The argument goes like this: if performance is built on lower levels of learning, then lower levels of learning should predict performance, and they are much easier to assess.

Recall can be measured with a high level of validity and reliability; either the learner remembers the answer or they do not. Higher levels of cognition are more difficult to test, but a range of formats aim to do so by requiring learners to apply general learning to solve specific problems. At the behavioural level we can assess controlled representations of practice using 'standardised' challenges. The Objective Structured Clinical Examination (OSCE), for example, employs this approach.

However, we have already seen from the work of Rethans and colleagues (1991), and Ram and colleagues (1999), that learners who do well in knowledge tests or in controlled representations of practice are no more likely to perform well in the workplace than those who do badly. Consequently, even the most reliable controlled assessments have no validity for the workplace.

A second option is to move the focus from content-dependent learning to content-independent traits. Traits were mentioned in the introduction. The argument goes like this: workplace performance varies from task to task, but traits are relatively stable. Perhaps traits predict future performance better than past performance does. To illustrate: who would you want to do your neurosurgical operation, an experienced surgeon who is also a concert pianist but whose last patient died, or a junior surgical trainee who can't even ride a bicycle but whose last patient survived? Are you more persuaded by their relatively stable traits, or by their most recent performance?

The first formal attempts to assess traits in medical education were directed at clinical reasoning. Arthur Elstein and colleagues assumed that clinical reasoning would function as a trait enabling some gifted clinicians to solve clinical problems more efficiently and safely than others, whatever the case. That is not, however, what they found. Reflecting on their seminal work 'Medical problem-solving: an analysis of clinical reasoning', Arthur Elstein and colleagues (1990, p 14) wrote:

> The research team that assembled for the Medical Inquiry Project believed it could contribute ... by identifying the strategies and intellectual operations — not contents — that separated expert from less expert physicians ... The finding of case specificity clearly challenged both assumptions. Clinicians who employed a perfectly successful strategy in one case often had difficulty in the next.

Most evaluations of trait-based assessment show this same highly variable performance. This suggests either that stable traits do not exist, or that traits are expressed in such a variable fashion that they are unmeasurable in practice. Van der Vleuten and colleagues (2010, p 705) write:

> The trait approach was a logical extension of psychometric theory, which had its origins in personality research. However, empirical research in education contradicted the tenets of the personality trait approach, revealing that the expected stability across content / tasks / items was very low at best.

In a review of the experimental psychology literature, Regehr and Norman (1996) make the point that learning mechanisms do not work in compartments, but rather by linking new learning to existing learning through content-linking. In other words, learners do not learn 'medical problem-solving' or 'communication skills'; rather they learn lots of medicine and lots of communicating, and they construct idiosyncratic connections to help them retrieve and generalise. Consequently, their performance in any given situation is determined by content and not by traits.

In summary, attempts to circumvent the variability of the workplace by focusing on the assessment of underpinning learning or relatively stable traits have both failed. If we can't circumvent variability, we must work with its advantages. That is the subject of the following sections.

Sampling how learners respond to unplanned factors

All assessment data show is that some learners perform better in nearly every challenge (ability), some learners perform consistently better on particular types of challenge (aptitude), and then there is lots of problem-to-problem performance variation (case-specificity). This means that a learner's performance in a single problem predicts their performance in the whole 'universe' of possible problems poorly, but a learner's performances in a sample of problems provide a better prediction (see Fig. 18.4). Crossley and colleagues (2002) describe how we can measure the variance in real assessment data to model how large a sample is required for a reasonable representation of the universe of performance.

All this is true of both controlled and workplace assessments, and is one of the reasons for sampling in WBA. However, there is also another reason. As Rethans and colleagues (1991) showed, controlled assessments fail to predict real workplace performance even when exactly the same cases are represented in exactly the same way. What can it be that affects learners' performance in the workplace if not the 'hard' variables of the case, such as the clinical problem? The answer is that the learners respond with variable success to unplanned personal and situational factors, such as time pressure, relational compatibility, complexity, uncertainty, cognitive anchoring, etc. These are the factors that Rethans and colleagues (2002) held responsible for the competence-performance gap, and summarised in the Cambridge model.

The 'controlled' approach regards these as sources of measurement error, but there is another way of viewing them. Croskerry and colleagues (2013) summarise the literature on medical error, and conclude that these are the very cognitive and affective factors that threaten safety in real-world practice. By that view,

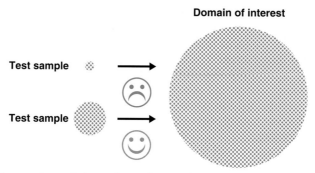

Figure 18.4: A visual illustration of the value of sampling

Source: reproduced with permission from Cees van der Vleuten.

we should be much less interested in how to control them out of assessments, and much more interested in how learners respond to them. Indeed, how learners handle these real-world factors should be the very focus of our assessment.

This is the second reason for sampling widely. It allows us to observe how the learner responds to more of the unplanned factors that critically influence real workplace performance and are missing from controlled assessments. To see the learner respond to these unplanned factors, however, we must do more than sample widely. We must also re-focus our assessments to examine the learner's reflection-in-action.

Focusing on meaningful variations in practice through reflection-in-action

Controlled assessment, like formal education, usually assumes that there are right and wrong solutions to a problem. In the workplace, however, this is far too simplistic. Sometimes there are several acceptable diagnostic formulations or management plans, and there are usually many reasonable pathways to reach them, depending on the nuances of the case. These are the situation-specific factors that define professional practice, according to Donald Schön (1983).

Together, these give rise to meaningful performance variation within a case. This means that we should examine not only the conclusions of the learner's case assessment, but also how the learner navigated the case. From an assessment perspective, this re-focusing offers three potential benefits:

- *Validity* — if we are concerned with how learners apply their learning to a unique situation in the real world, we should focus our assessment on their decision-making processes rather than just its outcomes.

- *Reliability* — the learner who can comment wisely on what they were doing and why is more likely to perform well in the future than a learner who just 'got it right this time'.

- *Educational impact* — the learner will develop by considering how and why they made the choices that they did.

Learner self-monitoring is a complex domain. Schön distinguishes between *reflection-on-action* (outside of the activity) and *reflection-in-action* (during the activity). Reflection-in-action requires continuous self-monitoring. This is how a practitioner moves between a relatively unconscious state of 'knowing-in-action' (*heuristic practice* or *system 1 reasoning*) and a more conscious state of options-appraisal. Eva and Regehr (2005) suggest that this is how practitioners deal with unplanned variables, and that makes it our focus of interest. So how do we go about assessing reflection-in-action?

First, we cannot rely on the many methods that focus on reflection-on-action. It appears that the two types of reflection are different things. Eva and Regehr (2011) studied university students taking a general knowledge test. They found that while self-assessment by reflection-on-action predicted performance poorly, measures of reflection-in-action (deferring an answer, delay in answering/deferring, and answer-specific confidence) predicted performance accurately. Therefore, portfolios, reflection templates and self-assessment templates are not the answer.

Secondly, we must understand that this is not a stable trait. Attempts to measure constructs related to reflection-in-action show context-specificity, leading Eva and Regehr (2005, p S52) to conclude: '…we must conclude from the metacognitive and self-efficacy literatures that self-assessment is not a stable skill, but one that that will vary by content, context and perspective'.

To tap into reflection-in-action, we must discover from learners how and why they did what they did. This is a central idea in the debrief literature. Rudolph and colleagues (2006) describe the clinical educator as a 'cognitive detective'. In their approach, for example, the educator makes an objective observation about a learner's performance ('I noticed that ...') followed by a genuinely curious question attempting to elicit the learner's reasoning ('Can you tell me why?'). Debrief techniques are the way to elicit reflection-in-action in WBA.

Unfortunately, most existing WBA lacks the required two-step observation-discussion process required. Even when observation is followed by discussion — for example, in mini-CEX — the discussion stage typically features evaluative feedback rather than analytical debrief. Conversely, those methods that promote analysis — for example, CBD — lack performance observation. As a result, the discussion tends to focus on relative certainties rather than the 'indeterminate zones of practice'.

But things are improving. One new version of the CBD, from the UK Royal College of Emergency Medicine (www.rcem.ac.uk), instructs the assessor to: 'Use the case discussion to probe the thinking behind the trainee's assessment and management; if there were any difficulties, try to understand why.' The assessor then uses that information to judge whether the learner: 'did not provide a safe evaluation', 'provided a safe evaluation', or 'understands the principles soundly enough to assess any similar case accurately'. This is using the learner's reflection-in-action to extrapolate the judgment beyond the index case. It provides a helpful indication of where WBA needs to develop in the future.

To summarise the learning from this section:
- Workplace performance is influenced by situational factors, personal factors and case-uniqueness.
- The traditional approach of trying to control such variation in the interests of reliability cannot solve the problem; controlled (competence) assessments fail to predict real workplace performance, and stable traits either don't exist or are unmeasurable.
- However, the way in which learners respond to situational factors, personal factors and case-uniqueness are at the heart of safety in healthcare, and tend to be lacking from controlled assessments.
- Therefore, rather than controlling them, it is better to sample them widely and to focus the assessment on the learner's reflection-in-action.
- Few existing WBA instruments yet do this well, because they have evolved from the outcome-based controlled assessment paradigm, but better examples are emerging.

The problems of subjectivity and authenticity in judgment-based assessment

> Problem 3: dealing with assessor subjectivity — optimise and unpack expert judgment
> - There is no substitute for judgment at the performance-assessment level.
> - Sample assessor judgment widely, as a window onto meaningfully different approaches.
> - Use clinicians' heuristics to optimise judgment.
> - Unpack clinicians heuristics to activate learning.
> - Allow for non-ordinal judgments.

In case study 18.1, practioners from St Peter's had complained about the unfairness of comparing assessments from different educators. Different educators appeared to have different standards — some easy to please (doves) and some hard to please (hawks). To make matters worse, each had a slightly different way of doing things, so that an approach to a clinical problem that one educator praised, another educator might criticise. Learners were afraid of being assessed as 'borderline' or 'poor', and tended to hide their weaknesses (fear of failure).

For their part, the educators didn't have great confidence in the judgment-based assessment process. In order to maintain their relationship with the learner, they felt a strong inclination to assess the learner as 'good' or 'excellent' (failure to fail). Sometimes the form seemed to miss a key element, so that an authentic performance didn't tick the form's boxes, and vice versa. These two concerns made the assessments seem futile to the educators, so they tended not to take them seriously.

It's easy to understand their concern; all assessments aspire to be systematic, fair and defensible, but relying on subjective assessor judgment doesn't seem fair. This is not just a problem for the case study; it's another one of the complaints many clinical educators and learners perceive with WBA. Furthermore, the data confirms that assessors do vary when judgment is involved (Wilkinson at al., 2008). Outside the workplace in formal educational settings, script concordance tests (SCTs) confirm that experienced clinicians take different approaches to the same problem, even in a short, written vignette. What is true of a written vignette, or an OSCE station, is even more true in real-world practice. Subjectivity is evident in workplace assessment scores.

How do we apply the golden rule to understand and solve this problem?

The need for judgment

When assessing procedural learning in the workplace, it is difficult to pre-define the complex integration and application decisions learners will make. Consequently it's difficult to pre-define particular behaviours as appropriate or inappropriate. This leaves assessors having to judge the appropriateness of what they see. These judgments are subjective, and vary from assessor to assessor.

One approach to this problem is to attempt to limit the assessors' judgment. There are two basic approaches to this: one is to constrain them to objective decisions on the assessment form, and the other is to train them. What does the evidence reveal about limiting assessor judgment?

Outside of the workplace, the traditional OSCE format determines a checklist of appropriate actions to be assessed objectively (e.g. 'the learner introduced him/herself'; 'the learner exposed the abdomen fully'). This is one reason for the OSCE's name (*Objective* Structured Clinical Examination); some authors call this 'objectification'.

To investigate objectification, Glenn Regehr and colleagues (1998) evaluated three parallel assessment formats in an OSCE examination: 1) an objective checklist; 2) a checklist alongside an overall subjective judgment; and 3) a subjective judgment alone. The third format was the most reliable. Their result is completely counter-intuitive. It means that assessors agreed better about whether they had just seen a good performance (subjective 'gut feeling') than about whether or not the learner had performed certain observable actions (objective reporting). This remarkable observation turns out to be true of all judgment-based assessment. The most likely explanation shouldn't come as any surprise after the previous section. In complex tasks, the whole is more than the sum of the parts. It is the success with which 'standard' behaviours are individualised to a particular situation that separates a good performance from a poor one.

Along with many others, Ringsted and colleagues (2003) call for more assessor training, suggesting that it will improve the reliability of judgment-based assessment. However, empirical studies of assessor training by Holmboe and colleagues (2004) and Cook and colleagues (2008) demonstrate a minimal or insignificant impact on assessor reliability even when theoretically informed training interventions are used.

In summary, measures designed to address assessor subjectivity by limiting or controlling it have proved to have a paradoxical effect of worsening consistency and fairness, rather than improving it. The following sections consider another approach to the problem, which dignifies rather than eradicates the expertise of the subjective assessor.

Judgment as a window onto meaningfully different approaches

With assessor variation, as with case variation, sampling improves 'average' representativeness. The view of one assessor about whether a learner is performing adequately may differ from the view of another assessor, but the views of 10 assessors are much less likely to differ from the views of a different 10 assessors. For this reason alone, sampling improves representativeness. But, as with case variation, there is another reason to sample widely.

From a theoretical perspective, Gingerich and colleagues (2014) describe three distinct ways of viewing assessors in relation to their differences: trainable (applying criteria wrongly), fallible (fundamentally poor at judgment), or meaningfully different (legitimate experienced-based experts). Schuwirth and van der Vleuten (2006, p 298) encourage us to seriously consider the third of these:

> We dismiss variance between observers as error because we start from the assumption that the universe is homogenous, where in fact the more logical conclusion would have been that the universe is more variant … We tend to extend the training of examiners to make sure all examiners are the same. We may

even eliminate outliers from the examiner role. Thus, we use a convergent strategy aimed at establishing homogeneity to assess whether a candidate is ready to work in a completely untrained, diverse and somewhat chaotic context.

If assessors are meaningfully different, then more judgments provide a wider sample of meaningfully different perspectives. These can help the learner understand the reasoning that underpins variations in practice, and the values, standards and evaluations that underpin professional differences.

To learn from professional variation, however, we must do more than sample widely. We must also re-design our assessments to show learners what their assessors are thinking.

Judgment in the language of the clinician

All traditional WBA assessment forms include some kind of ordinal response scale, enabling the clinical educator to register their judgment. (There may be a single summary scale, or multiple scales covering several domains of learning and performance.) An ordinal scale is a scale where any given point is more (or better) than a point below it, and less (or worse) than a point above it. There is a long research history of manipulating these scales to see whether it affects the reliability of judgments. However, in essence, no manipulation of the number of scale points, the scale design (visual analogue or ordinal categories), or the presence or absence of numbers has been shown to make any meaningful difference.

However, the scales must be anchored to an idea to give them meaning. In general, the scales have been anchored to merit (variations of 'poor', 'satisfactory' and 'excellent') or to educationally-based expectations ('below', 'at' or 'above' expectations for a given stage of learning). Using these types of anchors, typical WBA evaluations have found that 12 to 25 assessments are required to rank learners reliably, depending on the learning being assessed, the working context, the type of assessor, etc.

Marriott and colleagues (2010) evaluated a scale that was deliberately anchored to a different kind of idea. The new scale was anchored to the the learner's readiness for independent practice. Assessors were asked to register their judgment on a scale from 'unable to practise even under supervision' to 'competent to practise unsupervised'. The underpinning idea is very similar to ten Cate's (2006) notion of entrustability. The assessment data showed that the scale broke the usual rules of WBA reliability. It provided reliable rankings using just two observations per trainee. These high reliability figures were not achieved by controlling case variation, or by objectification, or by extensive assessor training. The strategy was to align the judgment format with a clinician's heuristic instead of providing clinicians with an educator's heuristic. Clinicians make entrustment judgments about learners in the workplace every day.

It appears that this is not just a surgical or technical skill phenomenon. Crossley and colleagues (2011), using a similar design, found that three mini-CEX observations and three CBDs were sufficient to rank the UK cohort of physician trainees reliably, compared with more than double that number of observations using conventional scales. A number of further studies have demonstrated similar dramatic increases in reliability.

Strikingly, then, it appears that WBA hasn't been hampered by assessor subjectivity. Assessors make remarkably consistent expert judgments about learners. The design of the forms has been masking that good judgment. The right solution is to improve the scales in order to tap into and optimise judgment.

Unpacking judgment to activate learning

Reliability is one thing, but wouldn't it be even better to unpack the implicit cognitive frameworks that clinical educators seem to share with one another, and make them explicit so that learners could also visualise progress? This is an example of the third kind of framework described by Pangaro and ten Cate (2013): a developmental framework. Crossley (2014, p 685) describes this as providing a learner with a roadmap: 'It must describe the pathway or pathways of development toward being a [practitioner] in ways that are both authentic to qualified [practitioners] and meaningful to learners.'

There are already examples in medical education. Pangaro (1999) was well ahead of his time when he developed the Reporter-Interpreter-Manager-Educator (RIME) framework, and the Accreditation Council for Graduate Medical Education (www.acgme.org) has described assessment milestones for doctors. However, the value of these maps or milestones depends on the level of granularity. The RIME framework and the ACGME milestones represent the extremes of coarseness and granularity, respectively. It is likely that learners also need frameworks of medium granularity to help them to see the next immediate step in their development.

In a converging development, other educators have borrowed the concept of 'word pictures' from the general education literature. The UK Royal College of General Practitioners (www.rcgp.org) describes learning progression using 'a series of word pictures that describe positive behaviours that doctors display in practice'. These word pictures typically depict learning as a developmental progression. For example, evolving communication and consultation skills are mapped as:

- Level 1: Develops a relationship with the patient, which works, but is focused on the problem rather than the patient;
- Level 2: Explores and responds to the patient's agenda, health beliefs and preferences. Elicits psychological and social information to place the patient's problem in context;
- Level 3: Incorporates the patient's perspective and context when negotiating the management plan.

Still others have recommended abandoning 'scaled' judgments altogether. For example, Govaerts and van der Vleuten (2013, p 1164) argue for entirely narrative assessment outcomes that reflect the traditions of qualitative research:

> *Basic principles of rigour specific to qualitative research have been established, and they can and should be used to determine validity in interpretivist assessment approaches. If used properly, these strategies generate the trustworthy evidence that is needed to develop the validity argument ... allowing for in-depth and a meaningful information about professional competence.*

They invite clinical educators to provide rich, unconstrained descriptions of performance that include an explicit articulation of the assessor's own criteria and values. This is surely the most extreme example of unpacking the assessor's rationale and judgment.

Somewhere between roadmaps/word pictures and pure narrative, Regehr and colleagues (2012) have investigated 'standardised narratives' constructed from interviews with experienced clinical educators. They have demonstrated that assessors can make reliable assessments using holistic narratives, even though they disagree about how to interpret learners' assessment scores. This raises the possibility that narrative scales might be used to capture some of the richness of free narrative, but preserve some of the utility of ordinal 'scoring'.

The place of non-ordinal judgments

So far we have considered what we might do to improve ordinal assessment scales in WBA. But is a linear ordinal scale the right way to represent everything we need to assess? It seems appropriate for most learning, as the learner attains successive stages in a reasonably predictable sequence. But some things that have a substantial impact on performance don't develop in this way, and it doesn't make sense to assess them using a linear ordinal scale.

Although traits are difficult to measure, clincians and educators continue to believe that some relatively stable characteristics have an important bearing on performance. The most widespread is probably professionalism. The vast majority of doctors whose licence to practise is called into question do not have a learning problem, it is their professional values and resulting conduct that are dysfunctional. To see whether professionalism is a stable characteristic, Papadakis and colleagues (2005) examined the student records of doctors coming before US state disciplinary boards. A student record noting 'serious irresponsibility', 'serious diminished capacity for self-improvement', 'impaired relationships' or 'anxiety/insecurity/nervousness' was associated with at least a threefold increase in disciplinary board action years later.

So, if professionalism is important and relatively stable over time, how do we assess it? Some of the professionalism scales draw on the personality literature, and assume that the ideal balance point lies somewhere between two extremes. Gauger and colleagues (2005, p 479) observed: 'It became evident that residents could "go too far" in some professional behaviours. Therefore, although a 7-point continuous ordinal scale forms the framework, a score of 7 does not necessarily indicate the ideal.' For example, their scale for 'responsibility' ranges from: 1 ('Complete lack of accountability; actively avoids responsibility'), to 7 ('So obsessed with performance that other aspects of their life are damaged').

Other characteristics relevant to workplace performance are likely to have a categorical rather than an ordinal nature (you've got it or you haven't). Obvious examples are social communication problems (autistic spectrum disorders), and personality disorders. Most clinical educators can bear witness to the serious impact that these can have on healthcare learners, the patients they treat, and the colleagues they work with. From time to time there are high-profile examples of healthcare professionals with personality disorders causing serious harm to their patients. Perhaps the best-known is Dr Harold Shipman from the United Kingdom. Should we assess these, and if so how? David Powis (2015, p 252) presents evidence from healthcare selection that the applicants in the 'best of the best' category are more likely to exhibit both social communication difficulties and obsessional personality traits. He suggests we should move from 'selecting in' to 'selecting out' in our selection assessments:

Perhaps it is time for a radical change in emphasis. Instead of endeavouring to differentiate among the top ranks of a pool of outstandingly qualified applicants, the selection effort might be better focused on identifying those potentially unsuitable in terms of their non-academic personal qualities to ensure they do not gain entry.

Finally, there is a group of learners and practitioners for whom neither learning progression nor stable characteristic is the right frame of reference for assessment. Learners who have been functioning adequately, but whose performance is deteriorating, may be identified as 'struggling learners' or 'struggling professionals'. They need a diagnostic assessment. Deterioration can be the result of situational factors like team dysfunction, social factors such as relationship difficulties or substance abuse, or cognitive factors such as intellectual deterioration or increased cognitive anchoring in older practitioners. Consequently, the UK General Medical Council (www.gmc-uk.org) guidance for assessing doctors in difficulty states: 'Remember poor performance is a "symptom and not a diagnosis" and it is essential to explore the underlying cause or causes.'

The point is this — not everything that influences workplace performance fits the developmental learning model. Bond and Fox (2001) point out that a key step in fundamental measurement is that the scale should reflect the characteristic. In the context of WBA, we must allow for the judgment of non-ordinal characteristics in our WBA designs. To help, here are four suggested categories of characteristics that matter in assessment:

- *distinctive ability* — a relatively stable 'helpful' trait, such as IQ;
- *dysfunction* — a relatively stable 'limiting' trait, such as social communication difficulty;
- *development* — an evolving learning domain;
- *deterioration* — a regressing learning domain.

The great majority of assessment should focus on developmental learning, and aligns well with ordinal judgment scales. However, it is a mistake to use ordinal scales for everything. If you need to assess for relatively stable characteristics, or investigate deterioration in a learner or practitioner, be prepared to use different formats that align with the characteristic.

To summarise the learning from this section:

- Judgment-based assessment is influenced by variable leniency (hawk versus dove), judgment preferences, and unaccountable residual variation.

- The traditional approach of trying to improve reliability by limiting assessor judgment through objectification or training often has the paradoxical effect of making reliability worse.

- However, differences between assessors are usually meaningful and can provide learners with a window onto the reasoning that underpins professional judgment, and the standards and values that underpin professional differences.

- Therefore, rather than controlling judgments, it is better to sample them widely and, where possible, to unpack the heuristics that clinical educators use to reach their judgments. This unpacking covers a spectrum from coarse developmental scales to open narrative judgments.

- While ordinal developmental scales are the best way to capture many learning assessments, WBA will sometimes need to focus on characteristics that don't fit this structure. To assess relatively stable charactertistics, or making diagnostic assessments of learners or practitioners in difficulty, we will require different approaches.

Applying theory to practice

Case study 18.1 (continued): Resolution

As assessment lead of the hospital multidisciplinary education team, it is your job to develop an assessment that will help the practioners to grow into the role, and reassure other staff, and the public, that the practioners can assess patients safely. Before reading this chapter, you were caught between two stools. The university assessments seemed reliable and fair, and they assessed all of the learning on the advanced practitioner training program (which should be the learning required for practice), but even the most successful graduates didn't appear or feel ready for practice. On the other hand, WBA, which seems to represent real practice, seems fraught with unreliability, and isn't liked by either the learners of the clinical educators.

Now that you have read the chapter, you think you know the way forward.

You understand that the university assessments were appropriate for assessing knowledge and competence in controlled situations (or declarative learning), and that these are important prerequisites for practice. However, real day-to-day practice rarely depends on whether a learner does or doesn't know something; it centres on how the learner integrates and applies their learning to solve unique problems (procedural learning). The evidence shows that declarative learning assessments don't predict procedural learning. So the university assessments are not wrong, they just don't measure the right thing. Controlled assessments and WBA are complementary, but WBA is definitely what you need to help with the hospital's current problem.

If you are going to plan a WBA strategy, the golden rule tells you that the first step is to define what you are going to measure. You now know that the framework you choose determines the kind of learning you will define. Because you are interested in the top of Miller's pyramid — what the learners can actually do as practitioners — you know that you will need a synthetic framework. You can forget breaking the learning up into knowledge, skills and attitudes. And you have seen enough examples of competency-based learning curricula to know that no two people mean the same thing by a 'competency'. Instead, you decide to define the learning in terms of FPAs, and you turn to Chapter 20 to discover more. You discover that the clinical educators in the emergency department can easily list eight essential clinical problems that the practitioners need to be able to manage without a supervisor's oversight.

You decide to start with mini-CEX observed assessments and CBDs based on these eight problems. You know from St Peter's that the practioners will be worried about unfairness, because some cases are more difficult than others, and some shifts are more pressured than others. You now know how you are going to handle that. You are not going to try to control it so that everyone has the same unhurried average case. Instead, you are going to explain to the clinical educators and the practitioners that you want the assessments to focus on how the practitioners handle the unpredictable variations in the real flow of work. Consequently, you want them to undertake as many assessments in as many different circumstances as possible. You include a box asking the educator to record whether this was an easy, average or difficult case, and a slow, average or busy shift, to make sure that the practitioners are getting the full range.

Looking at the existing mini-CEX and CBD forms, you feel that the assessment focuses entirely on whether the learner did the right thing. That is important, but you are convinced that it is equally important to discuss why the learner did what they did. The golden rule reminds you to design the form around its intended purpose/s, and you want this to be assessment *as* learning. So you re-design the form with instructions guiding both parties to discuss reflection-in-action, and including a template for recording this discussion. You can see that the clinical educators will need some training in preparation for their work assessing the practitioners, and you make a note to ask the simulation lead to train them in debriefing skills.

You also know from St Peter's that the assessors will struggle to use the forms. Sometimes the form will seem to 'miss the point', because a good performance won't tick all of the boxes on the form, and vice versa. They will also be strongly inclined to choose the 'good' and 'excellent' points on the judgment scale that these two forms use, to avoid difficult conversations. This will undermine the value of the feedback, and the ability of the assessment to detect problems. Because different clinical educators will take different positions on this, you design the strategy so that each learner is assessed by each of the educators.

You also re-design the forms. You realise that it doesn't work to constrain the assessors to objective observations. You have understood that experienced assessors can make excellent judgments if you choose a scale that is meaningful to them. You also like the idea of a developmental scale that will help the practioners to see where they are now and what they are trying to achieve next. You consider the RIME scale, but you think a bit more detail is needed. You convene a meeting with the clinical educators, and agree a 'roadmap' set of scales that describe the developmental benchmarks and the expected levels of supervision for the domains in the existing mini-CEX (medical interviewing, physical examination, communication, clinical judgment, professionalism and organisation). For example, the benchmarks for medical interviewing are:

1. *Novice historian:* The learner doesn't yet know or ask the components of a full 'generalist' history. (The educator will need to prompt or remind the learner about several aspects of a patient's story and will need to ask the patient some questions themselves.)
2. *Knows the questions:* The learner knows and asks the components of a full 'generalist' history. (The educator will be confident that all of the questions have been asked, but will need to help the learner to summarise and interpret what they have heard, and will need to clarify some points with the patient themselves.)
3. *Dependable history:* The learner clarifies, checks, sequences and follows leads, so that the presented history includes all of the information a doctor would need to make a clinical assessment of the patient. (The educator won't need to go back and retake the history, but will be confident to recommend the next steps — examination, investigations, management — based on the information provided, with a review later.)
4. *Diagnostic approach:* The learner gathers and organises the information purposefully, seeking to confirm or refute differential diagnoses, and to judge the impact on and views of the patient with a view to planning management. (The educator is confident that the next stage of management could commence, and need not review the patients unless asked.)

You recognise that some practioners will manifest problems that are not captured on these judgment scales and may not appear in the debrief notes. From experience with other learners, you know that resilience, relationships, taking responsibility, and insight are likely to be key areas of difficulty. These don't seem to fit a developmental pattern, so you simply add boxes asking the assessor to highlight concerns in any of these areas, stating that this will not prejudice the learner's progress, but will prompt a more diagnostic process to look into the concern.

You realise that you have developed an assessment system from first principles, and you feel satisfied that you have succeeded in applying the golden rule to your particular situation.

Potential directions for evaluation and research

Trait measurement

Currently, most educators doubt the existence of stable traits because of case-specificity. Nevertheless, personality traits and other distinctive strengths and limitations are commonly used for describing personal differences. Several investigators remain committed to the measurement of traits, either by careful revision of taxonomy (in search of a 'true' psychological taxonomy), or by developing better measures, or by more careful analysis of existing data, like Wimmers and Fung (2008). This fundamental question about the nature of learning remains an important field of psychometric research.

Reflection-in-action as an assessment focus

This chapter has argued that reflection-in-action is a crucial activity for learners and practitioners. At the same time, Eva and Regeher (2011) have shown that markers of reflection-in-action can predict performance. Furthermore Ginsburg and colleagues (2015) and others have drawn attention to how assessors 'read between the lines', and Hyde and colleagues (2014) have shown that assessors pay particular attention to 'fluency' as an indicator of attainment and 'disregard for error' as an indicator of concern. Taken together, these suggest that experienced assessors may well be focusing on inferred reflection-in-action rather than observed performance to make their judgments. This deserves further investigation.

Identifying and acting on indicators of dysfunction

The importance of learner and practitioner dysfunction in healthcare was clear even before Papadakis and colleagues (2005) demonstrated the persistence of early learner dysfunction. Even so, only a handful of investigators have shown an interest in the identification, diagnosis and remediation of these learners, and most of the work is relatively light on theory. Given the profound consequences of learner and practitioner dysfunction in healthcare, this field deserves more attention.

PRACTIAL TIPS FROM EXPERT PRACTITIONERS

Competence and performance

'As director of a postgraduate paediatric training program, I couldn't believe how often the very best trainees — the ones whom I would choose to care for my children — struggled with their exams and OSCEs. Meanwhile, trainees who had little depth or feel for clinical work were passing the assessments first time. I began to see that being competent doesn't make a trainee an effective clinician in the real world. That's why we began to develop "real-world" assessments based in the workplace.'

The limits of objectification

'Early in my career in assessment I developed a chronic and disabling illness. My rheumatologist was excellent. He negotiated management plans treating me as an equal. Then, one day, when I was feeling particularly defeated, he just said: "this is what we're going to do" — no negotiation at all! But I was so relieved because, at that moment, I needed someone else to take control. It occurred to me that his behaviour was completely inconsistent, but his care of me was utterly consistent. He would have failed the structured assessments I was designing. That's when I understood that the whole is more than the sum of the parts.'

Aligning judgment scales with clinicians' heuristics

'We implemented mini-CEX assessments for trainee anaesthetists eight years ago. We evaluated the scores and discovered that we needed more than 60 observations for reliability. The trainers were resistant and privately told me that they struggled to score a familiar trainee anywhere below "good", and the trainees moaned that assessors were not being frank with them. Two years ago we changed the scale to chart the trainees' progression towards autonomy. Now they say that it feels authentic and leads to meaningful conversations. What's more, just 7 observations give as much reliability as 60 did before. In retrospect it was stupid of us to take experienced clinician assessors and then ask them to use a scale that was bound to hide their judgments.'

Allowing for non-ordinal judgments

'I run a nurse education program. I was continually frustrated by mentors who told me that they had concerns about a student nurse — but their assessments were all "satisfactory". Then one of them pointed out that they were being completely honest. The students were satisfactory in terms of the assessment questions (basic care skills, record-keeping, etc.). That wasn't what my colleagues were worried about. They were concerned about personal resilience, "reading between the lines", and relationships. We started asking directly about "concerns" as well as learning progress and competencies, and now I can tell you that clinical supervisors have absolutely no difficulty raising concerns; all we had to do was ask!'

Conclusion

The fundamental principle for every assessment remains: choose or design an assessment process that is likely to measure the learning you are interested in, and has measurement characteristics consistent with the purpose of your assessment.

The workplace is currently the only setting in which it is possible to assess the end-point of all clinical learning: real work in the real world that affects real people — the pinnacle of Miller's pyramid.

Assessment in the workplace is not a cheap and chaotic version of controlled assessment. It is a different activity with entirely different affordances, and it is important to work with those affordances to make the most of workplace-based assessment.

- Sample cases widely because each is unique.
- Focus on reflection-in-action, not just 'hard' outcomes.
- Use (and try to unpack) the shared heuristics of clinician judges.
- Sample clinician assessors widely, because their differences are as meaningful as their similarities.
- Encourage assessors to highlight other observations that are not part of their developmental judgment.

Further reading

Introduction: assessment characteristics

Crossley, J., Humphris, G., & Jolly, B. (2002). Assessing health professionals. *Medical Education, 36*(9), 800–804.

Streiner, D., & Norman, G. (1995). *Health measurement scales: A practical guide to their development and use* (2nd ed.). New York: Oxford University Press.

Defining a focus: EPAs

ten Cate, O. (2013). Nuts and bolts of entrustable professional activities. *Journal of Graduate Medical Education, 5*(1), 157–158.

Accessing reflection-in-action: debrief methods

Sawyer, T., Eppich, W., Brett-Fleegler, M., et al. (2016). More than one way to debrief: A critical review of healthcare simulation debriefing methods. *Simulation in Healthcare, 11*, 209–217.

Judgment in workplace assessment

Crossley, J., & Jolly, B. (2012). Making sense of work-based assessment: Ask the right questions, in the right way, about the right things, of the right people. *Medical Education, 46*(1), 28–37.

References

Bloom, B. (1971). *Taxonomy of educational objectives: The classification of educational goals — Handbook 1: Cognitive domain.* New York: David Mackay.

Bond, T. G., & Fox, C. M. (2001). *Applying the Rasch model: Fundamental measurement in the human sciences.* Mahwah, NJ: Lawrence Erlbaum Associates.

Bruning, R. H., Schraw, G. J., & Ronning, R. R. (1999). *Cognitive psychology and instruction.* Upper Saddle River, NJ: Prentice-Hall.

Cook, D., Dupras, D., Beckman, T., et al. (2008). Effect of rater training on reliability and accuracy of mini-CEX scores: A randomized, controlled trial. *Journal of General Internal Medicine, 24*(1), 74–79.

Croskerry, P., Singhal, G., & Mamede, S. (2013). Cognitive debiasing 1: Origins of bias and theory of debiasing. *BMJ Quality and Safety, 22*, ii58–ii64.

Crossley, J., Davies, H., Humphris, G., et al. (2002). Generalisability: A key to unlock professional assessment. *Medical Education, 36*(10), 972–978.

Crossley, J., Johnson, G., Booth, J., et al. (2011). Good questions, good answers: Construct alignment improves the performance of workplace-based assessment scales. *Medical Education, 45*(6), 560–569.

Crossley, J. G. M. (2014). Addressing learner disorientation: Give them a roadmap. *Medical Teacher, 36*(8), 685–691.

Elstein, A., Shulman, L., & Sprafka, S. (1990). Medical problem-solving — A 10-year retrospective. *Evaluation and the Health Professions, 13*(1), 5–36.

Epstein, R. M., & Hundert, E. M. (2002). Defining and assessing professional competence. *Journal of the American Medical Association, 287*(2), 226–235.

Eva, K. W., & Regehr, G. (2005). Self-assessment in the health professions: A reformulation and research agenda. *Academic Medicine, 80*(10 Suppl.), S46–S54.

Eva, K. W., & Regehr, G. (2011). Exploring the divergence between self-assessment and self-monitoring. *Advances in Health Sciences Education: Theory and Practice, 16*(3), 311–329.

Gauger, P., Gruppen, L., Minter, R., et al. (2005). Initial use of a novel instrument to measure professionalism in surgical residents. *American Journal of Surgery, 189*, 479–487.

Gingerich, A., Kogan, J., Yeates, P., et al. (2014). Seeing the 'black box' differently: Assessor cognition from three research perspectives. *Medical Education, 48*(11), 1055–1068.

Ginsburg, S., Regehr, G., Lingard, L., et al. (2015). Reading between the lines: Faculty interpretations of narrative evaluation comments. *Medical Education, 49*(3), 296–306.

Govaerts, M., & van der Vleuten, C. P. (2013). Validity in work-based assessment: Expanding our horizons. *Medical Education, 47*(12), 1164–1174.

Holmboe, E., Hawkins, R., & Huot, S. (2004). Effects of training in direct observation of medical residents' clinical competence: A randomised trial. *Annals of Internal Medicine, 140*(11), 874–881.

Hyde, C., Lefroy, J., Gay, S., et al. (2014). A clarification study of internal scales clinicians use to assess undergraduate medical students. An oral presentation to ProReg Solutions conference, 27–29 April, Ottawa, Canada. Ottawa 2014 Conference Abstracts, 45.

McClelland, D. C. (1973). Testing for competence rather than for 'intelligence'. *The American Psychologist, 28*(1), 1–14.

Marriott, J., Purdie, H., Crossley, J., et al. (2010). Evaluation of procedure-based assessment (PBA) for assessing trainees' procedural skills in the operating theatre. *British Journal of Surgery, 98*(3), 450–457.

Miller, G. E. (1990). The assessment of clinical skills/competence/performance. *Academic Medicine, 65*(9 Suppl.), S63–S67.

Pangaro, L. (1999). A new vocabulary and other innovations for improving descriptive in-training evaluations. *Academic Medicine, 74*(11), 1203–1207.

Pangaro, L., & ten Cate, O. (2013). Frameworks for learner assessment in medicine: AMEE Guide No. 78. *Medical Teacher, 35*(6), e1197–e1210.

Papadakis, M. A., Teherani, A., Banach, M. A., et al. (2005). Disciplinary action by medical boards and prior behavior in medical school. *New England Journal of Medicine, 353*(25), 2673–2682.

Powis, D. (2015). Selecting medical students: An unresolved challenge. *Medical Teacher*, 37(3), 252–260.

Ram, P., van der Vleuten, C., Rethans, J. J., et al. (1999). Assessment in general practice: The predictive value of written knowledge tests and a multiple-station examination for actual medical performance in daily practice. *Medical Education*, 33(3), 197–203.

Regehr, G., Ginsburg, S., Herold, J., et al. (2012). Using 'standardised narratives' to explore new ways to represent faculty opinions of resident performance. *Academic Medicine*, 87, 419–427.

Regehr, G., MacRae, H., Reznick, R. K., et al. (1998). Comparing the psychometric properties of checklists and global rating scales for assessing performance on an OSCE-format examination. *Academic Medicine*, 73(9), 993–997.

Regehr, G., & Norman, G. (1996). Issues in cognitive psychology: Implications for professional education. *Academic Medicine*, 71(9), 988–1001.

Rethans, J., Norcini, J., Baron-Maldonado, M., et al. (2002). The relationship between competence and performance: Implications for assessing practice performance. *Medical Education*, 36(10), 901–909.

Rethans, J., Sturmans, F., Drop, R., et al. (1991). Does competence of general practitioners predict their performance? Comparison between examination setting and actual practice. *British Medical Journal*, 303(6814), 1377–1380.

Ringsted, C., Ostergaard, D., Ravn, L., et al. (2003). A feasibility study comparing checklists and global rating forms to assess resident performance in clinical skills. *Medical Teacher*, 25(6), 654–658.

Rudolph, J. W., Simon, R., Dufresne, R. L., et al. (2006). There's no such thing as 'nonjudgmental' debriefing: A theory and method for debriefing with good judgment. *Simulation in Healthcare*, 1(1), 49–55.

Schön, D. (1983). *The reflective practitioner: How professionals think in action*. New York: Basic Books.

Schön, D. (1987). *Educating the reflective practitioner*. San Francisco: Jossey-Bass.

Schuwirth, L. W., & van der Vleuten, C. P. (2006). A plea for new psychometric models in educational assessment. *Medical Education*, 40(4), 296–300.

ten Cate, O. (2006). Trust, competence, and the supervisor's role in postgraduate training. *British Medical Journal*, 333(7571), 748–751.

van der Vleuten, C. P., Schuwirth, L. W., Scheele, F., et al. (2010). The assessment of professional competence: Building blocks for theory development. *Best Practice and Research. Clinical Obstetrics and Gynaecology*, 24(6), 703–719.

Wilkinson, J., Crossley, J., Wragg, A., et al. (2008). Implementing workplace assessment across the medical specialities in the United Kingdon. *Medical Education*, 42(4), 364–373.

Wimmers, P. F., & Fung, C. C. (2008). The impact of case specificity and generalisable skills on clinical performance: A correlated traits-correlated methods approach. *Medical Education*, 42(6), 580–588.

Yule, S., Flin, R., Maran, N., et al. (2008). Surgeons' nontechnical skills in the operating room: Reliability testing of the NOTSS behavior rating system. *World Journal of Surgery*, 32(4), 548–556.

19

Ensuring assessment builds capacity for future clinical practice
Sustainable assessment in action

Rola Ajjawi and David Boud

Introduction

Workplace-based assessments (WBAs) are commonplace in health professions education. They were 'originally intended to inform learning and development by structuring effective observation-based feedback' (Barrett et al., 2017, p 138), but now play an important role in certification of learning. Several drivers for changes in WBAs within health professions education exist, including increased demand for accountability, changing needs of an increasingly diverse and aging population, concerns about health care quality, and calls for improved supervision and assessment of medical trainees (Holmboe et al., 2010).

In this chapter, we explore the challenges of WBAs for learners, for those designing assessments and those who implement them. Research suggests that WBAs are often ineffective in driving intended learning (Barrett et al., 2017) and so we argue that they need to be reconceptualised more productively as not only indicating *achievement* of particular competencies but also in *promoting trainees' capabilities* to judge their work for themselves. That is, in addition to contributing to formative and summative assessment, WBAs must exhibit characteristics of sustainable assessment through developing trainees' capabilities beyond the immediate task (Boud and Soler, 2016). Following this repositioning of WBAs we discuss how sustainable assessment can be operationalised in clinically-based assessment tasks. In doing so we examine the implications for the main parties involved. We use the term clinical educator to encompass clinical supervisor and preceptor (used differently across the health professions) to highlight the clinical and educational roles that need to be balanced. We also use the term trainee to encompass students and learners across the undergraduate to postgraduate continuum.

Establishing the problem

Despite trainees and educators acknowledging the potential learning value of WBAs, two systematic reviews concluded that WBAs do not result in demonstrable changes to practice (Miller & Archer, 2010; Overeem et al., 2007). Hence, although the stakeholders involved in these key educational interventions recognise they should be valuable for learning, their potential is not being realised. Two problems which face workplace assessments may be contributing to this effect. Firstly, they have considerable limitations due to the pressured circumstances under which they are conducted relative to the environments in which they are developed and tested. Secondly, if they were improved to be more practically useful, their psychometric value may be diminished. For example, a strong focus on reliability of the assessment approach (where all components are standardised including what questions may be asked) might compromise its authenticity and validity. While many of the issues related to the former are addressed in Chapters 18 and 20 they are pertinent for us to discuss here as they also influence assessments that seek to have an impact on learning in the longer term.

The challenges of work-based assessments in clinical environments

Clinical placements are widespread in undergraduate and postgraduate training programs and workplace assessments are commonly used in them. But, there are considerable challenges to effective learning and assessment within these environments. These challenges can be categorised based on whether they are related to the trainee, the clinical educator, the clinical environment or the tools themselves. First, trainees may be novices and not have the necessary skills or orientation to cues which enable them to regulate their own learning; this can also apply to experienced trainees in an unfamiliar setting. Trainees also report feeling like a burden to their busy supervisors who are first and foremost clinicians caring for patients and this may inhibit them actively utilising supervisors for learning (Urquhart et al., 2014). They may also feel conflicted about disclosing their 'weaknesses' or revealing uncertainties as their educators are also their assessors who will judge them, and potentially employ them. Many conceive of assessment and feedback as something done *to* them, rather than *with* them (Boud & Molloy, 2013). Further, trainees describe feeling significant anxiety when being observed, especially when expectations are unclear (LaDonna et al., 2017).

Second, clinical educators act as gatekeepers to learning opportunities within the workplace through facilitating patient encounters and involving trainees in particular clinical activities. They may struggle to balance their competing roles in clinical service, education and assessment (Sholl et al., 2017). Trying to balance patient care and education usually favours patient care with education activities being skipped or shortened (Fokkema et al., 2013). The demands of summative assessment are often imposed on clinical educators from the university or postgraduate training schemes, where they become perceived as acts of compliance rather than opportunities to embrace. They are often time-poor and do not necessarily understand (or agree with) the espoused purposes and processes of assessment and their material objects; for example, forms, scales and checklists (Massie & Ali, 2016). Clinical educators may not have the necessary training or educational capacity to optimise learning for their learners. They report a tension between supporting and promoting trainee development and providing summative judgments, a phenomenon Watling (2016) calls a 'tenuous balancing act'. Feedback within a summative assessment context, even 'low-stakes', can be distorted reducing its uptake by trainees, yet summative assessment is the dominant culture of medical education (Harrison et al., 2016). Clinical educators are likely also not to have been involved in the development of the curriculum and so may have limited knowledge of the location of the placement in relation to other elements of the curriculum and thus have limited awareness of what the trainee should be gaining from the placement. Despite the presence of competency frameworks generated by regulatory bodies, these standards are commonly interpreted and applied idiosyncratically in rater judgments (Govaerts et al., 2013).

Third, an affordance of the workplace is the opportunistic, informal learning that cannot be planned for or scripted. However, within a culture that values psychometric reliability at the cost of authenticity and contextual sensitivity, this can also be viewed as a drawback for assessment when learning experiences cannot be standardised. Learners are scheduled into rotations with multiple assessors and teams, leading to fragmentation of the learning experience and the time for assessors to make informed judgments about the safety and quality of a trainee's competence. The lack of continuity in both patient experience and time with educators for trainees in the current health professions education system makes longitudinal assessment and feedback very difficult (Holmboe et al., 2011). This fragmentation sets up a situation where each assessment task is seen as an isolated summative episode which compromises a developmental focus on trainees' subsequent work and professional identity formation. There is no collective memory beyond the trainee of what the trainee has been doing or has learned to date. Furthermore, when educators are not scheduled to work with the trainee again, this fragmentation leads to an inability to close feedback loops through identifying the effects on learners and seeing how agreed upon action plans are progressed.

Fourth, WBA tools have been implemented in a variety of ways with unintended consequences including a 'tick-box' approach to completion to merely fulfill requirements leading to concerns around relevance/ authenticity (Barrett et al., 2017; Bindal et al., 2011). The 'ticking boxes' approach, to meet requirements, is theorised to occur when there is a lack of alignment between the assessment processes and those of daily work (Elmholdt et al., 2016). Completing assessment documentation for both the educators and trainees becomes a form of compliance. These forms are often designed to meet university and course-specific requirements; a single educator may need to familiarise themselves with multiple documents and requirements for a limited number of trainee encounters. Further, they may drive unintended learning, for example in medical education the use of checklists to assess empathy and clinical communication, although reliable, seem to have detrimental value by driving comprehensiveness (and mindlessness) rather than expertise in skill development (Monrouxe & Sweeney, 2010), thus subverting the original intent of these assessment tasks. Typically, WBAs are designed to privilege the educator's judgment of performance, over and above peers' or self-judgments, thus setting up a system where trainees are dependent on their educators for information about progress.

In summary, trainees may have a very uneven experience with WBAs. There may be little facilitation of their learning, with pro forma assessments undertaken by personnel who have little commitment to or knowledge of trainees' wider trajectory but to whom the trainee is beholden for access to opportunities and information about progress. This creates considerable challenges for the design of workplace assessments and for trainees in managing their own learning.

While in an ideal world clinical placements may be refined to address some of their many limitations (e.g. length of rotation, continuity of supervisory relationships, skills of clinical educators, resources/dedicated time for education etc.), we have to start with a realistic view of what can be done given existing constraints with clinical cultures as they presently exist. The focus in this chapter is on assessment and the activities that surround it. We present ideas on what can be done to ensure WBAs make a positive contribution not only to making judgments on the capability of the learner to perform in the clinical environment, but also enabling the learner to navigate this environment and learn effectively from opportunities that present.

What do assessments need to do?

Trainees may gain considerable exposure to clinical situations, but this may not in itself equip them to 1) be effective practitioners within them, and 2) build their capacity to learn in clinical environments and assess for themselves what they need to learn and whether they have learned it?

What then are the needs of learning and assessment in clinical contexts? We suggest that they are:

1. the immediate need to learn and practice effectively and safely;
2. the need to demonstrate competence in order to move to the next stage;
3. the need to build capacity to continue to learn and practice when confronted with new challenges.

Assessment needs to contribute on all three fronts, but the first and second have been privileged in the literature and the workplace. Of course, the needs of the immediate task and competence standard should be addressed, but if that is all, then clinical experiences are not preparing a future practitioner. This is why a focus on sustainable assessment is necessary.

Sustainable assessment

Sustainable assessment builds on the notion of assessment *for* learning in that while it focuses on learning for the present learning task it extends it through preparing learners to meet their own future learning needs (Boud, 2000). Sustainable assessment focuses on building the capacity of trainees to make *evaluative judgments* of their own work and that of others through engagement in a variety of activities so that they could be more effective learners and meet the requirements of work beyond the point of graduation (Boud & Soler, 2016). This was proposed as a distinct purpose of assessment, as summative assessment typically meets the needs of other stakeholders (i.e. for grade generation and competence certification) and formative assessment is commonly limited to tasks within a particular course or course unit. Sustainable assessment design holds potential for promoting lifelong learning and is a high priority for professional programs such as those in health. Refocusing on the role of the trainee as active, engaged and responsible for driving learning from assessment can overcome the limitations of the fragmentation described above.

Refocusing assessment on developing trainees' evaluative judgments (Tai et al., 2017) puts them back in the driver's seat. Rather than trainees being passive recipients of tasks done to them (e.g. receiving feedback comments), sustainable assessment is mutually constructed between learners and educators (e.g. trainees engaging in self- and peer-assessment and feedback dialogue). Sustainable assessment cannot be limited to purely assessment tasks, but must permeate pedagogical preparation where trainees participate in opportunities to make judgments about the quality of their own work and that of others. It includes 'the capacity to evaluate evidence, appraise situations and circumstances astutely, to draw sound conclusions and act in accordance with this analysis' (Boud, 2007, p 19). Boud (2007) proposed five key elements of developing judgment for long-term learning from the perspective of the trainee as:

1. identifying oneself as an active learner;
2. identifying one's own level of knowledge and the gaps in this;
3. practising testing and judging;
4. developing these skills over time;
5. embodying reflexivity and commitment.

The focus on developing evaluative judgment is intimately wrapped up with lifelong learning; a cornerstone of professional practice. Campbell and colleagues (2010) describe a shift in the landscape from traditional continuing professional development (CPD) (e.g. listening to a speaker over a sponsored dinner) to competency-based CPD. This new form of CPD is premised on a set of competencies that depend on the trainee having agency and self-regulation of learning to undertake regular scans of the environment; to obtain peer observation and feedback; and to use informed self-assessment (Campbell et al., 2010). Hence, a focus on sustainable assessment throughout the continuum of education is necessary for safe and effective practice recasting 'the role of assessment as a professional expectation and obligation' (Campbell et al., 2010, p 657).

Becoming and being for the trainee

Developing evaluative judgment is about more that the acquisition of knowledge and skills (Ajjawi et al., 2018). Although these are important, making evaluative judgments is by necessity a contextual and disciplinary act. In learning to make evaluative judgments, trainees learn what disciplinary notions of quality looks like – for example, learning what constitutes a 'good' physical examination of a knee in physiotherapy. Making evaluative judgments and articulating these also enables trainees to take on the language and thinking of the discipline/profession and in so doing develop as a professional (Ajjawi et al., 2018). Thus, focusing on trainees' evaluative judgment introduces a dimension to assessment that brings in notions of professional identity. Becoming a professional involves the development of professional identities that are shaped (and reshaped) by multiple personal and contextual factors including the curriculum. Assessment is critical to this as it shapes professionals through providing powerful messages to trainees about what is important and what they should be learning. Through assessment tasks, trainees judge their own work in relation to necessary standards and criteria and plot their path to becoming a professional. Through suitable WBAs in particular they learn what it means to *be* a professional.

Assessment for learning in the workplace using a three-stage model

Workplaces present particular challenges for learning, not least because they are set up to fulfil the purposes of work with learning necessarily positioned as a secondary consideration. Nevertheless, we know a great deal about work environments that are more or less conducive to learning. One of the most important observations to come from research in this area is that suitable work environments create continual challenges that prompt learning and they allow enough agency on the part of the learner to both tackle the substantive work problems they face and to consciously learn from them (Boud & Rooney, 2014). In other words, there is sufficient space for trainees to engage in their own sustainable assessment and build their repertoire of good practice.

The key feature is preparing trainees to learn from assessments, especially when they are conducted in multiple contexts with multiple practitioners who may have no awareness of the wider context of trainees and their studies. The lack of educator continuity in clinical settings means that trainees have to manage more of the process than is commonly assumed, particular feedback aspects and educators need to accommodate this. There are various strategies to assist trainees in this process. One of the most useful is the development of learning plans negotiated with supervisors, organised by trainees and shared with educators/assessors (Anderson et al., 1996). These are drafted by the trainees in the light of the requirements of the course and form a plan for what they will do in a particular placement, what evidence they will need to demonstrate they have met their learning outcomes and how the process will be judged. In the undergraduate, or pre-service training context, this plan is approved by both a university representative and whoever has overall responsibility for their placement within the organisation. The plan enables trainees to collect evidence of meeting outcomes and prompts them to collect inputs from the various clinicians they will work with. These and any associated learning portfolios can provide the vehicle through which sustainable assessment can be managed (Clarke & Boud, 2016).

To help trainees manage their ongoing learning in placements, it can also be useful to introduce them to a model of learning from experience so they have some kind of conceptual framework through which to view the learning aspects of their work and thus facilitate learning at work. This complements the many different kinds of discipline-specific clinical frameworks they will be introduced to and utilise. The former is learning-focused, the latter are patient-focused. Here we apply Boud and Walker's (1990) model for promoting learning from experience to a sustainable assessment agenda (see Fig. 19.1). This model of learning from experience takes into account the social, cultural and material contexts of the workplace and considers the individual and relational (patient–trainee–educator) dimensions of the assessment task as composed of three stages: 1) activities and events prior to the assessment event; 2) during the assessement event; and 3) after the assessment event. These stages and the actions suggested within each act as prompts to clinical educators and trainees for optimising learning from assessment.

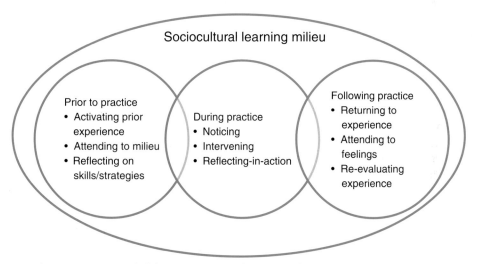

Figure 19.1: A three-stage model for promoting learning from experience
Source: Adapted from Boud, D., & Walker, D. (1990). Making the most of experience. Studies in Continuing Education, 12(2), 61–80.

Stage 1: Prior to the assessment event

The first stage is preparation for the assessment event (whether it be formative or summative). This is about activating prior experiences in order to build on existing knowledge and capabilities and to establish relations between acts of assessment; that is, enabling opportunities for feedback to be acted on, and preparing for clinical engagements. For example, if an aspect of practice such as eliciting a history is to be observed by the clinical educator as part of a formative mid-placement assessment, then the trainee might reflect on their relevant experiences to date with patients. In relation to the trainees, what feedback comments about their own capacity in history elicitation and establishing rapport might they bring to bear on this? They might reflect on their level of confidence, emotions, skills and experiences; plus personal learning goals and previously agreed-on relevant action plans. Trainees need to engage with the standards expected of them and upon which the assessment task will be judged in order to prepare for the assessment event. This might involve reading the expected learning outcomes and standards stipulated for the placement, considering which descriptor level are they aiming for. The trainee might also reflect on how familiar they are with the particular rules, expectations, demands of the assessment task itself and the context for action. For example, is there a checklist? What does it look like? Is there a time component? Who should initiate the assessment, choose the patient, check the patient's availability? How, where, when, for how long and using which 'model' might feedback be discussed? These expectations need to be discussed with the particular educator either at the beginning of the placement and/or prior to the assessment task itself. Trainees may wish to mentally rehearse the kinds of greetings they will use and the kinds of question they may wish to cover.

The clinical educator might also reflect on their knowledge of the trainee and experiences with and expectations around the assessment task. They also need to consider how much scaffolding the trainee needs in preparation for the assessment; for example, signposting the assessment criteria and rubrics. The educator may need to make time available in advance to discuss the expected standards given the trainee's level of experience, years of study, type and timing of the placement and their personal learning goals in order to develop shared goals, as well as attuning to the trainee's emotions or anxiety. This helping of trainees to unpack standards and quality criteria is necessary for developing evaluative judgment.

Stage 2: During the assessment event

The second stage of the model focuses on the assessment event itself. Three key elements here are noticing, intervening and reflecting in action. Assessment in the clinical workplace is important because it is an authentic opportunity for trainees to try on and practice their future professional roles. The milieu takes into account the physical spaces (e.g. consulting area, noise, interruptions); the materials (e.g. exercise equipment, monitoring devices, chairs, beds) and the social (e.g. interactions with individuals present including patients, their families, peers, colleagues, other health professionals). The learning milieu offers rich learning opportunities for trainees where they learn much of the hidden and unspoken rules, values and cultures. For example, trainees might learn how to talk with professionals from other disciplines through observing how the team interacts during a ward round. During the assessment task, the trainee might notice and pay attention to the assessor's and patient's responses and then intervene accordingly. For example, the trainee would actively listen to the answer a patient gives and so modify the next question accordingly. They may notice their assessor's and patient's facial experessions, intellectual and emotional responses. Reflection-in-action 'describes the process of working with, noticing and intervening to interpret events and effects of one's interventions' (Boud & Edwards, 1999, p 177). This has been equated to metacognition (Eraut, 2004). The extent to which there is time during the assessment for this will vary, but having this notion available can prompt reflexivity.

During this time the educator is also noticing through observing the trainee's actions, and interpreting the trainee's and patient's intellectual and emotional responses. The educator is constantly having to balance the interests of the patient with giving the trainee enough space, independence and autonomy to do and be the 'professional' demanded by the assessment task and its inherent rules/practices. If there is a question of patient safety being compromised the educator might intercede and stop the assessment task, and in some cases, such as in the emergency department or operating theatre, the educator may deem it necessary to step in and perform the task that forms the basis of assessment.

Stage 3: Following the assessment event

The third stage focuses on activities that occur after the assessment event either in the workplace or elsewhere once the placement is completed. Reflection-on-action following the assessment event is crucial for learning through recognising feelings generated, abstracting knowledge and developing action plans. Three key elements of this stage are: return to the experience, attending to feelings and re-evaluation of the experience. Trainees need to reflect on their performance in relation to the assessment criteria and be prepared emotionally and cognitively to engage in feedback dialogue relevant to the shared learning goals and any emergent issues or teaching moments. They may consider the following questions: What do they need to follow up on, how and with whom? How can they best prepare for their next encounter?

Immediately following an assessment event, educators might give the trainee opportunities to reflect on the experience. This space is also important to reflect on emotions and enable stress levels to drop. Observation of practice by seniors may be stressful for a trainee even in supposedly 'low-stakes' (formative) assessment events. The educator might prompt trainees to mentally revisit the experience – 'the what happened' – paying attention to their feelings. The educator should invite trainees to self-evaluate their performance in relation to the criteria, the outcomes for the patient and their own learning goals prior to having a feedback conversation. Feedback dialogue focusing on standards and criteria and the enactment of the trainee enables re-evaluation of the assessment event. Feedback comments might particularly be oriented towards gaps in the trainees' evaluative judgment; that is, ways in which the trainee misinterprets the qualities of their own performance. These discussions should further help to refine and build the trainee's conceptions of quality and standards for a particular task, within a particular social, cultural and material context. This could be extended further through considering aspects of quality given different dimensions of practice (e.g. different patient or setting). The educator might then engage the trainee in co-constructing action plans to address re-negotiated learning goals.

Implications of the model — learning from assessment

Many existing practices associated with WBAs may be modified or reconceptualised in order to meet the sustainable assessment purpose. Our intent in presenting the model is to link learning from experience with sustainable assessment. The emphasis is on how to shift the assessment from being solely a unilateral judgment by the educator on the trainee to one from which trainees can learn to make better judgments of their own performance on subsequent occasions. Evaluative judgment may be developed 'by providing direct authentic evaluative experience for learners' (Sadler, 1989, p 119); that is, involving them in making specific judgments about the work they have undertaken. The model divides each assessment event into three stages with particular prompts. Stage 1 urges consideration on how to prepare and equip trainees to learn from WBAs. Educators may utilise templates upon which to develop shared learning plans with prompts for discussing assessment criteria, learning goals and expectations. Three-way learning contracts are an ideal vehicle for documenting learning programmatically with opportunities for shared dialogue and understanding between the university mentor/clinical academic, the clinical educator and the trainee.

The activities that may form Stage 2 are diverse and not only rely on summative assessment tools applied formatively. Instead, opportunities for peer-review may be introduced. For example, trainees may be encouraged to work with a colleague or near-peer, to observe their performance with a patient and then to engage in feedback. They may be encouraged to view exemplars of practice through video or of their educator's practice and to discuss their evaluative judgments in relation to quality and competency frameworks.

Lately, there has been much attention dedicated to Stage 3 with the one-way information equated with feedback. Extensive critique of this transmission approach to feedback, highlights its limitations within a sustainable assessment agenda (Boud & Molloy, 2013). Instead, we advocate that trainees are prompted to qualitatively self-evaluate against the criteria and that feedback dialogue should be focused towards gaps in evaluative judgments. This dialogue becomes an opportunity for learners to calibrate their evaluative judgments of practice against an external source of feedback. What matters here isn't that they guess the grade or mark for each criteria but that they can articulate why a particular grade might be justified. Trainees can be invited to seek feedback about specific aspects of their performance to shape the dialogue in relation to their goals and needs but also those identified by the educator. Feedback that develops trainees' evaluative capacity should foster active engagement alongside an orientation towards seeking feedback (Boud & Molloy, 2013).

Designing sustainable assessments

What might be becoming apparent from the discussion so far, is that in order to refocus WBAs to develop trainees' evaluative judgment, their application needs to be purposeful, participatory and developmental. There are no recipes to inform this, but we do offer educational principles and their justification that might help educators and trainees to work towards a sustainable assessment agenda.

Characteristics to recognise if assessment is to be sustainable

Clearly any given assessment task must be appropriate for the subject matter, context, level and learning outcomes being pursued and feedback processes to be used. The design of assessment tasks and feedback activities is well covered elsewhere (see 'Online resources' section at the end of the chapter). But what particular features must we consider to ensure sustainable assessment requirements are met and trainees can develop their evaluative judgment? Six features are considered (see Practical strategies 19.1).

> **Practical strategies 19.1** Six features for the design of sustainable assessment
> - An active role for the trainee
> - Opportunities for clarification/dialogue
> - Assessment is oriented to subsequent action
> - Outputs of assessment decisions can be used
> - Trainees are equipped to learn from the assessment
> - A strong educational alliance is established

An active role for the trainee

Trainees need to be positioned so that they do not merely subject themselves to the judgments of others, but play an active role in managing the process and deciding what actions they should take.

- Trainee is asked for their learning goals.

- Trainee is asked to identify what they would like to have comments on.

- Trainee can add categories on which they wished to be judged.

- Trainees make their own assessment prior to that of assessor.

Much of the current research into assessment practices including those in the clinical setting highlight that trainees, particularly undergraduate ones, tend to take a passive role in WBAs. This sets up reliance on the educator to create learning and assessment opportunities. If trainees are to become independent, self-regulators they need to be increasingly able to judge the quality of their own work and to seek feedback from others to help them to calibrate these judgments. This by necessity requires an active approach from trainees.

Preliminary research across three countries, has identified that trainee engagement with feedback was enhanced by assessment cultures which promoted trainees' agency, by the provision of authentic and relevant assessment, and by appropriate scaffolding to aid the interpretation of feedback (Harrison et al., 2016). This research begins to highlight how through engaging learners in choice and agency in the context of assessment they become more receptive to feedback information. One possible explanatory mechanism we offer is the control-value theory which posits that if learners perceive they have control over the situation they are more likely to reframe the experience as positive and to see value in it (Pekrun, 2006). Asking trainees to elaborate their learning goals and identify which aspects they would like feedback about can give them some sense of control. Further, if a certain number of assessment events must occur within a rotation, then inviting trainees to drive forward when and where or to engage in a conversation about how and with whom, can give trainees more agency.

Opportunities for clarification/dialogue

A key element of having an active role in assessment is to be engaged with what counts as good work and clarifying expectations about goals, standards and criteria and being able to relate these to their own practice.

- Trainees' work is seen by educators and trainees have multiple opportunities in different contexts to dialogue with educators and other clinical staff about what constitutes good practice.

- Trainees can clarify with assessors what issues they identified and how they relate to expected standards.

Dialogue is crucial for establishing shared understanding. The language of standards may be difficult for novices to interpret because they are expressions of complex, integrative knowledge and practical know-how (Hager, 2000). The act of reading standards documents itself necessitates interpretation and negotiation of meaning based on the lenses or frames of reference the reader brings to the text and the relevant social, cultural and historical milieu. The trainee and educator must reach a shared understanding of the expected standard for any assessment event and for the placement overall if feedback interactions are to make sense. In addition, this shared understanding of standards then forms the context from which learning goals may be generated and future practice planned.

Trainees and educators are likely to have different goals for a particular assessment event which need to be uncovered and negotiated into a shared set of goals to frame dialogic feedback conversations (Farrell et al., 2017). Our model above highlights how goals should be continuously and iteratively explored, reassessed and re-negotiated; a finding supported by the research of Farrell and colleagues into goal-oriented feedback in the clinical workplace. By seeking out learners' frames of reference, their goals and action plans, the dialogue repositions the learner in the centre of the feedback interaction without giving the learner absolute control of the discussion content. Trainees' credibility judgments of their educators in the clinical environment influence their immediate and long-term behaviours such as feedback avoidance; for example, if they perceive that their educator doesn't have their interests at heart they tend to limit personal disclosure (Telio et al., 2016).

Assessment is oriented to subsequent action

Assessments should be driven by the need for each assessed task to contribute to ongoing learning and thus lead to new actions on the part of the trainee. Trainees need to know how to utilise the outcomes and feedback from the current assessment both in what they do next and in their longer-term learning plans. It helps then if trainees have an ongoing plan for what they aim to get out of any given placement which is continually revised as problems arise and opportunities present themselves. For any given act of assessment an action plan should be expected of the trainee which identifies what they need to do in the future and what they need to access to improve their performance.

Outputs of assessment decisions can be used

While some assessment activities later in a placement may be designed as summative only, the majority are oriented towards learning and reporting should follow this purpose.

- Trainees are not merely rated or graded but provided with information they can act on.
- Comments provided go beyond those necessary to justify a grade or classification to focus on desired behaviour or exemplars of good practice.

We cannot escape the fact that there are summative requirements that educators and trainees must comply with. How these requirements can be discharged while optimising learning is the challenge here. Both educators and trainees need to reconceptualise assessment so that developing evaluative judgments is a key purpose. This means that comments provided go beyond completing documentation for the institution to focus on desired behaviour or exemplars of good practice. Through improving a trainee's evaluative judgment, final summative decisions should not come as a surprise.

Trainees are equipped to learn from the assessment

Judgment itself is dialogic: it involves a conversation between what is observed and what are the appropriate standards to be applied in a given situation. People learn to make better judgments by making judgments and getting information about whether they are doing so effectively. This should prompt us to encourage trainees to judge their own performance and receive comments that enable them to refine their own judgment. This is not a matter of telling trainees what they did or didn't do, but eliciting from them their understanding of their performance and what they need to notice about it.

- Attention is given to helping trainees to elicit what are appropriate standards and criteria and how they are meeting them, it is not assumed that they know what these are from the start.
- Assessment is part of a plan which the trainee manages in order to navigate their placement activities and outcomes.

Engaging trainees in peer-assessment or encouraging them to work with colleagues who are more senior but closer to them on the trajectory or other health professionals, expands trainees' repertoires of practice (Blank et al., 2013; Tai et al., 2016). These opportunities may be maximised by utilising the model above.

A strong educational alliance is established

A key aspect of sustainable assessment is enhancing trainees' engagement and agency to seek feedback, develop goals and action plans, monitor progress and to drive assessment events. This can only occur within supportive clinical environments which are safe for learning. Clinical educators are in a position of power and authority in relation to the trainee, by virtue of seniority but also as they are often assessors too. However, perceptions of power can be softened within an interaction through the careful use of language, verbal and non-verbal communication; for example, always introducing trainees and patients and not referring to either in the third person when they are present (Rees, Ajjawi, & Monrouxe, 2013). Educators can set-up a learning culture through discussing expectations at the start of a placement, encouraging and modelling open dialogue, and inviting learner goals and self-evaluation. This dialogic approach fits with the proposition that for feedback information to be effectively utilised by trainees they must see their educators as engaged in an educational alliance, because it shows interest in the trainee as a person (Farrell et al., 2017). A strong educational alliance is where there are clear shared goals, shared action plans alongside trust and authenticity in the trainee–educator relationship (Telio et al., 2015). Within a strong educational alliance where trainees are given choice, and are engaged and respected as human beings, they might overcome their hesitations (or views that they are burdensome) and see their role as having agency despite the vertical hierarchical power structures at play within the clinical setting.

These issues are illustrated in case study 19.1 which draws attention to some of the practical implications of the issues discussed above.

Case study 19.1: Sustainable assessment in action

Sam is a clinical educator at a medium sized regional hospital. She has been in this role for a couple of years and is starting to feel comfortable with it. She takes on 2–4 students at a time from different universities. She currently has two students and is feeling irritated that the university has changed its assessment criteria and guidelines again. She checks herself thinking at least she got to chat with the academic liaison tutor to check her understanding of the new requirements and to establish how the placement fits within the revised curriculum.

Today she is conducting a mid-term formative assessment with one of her students, Frances, who is in her final year of study. Sam normally looks forward to these interactions as students seem to appreciate and learn from the observation and feedback sessions. Yet, Frances has been very quiet and difficult to engage in conversation despite having set expectations at the start of the rotation for open dialogue. She's found herself reverting to telling Frances what to do which comes easy to her as that's how she was taught. Sam fundamentally disagrees with this approach as students should be active in their own learning and so she has tried to be patient, to ask prompting questions and count to ten when there's silence after asking a question or making a comment.

Sam has prepared for today's session by reviewing the new assessment criteria and guidelines last night after putting her daughter to bed. She has asked Frances to read the assessment documents and to revisit the agreed learning plan. She's found the introduction of the learning contracts quite useful in facilitating a discussion about previous placements and students' learning goals and she plans to revisit this today. The learning contracts are aligned to the competencies set by the profession and the university and align with the learning outcomes for the placement which she herself has set. She also gave the students opportunities earlier in the week to work with each other as buddy pairs giving each other feedback using the assessment criteria. This she feels is important to give students experiences of what practice looks and feels like in relation to written standards which can be dry and difficult for students to understand.

Frances woke up with a sense of dread. Today is her mid-unit assessment and she doesn't like being observed. She feels nervous. She has done what the educator has asked of her in terms of reflecting on her learning and what she'd like to achieve. She finds these conversations awkward and in the past when she's gone quiet the educators have been happy to fill in the silence but Sam is different. She seems genuinely interested in her as a person and in her learning. She's made lots of effort to draw Frances out and so Frances is slowly feeling trust in her educator. Frances has also enjoyed the opportunity to observe her educator and to work with her colleague without being observed. She feels like she's getting a grip on what's expected of her in the placement and she reflects on what she's good at and where she needs to improve in order to not only pass but to do really well.

Sam has left some time before the patient arrives to talk with Frances about her goals for the session, to develop some shared goals and to answer any questions. She finds Frances more open and chatty today and discovers that the quietness was not ambivalence about the placement (or her) but related to the novelty of being genuinely asked to self-assess. It's also partly a natural shyness and homesickness as she is away from her partner and family. Frances mentions that she's not had much experience with younger patients and asks if that would that be possible today. She'd also like to know how she's tracking towards the final assessment — they agree that it's important for Frances to calibrate her ability to judge the quality of her own work. Sam agrees that these are relevant goals and adds one in relation to talking with family if they were going to see a young patient and given Frances' newly revealed shyness. They agree these would be their focus as these are natural progression points from the last round of feedback as documented in the learning plan.

During the assessment, Sam sits to the side to observe but not be in the patient's and Frances' direct line of sight. She introduces Frances to the patient and his family and seeks informed consent. Frances starts with her history after introducing herself. At some point she becomes acutely aware of the many sets of eyes on her and she gets flustered; her speech gets fast and she forgets the order of the tests which results in the patient getting confused with her instructions and having to change position several times. She notices the educator giving her an encouraging nod. She takes a big breath and slows down, revisiting the missing tests and engaging the patient and family in discussion of the treatment as previously signposted. During this Sam is making notes in the corner and notices the patient's family trying to catch her eye and trying to ask her questions. Sam avoids their eye contact and instead smiles and nods at Frances to subtly redirect the parent's gaze. She wonders briefly about intervening but the patient seems comfortable enough and changing positions won't hurt him. Sam notices that Frances recovers well but the session has taken 20 minutes longer than expected which will throw her schedule into disarray.

After the session, Sam asks Frances to complete her self-evaluation against each assessment criteria adding comments as to why she has made particular judgments. In the meantime Sam quickly goes to see the next patient who has been waiting. Upon her return, Sam asks Frances how she is feeling about the session and whether there's anything in particular she would like feedback on. Their judgments match for several competencies and they focus their discussion on gaps between their respective evaluative judgments. Although Frances had insight into some of the challenges, she wasn't sure on how to improve and so together they worked out new goals and agreed on a learning plan and a date for when these new goals would be revisited. Frances felt willing to disclose more about her anxiety as she feels safe with this educator who she trusts and who she feels is a credible practitioner. She is determined to work on the set goals and to monitor her progress in the next few weeks to achieve her goals.

Potential directions for evaluation and research

The exclusive emphasis on psychometrically driven research needs to be modified with a greater emphasis on the learning aspects of assessment. The following are fruitful areas to pursue:

- Tracking the development of trainee's evaluative judgment longitudinally within and across placements.
- Identifying the affordances of the clinical workplace setting on the development of evaluative judgment at the system (e.g. length of rotation), interpersonal (e.g. strength of the educational alliance), individual (e.g. feedback literacy, self-regulation), task (e.g. assessment task design), and technological (e.g. use of mobile apps) level. This would enable better assessment events to be designed and implemented appropriately.
- Exploring how issues of power and trust interplay with sustainable assessment. That is, to identify ways in which power relations inhibit the development of evaluative judgment.

Conclusion

In this chapter, we have highlighted that sustainable assessment shapes how trainees come to think about their practice and also equips them with the ability to continue to learn. This occurs through developing trainees' evaluative judgment: their capability to make judgments about the quality of their own work and that of others in order to improve practice. This means that it is not sufficient for assessments to merely judge whether trainees have attained a standard, they must also help them to be able to be better judges of their own work and learn from their own experience now and in the future. We have provided a framework to prompt educators and trainees to think about assessment in terms of three stages: before, during and after. The interplay between the individual, the relational (patient–trainee–educator) and the social, cultural and material are taken into account in this model. Refocusing the role of the learner as being active, engaged and responsible for driving learning from assessment can overcome the limitations of fragmentation and refocus on them managing their own learning through the complexities of many placements and supervisors. We position trainees and educators as collaborators within assessment processes with the focus of developing trainees' evaluative judgments for long-term learning.

Online resources

Assessment Design Decisions. Decisions Framework Website: www.assessmentdecisions.org.
Jisc feedback dialogue, University of Dundee: http://jiscdesignstudio.pbworks.com/w/page/50671082/InterACT%20 Project.
Monash University. Deakin University and Melbourne University: www.feedbackforlearning.org.
University of Technology Sydney. Overview: Assessment Futures: www.assessmentfutures.com.

References

Ajjawi, R., Tai, J., Dawson, P., et al. (2018). Conceptualising evaluative judgement for sustainable assessment in higher education. In D. Boud, R. Ajjawi, P. Dawson, et al. (Eds.), *Developing evaluative judgement in higher education: Assessment for knowing and producing quality work* (pp. 7–17). Abingdon: Routledge.

Anderson, G., Boud, D., & Sampson, J. (1996). *Learning contracts*. London: RoutledgeFalmer.

Barrett, A., Galvin, R., Scherpbier, A. J. J. A., et al. (2017). Is the learning value of workplace-based assessment being realised? A qualitative study of trainer and trainee perceptions and experiences. *Postgraduate Medical Journal*, 93, 138–142. doi:10.1136/postgradmedj-2015-133917.

Bindal, T., Wall, D., & Goodyear, H. M. (2011). Trainee doctors' views on workplace-based assessments: Are they just a tick box exercise? *Medical Teacher*, 33(11), 919–927. doi:10.3109/0142159X.2011.558140.

Blank, W. A., Blankenfeld, H., Vogelmann, R., et al. (2013). Can near-peer medical students effectively teach a new curriculum in physical examination? *BMC Medical Education*, 13(1), 165. doi:10.1186/1472-6920-13-165.

Boud, D. (2000). Sustainable assessment: Rethinking assessment for the learning society. *Studies in Continuing Education*, 22(2), 151–167. doi:10.1080/713695728.

Boud, D. (2007). Reframing assessment as if learning was important. In D. Boud & N. Falchikov (Eds.), *Rethinking assessment in higher education: Learning for the longer term* (pp. 14–25). London: Routledge.

Boud, D., & Edwards, H. (1999). Learning for practice: Promoting learning in clinical and community settings. In J. Higgs & H. Edwards (Eds.), *Educating beginning practitioners* (pp. 173–179). Oxford: Butterworth-Heinemann.

Boud, D., & Molloy, E. (2013). Rethinking models of feedback for learning: The challenge of design. *Assessment and Evaluation in Higher Education*, 38(6), 698–712. doi:10.1080/02602938.2012.691462.

Boud, D., & Rooney, D. (2014). What can higher education learn from the workplace? In A. Dailey-Hebert & K. S. Dennis (Eds.), *Transformative perspectives and processes in higher education* (Vol. 6, pp. 195–209). Dordecht: Springer.

Boud, D., & Soler, R. (2016). Sustainable assessment revisited. *Assessment and Evaluation in Higher Education*, 41(3), 400–413. doi:10.1080/02602938.2015.1018133.

Boud, D., & Walker, D. (1990). Making the most of experience. *Studies in Continuing Education*, 12(2), 61–80.

Campbell, C., Silver, I., Sherbino, J., et al. (2010). Competency-based continuing professional development. *Medical Teacher*, 32(8), 657–662. doi:10.3109/0142159X.2010.500708.

Clarke, J. L., & Boud, D. (2016). Refocusing portfolio assessment: Curating for feedback and portrayal. *Innovations in Education and Teaching International*, 1–8. doi:10.1080/14703297.2016.1250664.

Elmholdt, K., Elmholdt, C., Tanggaard, L., et al. (2016). Learning good leadership: A matter of assessment? *Human Resource Development International*, 19(5), 406–428. doi:10.1080/13678868.2016.1206362.

Eraut, M. (2004). Informal learning in the workplace. *Studies in Continuing Education*, 26(2), 247–273.

Farrell, L., Bourgeois-Law, G., Ajjawi, R., et al. (2017). An autoethnographic exploration of the use of goal oriented feedback to enhance brief clinical teaching encounters. *Advances in Health Sciences Education*, 22(1), 91–104. doi:10.1007/s10459-016-9686-5.

Fokkema, J. P. I., Teunissen, P. W., Westerman, M., et al. (2013). Exploration of perceived effects of innovations in postgraduate medical education. *Medical Education*, 47(3), 271–281. doi:10.1111/medu.12081.

Govaerts, M. J., Van de Wiel, M. W., Schuwirth, L. W., et al. (2013). Workplace-based assessment: Raters' performance theories and constructs. *Advances in Health Sciences Education*, 18(3), 375396. doi:10.1007/s10459-012-9376-x.

Hager, P. (2000). Know-how and workplace practical judgement. *Journal of Philosophy of Education*, 34(2), 281–296. doi:10.1111/1467-9752.00173.

Harrison, C. J., Könings, K. D., Dannefer, E. F., et al. (2016). Factors influencing students' receptivity to formative feedback emerging from different assessment cultures. *Perspectives on Medical Education*, 5(5), 276–284. doi:10.1007/s40037-016-0297-x.

Holmboe, E. S., Sherbino, J., Long, D. M., et al. (2010). The role of assessment in competency-based medical education. *Medical Teacher, 32*(8), 676–682. doi: 10.3109/0142159X.2010.500704.

Holmboe, E. S., Ward, D. S., Reznick, R. K., et al. (2011). Faculty development in assessment: The missing link in competency-based medical education. *Academic Medicine, 86*(4), 460–467.

LaDonna, K. A., Hatala, R., Lingard, L., et al. (2017). Staging a performance: Learners' perceptions about direct observation during residency. *Medical Education, 51*(5), 498–510. doi:10.1111/medu.13232.

Massie, J., & Ali, J. M. (2016). Workplace-based assessment: A review of user perceptions and strategies to address the identified shortcomings. *Advances in Health Sciences Education, 21*(2), 455–473. doi:10.1007/s10459-015-9614-0.

Miller, A., & Archer, J. (2010). Impact of workplace based assessment on doctors' education and performance: A systematic review. *BMJ (Clinical Research Ed.), 341,* c5064. doi:10.1136/bmj.c5064.

Monrouxe, L. V., & Sweeney, K. (2010). Contesting narratives: Medical professional identity formation amidst changing values. In S. Pattison, B. Hannigan, H. Thomas, et al. (Eds.), *Emerging professional values in health care: How professions and professionals are changing* (pp. 61–77). London: Jessica Kingsley.

Overeem, K., Faber, M. J., Arah, O. A., et al. (2007). Doctor performance assessment in daily practise: Does it help doctors or not? A systematic review. *Medical Education, 41*(11), 1039–1049. doi:10.1111/j.1365-2923.2007.02897.x.

Pekrun, R. (2006). The control-value theory of achievement emotions: Assumptions, corollaries, and implications for educational research and practice. *Educational Psychology Review, 18*(4), 315–341. doi:10.1007/s10648-006-9029-9.

Rees, C. E., Ajjawi, R., & Monrouxe, L. V. (2013). The construction of power in family medicine bedside teaching: A video observation study. *Medical Education, 47*(2), 154–165. doi:10.1111/medu.12055.

Sadler, D. R. (1989). Formative assessment and the design of instructional systems. *Instructional Science, 18*(2), 119–144.

Sholl, S., Ajjawi, R., Allbutt, H., et al. (2017). Balancing health care education and patient care in the UK workplace: A realist synthesis. *Medical Education, 51*(8), 787–801. doi:10.1111/medu.13290.

Tai, J., Ajjawi, R., Boud, D., et al. (2017). Developing evaluative judgement: Enabling students to make decisions about the quality of work. *Higher Education,* doi:10.1007/s10734-017-0220-3.

Tai, J. H.-M., Canny, B. J., Haines, T. P., et al. (2016). The role of peer-assisted learning in building evaluative judgement: Opportunities in clinical medical education. *Advances in Health Sciences Education, 21*(3), 659–676. doi:10.1007/s10459-015-9659-0.

Telio, S., Ajjawi, R., & Regehr, G. (2015). The 'educational alliance' as a framework for reconceptualizing feedback in medical education. *Academic Medicine, 90*(5), 609–614. doi:10.1097/ACM.0000000000000560.

Telio, S., Regehr, G., & Ajjawi, R. (2016). Feedback and the educational alliance: Examining credibility judgements and their consequences. *Medical Education, 50*(9), 933–942. doi:10.1111/medu.13063.

Urquhart, L. M., Rees, C. E., & Ker, J. S. (2014). Making sense of feedback experiences: A multi-school study of medical students' narratives. *Medical Education, 48*(2), 189203. doi:10.1111/medu.12304.

Watling, C. (2016). The uneasy alliance of assessment and feedback. *Perspectives on Medical Education, 5*(5), 262–264. doi:10.1007/s40037-016-0300-6.

20

Assessment through entrustable professional activities

H. Carrie Chen and Olle ten Cate

Introduction

The engagement and assessment of learners in the clinical workplace is a key component in the education of health professionals. Entrustable professional activities (EPAs) offer a framework for working with competencies that places them in the context of this workplace practice (ten Cate & Scheele, 2007). This framework defines competencies by first starting with the concrete activities that a health professional performs, and then works backwards to link these activities to existing competency domains. For instance, one concrete professional activity of a physician assistant is to perform an initial history and physical examination, which requires competence in such domains as medical expertise, communication and professionalism (Mulder et al., 2010). Therefore, EPAs are defined as units of essential professional practice (e.g. performance of the initial history and physical examination) for qualified professionals (e.g. physician's assistants, nurses, physicians) that require the integration of specific knowledge, skills and attitudes gained through training. They lead to recognisable outputs that are observable and measurable, and which in turn leads to concluding decisions about whether the activities (e.g. the initial history and physical examination) were well done or not.

Each EPA reflects important competency domains, and all the EPAs together constitute the core activities of the profession (ten Cate, 2005; ten Cate et al., 2015). Initially defined for the outcomes of postgraduate medical education, EPAs now have been used in a variety of health professions to define outcomes at different transition points, including the transitions from pre-clinical to clinical training, undergraduate to postgraduate education, and postgraduate education to further training or practice (Boyce et al., 2011; Chen et al., 2016; Duijn et al., n.d.; Pittenger et al., 2016; Wiersma et al., 2017; Wisman-Zwarter et al., 2016).

Because it grounds competencies in the everyday tasks of health professionals and incorporates the concept of entrustment and levels of supervision, the EPA framework reflects how members of the clinical workplace interact with learners. The clinical workplace, in contrast to the classroom, necessitates approaches to learning and assessment that include the expectation for the safe, effective, patient-centred care of patients. In their day-to-day practice, clinical educators balance supervision with learner autonomy to ensure both learner engagement and safe, quality patient care. They provide close direct supervision to learners who are learning a new task, and slowly provide more autonomy and less supervision as learners gain competence in completing the task. Determining the appropriate balance depends on the educator's trust of the learner to complete specific tasks successfully, and acceptance of the risk associated with that trust and its potential consequences (Holzhausen et al., 2017).

Assessments within the EPA framework focus on clinical educators' *entrustment decisions* about how much to supervise a learner's engagement with workplace activities. It asks clinical educators to use the routine supervision decisions they already make to provide information about learner competence. Instead of rating learner competence on various performance scales, clinical educators report how much supervision a learner requires for a specific task or professional activity, based on how much supervision they have been providing in their interactions with the learner. Assessments using the EPA framework therefore naturally align with clinical practice (Crossley et al., 2011).

Supervision and entrustment scales are published for use in both undergraduate and postgraduate education, and all include graded levels of clinical supervision/learner autonomy (Rekman et al., 2016). There are five key levels of entrustment that are commonly used, which can be further broken down into finer gradations for more junior learners. Learners reach full competence for a given EPA when they master the professional activity at a level that allows entrustment for future performance without supervision (level 4) (Chen et al., 2015; ten Cate et al., 2010). See Table 20.1.

TABLE 20.1: Entrustment and supervision scales: basic form and expanded form

Five-level entrustment and supervision scale	Expanded entrustment and supervision scale for undergraduate and postgraduate education

1. Not allowed to practise EPA	1. Not allowed to practise EPA
	  a. Inadequate knowledge/skill (e.g. does not know how to preserve a sterile field); not allowed to observe
	  b. Adequate knowledge, some skill; allowed to observe

2. Allowed to practise EPA only under proactive, full supervision	2. Allowed to practise EPA only under proactive, full supervision
	  a. As co-activity with the supervisor
	  b. With the supervisor in the room ready to step in as needed

3. Allowed to practise EPA only under reactive/on-demand supervision	3. Allowed to practise EPA only under reactive/on-demand supervision
	  a. With the supervisor immediately available, with all findings and decisions double-checked
	  b. With the supervisor immediately available, with key findings and decisions double-checked
	  c. With the supervisor distantly available (e.g. by phone), with findings and decisions promptly reviewed

4. Allowed to practise EPA unsupervised	4. Allowed to practise EPA unsupervised
	  a. With remote monitoring (e.g. next-day check-in for learner questions)
	  b. Without monitoring

5. Allowed to supervise others in the practice of EPA	5. Allowed to supervise others in the practice of EPA

In the literature, most EPA frameworks for programs or specialties are published or discussed using only their titles. However, it is important to note that a fully elaborated EPA description contains seven parts: 1) the EPA *title*; 2) *specifications and limitations*, describing the context and what is and is not included in the activity; 3) mapping of the EPA to the most *relevant domains of competence*; 4) the *required knowledge, skills, attitudes and experience* that are expected before learners can be trusted to carry out the EPA; 5) the *assessment information sources* to assess progress and ground summative entrustment decisions; 6) the *entrustment/supervision level expected at stages of training* (i.e. when learners are expected to reach what level of entrustment or supervision level for the EPA); and 7) an optional *expiration date* for when entrustment would drop if learners do not maintain competence (ten Cate et al., 2015). A clear description of what exactly is being entrusted, not just an EPA title, is necessary to avoid misunderstandings, especially if the decision leads to permission to act without supervision.

The goals of this chapter are to: 1) define EPAs and describe their applicability to workplace learning and assessment; 2) review the different theories that support their use; and 3) provide educational strategies for the practical application of EPAs in workplace-based assessment. The chapter opens with a case study of a clinical educator (Caroline) who supervises and must assess two learners (David and Amy) working with her in an outpatient clinic. Caroline is an experienced clinician and clinical educator (in medicine, but this could be any health profession), who has been asked to pilot a new assessment approach using EPAs, alongside the postgraduate program's traditional assessments of clinical performance.

Case study 20.1

Caroline is a clinical educator who works in a community clinic that serves as a required ambulatory clinical placement for medical students and paediatric residents from the local university. She has years of experience supervising learners in caring for patients, and is very familiar with the university's assessment forms. Recently, the paediatric residency program decided to pilot a new assessment approach using EPAs.

For the past several weeks, Caroline has had two first-year paediatric residents working with her in clinic. David performs at a level typical for an average first-year resident. He requests support in thinking through clinical cases, and frequently asks questions, both to ensure that he is providing appropriate care and to improve his learning. He is not lacking in confidence, but will point out his knowledge and skills gaps to focus Caroline's supervision and teaching. For instance, he will indicate when he is uncertain about a physical examination finding, and request that Caroline confirm that portion of the examination.

In contrast, Amy is a resident with an impressive fund of knowledge and clinical skills. Others describe her as a stellar independent first-year resident. In many ways, Caroline is inclined to agree, but she did have an experience with Amy last week that has made her uncomfortable. Amy had confidently presented a patient whom she had diagnosed with an upper respiratory infection. She told Caroline that she had already discussed her plans for supportive care with the family, and that Caroline just needed to send the family home. When questioned about the several days of fever and suspiciously worsening cough, Amy made light of the history, saying that the parents were just anxious and that the physical examination was normal. Caroline decided to re-examine the patient, despite Amy's annoyance, and discovered on auscultation, findings consistent with a diagnosis of pneumonia. When she attempted to use the findings to teach Amy auscultation technique, Amy responded that she had heard the same sounds on her examination but did not believe that they were important enough to mention.

Background theory

Assessment using EPAs with entrustment decisions is intimately embedded in the learning and work that occurs in the clinical setting. A variety of theoretical lenses, including those addressing learning in the workplace, workplace-based competency assessments, and entrustment, provide context for understanding EPAs and will be discussed in turn.

Learning as participation in the workplace

In health professions education (undergraduate and postgraduate), the workplace is an essential site of learning. Learners develop the knowledge and psychomotor skills required for the health professions through observation of, coaching by, and practice with experts in clinical settings. Learning about work arises out of the work itself, and learning can be reconceptualised from *learning as acquisition* to *learning as participation* (Billett, 2001; Collins, 2005; Morris & Blaney, 2013; Papa & Harasym, 1999; Strand et al., 2015). Two contemporary frameworks for understanding learning as participation in the workplace are *communities of practice* and *workplace learning*. Both derive from situated learning theory and offer a sociocultural perspective that acknowledges the interplay between learners and their environment, and puts equal emphasis on both (Billett, 2001; Durning & Artino, 2011; Lave & Wenger, 1991). They are particularly helpful for looking at the interactions between learners and clinical educators, and their impact on learning in the clinical workplace.

Communities of practice

The theory of situated learning argues that learning is social in nature and occurs through interactions with others and the environment. Learning is a product of the activity, context and culture in which the activity occurs, and both the learner and the environment are changed through the impact of the learner on their environment. From this perspective, Lave and Wenger contend that learning in the workplace is structured by work practices within a community and the learner's relationship with members of the community (e.g. clinical educators). They describe learning as an activity where learners are situated and participate in communities of practitioners, and where learning arises from acts of social participation (Lave & Wenger, 1991). A community of practice is a group of individuals who share a common goal and who share and develop a repertoire of common language, knowledge, beliefs, values, stories and practices to achieve that goal (Lave & Wenger, 1991; Wenger, 1998).

Learners, as new entrants to the workplace and its community of practice, gain the knowledge, skills and habits necessary to become full participants and members of the community by engaging in the community's activities and practices. Newcomers initially engage in peripheral yet legitimate activities of the workplace. Legitimate activities, such as EPAs, are those that make meaningful and valued contributions to the community of practice. This *legitimate peripheral participation* moves in a centripetal trajectory, becoming less and less peripheral until the learners' knowledge, skills and habits have progressed to allow full participation and membership in the community of practice (Lave & Wenger, 1991).

Many have applied the communities of practice framework to the healthcare setting to understand learner roles and experiences within communities of clinical practice (Daly et al., 2013; Dornan et al., 2007; Egan & Jaye, 2009; Gandamihardja, 2014; Jaye et al., 2010; Sheehan, 2011; Strand et al., 2015). For instance, the clinical educator role in the clinical community of practice is to welcome learners and help them understand the context of the clinical workplace. They provide opportunities and support for learner engagement in legitimate patient care activities (e.g. EPAs), and adjust the balance of supervision and autonomy to help learners safely move from peripheral to more central roles in the clinical community of practice.

Workplace learning

In his conception of workplace learning, Billett argues that the richness of learning in the workplace depends on the interactions and activities in which learners participate, and the degree of learner engagement in these interactions/activities (Billett, 2001). His framework of the workplace as a learning environment is similar to Lave and Wenger's community of practice, in that the workplace has the ability to structure and regulate learner participation (Billett, 2001; Lave & Wenger, 1991). It can either invite learner participation and sequence activities to support the participation of learners at different readiness-to-participate levels, or deny learners access to activities and interactions. Workplaces differ in their workplace *affordances*, or the situational factors (types of activities, interpersonal dynamics, rules and cultural practices) that invite and support learner participation (Billett, 2001, 2004). Clinical educators are an important part of these affordances and play a key role in influencing how learners experience the clinical workplace.

However, workplace affordances represent only one dimension of workplace learning, and are not the only determinants of learner participation. The second dimension is the learners. Learners are not passive, and can choose whether or not to engage, in which activities or interactions to engage, and their degree of engagement. They determine how and what they learn (Billett, 2001). Some learners are more agentic — setting out to learn actively and enthusiastically — than others, who may be reluctant and grudging in their participation. Learner *agency* determines how learners construe the affordances of the workplace. In turn, workplace affordances are likely to also influence learner willingness both to engage in activities and to seek guidance from others in the workplace to support their participation (Billett, 2004). In other words, while learner motivation is important and learners will vary in their willingness to engage, clinical educators can influence learner willingness. Clinical educators can help learners appropriately interpret the affordances and recognise opportunities for participation, provide meaningful activities, and encourage and support learner engagement.

Workplace learning, therefore, represents an interaction between the *affordances* of the workplace and the learner's *agency*. The clinical learning environment is negotiated by the learner and mediated by the practices of the clinical workplace. The clinical educator can be a powerful facilitator in these negotiations, interceding when necessary to maximise learner participation. An important goal underlying the EPA concept is to bring teaching and assessment efforts closer to clinical practice. EPAs are in fact legitimate clinical workplace activities. Entrustment with clinical responsibilities can be viewed as efforts both to provide affordances and to encourage learner agency. By entrusting learners with graduated levels of responsibility and autonomy, clinical educators can ensure learners feel welcomed and appropriately supported to participate in the workplace, and to move from peripheral to fuller participation and membership within the community of clinical practice. The reward of additional clinical responsibility and autonomy can also function as a powerful incentive for learners, impacting on their motivations, intentions and resultant behaviours.

Assessment of competence in the workplace

Competency-based education

The international movement towards competency-based education has been gaining momentum in health professions education since the 1990s. It calls for a greater emphasis on learner outcomes in designing and implementing curricula, as well as in learner assessment. Various competency frameworks (e.g. ACGME, CanMEDS) have been adopted in multiple countries to provide clear performance expectations for learners of health professions training programs. However, educators have expressed concerns that competency frameworks risk becoming a reductionist approach to learning and assessment (Touchie & Cate, 2016). If competencies lead to a tick-box approach to training, the whole (i.e. holistic view) of actually caring for patients may become lost. Mastery of individual competencies may not ensure the ability to integrate or apply them to patient care. Lastly, the ability to integrate and apply competencies in one context may not translate across different patient care contexts (Brooks, 2009; Frank et al., 2010; Lurie, 2012).

The EPA framework was introduced in an attempt to address some of these criticisms about how competencies have been adopted and applied to health education (Carraccio & Burke, 2010; ten Cate, 2013; ten Cate & Scheele, 2007). EPAs holistically integrate multiple competencies, translate them into clinical practice, and acknowledge the importance of context. Table 20.2 demonstrates this integration of

TABLE 20.2: Example of an EPA-competency matrix

CanMEDS competency domains	EPA 1	EPA 2	EPA 3	EPA 4	EPA 5	EPA 6
Medical expert	xx	xx	xx	xx		x
Communicator	xx	xx	xx	x	xx	xx
Collaborator		xx	xx	xx	xx	
Scholar			x	xx		
Leader				xx		xx
Health advocate			x	xx	xx	xx
Professional	x				xx	xx

EPA 1 = perform a venipuncture
EPA 2 = perform an appendectomy
EPA 3 = sign-over at morning report after a night shift
EPA 4 = develop and implement a patient management plan
EPA 5 = chair a multidisciplinary meeting
EPA 6 = request an organ donation
xx: competency is necessary for this EPA
x: competency is useful for this EPA

multiple competencies using sample EPAs and the CanMEDS competency domains (Frank et al., 2015). Note that successful achievement of EPA 1, 'perform a venipuncture', requires the integration of the medical expert, communicator and professional competency domains. By grounding competencies in patient care, the EPA framework helps ensure educators and learners focus on the care of patients, rather than mere achievement of competencies, as the end goal.

Validity challenges in workplace-based assessments

In addition to the question of what to assess (i.e. which competencies or frameworks to use), there have been concerns with the validity of workplace-based assessments. Assessment in the clinical workplace usually involves single learners, single assessors, and unique contexts (e.g. caring for a unique patient). Several authors have pointed to assessment problems arising from this. These include persistent psychometric problems, such as rater leniency bias or generosity error, halo effects, restriction of range, poor discrimination between learners, lack of documentation of deficits, and low intra-rater, inter-rater, and cross-occasion consistency (Albanese, 2000; Govaerts et al., 2007; Massie & Ali, 2016). From the perspective of the sources of validity evidence identified by the Standards for Educational and Psychological Testing, there is legitimate concern about *response process* (low accuracy and quality of the scoring), *internal structure* (low reproducibility), *relationship to other variables* (poor generalisability) and *consequences* (hardly any learner 'fails' a workplace placement) (AERA/APA/NCME, 2014). In attempting to capture elements of the workplace environment required for effective learning, many authors have realised that workplace-based assessments should not be treated the same as classroom assessments (Billett, 2006; Eraut, 2007; Teunissen, 2009). Workplace-based assessments must incorporate unique conditions critical to the workplace, such as the expectation for safe, effective and patient-centred care (Crossley & Jolly, 2012; Kogan et al., 2014). The inclusion of these expectations introduces a new way to think about consequential validity and its use in assessment, which is further explained in the next two paragraphs.

The consequential validity of tests is often explained from the perspective of avoiding unintended consequences caused by failing or passing someone who should not have failed or passed. Attention is typically directed at potential underrepresentation of the construct (i.e. not reflective of the relevant knowledge/skill of interest) and construct-irrelevant variance of scores (i.e. extraneous variables affecting assessment results) (AERA/APA/NCME, 2014).

Take for example, Caroline, our experienced clinical educator, and Amy, our learner from case study 20.1. After observing Amy's interaction with the patient with a cough, Caroline is asked to rate Amy in four areas using a 9-point scale: knowledge, psychomotor skill, communication ability and professional attitude (Norcini & Burch, 2007). Caroline may be unsure of what the consequences of her assessment will be, may be focused only on learner consequences, and may be influenced by a personal relationship with Amy. She may not know the significance and weighting of the four areas by the residency program, and may not be aware of the benchmarks against which to assess Amy on the scale. All of these variables add to the vagueness of ratings and the chances that Caroline could inadvertently introduce construct-irrelevant variance. Even with the best intentions, her construct for what should be included in her ratings of, for instance, communication ability, may differ from that intended by the residency program. Or worse, she may become less invested in careful rating due to the vagueness of the construct.

If, in contrast, Caroline is asked to recommend whether Amy should be allowed to perform this physical examination again tomorrow with another patient with a cough, *without direct supervision*, then her expert experience comes into play. The responsibility for safe care makes Caroline much more careful in weighing truly relevant features of Amy as a learner (ten Cate, 2006, 2017a). Instead of including criteria that lead to *construct-irrelevant* variance (weighing factors other than only learner competence), as often happens in traditional workplace assessments, in entrustment decision-making Caroline may actually include *construct-relevant* criteria. She may include criteria important for safe patient care that is not represented in the items on the rating instrument, and in doing so improve construct representation. These criteria, which could be unconscious and stem from gut feelings or intuition, can be particularly relevant in rapid decisions (Gigerenzer, 2007). The health professions education literature has shown that global ratings about learners are often more reliable than composite scores based on more complete checklist ratings of relevant observations (Ilgen et al., 2015; Regehr et al., 1998). In addition, the need to make a decision of entrustment may further add to the reliability of a global rating. Raters assess learners more accurately if the consequences of their rating are clear to them (George et al., 2014; Weller et al., 2014; Weller et al., 2017). Entrustment decisions, if viewed as assessments, represent clear intended assessment consequences for both the learner and the patient. They provide not just acknowledgments of learner competence, but permission for learners to act in the future with consequences for patient safety (Kogan et al., 2015).

Entrustment as a basis for assessment

Several authors have explained how different factors together determine whether a health professions learner will be entrusted with critical tasks in healthcare (Cianciolo & Kegg, 2013; Kennedy et al., 2008; Sterkenburg et al., 2010; Wijnen-Meijer et al., 2013b). Hauer covered a broad range of literature from several domains to arrive at a model of five factors that determine entrustment decisions: the context, the task, the supervisor/clinical educator, the trainee/learner, and their relationship (Hauer et al., 2014). A model borrowed by medical educators from the management literature stresses the significance of risk-taking by the trustor or clinical educator (Damodaran et al., 2017; Holzhausen et al., 2017; Mayer et al., 1995). By definition, trust involves taking risks. Clinical educators must consider the perceived risks of an activity as well as the perceived trustworthiness of the learner, further discussed below, for completing the activity. The perceived risk of the activity will include not only the activity, but the context of the activity (i.e. risks for complications of a tooth extraction in a healthy young adult versus a frail elderly person with a bleeding disorder). It can be easy to trust a learner with a task when the risks are small. However, entrustment decisions for tasks where errors may have severe consequences for the patient need to be grounded in knowledge of, and experience with, the learner.

To summarise, the broad categories that determine whether an entrustment decision is made depends on: (a) the learner's trustworthiness; (b) the clinical educator's trust propensity; (c) the perceived benefits of the decisions; and (d) the perceived risks of the decision (ten Cate, 2017b). Each of these can be broken down into multiple determinants.

- Trust in a learner's capability to perform a patient care task requires that the learner demonstrate trustworthiness for the task. Trustworthiness requires not just the *ability* (knowledge, skill, experience) to complete the task, but also *integrity* (truthfulness, benevolence), *reliability* (conscientiousness, consistency), and *humility* (observing limits, willingness to ask for help). In addition, a learner's adequate coping with unfamiliar situations can increase trust in them (Wijnen-Meijer et al., 2013a).

- The clinical educator's trust propensity may be partly a personality trait and partly determined by experience in patient care and in teaching. It can be affected by bad experiences, and potentially influenced by feedback and benchmarking against colleagues.

- Benefits include deliberate educational opportunities for learners; but also service demands can compel decisions to entrust learners with tasks.

- Risks include risks for patients, but also for the clinical educator, the healthcare team and the learner. Serious adverse events can affect all stakeholders.

- Both clinical educators and learners should be aware of these factors.

Finally, trust itself is not a uniform construct. Distinctions have been made between presumptive trust (Cruess & Cruess, 2014), initial trust and grounded trust (ten Cate et al., 2016). *Presumptive trust* is based on credentials only (diplomas, test results, documented prior experiences, recommendations). *Initial trust* (sometimes called *swift trust*) is based on first impressions of initial collaboration. *Grounded trust* develops over time, when cumulative experiences increase confidence in the learner. In health professions education, where learning experiences are often structured as a series of placements for a compartmentalised continuum, learners frequently transit to new environments that must rely on documented achievements. If these are EPAs with certified levels of entrustment/supervision, then presumptive trust is what the new location can use when starting with the learner. This happens most prominently with the transition from undergraduate to postgraduate education. After each transition, a new cycle of observations directed to new levels of achievement start, and grounding of trust is needed to support new entrustment decisions. Fig. 20.1 provides a graphic representation of the cycle of trust.

Summary

In summary, participation is key to learning in the clinical workplace, and the workplace can be viewed as a community of clinical practice. Learners identify with, gain membership in, and contribute to the community by engaging in legitimate patient care activities, initially peripherally, then more centrally. For learners to safely engage in these activities, clinical communities of practice need to have defined roles and activities

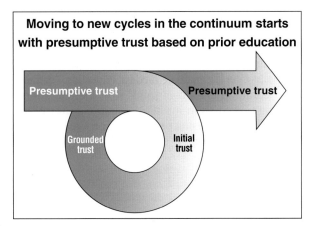

Figure 20.1: Trust cycle

for the learners, and trust in the learners' abilities to participate accordingly. It is also important that all members of the community (other clinical educators and health professionals as well as more senior learners) share a common understanding of learner competencies and appropriate activities for each level of learner. Thus EPAs become an attractive framework for defining the competencies of learners in relation to their participation in clinical workplace activities, and offer a useful approach for clinical educators to assist learners along their trajectory. They help inform diverse members of when and how learners may be invited into the communities of practice. Certification of learner attainment of entrustment for specific clinical activities can signal to the community that the learner is ready for safe participation in patient care. Similarly, EPAs help clarify for learners their roles in the clinical workplace, and how they can contribute meaningfully to the delivery of patient care.

Most importantly, assessments using the EPA framework maintain a clear focus on the assessment consequences for patients. With degrees of supervision and entrustment built into the assessment model, the goal for safe learner participation in patient care remains clear to clinical educators, and ensures their use of relevant criteria for learner assessment. It also reminds clinical educators that one consequence of assessment includes increasing learner responsibility and autonomy when learners demonstrate that they are ready for higher levels of entrustment. This link of increasing autonomy to learner progression may also help motivate learners and promote learner agency.

EPAs in educational and assessment strategy

Learner-level considerations

EPAs can be used to assess any level of learner in the clinical workplace environment. As noted at the beginning of this chapter, EPAs or outcomes can be defined for any transition point in undergraduate or postgraduate education. Although they were initially developed for postgraduate medical education, the key underlying principles of workplace-based learning/assessment and trust are applicable to all learners in the clinical workplace. Ideally, the same competency framework should be applied across the entire continuum of learner training within a particular health profession. However, the size and breadth of EPAs need to be appropriate for the type and level of intended learners, as well as the extent to which learners can be granted autonomy, or in other words, how much supervision they need for the specified EPA.

EPAs for junior learners will be of smaller size and scope; these smaller junior learner EPAs provide the foundation for, and nest up into, ones of larger size and scope for more senior learners. To illustrate, we will use an example from medical education, where EPAs have been defined for both postgraduate and undergraduate education. EPAs used for the transition from postgraduate medical education to practice include 'manage a complicated pregnancy' (obstetrics/gynaecology) and 'manage patients with acute common diagnoses' (paediatrics) with unsupervised practice (Carraccio et al., 2016; ten Cate & Scheele, 2007). These EPAs are at too high a level and too broad a scope to be practically useful for assessment in undergraduate medical education. Instead, learners at the transition from undergraduate to postgraduate medical education can be assessed on smaller EPAs such as 'gather a history and perform a physical examination' and 'document a clinical encounter in the patient record' with indirect supervision. Mastery of these professional activities provide the foundation for eventual mastery of 'manage care of complicated pregnancies' and 'manage patients with acute common diagnoses'.

Similarly, the EPAs at graduation from undergraduate medical education build on EPAs of even narrower scope from an earlier transition point in undergraduate medical education: 'gather a history from a cooperative, medically stable patient with a common chief complaint' with indirect supervision (Chen et al., 2016). This is analogous to how learning objectives in further training (e.g. nurse practitioner training) build on those from previous training (e.g. bachelor nursing programs). The size of a training program's EPAs (clinical placement, health professional school, residency, etc.) should align with the size of its end-of-program objectives. See Fig. 20.2.

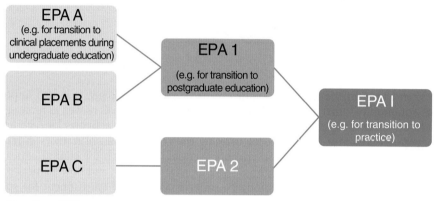

Figure 20.2: Nesting EPAs

In addition to requiring smaller EPAs that are narrower in scope, junior learners may require further adjustments to the entrustment/supervision scale. The initially published basic entrustment/supervision scale for use in postgraduate medical education is very useful in assessing learners in the final stages of training leading to unsupervised practice. To accommodate junior learners who may need smaller incremental changes in their required levels of supervision, the lower portions of this initial scale were expanded to include finer gradations in the various levels of direct and indirect supervision (Chen et al., 2015). See Table 20.1. One last consideration is that the goal or final expected achievement level for a junior learner will be lower than that of senior learners. A junior learner transitioning to additional training may appropriately be expected to achieve only up to an entrustment level of indirect supervision (level 3 in Table 20.1). In contrast, senior learners transitioning to practice (e.g. surgery residents or midwives) must reach an entrustment level of unsupervised practice (level 4) at completion of training.

In summary, the implementation of EPAs for any group of learners necessitates curricular attention to three elements: 1) choosing EPAs of the appropriate size and scope; 2) matching the chosen EPAs to an entrustment scale with enough gradations to allow reasonable assessment of progress; and 3) determining the expected level of entrustment that learners need to achieve by the completion of training. EPAs and variations of the entrustment/supervision scale continue to be defined and published for multiple health professions. These offer an excellent starting place for groups interested in adopting the EPA framework, and may be used to inform the development of new EPAs, or adapted to suit diverse professional or local contexts.

Questions often arise about the role or applicability of the EPA framework to classroom learning in the pre-clinical phase of health professions education. As EPAs by definition concern active contributions to the clinical workplace, they do not have a direct role in classroom learning. However, by defining the expected outcomes of health professions education in terms of EPAs to be mastered, they do provide curricular guidance and rationale for the pre-clinical curriculum. Classroom learning objectives should map to the knowledge, skills and attitudes that learners require to achieve the EPAs. As noted in the introduction, the elaborated descriptions for each EPA list these required knowledge, skills and attitudes. Here, EPAs can become a roadmap to guide learners in their learning, ameliorating the tendency for them to get lost in the multitude of learning objectives (Crossley, 2014). Also, health professional education programs increasingly are incorporating early clinical experiences, juxtaposing or threading workplace-based learning opportunities next to and throughout traditional classroom learning. In these circumstances, EPAs become relevant for learning and assessment throughout health professions education, rather than just the latter years of training.

Using entrustment for assessment

Elements of trust

In the EPA framework, a clinical educator's decision about how much supervision they must provide to a learner performing a specific patient care task is used as an assessment of that learner's competence with that task. As noted in the section on background theory, multiple learner factors impact on a clinical educator's decision about supervision. The clinical educator may first ask themselves whether the learner has the required knowledge, skills and experience (*ability*) to perform the task. This assessment of learner competence takes into account performance in specific competencies and associated milestones, and is consistent with traditional workplace-based assessments.

However, when making supervision decisions, the clinical educator goes further. Because they anticipate the possibility that each upcoming or future patient/situation may pose new challenges, the clinical educator asks a series of additional questions about the learner. 'Do I trust that the learner will have the best interests of the patient at heart, that the learner will be truthful about what the learner has or has not done?' (*integrity*). A learner who says that the potassium level is normal, rather than admit to not yet checking the patient's morning laboratories, demonstrates intentions that are favourable to oneself at the expense of the patient's safety. This erodes trust, and results in the clinical educator increasing rather than decreasing supervision. 'Do I trust the learner to be conscientious in their care of patients, to do what they say they will do, and to have consistent performance or predictable behavior from day to day?' (*reliability*). A learner with extreme good days and bad days that is reflected in wide fluctuations in their performance would not be reliable and would be difficult to trust. Lastly, 'Do I trust that the learner will recognise and heed their own limitations, and be willing to seek help as needed?' (*humility*). A clinical educator would have a difficult time entrusting a learner to evaluate the appropriateness of drug therapy of a future unknown patient if the learner cannot be trusted to know what they do not know and seek additional information or help. Therefore, assessment within the EPA framework necessarily takes into account not just ability, but integrity, reliability, and humility — the four learner conditions required for entrustment.

Every learner should know from the outset the expectations for the determination of entrustment and supervision. Clinical educators need to ensure learners realise that trust requires more than specific ability, and that learners will be supported in the behaviours expected of them. A learner who is not truthful about checking the patient's potassium level may be in an environment where it feels unsafe to be truthful about imperfect performance. Similarly, a learner may not acknowledge limitations or ask for help for fear of highlighting shortcomings that may be used against them. How often are learners applauded or rewarded for admitting to an oversight or requesting assistance? Clinical educators play an important role in not just explaining, but modelling, encouraging and supporting learners' demonstrations of integrity, reliability and humility, in addition to ability.

PRACTICAL TIP

Traditional assessments typically focus primarily on how well learners demonstrate the necessary knowledge and skills (ability). In contrast, assessments within the EPA framework focus on whether learners may be entrusted to safely perform patient care tasks in the clinical workplace. Four conditions must be met to allow entrustment; learners must demonstrate each of the following:

1. *ability* — knowledge, skills, experience;
2. *integrity* — benevolence, truthfulness;
3. *reliability* — conscientiousness, consistency;
4. *humility* — recognising limits, willingness to ask for help.

An explicit conversation with learners about these conditions at the beginning of health professions training may help raise awareness that EPAs assess the demonstration of more than just knowledge and skills.

Types of entrustment

There are two types of entrustment decisions that clinical educators make: ad hoc and summative. *Ad hoc* entrustment decisions are momentary decisions about the learner's readiness to participate, and are made every day in the field. They are deliberate decisions about supervision levels and trust in learner autonomy that apply to a specific case or circumstance. They are situation-dependent, and are confirmed each time. For instance, in case study 20.1, Caroline, our clinical educator, may decide to allow David, one of our learners, to perform, without direct supervision, an intravenous (IV) line insertion in a cooperative and stable 11-year-old child in the morning, but not for a 14-year-old with a highly anxious parent or low blood pressure later in the afternoon.

In contrast, *summative entrustment* decisions are formalised decisions that give permission for less supervision or less autonomy moving forward. Summative entrustment decisions are grounded in evidence, with sufficient information from multiple sources, including previous ad hoc decisions. They are more typically made by committee than by individual clinical educators. In this case, the multiple ad hoc entrustment decisions Caroline has made in regard to David's performance of IV line insertions will inform her summative entrustment recommendation in her final end-of-placement assessment of David's performance. Caroline's and other clinical educators' end-of-placement assessments of David's performance, as well as his performance on a simulated IV line placement station, will in turn help to inform the paediatric competency committee's decision about his readiness for entrustment for unsupervised IV placement in children.

The ultimate summative entrustment decision is the final awarding of a diploma, certificate or license. In an EPA-based training program, certification is awarded for individual EPAs as entrustment is achieved for each. Full certification or certification in all of the program's EPAs thus occurs over a period of time, typically during the latter half of the training program, rather than at a single point in time.

Entrustability scales and their validity evidence

Emerging evidence on the use of entrustment/supervision scales for assessment point to their ability to generate reliable and useful information about learner competence (Mink et al., 2017; Rekman et al., 2016; Warm et al., 2016; Weller et al., 2014). Clinical educators are able to achieve greater inter-rater reliability using these scales compared with typical performance scales, requiring fewer raters and fewer observations to achieve a reliable rating. There is also less 'grade inflation', with more learners identified as performing below expectations when using an entrustment/supervision scale (Weller et al., 2014). Clinical educators may feel more comfortable stating that a learner is not yet ready for less supervision than stating that a learner is performing poorly. The former is a neutral comment about a learner's developmental progression, whereas the latter could be perceived as a negative judgment about the learner's capabilities and/or person. Lastly, entrustment/supervision scales are able to measure incremental increases in entrustment and decreases in supervision as learners progress in training, providing evidence supporting their validity (Mink et al., 2017; Warm et al., 2016). This attribute nicely allows for the longitudinal tracking of individual learner performance as learners advance towards the goal of independent practice.

Gathering information for entrustment

While many instruments have been described for workplace-based assessment (Kogan et al., 2009; Norcini & Burch, 2007), the instruments recommended for informing entrustment decisions can be grouped into four categories as shown in Table 20.3 (ten Cate et al., 2015).

Short practice observations are assessments of a learner's mastery of an EPA, based on the learner's performance of the activity and their trustworthiness in the clinical workplace. Although direct observations of learner performance in practice (e.g. mini-clinical evaluation exercise [Mini-CEX], direct observation of procedural skills [DOPS] (Norcini & Burch, 2007)) are an important source of information, they are not the exclusive source of assessment information available in the workplace.

Entrustment-based discussions (EBDs), case-based discussion with a focus on entrustment, are 15–20-minute conversations following performance of an EPA (ten Cate & Hoff, 2017). They are particularly useful for estimating whether a learner is ready to be trusted under decreased supervision. As previously explained, summative entrustment decisions involve risks. A clinical educator must estimate whether the learner will be ready for the more general responsibility of the EPA in the future. The learner must know what to do if complications arise, if a history reveals relevant unexpected information, if laboratory tests show unusual results, if the patient is different from what the learner has encountered so far (co-morbidities, uncooperative

TABLE 20.3: Tools for assessment to inform entrustment decisions

Major tools for assessment	Explanation
Short practice observations	Sampled 15–20-minute observations of EPAs in practice, followed by a brief report and feedback; examples are Mini-CEX and DOPS
Entrustment-based discussions (EBD)	Resembles a chart-stimulated recall (CSR) and a regular case-based discussion (CBD). EBD has a particular focus on estimation of ability to cope with the EPA in different variations and contexts, supporting an entrustment decision
Longitudinal practice observation	Are particularly useful to capture integrity, reliability and humility. Multiple sources may be used, including clinicians, allied health personnel and peers. Reports are based on non-planned observations over a longer period of time (a night shift, a week, or longer)
Product evaluation	Includes entries into the electronic health record, presentations, QI products

or impaired, different language and culture), etc. A summative entrustment decision must be grounded sufficiently in a conviction that the learner can manage these situations and knows when to ask for help. Here is where EBDs can be particularly helpful. EBDs can be structured using four questions: 1) Can the learner explain what was done? 2) Does the learner show sufficient understanding of the background/underlying issues? 3) Does the learner show understanding of the potential risks and complications of what was done? and 4) What would the learner have done if the situation, patient or findings had been different? The latter two questions are particularly helpful for appreciating the risks of entrustment.

Longitudinal practice observations are observations in the natural course of clinical work over an extended period of time by whoever is in the position to observe. In contrast to short practice observations, they may or may not be planned for assessment purposes. Observers may be clinical educators, other health professional colleagues or staff, senior or peer learners, and even patients. The focus of observation is on the more general features that are important for trust (integrity, reliability, humility). Therefore, useful settings could include weekend or night shifts. Observers may be asked ahead to evaluate this behaviour and report with narrative comments, which can serve both as feedback and as an information source to inform summative entrustment decisions. Multi-source feedback is one example of longitudinal practice observations that exhibits a more planned, prolonged period of observation by selected observers.

Work products generated by everyday work or the workplace curriculum may provide additional insights into learner performance. For instance, clinical educators or competency committees can evaluate documentations of patient care (e.g. health record entries, discharge summaries, postoperative reports), self-reports of learning (e.g. activity logs, reflection reports, self-assessments and remediation plans), presentations, and results of clinical work (e.g. work quality/quantity, patient satisfaction).

Feedback

Feedback is an important part of any workplace-based assessment program. The EPA framework can help improve the quality of feedback by providing structure and focus to the feedback. Clinical educators often default to specific domains or activities on which they provide feedback (e.g. provider–patient communications, physical examination skills, or management plans). As a result, learners may not receive feedback on the breadth of professional activities expected of them. The EPAs can serve as a reminder to clinical educators to provide feedback on the breadth of all activities relevant to their workplace, and help identify opportunities for assessment and feedback (e.g. transitions of care responsibility, team collaboration, and identification of systems failures). More importantly, the entrustment scales help clinical educators focus on learner behaviours that allow progression to greater autonomy and patient care responsibility. This includes not just feedback to improve ability, but feedback to promote learner integrity, reliability and humility.

Finally, a brief note on terminology. While there is wide interest in the concept of entrustment decisions and EPAs, 'trustworthiness' is not the terminology to use in entrustment and supervision scales or in feedback. Labelling a learner as 'not (yet) trustworthy' leads to negative and incorrect connotations of character flaws and problems with the learner. Rather, we strongly advise using language that indicates placement along a trajectory of growth. We prefer *readiness* (i.e. 'not yet ready' or 'ready') for indirect supervision or unsupervised practice, or the AAMC Core-EPAs terminology of the 'pre-entrustable' and 'entrustable' learner (Englander et al., 2014).

Evaluating learner progression

Assessments within the EPA framework should lead to practical impact on learner responsibilities. As learners show that they can be trusted with activities, they should be rewarded with increasing responsibility and allowed to progress to greater autonomy. This should occur not just on a summative basis, when learners are formally advanced and awarded with a promise of greater autonomy for future clinical cases/ situations. It should also occur on an ad hoc basis, with individual clinical educators in specific contexts and with successive clinical educators in the same and/or different contexts.

To promote learner progression and enable the awarding of increasing responsibility by successive clinical educators, learner performance needs to be monitored and tracked over time, and this information made available to the learners and their future clinical educators. New cycles of clinical education (placements or programs) should rely on information that is passed forward to serve as a basis for establishing justified presumptive trust (see Fig. 20.1). Use of a portfolio system that employs technology to continuously collect, analyse, summarise and present data can greatly facilitate this process. It can provide a current overview of the learner's progression to all stakeholders, including learners, mentors/coaches, competency committees, clinical educators and other members of the clinical workplace.

Even in lieu of a comprehensive e-portfolio, learners can be awarded with 'badges' indicating summative achievement of certain entrustment levels for specific EPAs that may be shared with members of the clinical workplace, and clinical educators can hand learners off to successive educators with information about ad hoc entrustability for specific activities within certain contexts. These physical or electronic badges for EPAs are particularly helpful in healthcare settings, in which it is important for all stakeholders to know what learners are expected and allowed to do independently — a requirement of some healthcare accrediting agencies.

Aggregate data on the progression of all learners, which can be available within an e-portfolio system, can also be analysed at the programmatic level to inform curricular improvement efforts. Information should be used to determine gaps in the curriculum, the adequacy of learning/practice opportunities, and the best sequencing of these opportunities. Since published EPAs have been defined primarily through consensus methods, it is also important to determine from aggregate learner performance data whether the consensus entrustment expectations for specific EPAs are realistic and appropriate. Some EPAs may need to be adjusted after initial introduction, either up or down, in scope or in the expected entrustment level at completion of training.

Case study 20.1 (continued): Application to learning and teaching contexts

Returning to our case, David and Amy, the two learners, complete their clinical placement. Caroline, the clinical educator, sits down to complete the residency's new EPA-based assessment forms. Based on her experience with the previous assessment forms, she expects to give Amy higher overall ratings for her greater fund of knowledge and clinical skills. However, when Caroline applies the concept of entrustment and supervision levels using the EPA assessment form, she finds that she rates David more highly. Because David understands his limitations and appropriately asks for help when needed, she finds she can, and has been, providing him with more autonomy. In contrast, Caroline does not feel she can trust Amy to be reliable or willing to admit mistakes. In fact, she has been putting increasing limits on Amy's autonomy, and checking her work more than the work of the other residents. As Caroline submits the EPA assessment forms, she reflects that the EPA ratings represent well how she would prefer to staff the community clinic to ensure delivery of safe optimal care to her patients.

Caroline also realises that she ought to have discussed with Amy, and provided feedback about, the incident involving the child with a cough. Amy had commented that she discovered but did not report the findings on her examination because she did not believe they were important enough to mention. Was this Amy's way of saving face rather than admitting that she had missed the findings on physical examination? Did she leave out information in order to push forward her diagnosis? Or did she not recognise the significance of the lung findings? With an improved understanding of the underlying issue (lapse of ability, integrity, reliability or humility, versus a misunderstanding of expectations), Caroline could have focused the feedback on behaviours that would help Amy achieve greater autonomy and assume greater patient care responsibility. She should have helped Amy recognise that breaching the trust she had, by not reporting critical information, had set her back and required a restoration of trust, which takes more time and effort than she might realise.

Based on the lessons learned with Amy and David, Caroline realises she should change her approach to teaching. With the next cohort of learners, she takes the following steps:

1. Caroline welcomes the learners by setting clear expectations for the clinical placement, and talking explicitly about the concepts of trust and entrustment. She explains that her daily decisions about how to supervise their engagement in patient care activities, and her summative assessments of them at the end of their clinical placement, will be based on entrustment for specific activities. She describes the qualities of ability, integrity, reliability and humility, which all need to be in place to enable entrustment.

2. Caroline reviews the relevant EPAs for the clinical placement with the learners. She provides information on the typical learning trajectory and level of mastery learners usually reach at the end of the placement. She asks them about their experiences with the EPAs to date, and for their self-assessment of the supervision required for each EPA. Together they look at the elaborated descriptions to identify the requisite knowledge, skills and attitudes needed to master each EPA. Caroline uses this information to inform her teaching, and encourages the learners to bring to her attention opportunities they may identify for supporting their learning and progression to greater autonomy.

3. In addition, Caroline empowers the learners to own the feedback process. She encourages them to direct her attention to areas of individual need and to growth targets. She also charges them with the responsibility for ensuring that, over their time together, they receive feedback on each of the relevant EPAs.

4. As Caroline begins working with the learners, she remembers to use artifacts of the learners' work in the clinic to supplement her observations of their workplace activities. For instance, she reviews their documentation with attention to integrity and reliability as well as ability, and obtains multi-source feedback from others in the clinic community on the learners' reliability and humility. However, she is concerned that all of the recent patients have had uncomplicated, minor illnesses, and she needs to gain insight into whether the learners would be able to manage sicker patients. Caroline decides to use the technique of EBDs regularly to further push and explore the learners' knowledge. Even though the patient today had a mild cough and no fever, she asks the learners what they would have done differently if the patient had had five days of fever and/or had evidence of respiratory distress.

5. To increase the frequency of feedback to her learners, Caroline decides to limit the amount of feedback, focusing on just one EPA or issue in each feedback encounter. She also now frames her feedback around the behaviours she would like to see the learner demonstrate, so that she may provide the learner with greater responsibility and autonomy. She finds this allows her to talk about specific behaviours rather than provide general comments and ratings about performance (e.g. 'you are doing well'). She also finds that she can address issues beyond ability more easily (e.g. 'I would like to see you ask for help earlier. If I know you will come find me when you are uncertain, I would be more comfortable having you see less stable patients').

6. Caroline realises that for the learners to progress to greater responsibility and supervision, the learners need ad hoc opportunities to practise performing at these higher levels with her support. She therefore looks for opportunities to slowly increase the scope of activities (e.g. by varying the context, type of patients), and to incrementally decrease the level of supervision ad hoc. As the learners demonstrate their entrustability in these opportunities, she rewards them with continuing increases in responsibility and autonomy.

7. Lastly, Caroline ensures that she shares the learners' levels of entrustment for specific EPAs with other members of the clinic community. This allows other members of the clinic to engage or support the learners in their safe participation in patient care. The other clinic members are also able to provide information about the learners' performance and readiness for increased responsibilities.

The new cohort of learners in Caroline's clinic respond well to this new approach to their workplace learning. The EPAs and entrustment levels provide them with clear targets towards which to work. They are motivated by the ability to gain additional responsibility and autonomy, and proactively request observations and feedback in order to ensure their personal progression towards mastery of specific EPAs. They appreciate the behavioural focus of the feedback they receive, which provides more specific information on how they may be rewarded with greater responsibility. The learners are also appreciative of the positive feedback they receive when they acknowledge gaps in their knowledge and skills, and seek appropriate help. The learners feel safe in admitting oversights/mistakes, and are willing to engage in conversations about inconsistencies in their performance to improve their readiness for entrustment.

Potential directions for evaluation and research

The concept of EPAs is relatively new, and at the time of publication of this chapter (2018) most studies have focusd on the theoretical evidence supporting the use of EPAs in assessment, content validity evidence for different sets of EPAs for various disciplines and programs, early implementation studies, and studies on the use of entrustability scales and factors affecting entrustment decisions. Further validity evidence is emerging for internal structure, response process, relations to other variables, and consequences. Continued evaluation of EPAs for assessment will help inform best practices for implementation, including engagement of members of the clinical community other than the clinical educator in the assessment process, summative entrustment decision-making (who and upon what and how much evidence), and faculty development needs of clinical educators and other entrustment decision-makers.

EPAs have allowed stakeholders to clarify the expectations around transition points, such as between undergraduate and postgraduate education, and offer an assessment strategy for the realisation of true competency-based education with time-variable, competency-based advancement. The following are therefore important areas for additional research.

1. *Cohesion of the learning curriculum and experience throughout health professions training:* Are transitions during training, and from training to practice, improved? How do stakeholders on the receiving side of the transition view the credibility of the entrustment decisions made by those preparing learners for the transition?

2. *Competency-based advancement:* What are the advantages/disadvantages of time variability and the impact of time-variability on transitions along the training continuum? Are there strategies for achieving competency-based education within time-fixed programs?

3. *Educational design studies of EPA-based workplace curricula:* How does the performance of graduates trained with an EPA-based curricula compare with those trained with more traditional workplace curricula?

In addition to providing insights into assessments and curricula, these studies have the ability to contribute to theory-building while implementations are being carried out (Plomp & Nieveen, 2010).

PRACTICAL TIPS

1. *Encourage continuity to facilitate the development of trust.* Clinical educators need to have sufficient opportunities to develop trust in a learner. The longer the relationship, the better the entrustment decisions. However, curricular and workplace structures may not necessarily provide longitudinal clinical placements or consistent clinical educator–learner pairings. In these circumstances, clinical educators can employ alternative strategies to facilitate building relationships and trust. For instance, junior learners can be paired with senior learners on similar clinical placement schedules to provide alternative sources of continuity in learner supervision. Clinical educators can hand off or transfer responsibility for learners, similar to how they transfer responsibility for patients, to ensure continuity of supervision.

2. *Imagine having the learner as the healthcare provider for your family member.* Sometimes clinical educators may feel uneasy about granting a learner more responsibility or autonomy despite available evidence that may support a higher entrustment level for the learner. These gut feelings may be giving voice to the educator's unconscious processing of previous experiences with this learner or other similar learners. Because not everything can be easily measured or articulated, it is important that clinical educators listen to and reflect on their gut feelings, and examine the information they have on the learner's ability, integrity, reliability and humility.

3. *Adapt the language in the entrustment and supervision scale as needed to suit the local context of clinical educators.* The wording of published entrustment and supervision scales may not necessarily resonate with clinical educators in all contexts. The question of whether a learner is ready for reactive/on-demand supervision may be more difficult for an anaesthetist to answer than the question of whether they feel they can step out of the operating theatre to have lunch, leaving the learner a way to contact them as needed (Weller et al., 2017). Adapting language to local contexts may help support clinical educators' development efforts and the successful implementation of EPAs for assessment.

Conclusion

In this chapter, we introduced the concept of EPAs, a relatively new and exciting framework for the assessment of competencies in the clinical workplace. It places emphasis on safe patient care, and uses the entrustment decisions made about learner participation in the workplace to provide information on learner competence. Assessment using the EPA framework takes into account future performance with an unknown case, and addresses not just the learner's ability but also their integrity, reliability and humility. It makes clear the consequences of assessment for the learner and the patient/public, and includes permission for professional practice and expectations for safe and quality care of patients.

Over the past decade, EPAs have become increasingly popular among postgraduate and undergraduate medical education programs in several countries, including the United States, Canada, Australia/New Zealand, the Netherlands, Switzerland and others. They are also being actively developed for nursing, midwifery, physician assistant training, pharmacy, dentistry and veterinary medicine. As they are further developed and implemented, EPAs will likely affect the future of competency-based assessment and advancement in multiple health professions education programs and in many countries.

Further reading and online resources

Chen, H. C., van den Broek, W. E. S., & ten Cate, O. (2015). The case for use of entrustable professional activities in undergraduate medical education. *Academic Medicine*, 90(4), 431–436.

ten Cate, O. (2017). Competency-based medical education and its competency-frameworks. In M. Mulder (Ed.), *Competence-based vocational and professional education: Bridging the worlds of work and education* (pp. 903–929). Cham: Springer International Publishing Switzerland.

ten Cate, O., Chen, H. C., Hoff, R. G., et al. (2015). Curriculum development for the workplace using entrustable professional activities (EPAs): AMEE Guide No. 99. *Medical Teacher*, 37(12), 983–1002.

ten Cate, O., Hart, D., Ankel, F., et al. (2016). Entrustment decision-making in clinical training. *Academic Medicine*, 91(2), 191–198.

Animations created for instruction

College of Anaesthetists of Ireland [animation video of the EPA Team explaining EPAs]. <https://www.anaesthesia.ie/index.php/epa>; <https://www.youtube.com/watch?time_continue=118&v=ZW87vvc5Bgg>.

Dutch Federation of Medical Specialties [animation video explaining EPAs for postgraduate training]. <https://vimeo.com/178895320>.

University of Toronto [animation video explaining EPAs]. <https://www.youtube.com/watch?v=HS5BUiAMKW8>.

A search of YouTube using 'entrustable professional activities' will yield additional explanations from local, national and international conferences and webinars that can be helpful.

References

Albanese, M. (2000). Challenges in using rater judgements in medical education. *Journal of Evaluation in Clinical Practice, 6*(3), 305–319.

American Educational Research Association (AERA)/American Psychological Association/National Council on Measurement in Education. (2014). *Standards for educational and psychological testing.* (B. Plake, L. Wise, & others, Eds.). Washington, DC: AERA.

Billett, S. (2001). *Learning in the workplace: Strategies for effective practice.* Crow's Nest, NSW: Allen and Unwin.

Billett, S. (2004). Workplace participatory practices: Conceptualising workplaces as learning environments. *Journal of Workplace Learning, 16*(6), 312–324.

Billett, S. (2006). Constituting the workplace curriculum. *Journal of Curriculum Studies, 38*(1), 31–48.

Boyce, P., Spratt, C., Davies, M., et al. (2011). Using entrustable professional activities to guide curriculum development in psychiatry training. *BMC Medical Education, 11*(1), 96.

Brooks, M. A. (2009). Medical education and the tyranny of competency. *Perspectives in Biology and Medicine, 52*(1), 90–102.

Carraccio, C., & Burke, A. E. (2010). Beyond competencies and milestones: Adding meaning through context. *Journal of Graduate Medical Education, 2*(3), 419–422.

Carraccio, C., Englander, R., Gilhooly, J., et al. (2016). Building a framework of entrustable professional activities, supported by competencies and milestones, to bridge the educational continuum. *Academic Medicine, 92*(3), 324–330.

Chen, H. C., McNamara, M., Teherani, A., et al. (2016). Developing entrustable professional activities for entry into clerkship. *Academic Medicine, 91*(2), 247–255.

Chen, H. C., van den Broek, W. E. S., & ten Cate, O. (2015). The case for use of entrustable professional activities in undergraduate medical education. *Academic Medicine, 90*(4), 431–436.

Cianciolo, A., & Kegg, J. (2013). Behavioral specification of the entrustment process. *Journal of Graduate Medical Education, 5*(1), 10–12.

Collins, A. (2005). Cognitive apprenticeship. In R. K. Sawyer (Ed.), *The Cambridge handbook of the learning sciences* (pp. 47–60). Cambridge: Cambridge University Press.

Crossley, J. G. M. (2014). Addressing learner disorientation: Give them a roadmap. *Medical Teacher, 36*(8), 685–691.

Crossley, J., Johnson, G., Booth, J., et al. (2011). Good questions, good answers: Construct alignment improves the performance of workplace-based assessment scales. *Medical Education, 45*(6), 560–569.

Crossley, J., & Jolly, B. (2012). Making sense of work-based assessment: Ask the right questions, in the right way, about the right things, of the right people. *Medical Education, 46*(1), 28–37.

Cruess, R. L., & Cruess, S. R. (2014). Professional trust. In W. Cockerham, R. Dingwall, & S. Quah (Eds.), *The Wiley Blackwell encyclopedia of health, illness, behavior, and society.* Hoboken, NJ: John Wiley & Sons.

Daly, M., Roberts, C., Kumar, K., et al. (2013). Longitudinal integrated rural placements: A social learning systems perspective. *Medical Education, 47*(4), 352–361.

Damodaran, A., Shulruf, B., & Jones, P. (2017). Trust and risk: A model for medical education. *Medical Education, 51*(5), 892–902.

Dornan, T., Boshuizen, H., King, N., et al. (2007). Experience-based learning: A model linking the processes and outcomes of medical students' workplace learning. *Medical Education, 41*(1), 84–91.

Duijn, C., ten Cate, O., Bok, H. G. J., et al. (n.d.). Entrustable professional activities in competency-based veterinary education in farm animal health care. *Medical Teacher,* [accepted].

Durning, S. J., & Artino, A. R. (2011). Situativity theory: A perspective on how participants and the environment can interact. AMEE Guide No. 52. *Medical Teacher, 33*(3), 188–199.

Egan, T., & Jaye, C. (2009). Communities of clinical practice: The social organization of clinical learning. *Health, 13*(1), 107–125.

Englander, R., Flynn, T., Call, S., et al. (2014). *Core entrustable professional activities for entering residency: Curriculum developers' guide.* Washington, DC: Association of American Medical Colleges.

Eraut, M. (2007). Learning from other people in the workplace. *Oxford Review of Education, 33*(4), 403–422.

Frank, J. R., Snell, L. S., Cate, O. T., et al. (2010). Competency-based medical education: Theory to practice. *Medical Teacher, 32*(8), 638–645.

Frank, J., Snell, L., & Sherbino, J. (Eds.). (2015). *CanMEDS 2015 Physician Competency Framework.*

Gandamihardja, T. A. (2014). The role of communities of practice in surgical education. *Journal of Surgical Education, 71*(4), 645–649.

George, B. C., Teitelbaum, E. N., Meyerson, S. L., et al. (2014). Reliability, validity, and feasibility of the Zwisch scale for the assessment of intraoperative performance. *Journal of Surgical Education, 71*(6), e90–e96.

Gigerenzer, G. (2007). *Gut feelings. The intelligence of the unconscious.* New York: Penguin.

Govaerts, M. J. B., van der Vleuten, C. P. M., Schuwirth, L. W. T., et al. (2007). Broadening perspectives on clinical performance assessment: Rethinking the nature of in-training assessment. *Advances in Health Sciences Education: Theory and Practice, 12*(2), 239–260.

Hauer, K. E., ten Cate, O., Boscardin, C., et al. (2014). Understanding trust as an essential element of trainee supervision and learning in the workplace. *Advances in Health Sciences Education: Theory and Practice, 19*(3), 435–456.

Holzhausen, Y., Maaz, A., Cianciolo, A. T., et al. (2017). Applying occupational and organizational psychology theory to entrustment decision-making about trainees in health care: A conceptual model. *Perspectives on Medical Education, 6*(2), 119–126.

Ilgen, J. S., Ma, I. W. Y., Hatala, R., et al. (2015). A systematic review of validity evidence for checklists versus global rating scales in simulation-based assessment. *Medical Education, 49*(2), 161–173.

Jaye, C., Egan, T., & Smith-Han, K. (2010). Communities of clinical practice and normalising technologies of self: Learning to fit in on the surgical ward. *Anthropology & Medicine, 17*(1), 59–73.

Kennedy, T. J. T., Regehr, G., Baker, G. R., et al. (2008). Point-of-care assessment of medical trainee competence for independent clinical work. *Academic Medicine, 83*(10 Suppl.), S89–S92.

Kogan, J. R., Conforti, L. N., Bernabeo, E., et al. (2015). How faculty members experience workplace-based assessment rater training: A qualitative study. *Medical Education, 49*(7), 692–708.

Kogan, J. R., Conforti, L. N., Iobst, W. F., et al. (2014). Reconceptualizing variable rater assessments as both an educational and clinical care problem. *Academic Medicine, 89*(5), 1–7.

Kogan, J. R., Holmboe, E. S., & Hauer, K. E. (2009). Tools for direct observation and assessment of clinical skills of medical trainees: A systematic review. *Journal of the American Medical Association, 302*(12), 1316–1326.

Lave, J., & Wenger, E. (1991). *Situated learning. Legitimate peripheral participation.* Cambridge: Cambridge University Press.

Lurie, S. J. (2012). History and practice of competency-based assessment. *Medical Education, 46*(1), 49–57.

Massie, J., & Ali, J. M. (2016). Workplace-based assessment: A review of user perceptions and strategies to address the identified shortcomings. *Advances in Health Sciences Education: Theory and Practice, 21*(2), 455–473. doi:10.1007/s10459-015-9614-0.

Mayer, R. C., Davis, J. H., & Schoorman, F. D. (1995). An integrative model of organizational trust. *Academy of Management Review, 20*(3), 709–734.

Mink, R. B., Schwartz, A., Herman, B. E., et al. (2017). Validity of level of supervision scales for assessing pediatric fellows on the common pediatric subspecialty entrustable professional activities. *Academic Medicine,* doi:10.1097/ACM.0000000000001820.

Morris, C., & Blaney, D. (2013). Work-based learning. In T. Swanwick (Ed.), *Understanding medical education: Evidence, theory and practice* (pp. 97–109). Edinburgh: Association for the Study of Medical Education.

Mulder, H., ten Cate, O. T., Daalder, R., et al. (2010). Building a competency-based workplace curriculum around entrustable professional activities: The case of physician assistant training. *Medical Teacher, 32*(10), e453–e459.

Norcini, J., & Burch, V. (2007). Workplace-based assessment as an educational tool. AMEE Guide No. 31. *Medical Teacher, 29*(9), 855–871.

Papa, F. J., & Harasym, P. H. (1999). Medical curriculum reform in North America, 1765 to the present: A cognitive science perspective. *Academic Medicine, 74*(2), 154–164.

Pittenger, A. L., Chapman, S. A., Frail, C. K., et al. (2016). Entrustable professional activities for pharmacy practice. *American Journal of Pharmaceutical Education, 80*(4), 57.

Plomp, T., & Nieveen, N. (Eds.), (2010). *An introduction to educational design research: Proceedings of the seminar conducted at the East China Normal University, Shanghai (PR China), November 23–26, 2007.* Enschede: SLO — Netherlands Institute for Curriculum Development.

Regehr, G., MacRae, H., Reznick, R. K., et al. (1998). Comparing the psychometric properties of checklists and global ratings scales for assessment performance on an OSCE-format Examination. *Academic Medicine, 73,* 993–997.

Rekman, J., Gofton, W., Dudek, N., et al. (2016). Entrustability scales: Outlining their usefulness for competency-based clinical assessment. *Academic Medicine, 91*(2), 186–190.

Sheehan, D. (2011). Clinical learning within a community of practice framework. *Focus on Health Professional Education: A Multidisciplinary Journal, 12*(3), 1–16.

Sterkenburg, A., Barach, P., Kalkman, C., et al. (2010). When do supervising physicians decide to entrust residents with unsupervised tasks? *Academic Medicine, 85*(9), 1408–1417.

Strand, P., Edgren, G., Borna, P., et al. (2015). Conceptions of how a learning or teaching curriculum, workplace culture and agency of individuals shape medical student learning and supervisory practices in the clinical workplace. *Advances in Health Sciences Education: Theory and Practice, 20*(2), 531–557.

ten Cate, O. (2005). Entrustability of professional activities and competency-based training. *Medical Education, 39*(12), 1176–1177.

ten Cate, O. (2006). Trust, competence, and the supervisor's role in postgraduate training. *British Medical Journal, 333*(7571), 748–751.

ten Cate, O. (2013). Competency-based education, entrustable professional activities, and the power of language. *Journal of Graduate Medical Education, 5*(1), 6–7.

ten Cate, O. (2017a). Entrustment decisions: Bringing the patient into the assessment equation. *Academic Medicine, 92*(6), 736–738.

ten Cate, O. (2017b). Managing risks and benefits: Key issues in entrustment decisions. *Medical Education, 51*(9), 879–881.

ten Cate, O., Chen, H. C., Hoff, R. G., et al. (2015). Curriculum development for the workplace using entrustable professional activities (EPAs): AMEE Guide No. 99. *Medical Teacher, 37*(12), 983–1002.

ten Cate, O., Hart, D., Ankel, F., et al. (2016). Entrustment decision making in clinical training. *Academic Medicine, 91*(2), 191–198.

ten Cate, O., & Hoff, R. (2017). From case-based to entrustment-based discussions. *The Clinical Teacher, 14*(6), 385–389.

ten Cate, O., & Scheele, F. (2007). Competency-based postgraduate training: Can we bridge the gap between theory and clinical practice? *Academic Medicine, 82*(6), 542–547.

ten Cate, O., Snell, L., & Carraccio, C. (2010). Medical competence: The interplay between individual ability and the health care environment. *Medical Teacher, 32*(8), 669–675.

Teunissen, P. W. (2009). *Unravelling learning by doing.* (Doctoral dissertation. Amsterdam, VU University).

Touchie, C., & ten Cate, O. (2016). The promise, perils, problems and progress of competency-based medical education. *Medical Education, 50*(1), 93–100.

Warm, E. J., Held, J. D., Hellmann, M., et al. (2016). Entrusting observable practice activities and milestones over the 36 months of an internal medicine residency. *Academic Medicine, 91*(10), 1398–1405.

Weller, J. M., Castanelli, D. J., Chen, Y., et al. (2017). Making robust assessments of specialist trainees' workplace performance. *British Journal of Anaesthesia,* *118*(2), 207–214.

Weller, J. M., Misur, M., Nicolson, S., et al. (2014). Can I leave the theatre? A key to more reliable workplace-based assessment. *British Journal of Anaesthesia, 112*(March), 1083–1091.

Wenger, E. (1998). *Communities of practice: Learning, meaning, and identity.* Cambridge: Cambridge University Press.

Wiersma, F., Berkvens, J., & ten Cate, O. (2017). Flexibility in individualized, competency-based workplace curricula with EPAs: Analyzing four cohorts of physician assistants in training. *Medical Teacher, 39*(5), 1–5.

Wijnen-Meijer, M., van der Schaaf, M., Booij, M., et al. (2013a). An argument-based approach to the validation of UHTRUST: Can we measure how recent graduates can be trusted with unfamiliar tasks? *Advances in Health Sciences Education: Theory and Practice, 18*(5), 1009–1027.

Wijnen-Meijer, M., Van der Schaaf, M., Nillesen, K., et al. (2013b). Essential facets of competence that enable trust in graduates: A Delphi study among physician educators in the Netherlands. *Journal of Graduate Medical Education, 5*(1), 46–53.

Wisman-Zwarter, N., van der Schaaf, M., ten Cate, O., et al. (2016). Transforming the learning outcomes of anaesthesiology training into entrustable professional activities: A Delphi study. *European Journal of Anaesthesiology, 33*(8), 559–567.

21

Reworking feedback to build better work

Elizabeth Molloy and Monica van de Ridder

Introduction

For healthcare practitioners, feedback seems to pervade all aspects of daily work. Colleagues in the emergency department will observe a procedure and offer advice on how to better stabilise the intubating tube. One colleague may congratulate another colleague during closure of a surgical procedure and comment on the factors that made it so successful. A physiotherapist may press on a segment of the spine and gauge the haptic feedback that tells them whether a joint is hypo- or hypermobile. Or a patient may come back to the consulting rooms and state that they did not really understand the instructions about what to do, and what to avoid, after their operation. In healthcare work there are also more formalised channels for feedback, such as filming of simulated procedures where the tape is rolled back and a debrief ensues on aspects of practice that could be improved at the next attempt. There are also mandated annual performance development sessions where goals are set for the coming year, and, for those involved in research, regular feedback is received from peers about the quality of their submitted work. Although feedback is ubiquitous in the working lives of practitioners, surprisingly little time is spent in formal education programs dealing with what it is, how it can work for the learner and how learners might apply these skills in giving and receiving feedback in their future working lives as practitioners (Molloy & Boud, 2014).

Students often build their understanding of the job that feedback is designed to do through exposure to assessment in their programs (Watling et al., 2013); that is, through exams and assignments in the classroom setting, and through case presentations, work-based assessments and longitudinal assessments in clinical placements. Feedback is often seen by students as comments from teachers that help to explain the mark allocated (Boud & Molloy, 2013a; Carless et al., 2011). The early adoption of this narrow notion of feedback, including students' perceptions of their role within the process, continues to be reinforced in work-based learning where supervisors typically 'tell' learners what went well and what went wrong in the observed performance (Molloy & Boud, 2014; Molloy, 2009; Fernando et al., 2008; Ende et al., 1995). With these types of unidirectional rituals, it is of little surprise that students are dissatisfied with feedback, and see feedback as information they are subject to, rather than a process that they drive for their own benefit.

Given the dissatisfaction with feedback from both learner and educator perspectives (Carless et al., 2011), there has been an increasing focus over the last five years on conceptualising feedback from a constructivist perspective where learners actively participate in the process (Eva & Regehr, 2005; Boud & Molloy, 2013a; van de Ridder, McGaghie et al., 2015). To help learners to take a proactive role in the feedback dialogue, *feedback literacy* is necessary. There is a growing body of literature devoted to building feedback literacy in learners (Winstone et al., 2017; Esterhazy & Damşa, 2017). This notion of feedback literacy builds on the work of Smith and colleagues (2013) with their exploration of assessment literacy in higher education. Assessment literacy is described as learners' induction into the roles and processes of assessment. Similarly, feedback literacy is about learners and providers gaining a theoretical and embodied understanding of the role, processes and results of feedback. Winstone and colleagues (2017) use the term 'proactive recipience' to depict the learner's active engagement with feedback processes, which necessarily involves the contribution and responsibility of the learner. 'There is increasing consensus that a critical determinant of feedback effectiveness is the quality of learners' engagement with, and use of, the feedback they receive' (Winstone et al. 2017, p 17). Others in the higher education literature have described this 'front-foot learner stance' as learner-centred feedback (Archer, 2010; van de Ridder, McGaghie et al., 2015), 'agentic engagement' (Reeve & Tseng, 2011) or Feedback Mark 2 (Boud & Molloy, 2013b). The aim of this type of feedback is, of course, to improve the quality of the immediate task and importantly, build a practitioner disposition for seeking, providing and using feedback within the workplace. This rationale feels more compelling than the alternative of 'listen to what you are told', which places a high degree of responsibility on the clinical educator who must carefully generate the comments, and a high degree of crossing the fingers in the hope that learners will respond to messages in predictable ways.

This chapter discusses *why feedback is important* in learning in clinical contexts, and highlights key recent studies that have examined what works and through what mechanisms. Results of observational studies are synthesised to illuminate what is *not working in the feedback process* for learners, patients and clinical supervisors. Based on the literature, we examine alternative ways to see feedback as a set of processes that learners can design, engage in and use for their short-term as well as longer term advantage. In particular, we draw on the model Feedback Mark 2, with its roots in constructivism, as a sensitising agent to alert us to the notion that verbal feedback in the workplace is a relational activity and an activity in which the learner benefits from actively playing a part.

For too long, clinical educators have engaged in faculty development short courses on feedback where the emphasis is purely on *feedback providing*. In many courses, the role of the learner is underemphasised, as are techniques on how to foster a *feedback dialogue that has an effect*. With this premise, it is not surprising that feedback in clinical education has been found to be problematic. We argue that it may be the lack of consideration of context and relationships that have rendered feedback as one of the most problematic aspects of the student experience (Molloy & Boud, 2013a, Winstone et al., 2017).

Why is feedback important?

Review studies by Kluger and DeNisi (1996), Hattie and Timperely (2007) and Shute (2008) highlight the benefits of feedback for student learning. Feedback, under the right conditions, can help learners to see the strengths and deficits in their performance, and help learners to try different strategies to further improve their work (Archer, 2010; van de Ridder, McGaghie et al., 2015). Ironically, the very need for feedback is that we all have blind spots when it comes to our behaviour. Engagement with externally generated feedback is an important mechanism that helps us to calibrate our judgment about the quality of our work and the work of others, known as evaluative judgment (Tai et al., 2015; Ramani, Konings et al., 2017). This dialogue with 'the other' (peer, patient or teacher) helps orient the learner to what constitutes good work and helps the learner to sharpen their own 'internal radar' for times when external input cannot be sought (Boud & Molloy, 2013b; Ramani, Konings et al., 2017; van de Ridder, Berk et al., 2015). These necessary components for effective feedback were described in Sadler's (1989) seminal paper on feedback in higher education, where he stated that learners needed to understand the goal of performance, the actual performance undertaken and how to bridge the gap between the two. Helping learners to understand these three processes would place the learner in a better position to self-regulate their practice in the clinical setting.

Feedback serves a number of functions. Often when we think of the functions of feedback we relate this to the *learner* and we underestimate the function of feedback for *patient care*, *collaboration* with other healthcare providers and the *feedback providers*. The functions of feedback, as described by the literature, are highlighted below.

Teaching and correcting learners

When thinking about feedback we mostly think about feedback as a *teaching* tool to help bring the learner closer to the practice goal (Irby, 1995; Norcini & Burch, 2007; Veloski et al., 2006). Feedback, specific information about a comparison between the learner's observed behaviour and a standard given with the intent to improve the learner's performance (van de Ridder et al., 2008), can be used to *correct* learners and to *transfer* knowledge or skills: 'When you are exploring patient's history, don't forget to use open questions, because …' 'Wash your hands after leaving the patients room, to avoid spreading germs.' The goal of this type of feedback is teaching learners how to become better healthcare providers. Ideally, learners and feedback providers can together engage in a discussion about the performance. However, when a learner is performing a surgical procedure and is about to make an incision in the wrong place, a unidirectional correction from the clinical educator is the most appropriate response.

Revealing learners' blind spots

Help from people or artefacts around us — be it from patient, teacher, colleague, peer or equipment — is key to improving performance. Learners cannot rely on their own self-evaluation alone as a trigger for improvement (Kruger & Dunning, 1999; Kent & Molloy, 2013; Ramani, Konings et al., 2017; van de Ridder, Berk et al., 2015). The information from an external source can inform the learner about their own blind spots. A blind spot is defined as an area that is hidden for ourselves but known to another (Ramani, Post et al., 2017; Stone & Heen, 2015). Learners at all points along the spectrum of expertise (including senior experienced consultants) need to have people around them who have an eye for quality practice and an eye out for blind spots. They not only need to have an eye for this, but also need to engage in a dialogue about these blind spots, making the learner aware of them. Being aware of our blind spots is the first step to changing or working on them.

Reinforcing learners

Another function of feedback is to reinforce to learners when they are demonstrating desirable behaviour, knowledge or attitudes (Ilgen et al., 1979). Sometimes learners are not aware that they show 'good' behaviour. They may exhibit the target behaviours deemed to be part of competence, but do not know that they have demonstrated these characteristics, or the reasoning behind it. Examples might be certain reactions in conversations that learners did not plan to give, but they happen. By making these actions that the learner is not aware of explicit, and explaining *what* worked well and *why* this reaction worked so well in a given situation, the feedback is helpful, reinforcing the learner to keep this reaction. Another situation might be where a learner is not sure about their behaviour. By explaining to the learner what did go well and why it went well, the process can help overcome the learner's insecurity and this serves to reinforce the learner's productive approaches to clinical practice (Batista, 2013; Feys et al., 2011).

Motivating learners

Feedback can also function to motivate the learner (Ilgen et al., 1979; Kluger & DeNisi, 1996). Feedback that has a motivational function is given to encourage the learner to have a go and try more complex tasks. In this case, it is important that the feedback provider and the learner know what is motivating. Some learners with an external feedback preference (Herold et al., 1996) might be motivated when they hear what they can improve and how. It can be motivating when learners notice that a supervisor is really paying attention to them and that their practice and development matters to this person. Other students need to hear what is going well and why (Batista, 2013; Feys et al., 2011). It is hard to say what type of feedback is motivating for a learner, because this is so dependent on the learner's history, feedback preferences and learning approaches, as well as on the task they are performing. Therefore, it is important that both the feedback provider and the learner have a conversation at the start of the placement about what works and what doesn't (Ajjawi et al., 2017; van de Ridder, Berk et al., 2015). Observing for the effect of feedback conversations on learner performance is another way to gauge what works for the learner in terms of the conversational approach.

Identifying the gap between the learner's goal and performance

Feedback processes help the learner to see the difference between actual performance (knowledge, skills and attitudes) and the goal of performance (Ilgen et al., 1979; Sadler, 1989; van de Ridder et al., 2008). Used in this way, feedback can inform learners about the distance they need to travel, and the directions they might take to achieve their goal.

Improving patient safety and patient care

When feedback is given in an honest way and learners and the team act on the feedback and follow through, skill acquisition can be accelerated. Learners are entrusted to take on certain tasks, depending on their prior performance and perceived level of capability in the particular domain of practice. If the feedback information affects the learning curve and reveals that learners are improving quickly, it may help improve patient care. Instead of trying five times on the same patient to insert an intravenous line, with focused observation and specific feedback, the learner may be able to master the skill sooner, meaning that the patient's experience and recovery may be improved (van de Ridder, Berk et al., 2015; Veloski et al., 2006).

Collaboration with peers and other healthcare providers

Peers and colleagues in the workplace are important sources of feedback. When a learner receives honest feedback and the learner is able to apply the information to improve subsequent practice, this can improve collaboration among healthcare providers and is more likely to result in an open and rich feedback culture. When it becomes clear that learners are able to act on feedback and show improvement in performance, or if they show the willingness to become better in areas they are not good at, this can establish trust within a team. Trust, in turn, has been shown to perpetuate a positive learning culture (Batista, 2013; Brown & Porter, 2006; Slootweg et al., 2014).

Benefits to the feedback provider

When the relationship between the feedback provider and the learner is healthy, and both parties respect each other, the feedback provider can reflect with the learner on the feedback that was generated. The feedback provider can ask for feedback on their feedback (in addition for observing for the effect of feedback). This makes the feedback situation a learning situation for the feedback provider as well (van de Ridder, Berk et al., 2015). A feedback provider who is interested in learners will also gain a lot of information about the learning process in itself, being watchful for how information is processed and which type of information may, or may not, have an effect. The other key advantage for the feedback provider is that, through engagement in the feedback process, they are forced to consider standards of practice, some of which are more implicit than others. Feedback providers are not always aware of the implicit norms and values they hold as a standard. Through asking questions as part of a dialogue, learners can help to make these implicit norms and values explicit. This is an important, and less examined, function of feedback (van de Ridder, Berk et al., 2015).

What's wrong with current feedback practices in the workplace?

Feedback has been reported as one of the steepest challenges facing higher education (Winstone et al., 2017; Esterhazy & Damşa, 2017). Students feel that they do not get enough feedback, and that when they do receive feedback, it is difficult to use for their benefit. These findings are also reflected in studies within the health professions education literature. Observational studies in clinical education have demonstrated that feedback is often delivered in a didactic way from clinical educators to students (Ende et al., 1995; Molloy, 2009; Johnson et al. 2016). A study by Molloy (2009) highlighted that when students were exposed to these didactic forms of feedback, they had little opportunity to evaluate their own performance and very little investment in goal-setting and planning for future tasks. The other finding in this observational study was that learners, when interviewed after the formal feedback session, had very different 'take-home points' compared with what clinical educators' reported when they were interviewed about the outcomes of the feedback session. Without an invitation to summarise the take-home messages from the discussion, there is no avenue for both parties to check for shared understanding of the discussion, including plans for future practice and observation.

Feedback as monologue

The unidirectional nature of feedback discussions may help to explain the phenomenon that even when supervisors are crafting detailed messages about learners' performance in the workplace, learners often don't act on the advice. Sadler (1989, p 119) pointed out the 'common but puzzling observation that even when teachers provide students with valid and reliable judgments about the quality of their work, improvement does not necessarily follow'. If learners have an active role in the discussion about their own performance, if their own perspectives are sought, and responded to, and if they are encouraged to work within conversations to devise goals that might work for them, we may see more translation of strategies for improvement into practice (Boud & Molloy, 2013a).

The literature tells us that students respond differently to feedback information depending on the circumstances and what they bring to the occasion, including their knowledge of, and prior experience with, feedback (Winstone et al., 2017; Kluger & DeNisi, 1996).

Underestimating the learner–teacher relationship in feedback

There is also a groundswell of evidence suggesting that the relationship between learner and clinical teacher has a strong influence on the learning that takes place through feedback processes (Telio et al., 2015; Telio et al., 2016; Urquhart et al., 2014; Pugh & Hatala, 2016; Ross et al., 2016; Wearne, 2016). Telio and colleagues' (2015) description of the 'educational alliance' has roots in the therapeutic alliance between patient and therapist. If the learner feels that the supervisor has their best interests at heart, and if they have an established trusted relationship, they are more likely to 'hear' and respond to the feedback message, regardless of whether it is positive or negative in direction. Establishing trusted relationships between learner and clinical educator is further challenged by the current climate of clinical training characterised by shorter rotations and fewer opportunities for direct observation of performance (Ajjawi et al., 2017).

The importance of this relationship in feedback exchanges does not come as a surprise given that feedback is inherently an emotional business. Learners, at all points of expertise (from undergraduate students through to experienced practitioners), are typically invested in their work and their identity as a practitioner. If they receive information that challenges the stability of their views about themselves in work, this can create a sense of turbulence and discomfort. Researchers exploring the intersection between emotion and feedback report on the tendency of learners to feel defensive when they receive 'negative feedback' (Molloy et al., 2013). Butler and Winne (1995) and Watling and colleagues (2013) have described a range of maladaptive responses to feedback that serve to deflect the responsibility of the learner to act on the advice and instead challenge the viewpoint of the feedback provider or challenge the very credibility of the provider themselves.

Not only can students find feedback difficult 'to take', but supervisors can also find feedback difficult 'to give' (Molloy, 2009). Supervisors have reported feeling attune to learners' emotions, and often get themselves linguistically tangled, in anticipation of the emotional response that may be triggered through difficult conversations. This 'mealy mouthed' (Molloy et al., 2013) approach to feedback has also been described by Ende (1983) as 'vanishing feedback' because the message, for the learner, disappears in the supervisor's attempt to construct a conversation that is sensitive to the learner's feelings. Again, this supervisor effort in 'delivery' or 'monologue construction' or 'sweetening the pill' seems to be rather displaced. What would a feedback culture look like in the workplace if more effort was expended up front in orienting all parties to the ideal processes of feedback? Making role expectations clearer, and expending energy on developing positive relationships where trust is a central tenet, would seem a smarter strategy (Molloy et al., 2013; Watling et al., 2013; van de Ridder, Berk et al., 2015).

There is a fear that feedback can harm the relationship between the learner and the supervisor, and the world of clinical practice is a small one. Both parties are afraid of this (Audia & Locke, 2004). This is one of the reasons why feedback providers struggle to be honest with the learner and why they deliver models of feedback such as the feedback sandwich or 'sugar coated pill' (Molloy et al., 2013). This is also one of the reasons why the learner finds it difficult to explain to the feedback provider why certain feedback was not helpful.

Feedback that does not lead to improvement

Feedback can be detrimental to performance (Kluger & DeNisi, 1996). Some studies have shown that the learner focuses on part of the task and is not able to pay attention to the task as a whole. The specific element on which the feedback was given could be improved, but the task as a whole did not improve. Another explanation is that there might not be sufficient time for the feedback information to sink in. It needs to be processed and this takes varying amounts of time depending on the learner and the context of learning (Arora et al., 2010). The outcomes might not be visible on the level that the feedback provider and the learner anticipate. For example, the feedback might have led to increased awareness, which may manifest as a request for more support during the next task attempt, and potentially performance improvement on subsequent task attempts. The feedback conversation is effective in inviting change, but the change may not be captured at the level that the outcomes are measured.

Tokenism

Another reason why feedback may not have an effect is in the circumstance where both the learner and the supervisor engage in a feedback episode because it is seen as a requirement, instead of a learning opportunity. When feedback is seen as a requirement, the feedback can become a set of hollow sentences without adding value. This tokenistic approach to feedback is a serious threat to a healthy feedback culture in the workplace. The tension implicit in summative assessment and developmental feedback also means that students may 'game' the feedback discussions to present 'their best selves' and preserve face (Molloy & Boud, 2013a). This student reluctance to expose their own deficits in performance can represent a loss in the potential of feedback for learning.

Case study 21.1: Feedback in a neurological rehabilitation placement

The clinical supervisor

Julia is an experienced neurologist working in a rural rehabilitation hospital. She has many years of experience working with patients with degenerative neurological conditions such as multiple sclerosis and Parkinson's disease. Earlier this year, the rehabilitation hospital signed a contract with the university and now has 'teaching hospital status' in taking a group of four undergraduate medical students for a six-week clinical placement in neurology. Julia is pleased when the contract is signed as she has had what seems like a lifetime of experience in work-based training, and she feels she understands the benefits to the health service, patients and the supervising clinicians themselves in having students on clinical placement. At the same time, a week before commencement of the first wave of students, Julia does feel some apprehension about the new commitment: 'How much time will the students take up? Who will take the lead in supervising the students on a Tuesday morning when I head up to the city for the case review meeting? Am I up to the task in terms of filling out all the paperwork for the university and running the six work-based assessments per student that are stipulated for the six-week placement?'

Julia has worked with postgraduate trainees on the neurology training program but it has been years since she has worked with pre-service medical students. Julia is most concerned about giving feedback to students. To do this, she knows she needs to be able to judge what's good and what's inadequate for a student at this level of experience.

The learner

Pearl is in her final year of medical school and so far she has performed well in her studies. At university, her marks were excellent and most of her work-based assessments in clinical placements have been good during her rotations in cardiology, surgery and general practice (primary care). This is Pearl's first exposure to a rehabilitation facility. Based on advice from peers who have already cycled through this rehabilitation placement, Pearl anticipates that the pace will be slower in the rehab setting, and that the need for diagnostic skills will be reduced, as referrals would arrive from acute hospital wards, stipulating the patient's condition. Contrary to her expectations, five days in, Pearl feels as if she is at sea. She realises that assessment and care of patients at this point in their recovery is just as complex as in acute care, and that her understanding of anatomy and physiology is not adequate for the demands of the job. Not only does she feel her knowledge is down, but her reflex, muscle and sensation testing, and functional assessments don't seem to be as advanced as her peers. During the week, her supervisor, Julia, watched her complete a full assessment of a patient with Parkinson's disease and all these deficits were pointed out to her, including the fact she was flustered. The informal feedback didn't help Pearl's confidence or performance, and all weekend she has had a knot in her stomach, anticipating the second week of placement.

Feedback as seen through a constructivist lens

How we look at feedback is determined by the theoretical lens we use. In the literature, feedback has been viewed through many different lenses such as functionalism, behaviourism, cognitivism and constructivism (van de Ridder, 2015a). Kanselaar and colleagues (2000) point out that constructivism is not one concept but consists of a series of beliefs about the nature of reality, the nature of mind, and educational beliefs on how to support learning. What do we mean by these beliefs and how do they affect our beliefs about, and practices in, feedback?

Nature of reality: reality is constructed in the mind of the learner

All humans experience the real world, but every individual will ascribe a different meaning to this experience (Ponterotto, 2005). Because meaning is rooted in an individual's experience, there is not only one correct meaning. Knowledge and reality can therefore only be constructed by the learner (Kanselaar et al., 2000) through interaction with the environment. This means that there are *multiple* realities. This is an important notion for feedback. Based on an observation of the learner's performance, both the learner and the feedback provider may have two different realities. The feedback provider does not know the learner's reality, and vice versa. Therefore, exploring each other's thought processes is important: getting to know each other's reality and trying to understand it. The dialogue is crucial. Questions from the feedback provider for the learner could be: What was your sense of the consultation this morning? What was your approach and what are your thoughts behind this? Questions for the feedback provider from the learner could be: Can you explain why this is so important for me to change? Are there any other alternatives to the approach you suggest?

Nature of mind: learning as construction of own knowledge

Every person has different experiences, a different frame of reference and different knowledge. Based on our previous experiences, the knowledge we have and our frame of reference, we construct our reality. We relate our experience to previous experiences, we merge new knowledge with our existing knowledge, and our frame of reference determines how we perceive and label our observations. In this way we construct our knowledge. Because every learner and every feedback provider has different anchor points (knowledge, experience and frame of reference), the knowledge construction from both the learner and the feedback provider will be different. This knowledge resides in an individual's internal state and is not always apparent to others (Anderson et al., 1999). Instead of making assumptions about the knowledge and the learning process of the learner, active enquiry is crucial in the feedback process. An example is asking the learner during the feedback exchange: What did you learn from the discussion? What are you going to apply in practice? How? (van de Ridder, 2015b). Furthermore, it is important for feedback providers to consider that using the same feedback messages and approaches for different learners — even if they are in the equivalent stage of their course/training — might have different effects. Anticipating that giving 'good feedback' might not lead to the effect you expected is important.

Educational beliefs on how to support learning: interaction with learning materials and others is crucial

The learning environment provides stimuli and tools for engaging in this knowledge construction process (Duffy & Jonassen, 1991; Phye, 1997). Meaningful interactions between the learner and the context need to be sought (Anderson et al., 1999). These interactions — including engagement with patients, teachers, peers, teaching materials, teaching activities and the workplace culture — lead to knowledge construction. Authentic activities, considered to be meaningful and purposeful, are important for learning. Because every learner has their own reality and constructs their own knowledge, knowing the learner's goals is key to the feedback process. What would they like to learn? How can this learning be best facilitated? Through what means might the learner gain improvement? Could the learner practise on standardised patients, take a course, have access to certain reading materials? Observe certain practitioners on the wards? How much scaffolding should be offered to the learner?

In feedback dialogues, clinical educators often reach for these suggested processes when helping the learner to devise their follow-up plan. Not all suggestions will work, because each individual has their personal learning experience. The most important aspect is that the feedback needs to be tailored to the learner's individual needs (van de Ridder, 2015b). With increasing focus on learning objectives, standards of performance and equity in access to learning materials, feedback is one of the only modalities in education that can be tailored specifically to the individual learner. For the learner it is important to realise that feedback providers differ from each other. Based on their experience they give suggestions on how knowledge, attitudes and behaviour can be changed. Some feedback will be useful; other feedback might not be useful. Here the learner uses their own judgment about the credibility of the teacher and their own knowledge about the relative effect of the teacher's advice on the quality of their work (Watling et al., 2013).

> **Case study 21.1 (continued):** Formal feedback episode between learner and supervisor
>
> At the end of week three, Pearl and Julia meet for their scheduled half-way feedback session to discuss progress so far. Julia says she is going to use the medical school competency form (based on CanMEDS standards) to guide the discussion. Pearl is nervous about the discussion and does not pick up that Julia, too, despite her seniority, is not comfortable in approaching the feedback session. Julia can see that Pearl is a keen student and that her anxiety seems to be negatively affecting her performance. Julia is very mindful that she does not want to come down hard on Pearl, because Pearl already seems hard on herself. When they first sit down in the student interview room Julia asks Pearl 'How do you think you're going so far?'
>
> Pearl responds: 'Not bad, but probably not good enough.'
>
> Julia extends another probe to follow up on Pearl's statement: 'Tell me, what you mean by that?'
>
> Pearl responds: 'Well it's such a different way of thinking in neuro rehab, and I'm not sure I have the knack. I'm used to differential diagnosis and finding out what the problem is and then prescribing the fix. And in most cases in my last placements my ideas seemed to be fairly much in line with my supervisor's approach. Here, I just don't know what the fix is. It sort of ... it sort of feels like the patients have this depressing level of impairment, and that this functional impairment is not going to get better, and I don't want to throw my hands up and say "we can't do much for you" and I don't want to say "I know just the thing that's going to work for you", so I'm sort of struggling to work out the goals of treatment, let alone how I would go about communicating these in a sensitive way to the patient.'
>
> Julia doesn't respond to Pearl's concerns here, and instead signals that she wants to talk about a patient interaction she observed Pearl undertake in week one (a full assessment of a patient with late-stage Parkinson's disease). Even though Julia is thorough with her explanations of what she observed, Pearl finds herself feeling distracted and angry that of all examples, Julia has chosen to draw on this one where she performed particularly poorly. Pearl has lost the thread of the conversation. They finish the feedback session after 25 minutes (Pearl hasn't spoken since the 5-minute mark) and Julia mentions that she will follow up with Pearl early in the week to see how the progress is going. Pearl feels that her suspicions are confirmed, that she's not cut out for this type of work and, if anything, she feels more at sea than before the feedback session.

Feedback evolution from behaviourism to constructivism

Feedback Mark 0, Mark 1 and Mark 2

Models of feedback have been presented by Molloy and Boud (2013b) to describe ways that feedback is enacted in learning and teaching contexts. Feedback Mark 2 builds off the more behaviourist-informed Feedback Mark 1 and re-conceptualises feedback as a set of processes driven by learners and teachers together, rather than an act of 'telling' imposed on learners. Below, we highlight the key features of Feedback Mark 0, Mark 1 and Mark 2 and how they might manifest in clinical education.

Feedback Mark 0: hopefully useful information

Feedback Mark 0, as its name suggests, is equivalent to zero feedback. Alarmingly, it represents much of the feedback observed in workplace learning. It comprises clinical educators telling learners what they need to improve on, and the process ends on the telling (Molloy, 2009). With no follow-up, there is no way to establish whether the feedback has an effect. There is no collaborative development of strategies for improvement, and no opportunities set up for learners to put into effect the new strategies devised through dialogue. Very often, the unpredictable nature of clinical education, with little control over the setting up of experiences with certain qualities, including the presentation of patients with certain characteristics, means that students may have little opportunity to improve their work. Without opportunities 'for another try' in close succession, students may feel less inclined to make meaning from the comments they receive. Another reason students might not engage with comments is that they do not understand the meaning within the educator's monologue. A study by Molloy (2009) found that learners' understanding of key messages after a feedback session was very different from the supervisor's interpretation of what was discussed. Without an opportunity for dialogue there is little opportunity for clarifying, meaning-making or ownership/investment in ideas. In summary, feedback that resembles Feedback Mark 0 is 'hopefully useful information' at best.

Feedback Mark 1: inputs and outputs

Feedback Mark 1 represents an improvement on Feedback Mark 0, in that feedback is designed to have an effect. The model of feedback in clinical education is equivalent to an engineering model of feedback, such as the thermostat (Molloy & Boud, 2013b), where there is a designated set point (or standard, such as 18°C), an input (detection of current room temperature) and an output (either heating or cooling as required to achieve the set point). In applying this model of feedback to clinical education, learners and clinical educators have a shared understanding of the standard of clinical practice (set point), the educator provides comments for improvement (input) and then there is engagement in a subsequent overlapping task that enables the feedback to have an effect (the output). The important facet of this model is that task design is important, including the fact that the subsequent tasks must have some overlapping features to the prior tasks to enable demonstration of effect.

Not only does the learner benefit from this model, through improved clinical performance, but the educator also benefits in that they have a chance to monitor the influence of their comments on the learner's performance. That is, observation of the effect on the next task helps educators to calibrate their own capacity to generate useful comments. If there is a change in a positive direction, educators are encouraged to continue with the feedback approach; and if there is no change, or there is deterioration in student performance, there is an impetus for the educator to reconsider their feedback approach (content of comments, process, timing, complexity of task selected etc). The feedback loop, as depicted in Fig. 21.1, therefore benefits both the learner and the educator.

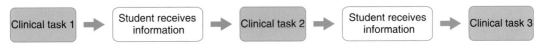

Figure 21.1: Feedback Mark 1: looking for effect
Source: Adapted from Molloy, E., & Boud, D. (2013). Changing conceptions of feedback. In D. Boud & E. Molloy (Eds.), Feedback in higher and professional education (pp 11–33). London: Routledge.

Feedback Mark 2

Feedback Mark 1 would be quite sufficient if learners were machines and displayed similar characteristics to thermostats. We know with certainty, however, that different learners respond differently to the same input, depending on their prior experiences, knowledge base, skills, motivations and relationship with 'the other' in the learning context (Esterhazy & Damşa, 2017). This means that we need to move beyond behaviourism and view feedback from a constructivist lens where learners and 'others' (teachers, peers, patients) co-construct meaning from experience and dialogue. Through identifying their own needs and practice goals, learners are more likely to assimilate the strategies devised for improvement. This dialogic form of feedback not only acknowledges the agency of the learner within a feedback encounter or within a clinical placement, but also, if practised enough, may generate reflective patterns within learners. Developing self-regulatory capacities in the learner is desirable, but this requires displays of vulnerability and establishment of trust between parties. 'By playing active roles in the feedback process and engaging with the comments they receive, learners can develop the skills to self-regulate their learning, meaning they will not always be dependent on others for appraisal' (Winstone et al., 2017, p 18).

Fig. 21.2 illustrates the key components of Feedback Mark 2. Engagement of the learner within all of the processes is a hallmark of Feedback Mark 2, particularly when it comes to privileging the learner's evaluative judgment within the dialogue. It is also important to note that the 'looking for effect' characteristic of Feedback Mark 1 is maintained in this model (depicted by Activity 1 and Activity 2 in the model), meaning that task selection, timing of information and task engagement remain important features in the feedback model. The definition that accompanies Feedback Mark 2 is: 'Feedback is a process whereby learners obtain information about their work in order to appreciate the similarities and differences between the appropriate standards for any given work, and the qualities of the work itself, in order to generate improved work' (Boud & Molloy, 2013a, p 6). Along with privileging the notion that feedback is only feedback if it has an effect, this definition positions the learner as the seeker, generator, interpreter and user of information. It is a significant contrast to behaviourist-informed notions of feedback where learners are positioned as passive recipients of information. Ironically, this passive positioning in the workplace is often reinforced through curriculum in higher education where students have little agency within feedback.

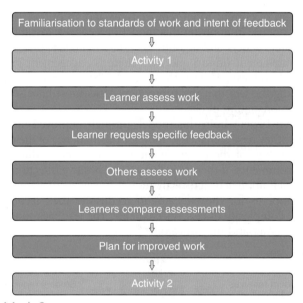

Figure 21.2: Feedback Mark 2

Source: Adapted from Molloy, E., & Boud, D. (2013). Changing conceptions of feedback. In D. Boud & E. Molloy (Eds.), Feedback in higher and professional education *(pp 11–33). London: Routledge.*

Feedback culture

Case study 21.1 outlined above reflects the constructivist principles of Feedback Mark 2. Both the learner, Pearl, and the educator, Julia, have a high degree of feedback literacy, a notional and embodied understanding of the role, processes and results of feedback in learning (Winstone et al., 2017). Table 21.1 depicts the hallmarks of different feedback cultures that manifest in clinical education. Case IV, 'Feedback as output: closing the loop' exemplifies a rich feedback culture where both parties are aware of their role in feedback, both parties engage in the processes, and the outputs extend beyond immediate performance improvement to include gains in evaluative judgment.

Case study 21.1 (continued): How the feedback interaction would look if guided by Feedback Mark 2

If Julia and Pearl had shared expectations about feedback as a process whereby they both had responsibility to contribute, the process might have yielded more productive outcomes. This is a 'take two' scenario, based on Feedback Mark 2.

Pearl starts her neurological rotation, and her clinical educator, Julia, suggests that they devote an hour to discussing Pearl's learning goals for the six-week placement. In this discussion, Pearl highlights the rotations she has experienced so far that year, the types of challenges she has found with her learning and performance, and the strategies that seem to have worked well for her (e.g. at the close of each day, if Pearl writes down a patient list with priorities for the next day on the ward, it helps to set her up and guides her study priorities for that evening). In this learning needs discussion, Julia extends an invitation for Pearl to express any concerns she has about the upcoming placement, and about neurology in general. Pearl is able to express that she is unclear about the sorts of demands of this rehabilitation environment (it is her first experience) and that the only cues she has received are from peers who have found the pace to be slower and therefore less intimidating than acute hospital environments where the stakes might be higher.

This open dialogue provides a platform for Julia to express some of her experiences in acute versus rehabilitation-based care, and to challenge the myth that rehabilitation is less demanding on doctors. Julia gives an example of a patient with end-stage multiple sclerosis and talks about both the medical demands of catheterisation, pain management and managing sleep quality, as well as end-of-life decision-making, goal-setting for the patient in the home or hospital, and support for the family in both of those scenarios. Immediately, this description gives Pearl more insight into what good practice might look like in neurology and palliative care.

They have a discussion about workplace-based assessments as part of the university requirement. Pearl is able to select the patient/condition for these assessments, and Julia discusses the merits of undertaking assessments early, so that feedback can be taken up and incorporated into Pearl's practice throughout the placement. They both have a laugh at the futility of completing the assessments in the last week (in an attempt to look good with more experience under the belt) — basically driving feedback out of the system!

Julia asks Pearl about her experience with feedback, and the type of information and the nature of the interactions she has found most valuable to date. She is interested to hear that Pearl is a pianist and has had a lot of feedback from teachers and examiners through her musical career. They draw parallels to feedback in the workplace, and how important it is for Pearl to be directly observed either by a supervisor (there are three in the department and they will all have different, but hopefully useful, perspectives on Pearl's clinical practice) or by peers (two additional peers on placement). Julia offers her own experience of receiving 'difficult to hear' feedback in her practice (still happens now, even though she is senior) and talks about the merits of self-evaluation, and also allowing time for sometimes confronting, or unexpected, news to marinate.

Throughout the placement, Pearl is committed to asking supervisors to watch for certain aspects of her performance (e.g. 'do you mind watching for my reflex testing in this patient assessment?') and again asks for feedback after encounters if it is feasible. Although self-evaluation is initially confronting, Pearl learns very quickly that all supervisors have an expectation that learners need to 'explore their own mind' before the external opinion is offered. It becomes less intimidating over time, and even when Pearl doesn't perform in line with her own high expectations, there is something comforting about being able to identify where you think you went wrong, before the educator states their observation. Pearl feels it's a bit like a 'cross for performance' but a 'tick for insight', and this makes her feel like things are going to keep progressing in the right direction. Pearl has had a positive and open relationship with Julia from the start of the placement and she trusts that the feedback, even if it might be difficult to hear, is coming from the right place and hits the right place in that the suggestions they discuss seem to reap positive results. Pearl observes that whenever there is a discussion about improvement, both Pearl and Julia work hard to create a situation where Pearl can have another go at a similar task.

TABLE 21.1: Features of common feedback cultures in the clinical workplace

Case	Case I No news is good news	Case II One way: feedback as input	Case III Dialogue: interaction	Case IV Feedback as output: closing the loop
Description of culture	No 'need' for feedback, if it is needed it is seen as 'a shame'	Feedback as a monologue: what the feedback provider does is most 'important'	Feedback as a dialogue: learner opinion highly valued, eye for the feedback process	Feedback is accessible and embedded in daily activities. Feedback seeking is stimulated. Feedback is normal and part of lifelong learning and practice
Literacy of educators	Educator skills are instruction-based. Feedback reserved for poor performance only: 'pulling up the student'	Educator as observer, diagnostician and crafter of comments. No attention for feedback perception and reception	Educator asks the learner to self-evaluate and validates or contests this with their own view based on observed performance	Feedback is more than comments; through engaging in feedback processes, students gain confidence in their own evaluative judgment and educators further develop their evaluative judgment
Literacy of learners	Not experienced in receiving feedback. Asking for feedback is a sign of weakness or a sign of challenge. Keeping under the radar is a good attribute	Student is the 'thirsty learner', keen for the expert's diagnostics about what to improve	Learners are aware of their role in seeking feedback on performance and in articulating their own perspective on aspects of performance that went well and aspects that need improvement	Learners seek information internally as well as externally from peers, patients and educators to help build a picture of their performance relative to standards. A plan for improvement is made, and there is shared responsibility to follow up on the effects

Feedback cultures in health professions education can differ from country to country, from hospital to hospital and from department to department (van de Ridder, 2015c). Watling and colleagues (2013) compared the medical education training culture with the culture in teacher education and music, and concluded 'medicine's current training culture is not, in fact, a feedback culture'. Credibility and constructiveness of feedback are the vulnerable aspects in our training culture.

Ramani, Post and colleagues' (2017) study describes five aspects of feedback cultures in medical education that could be improved. In many departments there is lack of clear expectations and messages around feedback. Departments frequently have a culture of 'niceness' that can prohibit honest feedback. Bidirectional feedback is not part of the culture. Feedback to learners is common, but there is little 'upward' feedback to faculty. Also the hierarchy in the faculty–resident relationship is not helpful, impacting learner receptivity to feedback (Ramani, Post et al., 2017; Warman et al., 2014). The need for lifelong learning and professional growth needs to be more established.

Feedback culture can be described as 'the organisation's support for feedback, including non-threatening, behaviourally-focused feedback, coaching to help interpret and use feedback, and a strong link between performance improvement and valued outcomes' (London & Smither, 2002, p 2). The literature describes examples of why a supportive feedback culture is important. It improves the likelihood that feedback will be sought, generated and acted upon, and it communicates that learning and development are supported in the organisation (London & Smither, 2002; Rougas et al., 2015). Courses for both feedback providers and receivers to increase feedback literacy are such an example of investing in a strong learning culture (Archer, 2010).

Feedback providers also play an important role. The feedback source needs to be credible (Steelman et al., 2004; Watling et al., 2013). Feedback providers who are honest, observe the learners and have expertise in the area of the feedback reap better results in learners (van de Ridder, Berk et al., 2015). They deliver feedback information tactfully and with respect for the learners (Steelman et al., 2004). A crucial aspect reported is the feedback provider's personal accountability. The leaders and feedback providers need to show that they 'walk the talk'. Educators need to be transparent about their own endeavours in improving their own feedback seeking, feedback reception and feedback giving skills (Batista, 2013).

There is an expanding body of work investigating the role of feedback seeking in building a positive feedback culture. Both learners and feedback providers actively seek feedback opportunities and ask for comments on certain aspects of their performance. This behaviour is encouraged by both learners and faculty (Archer, 2010; Batista, 2013; Sargeant et al., 2010). The feedback opportunities in a strong feedback culture are embedded in all activities in the clinical setting, and the feedback conversation goes both upwards (student gives feedback to faculty) and downwards (faculty gives feedback to students) (Archer, 2010).

Dudek and colleagues (2016) demonstrate in a qualitative study that a feedback culture serves as an enabler for residents to give upward feedback to faculty in a non-anonymous way. The learners feel safe to do this. Embo and colleagues (2014) point out that a healthy feedback culture is necessary because it will not only stimulate students to seek and strive for positive feedback, but also help them to deal with 'negative feedback' or aspects they can improve on. Outside medical education, Levy and Williams (2004, p 895) describe the impact of the feedback culture on annual reviews or 'performance appraisals' in organisations: 'the feedback culture of the organization should play a vital role in how feedback is sought, perceived, processed, accepted, used, and reacted to'. A feedback-rich culture has been found to improve work-related outcomes and success in the market (Baker et al., 2013).

In this chapter, we have problematised feedback, described an alternative way of viewing feedback from a constructivist frame, and drawn on findings from observational studies of feedback in work-based education where learners have played an active role in the process. We hope that through presenting case studies of both unproductive and rich feedback encounters we have helped illuminate conditions and properties that may contribute to more positive outcomes in feedback. Below we present some practical tips for clinical educators wanting to facilitate productive feedback exchanges.

PRACTICAL TIPS

Feedback, when viewed from a constructivist lens, acknowledges the importance of the active role of the learner within the process. Important elements in creating a rich feedback culture include: 1) setting expectations for feedback and the goals of the placement/work; 2) establishing trust, which in turn creates a culture of open disclosure of evaluative judgments and increases the value of messages from others (credibility judgments); and 3) sequencing of tasks to enable closing of the loop (observing for learning outcomes). Tips include:

- Explain that the intention of feedback is for learner improvement (orientation to purpose) and set expectations about the process over the placement (orientation to feedback process).
- Understand that direct observation is at the heart of feedback.
- Be aware that multiple sources of feedback are helpful, including patients, peers and practitioners from different disciplines and professions.
- Seek the opinion of the learner; the learner needs to search their mind too.
- Reinforcement is important (it's not about flattering the ego: the learner might not know they have attained the standard, or know how they got there).
- Know the goals of the learner.
- Tailor the messages to these goals and prioritise the messages. Stick to the big rocks, no need to pack in all the pebbles; the cognitive load of the learner should be considered.
- Check learner perceptions throughout the process: What does the learner see as the priorities? What are the learner's goals going forward? (Encourage the learner to write down the key discussion points and plan for action!)
- Task design is also at the heart of the feedback process. Set up the 'right task' to stretch a learner, and help to set up a subsequent task attempt so the loop can be closed.
- Faculty development has typically focused on educators picking up new techniques for communication of a message, rather than design of the process and culture.
- Learner feedback literacy is key to effective feedback, so students can recognise the opportunities, and have the skills and language to engage in opportunities for learning.
- Feedback giving and receiving are skills that can be acquired through deliberate practice (including feedback on feedback).

Future directions for research

The rationale for looking to a different conception of feedback in the clinical workplace is a compelling one given that research reflects a culture of 'feedback as telling', with little effect on students' learning. The next step is to critically examine the effect of these newer approaches to feedback, where relational and contextual features are acknowledged as important ingredients for learning. Researchers are claiming that a key determinant of feedback quality is in fact the quality of learners' engagement with, and use of, the feedback comments they seek. For this reason, we see one of the research priorities in this field as examining the impact of feedback literacy training on students' performance in the workplace. We anticipate that longitudinal study designs will be employed to trace immediate effects of feedback on study strategies and work, along with students' capacity to self-evaluate and self-regulate as they gain more experience in the workplace.

Acknowledgment of context has been a key missing ingredient in feedback research to date. We expect that observational studies, particularly those using video reflexive ethnography (Iedema, 2011), will feature more in this field. Video-based observation, coupled with reflections by participants, may help to further illuminate the influence of trust (Telio et al., 2016; Watling et al., 2013) and reciprocal vulnerability (Molloy et al., 2013; Bearman & Molloy, 2017) on feedback encounters.

Conclusion

When certain conditions are established, feedback has been shown to be a potent mechanism in learning. However, research in workplace settings indicates that feedback rarely fulfils its job in improving students' performance. In this chapter, we argue that part of the problem with feedback is that we have taken it to be a rather shallow version of its original manifestation in biology and engineering. That is, rather than seeing feedback as a process involving an input and an output, it has been diminished to a ritual whereby the educator comments on the student's performance. From a constructivist viewpoint, feedback is not 'an act' but rather a 'set of acts' extended over time, involving the learner and other parties who are deemed to have a stake in the learner's performance. In order to have an effect, students need to have an opportunity to engage in similar tasks that triggered the 'feedback cascade', thereby enabling a closing of the loop. Looking for an effect helps not only the learner, but also the 'other party' (e.g. the supervisor) in evaluating their own feedback approaches (i.e. if the feedback is working, educators or peers who have contributed to the dialogue are likely to continue to employ similar strategies, and vice versa when the effect is negative).

Creating a culture where student engagement in feedback processes is valued is the key to success. We argue that culture change requires feedback literacy (understanding and doing) on behalf of both learners and clinical educators, and ideally this literacy would be developed progressively throughout professional programs, from day one, year one. Ironically, engaging students in dialogic feedback should help them to build self-regulatory capacities so they can wean themselves off expert-generated comments. Explicit discussions around learning needs and feedback expectations, and establishing professional trust and a shared commitment to follow up on tasks (to look for the effect of feedback), may be important factors in building a rich feedback culture in the workplace.

Acknowledgment

We would like to thank Lyndall Molloy (Liz's mum, 1945–2017) and Otto van de Ridder (Monica's dad, 1942–2017) for their wonderful skills in teaching and feedback. We lost our great mentors during the writing of this chapter, and we would like to dedicate this work to them.

References

Ajjawi, R., Molloy, E., Bearman, M., et al. (2017). Contextual influences on feedback practices: an ecological perspective. In D. Carless, S. Bridges, C. Chan, et al. (Eds.), *Scaling up assessment in higher education* (pp. 129–143). Singapore: Springer.

Anderson, J. R., Rede, L. M., & Simon, H. A. (1999). *Applications and misapplications of cognitive psychology to mathematics education*. ERIC Clearninghouse.

Archer, J. C. (2010). State of the science in health professional education: effective feedback. *Medical Education*, 44(1), 101–108. doi:10.1111/j.1365-2923.2 009.03546.x.

Arora, S., Sevdalis, N., Nestel, D., et al. (2010). The impact of stress on surgical performance: a systematic review of the literature. *Surgery*, 147(3), 318–330, 30 e1–6.

Audia, P. G., & Locke, E. A. (2004). Benefiting from negative feedback. *Human Resource Management Review*, 13(4), 631–646.

Baker, A., Perreault, D., Reid, A., et al. (2013). Feedback and organizations: feedback is good, feedback-friendly culture is better. *Canadian Psychology-Psychologie Canadienne*, 54(4), 260–268. doi:10.1037/a0034691.

Batista, E. (2013). Building a feedback-rich culture. *Harvard Business Review*, https://hbr.org/2013/12/building-a-feedback-rich-culture.

Bearman, M., & Molloy, E. (2017). Intellectual streaking: the value of teachers exposing minds (and hearts). *Medical Teacher*, 39(12), 1284–1285. doi:10.1080/0142159X.2017.1308475.

Boud, D., & Molloy, E. (2013a). What is the problem with feedback? In D. Boud & E. Molloy (Eds.), *Feedback in higher and professional education* (pp. 1–10). London: Routledge.

Boud, D., & Molloy, E. (2013b). Rethinking models of feedback for learning: the challenge of design. *Assessment & Evaluation in Higher Education*, 38(6), 698–712.

Brown, D. S., & Porter, T. (2006). Enhance individual, team and firm performance by creating a feedback culture. *CPA Practice Management Forum*, 2, 14.

Butler, D. L., & Winne, P. H. (1995). Feedback and self-regulated learning: a theoretical synthesis. *Review of Educational Research*, 65(3), 245–281.

Carless, D., Salter, D., Yang, M., et al. (2011). Developing sustainable feedback practices. *Studies in Higher Education*, 36(4), 395–407.

Dudek, N. L., Dojeiji, S., Day, K., et al. (2016). Feedback to supervisors: is anonymity really so important? *Academic Medicine*, 91(9), 1305–1312. doi:10.1097/acm.0000000000001170.

Duffy, T. M., & Jonassen, D. H. (1991). Constructivism: new implications for instructional technology? *Educational Technology*, 31(5), 7–11.

Embo, M., Driessen, E., Valcke, M., et al. (2014). A framework to facilitate self-directed learning, assessment and supervision in midwifery practice: a qualitative study of supervisors' perceptions. *Nurse Education in Practice*, 14(4), 441–446. doi:10.1016/j.nepr.2014.01.015.

Ende, J. (1983). Feedback in clinical medical education. *JAMA: The Journal of the American Medical Association*, 250(6), 777–781. doi:10.1001/jama.1983.03340060055026.

Ende, J., Pomerantz, A., & Erickson, F. (1995). Preceptors' strategies for correcting residents in an ambulatory care medicine setting: a qualitative analysis. *Academic Medicine*, 70(3), 224–229.

Eva, K., & Regehr, G. (2005). Self-assessment in the health professions: a reformulation and research agenda. *Academic Medicine*, 80(10), S46–S54.

Esterhazy, R., & Damşa, C. (2017). Unpacking the feedback process: an analysis of undergraduate students' interactional meaning-making of feedback comments. *Studies in Higher Education*, doi:10.1080/03075079.2017.1359249. August.

Fernando, N., Cleland, J., McKenzie, H., et al. (2008). Identifying the factors that determine feedback given to undergraduate medical students following formative mini-CEX assessments. *Medical Education*, 42(1), 89–95.

Feys, M., Anseel, F., & Wille, B. (2011). Improving feedback reports: the role of procedural information and information specificity. *Academy of Management Learning & Education*, 10(4), 661–681.

Hattie, J., & Timperley, H. (2007). The power of feedback. *Review of Educational Research*, 77(1), 81–112.

Herold, D. M., Parsons, C. K., & Rensvold, R. B. (1996). Individual dirences in the generation and processing of performance feedback. *Educational and Psychological Measurement*, 56(1), 5–25.

Iedema, R. (2011). Creating safety by strengthening clinicians' capacity for reflexivity. *BMJ Quality & Safety*, 20(Suppl. 1), i83–i86.

Ilgen, D. R., Fisher, C. D., & Taylor, M. S. (1979). Consequences of individual feedback on behavior in organizations. *Journal of Applied Psychology*, 64(4), 349.

Irby, D. M. (1995). Teaching and learning in ambulatory care settings: a thematic review of the literature. *Academic Medicine*, 70(10), 898–931.

Johnson, C., Keating, J., Boud, D., et al. (2016). Identifying educator behaviours for high quality verbal feedback in health professions education: literature review and expert refinement. *BMC Medical Education*, 16(1), doi:10.1186/s12909-016-0613-5.

Kanselaar, G., de Jong, T., Andriessen, J., et al. (2000). New technologies. In R. J. Simons, J. van der Linden, & T. Duffy (Eds.), *New learning* (pp. 55–81). Dordrect: Kluwer Academic.

Kent, F., & Molloy, E. (2013). Patient feedback in clinical education: a mixed methodology study. *Focus on Health Professional Education*, 14(2), 21–34.

Kluger, A. N., & DeNisi, A. (1996). The effects of feedback interventions on performance: a historical review, a meta-analysis, and a preliminary feedback intervention theory. *Psychological Bulletin*, 119, 254–284.

Kruger, J., & Dunning, D. (1999). Unskilled and unaware of it: how difficulties in recognizing one's own incompetence lead to inflated self-assessments. *Journal of Personality and Social Psychology*, 77(6), 1121–1134.

Levy, P. E., & Williams, J. R. (2004). The social context of performance appraisal: a review and framework for the future. *Journal of Management*, 30(6), 881–905. doi:10.1016/j.jm.2004.06.005.

London, M., & Smither, J. W. (2002). Feedback orientation, feedback culture, and the longitudinal performance management process. *Human Resource Management Review*, 12(1), 81–100.

Molloy, E. (2009). Time to pause: feedback in clinical education. In C. Delany & E. Molloy (Eds.), *Clinical education in the health professions* (pp. 128–146). Sydney: Elsevier.

Molloy, E., Borello, F., & Epstein, R. (2013). The impact of emotion in feedback. In D. Boud & E. Molloy (Eds.), *Feedback in higher and professional education* (pp. 50–72). London: Routledge.

Molloy, E., & Boud, D. (2013a). Seeking a different angle on feedback in clinical education: the learner as seeker, judge and user of performance information. *Medical Education*, 47(3), 227–229.

Molloy, E., & Boud, D. (2013b). Changing conceptions of feedback. In D. Boud & E. Molloy (Eds.), *Feedback in higher and professional education* (pp. 11–33). London: Routledge.

Molloy, E., & Boud, D. (2014). Feedback models for learning, teaching and performance. In M. Spector, D. Merrill, J. Elen, et al. (Eds.), *Handbook of research on educational communications and technology* (pp. 413–424). New York: Springer.

Norcini, J., & Burch, V. (2007). Workplace-based assessment as an educational tool: AMEE Guide No. 31. *Medical Teacher*, 29(9–10), 855–871.

Phye, G. D. (1997). Epilogue: classroom learning, looking ahead. In G. D. Phye (Ed.), *Handbook of academic learning: construction of knowledge* (pp. 593–596). San Diego: Academic Press.

Ponterotto, J. G. (2005). Qualitative research in counseling psychology: a primer on research paradigms and philosophy of science. *Journal of Counseling Psychology*, 52(2), 126.

Pugh, D., & Hatala, R. (2016). Being a good supervisor: it's all about the relationship. *Medical Education*, 50(4), 395–397.

Ramani, S., Konings, K., Mann, K. V., et al. (2017). Uncovering the unknown: a grounded theory study exploring the impact of self-awareness on the culture of feedback in residency education. *Medical Teacher*, 39(10), 1065–1073. doi:10.1080/0142159x.2017.1353071.

Ramani, S., Post, S. E., Konings, K., et al. (2017). 'It's just not the culture': a qualitative study exploring residents' perceptions of the impact of institutional culture on feedback. *Teaching and Learning in Medicine*, 29(2), 153–161. doi:10.1080/10401334.2016.1244014.

Reeve, J., & Tseng, M. (2011). Agency as a fourth aspect of student engagement during learning activities. *Contemporary Educational Psychology*, 36, 257–267. doi:10.1016/j.cedpsych.2011.05.002.

Ross, S., Dudek, N., Halman, S., et al. (2016). Context, time, and building relationships: bringing in situ feedback into the conversation. *Medical Education*, 50(9), 893–895.

Rougas, S., Clyne, B., Cianciolo, A. T., et al. (2015). An extended validity argument for assessing feedback culture. *Teaching and Learning in Medicine*, 27(4), 355–358. doi:10.1080/10401334.2015.1077133.

Sadler, D. (1989). Formative assessment and the design of instructional systems. *Instructional Science*, 18(2), 119–144.

Sargeant, J., Armson, H., Chesluk, B., et al. (2010). The processes and dimensions of informed self-assessment: a conceptual model. *Academic Medicine*, 85(7), 1212–1220.

Shute, V. J. (2008). Focus on formative feedback. *Review of Educational Research*, 78(1), 153–189. doi:10.3102/0034654307313795.

Slootweg, I. A., Lombarts, K. M., Boerebach, B. C., et al. (2014). Development and validation of an instrument for measuring the quality of teamwork in teaching teams in postgraduate medical training (TeamQ). *PLoS ONE*, 9(11), doi:10.1371/journal.pone.0112805.

Smith, C., Worsfold, K., Davies, L., et al. (2013). Assessment literacy and student learning: the case for explicitly developing students 'assessment literacy'. *Assessment & Evaluation in Higher Education*, 38(1), 44–60. doi:10.108 0/02602938.2011.598636.

Steelman, L. A., Levy, P. E., & Snell, A. F. (2004). The feedback environment scale: construct definition, measurement, and validation. *Educational and Psychological Measurement*, 64(1), 165–184.

Stone, D., & Heen, S. (2015). *Thanks for the feedback: the science and art of receiving feedback well (even when it is off base, unfair, poorly delivered, and frankly, you're not in the mood)*. New York: Penguin.

Tai, J., Canny, B., Haines, T., et al. (2015). Building evaluative judgement through peer-assisted learning: opportunities in clinical medical education. *Advances in Health Sciences Education*, 21, 659–676.

Telio, S., Ajjawi, R., & Regehr, G. (2015). The 'educational alliance' as a framework for reconceptualizing feedback in medical education. *Academic Medicine*, 90(5), 609–614.

Telio, S., Regehr, G., & Ajjawi, R. (2016). Feedback and the educational alliance: examining credibility judgements and their consequences. *Medical Education*, 50(9), 933–942.

Urquhart, L., Rees, C., & Ker, J. (2014). Making sense of feedback experiences: a multi-school study of medical students' narratives. *Medical Education*, 48(2), 189–203.

van de Ridder, J. M. M. (2015a). General introduction. In *Feedback in clinical education* [Thesis] (pp. 11–46). University of Utrecht.

van de Ridder, J. M. M. (2015b). Conclusion and discussion. In *Feedback in clinical education* [Thesis] (pp. 133–162). University of Utrecht.

van de Ridder, J. M. M. (2015c). Measuring trainee perception of the value of feebback in clinical settings (P-FiCS). In *Feedback in clinical education* [Thesis] (pp. 83–102). University of Utrecht.

van de Ridder, J., Berk, F. C. J., Stokking, K. M., et al. (2015). Feedback providers' credibility impacts students' satisfaction with feedback and delayed performance. *Medical Teacher*, 37(8), 767–774. doi:10.3109/ 0142159X.2014.970617.

van de Ridder, J., McGaghie, W. C., Stokking, K. M., et al. (2015). Variables that affect the process and outcome of feedback, relevant for medical training: a meta-review. *Medical Education*, 49(7), 658–673. doi:10.1111/ medu.12744.

van de Ridder, J., Stokking, K. M., McGaghie, W. C., et al. (2008). What is feedback in clinical education? *Medical Education*, 42(2), 189–197.

Veloski, J., Boex, J. R., Grasberger, M. J., et al. (2006). Systematic review of the literature on assessment, feedback and physicians' clinical performance: BEME Guide No. 7. *Medical Teacher*, 28(2), 117–128. doi:10.1080/01421590600622665.

Warman, S. M., Laws, E. J., Crowther, E., et al. (2014). Initiatives to improve feedback culture in the final year of a veterinary program. *Journal of Veterinary Medical Education*, 41(2), 162–171. doi:10.3138/ jvme.1013-142R.

Watling, C., Driessen, E., van der Vleuten, C. P., et al. (2013). Beyond individualism: professional culture and its influence on feedback. *Medical Education*, 47(6), 585–594. doi:10.1111/medu.12150.

Wearne, S. (2016). Effective feedback and the educational alliance. *Medical Education*, 50(9), 891–892.

Winstone, N., Nash, R., Parker, M., et al. (2017). Supporting learners' agentic engagement with feedback: a systematic review and a taxonomy of recipience processes. *Educational Psychologist*, 52(1), 17–37. doi:10.1080/ 00461520.2016.1207538.

Section 4

Leadership and faculty development in health professions education

22

Faculty development
Becoming a 'clinician as educator'

Gabriel Reedy and Anna Jones

Introduction

The idea of 'doctor as teacher' (General Medical Council, 2012) or 'clinician as educator' is a familiar one to clinicians across the health professions, and the key impetus for this book. Many clinicians recognise that a teaching role is integral to their work caring for patients, and so engage in peer teaching, and teaching of students, juniors and patients in both informal and formal settings. However, while the *act* of teaching is commonplace, the work of *becoming* and *being* an educator is an often underexplored aspect of clinical practice. Unlike the rhetoric of evidence-based care on which clinical practice is based, practice as a clinical educator is rarely underpinned by a well-grounded understanding of pedagogical theory and practical applications. Because educational theory is founded on a different epistemology from much of formal medical training (although, we argue, not necessarily different from *good* clinical practice), the ways of thinking that underpin educational theory may seem, at first glance, quite foreign to clinicians (Kneebone, 2002).

This chapter explores what is needed in order to become a 'clinician as educator'. We argue that this needs to be well-grounded in educational theory, clearly applicable to practice and supported by infrastructure. Moreover, we understand that despite the apparent epistemological contradictions, an understanding of pedagogical theory is complementary and enriching to an understanding of clinical practice. We suggest that traditional delineations between learning and teaching, and clinician and teacher, are unhelpful. We argue that the traditional roles of clinicians can be reframed within a faculty development environment so that teachers become less custodians of knowledge and more facilitators of learning.

In clinical professions (unlike in some other fields) there is less bifurcation between clinician and teacher — education is not seen as a lesser activity but rather as central to professional identity. However, we argue that there is a need for education to be seen not as a 'commonsense' activity but rather one that requires careful thought, rigorous intellectual reasoning, a clear conceptual underpinning and the commitment to make intentional decisions. It is through fostering this that faculty development can enable clinicians to become educators.

In this chapter, we explore the development of 'clinician as educator' using two theoretical frameworks drawn from educational theory: threshold concepts (Meyer & Land, 2003, 2006) and signature pedagogies (Shulman, 2005). We believe that these theories can help to conceptualise, explore and more fully understand the ways in which clinicians shape their own career paths to enable them to become educators within their profession, and the ways in which all of us who participate in the endeavour can make the process more useful, engaging and meaningful. We suggest that in this case the 'learner' is clinical faculty, and we outline some of the threshold concepts associated with becoming an educator and the signature pedagogies associated with the health professions.

Threshold concepts (Land, Meyer & Flanagan, 2016) are the set of concepts that are key to mastery of a given discipline or subject area. These concepts are 'threshold' because they share a set of common features and are the gateway to mastery. The elements of acquiring a threshold concept are:

- *transformative*, which involves epistemological, conceptual and ontological shifts for the learner through a *liminal* space;

- *bounded*;

- *integrative, discursive and reconstructive*, enabling the learner to see relationships within the larger conceptual framework within which the concept resides, and to make deeper connections;

- *troublesome knowledge*, since they challenge previously held understandings and assumptions and 'commonsense' knowledge;

- *irreversible*, as they are usually not forgotten once acquired.

Threshold concepts require the learner to enter a 'liminal space' in the process of mastery. In this process the learner enters a phase of doubt, possible misunderstanding and confusion. The learner often needs to mimic and reiterate before they are able to fully grasp, understand and integrate the concept. This process requires a stage of rehearsal and can be sporadic and recursive, until the learner has transformed their own understanding. The liminal space is rarely linear, but rather spiral, and involves progressive advances and regressions.

Signature pedagogies are the particular ways in which each discipline or profession draws in newcomers to the 'critical aspects of the three fundamental dimensions of professional work — to think, to perform, and to act with integrity' (Shulman, 2005, p 52). Signature pedagogies are significant in helping to understand both the content and the process — the 'what' and the 'how' — of how people develop from being a newcomer to a fully functioning member of a profession. Importantly, the conceptual basis of signature pedagogies is that educating members of a profession is fundamentally different from educating in disciplines or domains of knowledge.

Importantly, some of the ways in which clinicians, and perhaps doctors in particular, are educated is traditionally based in a different set of epistemological assumptions, compared with the ways in which educators (who are typically steeped in the applied social sciences) view the world. Although binary characterisations are generally unhelpful when trying to tease apart complex and nuanced work such as that of the clinical educator, traditional and didactic teaching approaches that have dominated the education and training of clinicians are often framed as oppositional to the more constructivist pedagogies proffered by those in the applied social sciences. In that sense these two frameworks — threshold concepts and signature pedagogies — are, we argue, particularly useful. A clinician's professional journey as an educator could be characterised as reconciling the signature pedagogies of their training (often fact-based and grounded in a positivist worldview and epistemology) with more transformative signature pedagogies. Furthermore, this occurs through a conceptualisation of teaching and learning that is grounded in an understanding of the key ideas in education theory and associated practice. Therefore, in developing the skills of 'educator as clinician', they must potentially find ways of embracing signature pedagogies that seem divergent but that, once mastered, can provide a rich and integrated set of conceptual frameworks for understanding, critiquing and changing practice.

In the remainder of this chapter, we briefly explore and argue for the importance of considering these two theoretical approaches for health professions. We then present a case study, drawn from our own work as educators of clinicians, which we believe highlights some of the ways in which these theories can help to explore, unpack and enlighten the process of becoming (and eventually, being) a clinical educator. Finally, we make the case for specific approaches to faculty development that are grounded in theory and in our own practice, which we believe can be helpful in creating an environment where those who seek to can grow and flourish as clinical educators.

Threshold concepts in clinical education

'Threshold concepts' is a useful framework for helping to understand and explore the process of becoming and being an educator. While it does not provide a clear set of steps for the acquisition of educational skills and understanding, it outlines the process and the idea of key (or threshold) concepts that learners need to 'break through' in order to begin to develop as educators and to integrate this understanding into their thinking as clinicians. Without an integrated understanding of the educational threshold concepts, we argue that clinicians cannot fully become clinical educators — and this process is transformative, both epistemologically and ontologically (Meyer & Land, 2003). Meyer and Land (2005) proposed that threshold concepts are characterised as transformative, reconstructive, troublesome, irreversible, integrative, bounded, discursive and liminal (Land et al., 2005; Meyer & Land, 2006; Cousin, 2006). For the sake of clarity, each of these is outlined separately below. Threshold concepts are:

- *transformative*, because the learner's view of the discipline is changed as a result of an emerging understanding of a concept; this enables the forging of a deeper understanding, the ability to make sense of key principles and the ability to make connections;
- *reconstructive*, since by enabling a learner to deconstruct and then reconstruct knowledge, a threshold concept allows a new and different understanding; thus a threshold concept is not just new knowledge but a changed and restructured way of thinking, enabling new insights;
- *troublesome*, since threshold concepts are difficult, sometimes counterintuitive and complex; often they run counter to the set of prior understandings and assumptions — as such, they can take effort on the part of both the teacher and the learner;
- *irreversible*, since once acquired, the learner is permanently transformed by a threshold concept — they shape the ways in which the learner thinks and possibly learns; once a threshold concept is learned, the learner will never again be able to return to a state of 'not knowing' and so will be permanently changed;
- *integrative*, which means that once a threshold concept is understood by a learner, it provides the tools to make connections and to integrate previously divergent concepts, thus enabling links and networked thinking;
- *bounded*, in that they are discipline-specific since they form the key ideas for a particular discipline and may not be of significance in other disciplines or fields or may not be conceptualised in the same way (although many concepts overlap several disciplines);
- *discursive*, because a threshold concept means that the learner can begin to come to terms with the disciplinary epistemology; the concepts provide a language and structure, with vocabulary and grammar within which learners can discuss and interrogate the discipline itself;
- *liminal*, because threshold concepts require a state of confusion, disorientation and misunderstanding before understanding can be reached and this process will be continual and recursive.

Threshold concepts are so important because in the process of acquisition, the learner changes both how they think and how they *are*. As Cousin points out: 'Grasping a threshold concept is transformative because it involves an ontological as well as a conceptual shift. We are what we know. New understandings are assimilated into our biography, becoming part of who we are, how we see and how we feel' (Cousin, 2006, p 4).

In the case of clinical education, by seeing education as not just a set of practical skills but also a discipline, underpinned by complex theories, debates and key concepts, clinical educators can encounter new ways of thinking and teaching. This is conceptual and theoretically and empirically based, rather than a 'tips and tricks' or technical skills approach to teaching. However, this requires carefully planned education programs that address both pedagogical theory and its application to clinical contexts, career rewards and infrastructure in the form of support, such as professional recognition from societies such as the Academy of Medical Educators (AoME). Threshold concepts can provide new perspectives and a framework for curriculum design and teaching (Neve et al., 2016). Through the process of wrestling with a new way of thinking the clinician can not only gain a rich, discursive and integrated understanding of education but also use this knowledge to interrogate their own practice as an educator and that of their profession more generally. They gain new insights into their own work and sometimes into their own identity.

Signature pedagogies and the clinical professions

Educational psychologist Lee Shulman (2005) developed a theoretical model of professional education, based on extensive research with members of various professions, known as signature pedagogies. Taking the idea of pedagogy — which itself combines both the process and the content of education — as the starting point, Shulman argues that a signature pedagogy in a profession has some central dimensions that vary from profession to profession and that are useful to consider. The first is the surface structure, which is the overt and concrete aspects of teaching with which we are probably most familiar. The second is what he refers to as the deep structure: the set of assumptions about knowledge and skills and activity that comprise the profession. Third, Shulman posits what he refers to as the implicit structure of a profession, which includes the moral codes, beliefs and professional values that it encompasses. And finally, a signature pedagogy is notable for what it does not include or impart, often unintentionally so.

However distinctive signature pedagogies might appear when viewed through the lens of a profession, Shulman argues that they also share a number of features that span across various professions. In examining how we bring newcomers into the world of clinical practice, from allied health professions to medicine to dentistry, these features consistently appear in the ways in which we teach and train. If they are not present, Shulman argues, the professional education experience becomes less meaningful, less effective and over time less valuable for both the individual learner and the profession (not to mention the larger society of which our professions are a key part).

Signature pedagogies are pervasive and routine

Shulman (2005) argues that one of the important aspects of a signature pedagogy is that it cuts across the various contexts in which we teach and train professionals, and indeed the settings in which they learn, such that they become both pervasive and routine. This is important and necessary in the context of teaching and learning to become a fully-fledged member of a profession, because professional practice is so complex, nuanced and difficult to achieve that it requires some standardised ways of teaching and learning that can help to enable that transition. In learning to become a clinician, for example, routine approaches to teaching and learning such as bedside teaching 'simplify the dauntingly complex challenges of professional education, because once they are learned and internalised, we don't have to think about them: we can think with them … the routine cushions the burdens of higher learning' (Shulman, 2005, p 56). The routine lowers the cognitive load of an already potentially overwhelming learning situation, and the pervasive nature of the pedagogical approach means that learners can go into a variety of clinical settings knowing what to expect, how to act and what they might be expected to learn from the situation. As such, Shulman notes that these habits of teaching and learning can 'shift new learning into our zones of proximal development, transforming the impossible into the merely difficult' (2005, p 56).

Signature pedagogies involve public performance as a learner

Again, unlike in purely discipline-based teaching, pedagogy in the professions consists of students' active performance of their newly acquired skills and professional competencies (and with it, the continued development of skills under acquisition). For the health professions, this is a fundamental part of the educational experience, even if the nature, scope and scale of this public performance may differ across various professions and educational contexts. Traditionally, medical education is bifurcated into 'pre-clinical' and 'clinical' stages, and academic study in nursing is often divided similarly. However, some dental curricula require students to begin to engage actively with patients during their first year of study, with the tasks students perform developing hand-in-hand with their conceptual knowledge. In almost all cases, the clinical but pre-qualification performance in professional training serves to translate the required conceptual knowledge into the messy reality of professional practice settings, while also exposing learners to the gaze and associated accountability of their teachers, peers and patients.

Regardless of structure, the point of such public performance is clear: to begin to appreciate the uncertain, unpredictable and varied nature of what will be their eventual professional practice. Shulman notes that this 'uncertainty, visibility, and accountability inevitably raise the emotional stakes of the pedagogical encounters … producing both excitement and anxiety' in learners (2005, p 56). As such, these experiences are central in developing professionals who have the character and integrity to make difficult judgments in uncertain situations.

Signature pedagogies are balanced

Finally, in order for a signature pedagogy in the professions to be valuable, it must give due attention to the holistic attributes of what it means to function as a member of the profession. The intellectual component of practice is where most professional training programs begin, and when most people think about what it means to be a health professional, the 'content' is the starting point. One must, after all, know quite a lot about a number of subjects to function as a health professional. The technical skills of professional practice usually follow on from this starting point — and again, this is often reflected in the structure of the curriculum, with pre-clinical learning focusing on bioscience content and clinical experiences focusing on the development of technical competencies. Woven among these in most clinical professions is what Shulman (2005) calls the moral dimension of practice. The tension present in balancing these aspects in a curriculum mirrors the tensions of balancing them in day-to-day clinical practice as a clinician; therefore, attention must be paid to a thoughtful engagement with each. According to Shulman, the effectiveness of pedagogy is compromised when one of these dimensions is subordinated to the others.

Signature pedagogies are resistant to change

Because signature pedagogies are reflective of, emergent from and focused on the professions they represent, they are quite persistent and do not change easily. Rather, Shulman (2005) argues that quite significant changes are required in order to shift the ways in which we train and develop health professionals. Drastic changes in professional practice are one such way of changing signature pedagogies, and one that is starting to have quite a significant impact in the health professions especially. Changes in technology that impact practice, or in technology more generally, can also have an impact on signature pedagogies. Finally, societal shifts and challenges to the legitimacy or sanctity of professional practice can make signature pedagogies change rather dramatically.

Traditional — and emerging — signature pedagogies

Even though professions, and the pedagogies that bear their signatures, are generally resistant to change, the rapid changes in science and medicine and the subsequent changes to clinical practice over the last two generations have generated some significant changes to the way health professionals are trained. The traditional approach to the imparting of clinical knowledge in the health professions was a didactic one that privileged a fixed body of knowledge and mastery of technical skill, and this is embodied in the pre-clinical/clinical practice bifurcation of medical and nursing curricula. Problem-based learning, which emerged in Canada in the 1960s and has spread worldwide since, sought to take a different approach in an effort to rebalance the curriculum and better reflect the nature of the skills and knowledge required by doctors practising in an era of specialised medicine and rapid emergence of scientific knowledge (Davis & Harden, 1999). The approach seeks to situate the learner at the centre of medical training, and to tap into their motivation and enthusiasm to seek out and find the information they need to diagnose and treat patients. In doing so, trainee doctors develop the habits of mind that are required of them as practising professionals. As the approach has gained currency over time, it has achieved a signature status in medical training. Though not universally adopted, it is pervasive across Western medical school contexts and seems to produce practitioners who are both competent and engaged in their training while also being able to effectively treat patients once qualified (Wood, 2003).

Similarly, the bedside teaching approaches that have traditionally been associated with training clinicians in hospital settings have become more difficult to maintain in the context of patients spending less time in hospital and having more care as outpatients or in community care settings. Simultaneously, the time available for training has been decreasing. One answer to this challenge has come with the technological innovations enabling healthcare practitioners to learn in highly realistic simulated settings, using mannequins and skills-based trainers, that can reflect conditions and scenarios that may be rare or challenging for trainee clinicians to handle. Though simulation as a core part of healthcare training has emerged relatively recently, it has quickly become a part of training for clinicians across health professions in many contexts worldwide (Long et al., 2012). Many of the features of a simulation-based approach to healthcare pedagogy reflect the deep, surface and implicit features of a signature pedagogy, and mark a change in the ways in which health professionals learn.

Case study 22.1 Becoming a clinical educator

Maria, an emergency medicine trainee, was an enthusiastic and capable doctor who was comfortably on track for finishing her training and was looking forward to her career as a consultant. She had had some negative experiences as a medical student, and as an early-career trainee, but she also had plenty of quite positive ones that left her motivated and keen to do her best. Furthermore, she came from a family of teachers, so teaching was something she was comfortable with, committed to and interested in. She had very positive learning experiences in simulation, and had seen how valuable the learning was for her own clinical practice as an emergency medicine doctor. Some of her other powerful learning and practice experiences were those where she worked out-of-hospital, such as serving as a medical officer for equestrian events, cycle races and marathons. She knew that she wanted these aspects, along with a clear role supporting medical students and trainees, to be among those that would make the varied career in emergency medicine that she was hoping for.

Maria's decision to pursue her specialty training in emergency medicine had as much to do with her clinical interest as it did with her growing self-identity. For Maria, the identity of 'doctor as teacher' took shape and form in emergency medicine in a way that it had not in her other early training experiences. She began to see what her colleagues and seniors did in emergency medicine as primarily an educative endeavour, because there were constant opportunities to teach, and to learn: collegially with other doctors both within and across the hospital (and beyond, into the community and mental health); across the professions and with the skilled paraprofessionals in the emergency department and the other areas of the hospital; and not least, both from and with patients and their families. The more she spoke with colleagues in emergency medicine, and the further she got into her training, the more her thinking and her identity as an educator developed. She could no longer conceptualise emergency medicine as just any other speciality. It was, for Maria, a new way of seeing herself and her work.

After a few years of training, and spurred on by her burgeoning identity as an educator, Maria applied for and was appointed to a one-year medical education fellowship at a large teaching hospital, which had an organised program of support and development focused around her work as an educator. By design, the fellowship allowed her to continue her specialty training in emergency medicine while she developed her educational work, so she alternated weeks in emergency medicine and teaching in the simulation centre.

One part of the fellowship program was a subsidised postgraduate degree in medical education, which was offered through the university. Maria approached it with enthusiasm, and relished what she spoke about as the challenge of making sense of the concepts and ideas that were occasionally quite different from ways of thinking she was used to from the natural sciences. Maria conceptualised the course as helping to fill in some of the theoretical and empirical bases for what she was doing in her simulation teaching, but over the course of her year she found that it was also bleeding into her thinking about her clinical work.

By having dedicated time for each aspect of her training, and doing them in parallel, Maria began to quickly realise the synergies between the two roles and how she was making significant strides in both domains. Her time in the simulation centre was helping her to become a better emergency medicine doctor, and her time on 'the shop floor' gave her a lot of practical day-to-day experience to discuss in the course and to inform how to make her simulation teaching more relevant. Her fellowship experience offered her an entrée into a team of people who were doing medical education practice and scholarship, and so as she began to grow into the role she also began to grow into the culture associated with it. She worked on teams to draw together conference posters and presentations of their shared work, and to put in place plans for scholarly projects that would take weeks or months to come to fruition. All of which was very different, she noted, from the immediate nature of her work, its impact and feedback on it, which she received in the emergency department.

In developing herself as a simulation educator, Maria noticed the importance of practising and asking for feedback on her debriefing skills. She began to shift, slowly but certainly, away from what she called her natural didactic teaching pose towards what she referred to as a more facilitative stance: she began to see from some more experienced colleagues that providing a supportive space for learners to explore their practice and their ideas was potentially much more powerful than them being 'told the right answer'. She began to conceptualise that her role as an educator was to provide something much more than her trainees could get in a book, and therefore required more from her than just knowing content. Her extensive experience as a senior emergency medicine registrar provided something so much more: the ability to help trainees consider *why* to make care and treatment decisions, rather than simply *what* care or treatment to provide.

Over the course of the year, Maria grappled with one of the most common things asked of healthcare professionals: how to be 'reflective' in her training as a clinician and educator, and what the process of reflection means for her professional life. She identified it as an issue early in her training, noting with annoyance that she was *required* to reflect by any number of workplace-based assessments. Surely, she argued, that is a paradox: being reflective should be an internal and self-generated process, and any requirement to do so obviously negates the value of it. By identifying her concern and talking through it with colleagues in the emergency department and on the course, with her tutors and with her own trainees, she began to think more carefully and critically about this concept as she developed her thinking and practice over the year. She took the opportunity to write about reflection as one of her course assessments, considering how reflection was related to theory and evidence in professional education. By the end of the year, she came to conceptualise reflection in a very different way: it was, she determined, core to what she did on a day-to-day basis as a senior trainee who was on the cusp of a consultant post. It was, she determined after talking it through extensively with her consultant mentors, central to their practice as well. She also found that in debriefing simulation-based education, guiding trainees and colleagues towards reflection helped them to think carefully and critically about how to improve their own practice. She began to reframe reflection from a required activity to something that, for her, is central to the role of an emergency medicine consultant. The job requires that she constantly consider her actions and interactions based on her previous knowledge and experience, and what she might change or maintain about her practice on an ongoing basis. In her work as an educator, Maria realised that helping trainees to reflect on their practice gave her new insight on reflecting on her own practice.

By the end of the year, Maria was articulating her career trajectory differently. She began to talk about herself as a teacher of other teachers — 'a faculty developer, I guess you might say' — and imagined herself as someone who would go on to use the theory, evidence and scholarship of education to change the way she worked with trainees, colleagues and patients.

Unpacking the case study: becoming a clinical educator

Two key points arise from case study 22.1:

- Maria spent time 'doing' education and immersed herself in the role of an educator.
- She was part of a supportive team that helped her to see the value of what she did and encouraged her to think about her practice as an educator.

Key changes that can be identified are:

- Maria shifted her viewpoint from education as an immediate gain to seeing the longer term impact and to understand how long it can take to affect change.
- She shifted from a didactic approach to a more facilitative approach.
- She changed her view of education, now seeing it as more than 'facts'.

- She no longer wanted to teach as she was taught, but to think about the rationale.
- She saw theory as central to her teaching.
- Her conceptualisation of reflection changed, for herself, her work and her role as a consultant and as an educator.
- She now described herself as a 'teacher of teachers'.

This case study clearly illustrates three points. First, there were a number of threshold concepts that fundamentally changed both Maria's thinking and her practice as a clinical educator; second, Maria moved to an understanding of the signature pedagogies of medical education as distinct from medicine itself; and third, she needed a particular set of 'conditions' in order to foster this.

Maria's focus began to be driven by signature pedagogies that put the learner at the centre and drew on learners' motivation to seek out the information they need. In her teaching, she looked to develop in her learners the habits of mind of a practising professional. She had started to grapple with threshold concepts, and in so doing had changed not only how she *thinks* but also how she *is*. In her discussions about her teaching, she was now much more aware of key concepts such as the importance of context, uncertainty and multiple perspectives, and of the ways in which people learn and the factors that can shape this.

Maria's view of herself became one of 'doctor as teacher' and, for her, there was no tension between herself as an educator and her role as a doctor. She had not simply acquired a few helpful teaching techniques, but rather had transformed her view of herself and her career. Not only did she now think differently about teaching, but she also had a desire to ground this thinking in theory. Her driver was to teach intentionally, focusing on 'why' something was important rather than 'what'. Her move from didactic teaching to a more facilitative approach is indicative of her consideration of a number of key constructivist educational concepts, such as learners building their own mental models, the social nature of learning, encouraging learners to engage with ideas and to articulate their own thinking, and dealing with uncertainty and ambiguity.

One fundamental change for Maria was her new focus on critical reflection. Her struggle with this was a move from resentment at the forced and formalised nature of reflection, to an awareness of the power of serious reflection to improve and guide her own clinical practice. As part of this, Maria engaged with the literature through formal course work in education, and the associated assessment. Not only did Maria now use reflection in her own practice as an educator and a clinician, she sought to teach others to think in this way too. She had wrestled with the ideas and come out the 'other side' with different perspectives. This is a clear illustration of the elements of threshold concepts. The idea of critical reflection was initially very troublesome, and Maria went through the liminal stage, characterised by confusion. However, once grasped, the concept of reflection was one that was transformative. It was integrative and reconstructive in that it provided Maria with ways of making connections between other ideas and seeing things in new ways, and was discursive in that it provided her with a means of explaining her thinking and structuring her teaching.

This case study also illustrates that what Maria needed was an environment that was conducive to fostering learning, and in that environment she began to experience the signature pedagogies of a different discipline. Not only did she spend time 'doing' education, but it was also done in a deliberate and focused way. She was not just teaching in opportunistic situations or teaching 'on the fly' as part of a busy clinical day, she was teaching in an education-centric setting where thinking about teaching and learning were deliberate, explicit, surfaced and clear.

Maria was part of a team and so had the opportunity to work with others — some who were very experienced educators and others who, like herself, were less experienced. As such, she had opportunities for discussions about education and to articulate her own developing thinking. She had encouragement, feedback and challenge. In addition, Maria was doing a formal education course, and so was exposed to current scholarly thinking about education. This meant that she had a structured underpinning to her thinking about education and was challenged to develop her intellectual understanding, her reasoning and her understanding of the decisions that she and others made about teaching. Moreover, a formal education course gave her an understanding and a means for articulating her thinking. As she explored and continued this process, the constructivist and explicit pedagogies of education began to change the way she thought about the signature pedagogies of her original profession. Opportunities to merge the two ways of thinking, and forge what she envisioned as a new pedagogy for her profession, came onto her horizon.

This case study highlights that a number of things can be central to a clinician's development as an educator. These include a solid theoretical underpinning, clearly grounded in practice, and opportunities to teach and to do so in a supportive environment, to think critically about education and to engage with others (both experienced educators and novices), and to think about and discuss one's practice as an educator. Furthermore, it importantly includes aspects of pedagogy that are signatures of an educator but have often not been present in the signature pedagogies of the health professions — although they *are* signatures of good clinical practice. These include an explicit articulation of the decisions that are made, the rationale behind the decisions and the consequences of each decision, and the opportunity to be both supported and challenged.

As this case study illustrates, faculty development can provide a 'way in' to education. It can provide the opportunities to think about education and to consider the scholarship and research underpinning the discipline. It can provide an environment in which conversations about education are surfaced, sometimes for the first time. What faculty development does, when done well, is it problematises education. Rather than teaching being a 'commonsense' activity that can be done by anyone who knows their own discipline, faculty development encourages us to think critically about education and to question the decisions (tacit as well as overt) that are made. And it encourages us to find a thoughtful, well-grounded rationale for the decisions that we make.

Implications for developing faculty in the health professions

Faculty development is not an ad hoc activity, but rather one that promotes good education by doing so in careful, planned and structured ways. As the case study on Maria illustrates, change can happen and people can be transformed as educators and go on to inspire others. It requires on the part of those responsible for faculty development an understanding of the signature pedagogies and of the threshold concepts underpinning this. And it requires a commitment to work towards this. What this means is a multi-faceted approach.

Formal education

Formal qualifications in medical or clinical education are essential, as they provide an in-depth understanding of the literature and its application to practice, as well as a way into the discipline that is guided, structured and supported. A course such as a postgraduate certificate or diploma can provide a well-organised, carefully structured introduction to scholarship and research in the field of education and an entry into 'thinking like an educator'. Ideally this is done in the company of other learners, so that each person can learn from others, challenge and encourage each other.

Opportunities to develop

This can be in the form of workshops, conferences, journal clubs, seminars and other opportunities to develop one's thinking and critically reflect on one's own practice as an educator in ways that allow for the possibility of change. These opportunities expose clinicians to others who are thinking seriously about education and so it challenges their own thinking and practice and can provide opportunities for meeting others, observing, sharing ideas and being part of a community of educators.

Career structure

For some professions, teaching students and supervising trainees has long been overlooked as a legitimate component of day-to-day work, and was not considered as part of a longer term career plan. As this gradually changes and teaching becomes legitimised, the role of 'clinician as teacher' becomes more visible. Rewarding teaching gives it status and provides an impetus to think seriously about education, to learn more, to document one's achievements and to possibly gain a qualification.

Professional frameworks

Emerging frameworks of professionalism for those who teach, supervise and support clinicians in their training provide a grounding for what it means to practise as a clinical educator. One such framework comes from the Academy of Medical Educators (2014), and provides guidance on expectations of professional practice and recognition of consistent performance against those standards in the form of membership and fellowship. Such resources enhance teaching and learning by providing a formal structure and recognition and by articulating what the community values in teaching and learning. Moreover, these raise the profile of education and thus provide impetus for ongoing faculty development.

Strategy

Higher education institutions that train pre-registration health professionals, and hospitals and other healthcare institutions that sponsor clinical placements, need clear faculty development strategies which set out their priorities and approach. The importance of articulating this in a clear and public way conveys a commitment to developing teaching as a meaningful and explicit part of the clinician's role.

Teaching fellowships

Teaching fellowships provide clinicians with the opportunity to engage in the 'doing' of education in a focused and well-supported way, and allow clinicians to critically reflect on their own practice as both educators and clinical practitioners. If this is done as part of a supportive team that is committed to thoughtful and intentional education practice, the clinician can simultaneously develop their own skills and go on to 'infect' others with their enthusiasm and knowledge.

Interdisciplinary involvement of educators and clinicians

Interdisciplinary collaboration between those trained in the field of education and those trained in medicine can provide fruitful thinking and development on each side. In the case study, for example, Maria found inspiration from the research and scholarship collaboration that occurred in her simulation centre.

Research and scholarship

Grounding education and faculty development means that it is possible to provide a solid and integrated theoretical and conceptual foundation and framework for educational work and the discursive capacity for interrogation and critique. It also means that through ongoing research our understanding of clinical education can be further stretched and developed.

Conclusion

For clinicians, educational ways of thinking can push against the traditional view of teaching and learning and against the ways in which people have themselves sometimes been taught. In this way, they can provide new insights, new understandings and hence the possibilities for reflection. Kneebone (2002) very eloquently describes his own experience in encountering the world of education and his initial confusion and even dismay. Using a case study in this chapter, we considered the ways in which faculty development can provide a 'way in' to educational ways of thinking. We then examined the ways in which faculty development needs to be carefully structured and provide an extensive and multi-faceted approach that is scholarly, grounded in pedagogical theory, applicable to practice and supported by infrastructure.

We argue that education does not provide a 'better' way of thinking but a different one. Normative judgments about the 'value' of each epistemology are futile at best. By allowing clinicians an opportunity to engage meaningfully with a new way of thinking, we provide an alternative dimension, well-grounded in research and serious scholarship in pedagogy. Using the frameworks of threshold concepts and signature pedagogies, we can start to view faculty development as a 'way in' to the complex and transformative thinking about clinical education. This can provide an integrative way of understanding clinical education that takes account of the context, the pressures and priorities, and yet provides a conceptual underpinning.

Good faculty development programs take account of education or pedagogy as a threshold concept by tackling pedagogy head on. This means acknowledging that it is 'troublesome knowledge' and that much of what we present will initially be seen as counterintuitive. By acknowledging, but not shying away from, our confidence in our own discipline, we are able to present educational thinking in a way that is scholarly and well-grounded in research. Rather than presenting teaching as a set of technical skills, it is conceptualised in the context of the underpinning thinking, providing a rationale for what we do as educators. This can be an experience of a conceptual threshold for some clinicians: we acknowledge the liminal space that people will enter when acquiring these threshold concepts. However, in building effective faculty development we also use the integrative and discursive nature of these concepts.

In exposing clinicians to the signature pedagogies of the social sciences, and articulating why and how they help to create educators who think differently about their work, their students and themselves, we similarly invite clinicians to re-engage with the pedagogical approaches that are signatures of their own professions. As faculty are developing their understanding of pedagogy, they are developing the ability to make sense of their teaching, to articulate this understanding in increasingly sophisticated ways and to make links between ideas that were previously seen as disconnected. The potential opportunity here is, we argue, significant: by drawing on the signature ways of thinking in the social sciences and applying them to the pedagogies of the clinical sciences, pedagogical settings that retain some of the features of the old signature pedagogies can be refashioned into more meaningful and powerful learning opportunities. Furthermore, new signature pedagogies (e.g. problem-based learning, simulation-based education) can emerge.

A well-designed program of faculty development will build on these ideas, and will take opportunities to continually re-engage with and revisit clinical educational concepts with increasing complexity and in terms of the dynamic links between theory and practice. One way of conceptualising the success of a faculty development program is by the ways in which it is transformative, itself one of the key elements of a threshold concept. If faculty tell us that they now see their teaching (and perhaps even their practice as clinicians) in new ways, then we have succeeded in creating a setting that encourages clinicians to both become and be educators.

References

Academy of Medical Educators (2014). *Professional standards* (3rd ed.). Cardiff: Academy of Medical Educators.

Cousin, G. (2006). An introduction to threshold concepts. *Planet, 17,* 4–5.

Davis, M. H., & Harden, R. M. (1999). AMEE medical education guide number 15. Problem-based learning: a practical guide. *Medical Teacher, 21,* 130–140.

General Medical Council. (2012). *Working with doctors, working for patients.* London: GMC.

Kneebone, R. (2002). Total internal reflection: an essay on paradigms. *Medical Education, 36,* 514–518.

Land, R., Cousin, G., Meyer, J. H. F., et al. (2005). Threshold concepts and troublesome knowledge (3): implications for course design and evaluation. In C. Rust (Ed.), *Improving student learning: diversity and inclusivity. Proceedings of the 12th Improving Student Learning Conference* (pp. 53–64). Oxford: Oxford Centre for Staff and Learning Development (OCSLD).

Land, R., Meyer, J. H. F., & Flanagan, M. T. (Eds.), (2016). *Educational futures: rethinking theory and practice* (Vol. 68). Rotterdam/Boston/Taipei: Sense Publishers.

Long, T. L., Breitkreuz, K. R., Diaz, D. A., et al. (2012). Competence and care: signature pedagogies in nursing education. *Exploring More Signature Pedagogies: Approaches to Teaching Disciplinary Habits of Mind,* 171–187.

Meyer, J. H. F., & Land, R. (2003). Threshold concepts and troublesome knowledge: linkages to ways of thinking and practising. In C. Rust (Ed.), *Improving student learning: theory and practice ten years on* (pp. 412–424). Oxford: Oxford Centre for Staff and Learning Development (OCSLD).

Meyer, J. H. F., & Land, R. (2005). Threshold concepts and troublesome knowledge (2): epistemological considerations and a conceptual framework for teaching and learning. *Higher Education, 49*(3), 373–388.

Meyer, J. H. F., & Land, R. (2006). *Overcoming barriers to student understanding: threshold concepts and troublesome knowledge.* London: Routledge.

Neve, H., Wearn, A., & Colett, T. (2016). What are threshold concepts and how can they inform medical education? *Medical Teacher, 38*(8), 850–853.

Shulman, L. S. (2005). Signature pedagogies in the professions. *Daedalus, 134*(3), 52–59.

Wood, D. F. (2003). Problem based learning. *British Medical Journal, 326,* 328.

23

Leadership in health professions education
What does it mean?

Jennene Greenhill and Judy McKimm

Introduction

Every educator involved in health professions education is to some extent both a leader and a manager. This chapter presents a new approach to management and leadership and will be useful to health professional educators working at different levels in a variety of contexts. The chapter is designed to provide theory and practical strategies for leadership for changing times. The aim is to promote an understanding of the application of a range of contemporary leadership theories to help educators as leaders to become more effective agents of change.

Educators are curators of ideas, information and knowledge — and in complex adaptive systems, ideas constantly emerge. Leaders who are also good followers can sense the tide, and synthesise ideas and information to make people feel they are contributing, so creating an inclusive culture for change. Working collaboratively within and between organisations, 'educator leaders' can help steer the co-creation of a culture for continuous learning.

This chapter introduces key aspects of leadership and management for healthcare educators who would like to develop a deeper understanding of leadership theory and gain an evidence base to help them to become more effective leaders. We synthesise contemporary leadership theory with a focus on change and complexity and the art of followership in the context of health professions education that aims to build a knowledgeable, skilled and resilient health workforce ready to deliver ever-changing healthcare. Health professions education is complex and dynamic, embodying inherent tensions due to its positioning in university/academic and health provider settings. Individual educators and their teams have to manage such tensions through both leading and following, depending on context and situation; we therefore provide examples relating to various aspects of this complexity.

We conclude with a case study that brings together the concepts, issues and challenges discussed. The case study considers an educator who has been asked to establish a new program to educate the next generation of health professionals in an underserved community. We raise typical issues that confront educational leaders and explore topics including:

- leadership, management and followership theory and practice;
- change and complexity theory — models and frameworks that help stimulate and generate change in a complex world;
- adaptive leadership for complex systems — how to use VUCA (volatility, uncertainty, complexity and ambiguity) and RUPT (rapid, unpredictable, paradoxical and tangled) approaches in leadership and management;
- inclusive and person-centred leadership — putting people at the heart of what we do, working with diversity, and recognising and addressing unconscious bias;
- resilience, grit and emotional intelligence — key personal qualities for effective leadership;
- influencing skills;
- setting personal goals and action planning.

Leadership is as important to providing quality education as clinical knowledge and skills are to healthcare delivery. Educational leadership in health service contexts needs to reflect and promote practices that develop health leaders who can:

- design and implement integrated models of care;
- continuously adapt practices and improve systems and processes;
- promote teamwork;
- establish an inclusive, respectful culture;
- manage the workforce to meet community and patient needs.

Health professional educators are curators of ideas, information and knowledge, and they draw (explicitly and implicitly) on a range of leadership theories and strategies to develop clinicians' leadership skills. A recent study of the leadership literature over a 14-year period found that six leadership approaches are most often used in health professional contexts: transformational leadership, charismatic leadership, strategic leadership, leadership and diversity, participative/shared leadership, and the trait approach to leadership (Meuser et al., 2016). Adaptive leadership and followership are also prominent and Meuser and colleagues (2016) found that there is considerable overlap between leadership approaches. They suggest that integrated approaches, which draw on multiple concepts from the leadership literature, are becoming more common.

Healthcare education leaders work in ever-changing, complex, adaptive systems in many different contexts. They often have a wide range of responsibilities, and those working in more senior positions particularly have the ability to influence all levels of the health and education systems. This chapter proposes that taking an integrative approach to leadership (using a range of concepts and theories) will help create collaborative working relationships between educators, health professionals, policymakers, politicians and multidisciplinary teams. For example, many educators are grappling with ways to design an interprofessional curriculum and develop innovative education programs for new models of care. An integrated leadership approach draws from several complementary leadership theories and thus helps leaders to work with others to co-create health and education systems that are adaptive to new technologies and responsive to the needs of communities.

Leadership theories for changing times

Leadership is critical to successful education and health service management (Dzau et al., 2015; West et al., 2014; West et al., 2015). A range of complementary approaches have been identified as being most relevant for leadership in complex health and education systems. These include transformational, collaborative, collective, compassionate, inclusive, person-centred, distributed and servant leadership (West et al., 2015; McKimm et al., 2017). Here we examine two commonly used approaches that go hand in hand: transformational leadership and collaborative leadership. At the organisational or system level, transformational leadership is a process that encourages people to move out of their comfort zone and to collaboratively implement organisational change, with the aim of ultimately embedding or integrating change into the system. In health professional education, transformational leadership is particularly useful in distributed organisations with a social mission that involves navigating multiple stakeholders and relationships, and aims to influence healthcare at a systemic level.

At the team or individual level, transformational leaders work collaboratively to improve performance through motivating and improving morale, and by involving and developing others' expertise and leadership skills. They do this through identifying changes that are aligned to certain values and creating a shared vision which enthuses and inspires others. Transformational leaders therefore act as role models to promote a sense of identity for the workforce aligned with the future direction of the organisation. Bass and Riggio (2006) identify four components of transformational leadership:

- idealised influence — leaders act as role models;
- inspirational motivation — leaders inspire and motivate employees;
- individualised consideration — leaders are aware of their employees' individual needs and feelings;
- intellectual stimulation — leaders encourage innovation and creativity.

In the healthcare setting, an example of where a transformational leadership approach is relevant would be the view that the rising cost of healthcare means that health services must make transformative changes. Leaders must reform systems, models of care delivery and financing to improve productivity and must foster innovation and implement strategies that can reduce costs or increase revenue (Dzau et al., 2015). They will need to mould the internal culture and structures to adapt to newly emerging changes in the external environment to create new growth (Austin et al., 2016). For education leaders this means that they must identify longer term, transformative opportunities (such as developing new or extended practitioner roles) to deal with future uncertainty around workforce needs, education and training while balancing short-term requirements to deliver existing programs.

Within any health system, patients (and consequently learners) move between different contexts: home, primary care, secondary care, social care. These contexts often act as silos, with little integration and a consequent lack of quality, efficiency and continuity. As a result, in many settings, a more integrated approach to service provision is being taken. The leader's role is to create and nurture relationships between hospitals, primary care and social care to provide services that work together across the entire spectrum of care and enable patients to access care appropriately. Developing and providing integrated services is a huge challenge, in terms of the management systems needed and in training and designing the health workforce. Integrated information systems that link electronic health records to decision-support systems, patient and work-flow management are essential. Interprofessional education (IPE) and collaborative practice have the potential to improve health outcomes within such integrated services, but require a redesign of the health workforce and greater connectivity between education and clinical practice (Cerra & Brandt, 2015). A transformational and collaborative leadership approach will promote, encourage and facilitate relationship-building and collaborative practices, developing a culture in which all staff and learners feel valued. This may involve different approaches to program design and developing new or extended health practitioners (e.g. doctors' associates or nurse consultants) who can work across and within systems in a different way to meet patients' needs.

Followership theory and practice

Until relatively recently, the main focus of attention was on the leader and how individual leaders influence and promote change. However, effecting and sustaining change is not simply a one-way linear activity in which the leader 'commands' and others follow blindly and without question. The leader–follower relationship is complex. It involves a dynamic interchange and co-creation of ideas between leaders and those who they aspire to lead, and movement between who leads and who follows depending on the situation or context. Uhl-Bien and colleagues (2014) suggest that our understanding of leadership is incomplete without an understanding of followership, and that followership has been largely missed in the leadership literature.

The followership literature can help leader-educators in three ways. First, from a leadership perspective, understanding the influence and needs of followers will help leaders to work out ways in which they can build trust and engage others in implementing changes, as well as providing them with an appreciation of how changes will impact on the team. Depending on the context and the psychological and physical needs of followers (identified through observation and trustful and respectful conversations) leaders can adjust and adapt their style and behaviour. An active consideration of followers (colleagues and learners) will help health education leaders to provide leadership that is calm, empathic, inclusive and compassionate. While charismatic or authoritative leadership may be required in some situations (e.g. where there are tough decisions to be made or the program needs a 'front face' leader to communicate the vision), the day-to-day work of clinical education is much more about leadership being distributed throughout the organisation and people striving collaboratively to provide excellent education or training. Individuals (including leaders) engage in followership in a variety of ways through 'doing following', 'standing by' or 'resisting following'. Followers and leaders do not necessarily remain in one category but may move between categories depending on the situation (Kean et al., 2011).

The second way that the followership literature can help leader-educators is by considering followers as equally influential on leaders as leaders are on followers. No-one leads all the time — even senior leaders and managers are required to be accountable to and meet the demands of those above them. Also, it may be more relevant for a 'follower' to take the lead and step up in a situation where they have more expertise or experience than someone in a higher leadership position. So, followership (like leadership) is not necessarily tied to a role but rather is a set of behaviours within a dynamic, co-constructed relational process. As we have already mentioned, there are increasing calls for healthcare professionals to work more collaboratively to provide and improve healthcare. Education institutions have responded by adopting IPE in an attempt to produce health professional graduates who understand one another's roles and are ready to work collaboratively. This implies that all health professional educators need to not only educate people who are skilled and knowledgeable about their own profession but also create a shared identity as health professionals within an interprofessional team.

Interprofessional teams working in various clinical contexts will have different ways of working together. To be effective they have to share responsibility for patient care and work together to improve the system. This interaction between professional and personal identity, power relations and leadership and followership suggests that new understandings of these concepts are needed to influence the educational preparation of students in the health professions (Barrow et al., 2011). Research on a team process model of action and planning phases in collaborative work discusses leadership and followership, including how locus (a leader's integration into a team's usual work) and formality (a leader's responsibility conferred by the traditional hierarchy) can influence team functions (Dow et al., 2013). Leadership researchers also describe 'dynamic delegation' as an approach to conceptualising escalation and delegation within healthcare teams. They identify competencies to improve collaborative practice, including specific knowledge, attitudes and behaviours that can be included in curricula. They suggest that gaining an understanding of these principles will prepare students as team leaders with the skills to analyse team performance and adapt behaviours that improve collaboration and lead to improved clinical outcomes (Dow et al., 2013).

The question remains, what kind of curriculum enables students to learn about professional power, leadership and followership? There is a gap between theory and practice that indicates a need to understand the meaning of leadership and followership in interprofessional healthcare workplaces (Gordon et al., 2015). Perhaps an understanding of leadership and followership should be scaffolded throughout the curriculum. Attention could be paid to interactions happening at the team, organisational and systemic levels among different leaders, followers and external actors. Clinical educators who have an understanding of followership can play a key role in facilitating these interactions beyond the patient–clinician dimension. Developing IPE curricula that strengthen collaborative practice across professions can be challenging. A theoretical basis for understanding collaborative practice in healthcare settings is needed to guide curriculum design and support the team-based delivery of care. IPE should incorporate theory-based educational methods that build skills for effective collaboration.

The third way that followership literature can help leader-educators is through highlighting the role of followership within complex dynamic systems. Followership theory views leadership as a group process, which should be distributed across all levels of healthcare organisations. Most health services and organisations are hierarchical in their structure and usually those working at lower levels have less power to implement change. Followers have influence in the system because they are active and dynamic unpredictable agents who process information and have their own perspectives. Clinical educators typically act as role models for students and inexperienced clinicians and can have huge influence through using their 'soft power' within the organisation and wider system.

Complexity theory and adaptive leadership for complex systems

A consideration of followership within complex systems leads us on to another theory in this integrated approach to leadership: complexity theory. Complex adaptive systems are constantly responding and adapting to changes internally and externally. The term 'complex' does not mean the same as 'complicated'. A complicated system has individual components or constituents that can be differentiated such as a computer or aircraft. A complex system is dynamic and changing with interacting relationships between components that are unpredictable; for example, the weather or people moving round a city (Cilliers, 1998).

Many researchers characterise healthcare systems as complex adaptive and when health professional education is included, the 'system' becomes even more complex. New ideas, people and technologies are constantly emerging and evolving in unpredictable ways and these interactions dynamically reshape organisational structures and processes. To meet the challenges in managing health professions education within complex adaptive organisations, education leaders need to constantly adapt their approach, which is what theorists determine as 'complex leadership'. Complex leadership principles augment other competencies that healthcare and education scholars recognise and recommend as necessary for future leaders. Complex leader theory is derived from complexity science, a growing body of literature that investigates the underlying logic of complex adaptive organisations.

Complexity theory generates new, innovative practices and principles in leading and managing these ever-changing organisations (Ford, 2009). For example, Sturmberg and colleagues, in their review of the application of complexity science to general practice, suggest that: 'systems and complexity thinking was embraced as a transformational tool to link the specific with the particular of whole-person care — the patient as a subsystem of larger systems such as family, community, society, and the healthcare system. Not surprisingly, this approach resonates well with general and family practitioners as it much more accurately describes the high degree of variability they encounter among patients presenting with the same condition' (Sturmberg et al., 2014, p 73). However, healthcare leadership education continues to focus on the training and competence of individuals and little attention is paid to the interprofessional workplace and how its inherent complexities might contribute to the emergence of leadership.

As we have discussed, traditional views of leadership primarily regard success as dependent on the individual power of a leader or leadership team that sets strategic goals. However, such approaches have been critiqued, particularly with the emphasis on the charismatic solo leader as the leader of the transformational process. Individual leaders with too much power and too little emotional intelligence can become toxic and destructive. A toxic leader can infect the culture of an organisation in a negative way, especially when they are surrounded by 'yes people' and passive followers who feel they cannot challenge the leader. This can result in people taking subversive strategies to 'get round' or 'work against' the toxicity, instead of everyone pulling together towards a shared vision and goals in a spirit of collaboration. A good leader (and followers) takes the cultural temperature often, to ensure that people feel included, valued, engaged and involved in key activities.

Current thinking asserts that leadership should be (and, in reality, is) distributed across many levels of healthcare and educational organisations (Bolden, 2011). Complexity leadership suggests that under conditions of knowledge production and human interactions, informal network dynamics should be enabled, not constrained and controlled. Leaders should create the conditions for communication, develop that organisational capacity and leave the system essentially alone so that it can generate positive emergence. This type of change process is known as 'emergent' and is intrinsically different from a managed, planned change process such as a top-down program development approach or building a hospital.

Complexity theory suggests that most complex systems are underpinned by a few key ('simple') rules. For example, a review by Schneider and colleagues (2014) of Canadian experiences with primary healthcare reforms identified five simple rules of successful large-system transformation. They were:

1. a mix of designated leadership with distributed leadership in the change process;
2. the presence of feedback loops;
3. paying attention to past system history;
4. engaging front-line/powerful providers;
5. engaging end users (families and communities).

These simple rules emphasise collective or distributed leadership, which means that change processes should not only be driven by top managers, but also be inclusive of staff at all levels. Staff at the coal-face of systems actually implement policy and they may have very different interests and perspectives than managers. In education, a complex systems approach could be taken in curriculum development. Here, a leader could put the conditions for emergent change in place by setting some simple rules (as above) but with additional boundaries such as the number of years the program should run for, the resources available and a timeframe for the development process. They might also specify the number of hours to be spent on university and clinical learning. Then they would give their teams time and space to generate ideas about the principles, shape and structure of the new program, prior to reaching agreement on the final design. Once this has been agreed, the change will need to be managed through more linear change management models to translate the ideas and vision into a real-life curriculum. Of course, in practice the process is much more iterative than this, and any leader needs to be very clear about the project scope and boundaries and the roles and responsibilities of individuals within the curriculum development process.

Another example of complex leadership in health systems is a study from the North West Province of South Africa to implement a whole-system intervention drawing on concepts from complexity theory. The province was an early adopter of a national primary healthcare (PHC) strategy that included the establishment of PHC outreach teams of community health workers. Implementation of the PHC outreach team strategy was characterised by the following features:

- a favourable provincial context of a well-established district and subdistrict health system and longstanding values in support of PHC;
- the forging of a collective vision for the new strategy that built on prior history and values and that led to distributed leadership and ownership of the new policy;
- an implementation strategy that ensured alignment of systems (information, human resources) and appropriate sequencing of activities (planning, training, piloting, household campaigns);
- the privileging of 'community dialogues' and local manager participation in the early phases;
- the establishment of special implementation structures — a PHC task team (chaired by a senior provincial manager) to enable feedback and ensure accountability, and a non-government organisation (NGO) partnership that provided flexible support for implementation (Schneider et al., 2014).

Complexity theory can help to explain and inform how interprofessional teams can enact micro-level leadership through influential, dynamic and adaptive acts of organising. For example, if a new program for doctors' associates was being introduced, a team comprising university and clinical teachers from different professions and disciplines would have much more soft power and influence on stakeholders who might be resistant, due to their numerous connections and interconnections, than, for example, a team of doctors. Leadership training should give participants an opportunity to discuss and analyse everyday leadership practices and challenge deeply entrenched values, beliefs, practices and assumptions about healthcare leadership (Gordon et al., 2017). In complex systems, it is unhelpful to act as if outcomes can be completely controlled or engineered as there are too many influencing variables and too much unpredictability. Leaders therefore need to move beyond setting a vision and strategic plans to identifying a few long-term strategies and setting the conditions for change, especially those that facilitate interactions among people and enable them to self-organise. Taking a 'systems thinking' approach is challenging as it requires leaders to stop operating as solo leaders and change their perspective of the organisation as a complex adaptive system that fluctuates and emerges. This can feel as if control is being lost or given away; however, leadership and change emerge out of interactions and events, out of the interactive spaces between people and ideas.

How to use VUCA and RUPT in leadership and management

In a complex world, established procedures and approaches are not always effective and taking a systems or complexity thinking approach can help leaders and others to navigate through and influence the dynamics of a complex system. We have suggested that leaders need to 'simply' set the conditions for change, and while change will emerge, it is not always clear or certain what the change will be. Leaders therefore need to become comfortable working with ambiguity and uncertainty. VUCA (volatility, uncertainty, complexity and ambiguity) is a military acronym that is now widely used in various settings, including healthcare (Till et al., 2016). The acronym describes four distinct types of challenge found in complex systems, each of which requires a different response. George (2017) has extended the original VUCA concept into VUCA 2.0 to incorporate four leadership skills or actions (vision, understanding, courage and adaptability). Box 23.1 sets out the two VUCA models and their characteristics, and links them with approaches that leaders might take when working with their 'followers'.

Box 23.1: VUCA characteristics and approaches

Volatility

Characteristics. Leaders face challenges that, while not necessarily hard to understand, may be unstable or unexpected or last for an unknown duration.

Approach. Leaders should prepare supplementary resources and mitigation in all domains: financial performance, intangible performance and leadership, according to the extent of registered risk. The leader's role is to work with followers to prepare practical contingency plans.

Vision. Leaders need to define the vision clearly to followers, and maintain clarity and purpose to ensure that the vision is translated into reality through defining the mission, values, strategy and tactics that will achieve the vision.

Uncertainty

Characteristics. Leaders face challenges where the basic cause and effect are known but the lack of supplementary information shrouds the change management process.

Approach. Leaders should work with followers to invest in information systems and predictive analytics to collect, interpret and share information to reduce uncertainty. They should provide as much certainty as is possible about specific elements within the system.

Understanding. Leaders need in depth understanding of their organisation's capabilities and to take advantage of rapidly changing circumstances by playing to their strengths while minimising their weaknesses. They need to listen and engage widely to gather views from inside and outside the organisation.

Complexity

Characteristics. Leaders face challenges with a multitude of interdependent variables across and beyond the boundaries of their system.

Approach. Leaders should optimise and develop resources with the structure and specialism to address the complexity. Again, leaders need to simplify this complexity for their followers by helping people work towards agreement and/or certainty (Stacey, 2007).

Courage. Leaders need to face challenges, take (considered) risks and take their followers with them.

Ambiguity

Characteristics. Leaders face challenges of 'unknown unknowns' where there are unclear relationships between cause and effect.

Approach. Leaders should firmly embed systems of quality improvement throughout the organisation to test hypotheses, learn and spread sustainable change according to strategic objectives. Leaders should help followers to work within ambiguity by discussing and defining options and possibilities and collaborating to find a path through the ambiguity.

Adaptability. Leaders need to be flexible in their own approach, but also build flexibility into the system, curriculum or processes. Adaptability to changing circumstances helps an organisation not only to survive, but also to thrive.

Source: Adapted from Till A, Dutta N, McKimm J. Vertical leadership in highly complex and unpredictable health systems. *Br J Hosp Med (Lond)*, 2016 Aug 2;*77*(8), 471–475. doi: 10.12968/hmed.2016.77.8.471.

Another model that assists leaders to find their way through complexity, developed by the Center for Creative Leadership (CCL), introduces the concept of a RUPT (rapid, unpredictable, paradoxical and tangled) environment (Magellan Horth, 2016a).

- *Rapid.* Leaders face overlapping challenges, in multiple domains, which occur and should be overcome at pace — this requires leaders to have energy and direction.

- *Unpredictable.* Leaders face unexpected challenges, which despite thorough strategies and governance, can rapidly challenge assumptions and cause them to reframe their thinking — leaders need to be prepared to change their minds and be open to others' perspectives.

- *Paradoxical.* Leaders face challenges in polarity. Rather than providing one solution, challenges should be embraced as polarities to be leveraged both in the short and long term — leaders need to use management tools and engage with a wide group of people to generate options.

- *Tangled.* Leaders face interdependent challenges across and beyond the boundaries of their system — leaders need to be aware of both their internal and external environments, to horizon scan and gather multiple intelligences.

In such volatile and tangled worlds, leaders need 'learning agility'. Learning agility is the single best predictor of long-term leadership success and without this, leadership either freezes or becomes derailed from its strategy through subjective reactionary responses to the challenges faced (De Meuse et al., 2010; Magellan Horth, 2016b; Till et al., 2016). This approach has echoes of adaptive leadership (Heifetz, 2009), and reflects aspects of resilience that emphasise flexibility and 'bounce-back', and Senge's 'learning organisation' (Senge, 1990).

The CCL has also developed a model for leadership development that combines elements of formal leadership development (what is termed 'horizontal leadership') with those learned experientially ('vertical leadership') (Petrie, 2014). McKimm (2017) identifies three ways of learning in her 'leadership in three's model': learning about theories, models and evidence about 'what works, when and why' (for educators, this would also include educational theory and evidence); learning through deliberate, focused practice, obtaining constructive feedback and reflection (on both educational and leadership practice); and learning through experience and the development of practical wisdom — what Aristotle calls 'phronesis' — about how to behave and function in different situations and contexts.

Using these approaches, leaders can learn from VUCA and RUPT experiences, by applying leadership and management models to practice as well as using significant events or challenging situations as learning lessons (McKimm & Till, 2015). Petrie suggests that through the process of vertical development (which will vary among individuals), leaders will be better able to adapt and think creatively in more complex, systemic, strategic and interdependent ways. There are three elements in the process, which are outlined in Box 23.2.

Box 23.2: Vertical leadership development

Heat experiences are opportunities that disrupt a leader's habitual thinking and should be designed, within their competency levels, to stretch the leader beyond their comfort zone and into new, more advanced models of thinking. Examples of heat experiences might be leading a difficult meeting, taking on a challenging or new project or working with a very diverse multidisciplinary team. The heat experience is a situation that leaders put themselves in to provide a way of developing new skills and understanding.

Colliding perspectives occur within 'heat experiences' to develop the leader's thinking further. Ideally, these should focus on exposure to professionals and others with different views, backgrounds and thinking. This is vital within healthcare where leaders often interact with wide ranging multidisciplinary teams across organisational boundaries. As in inclusive leadership which celebrates and welcomes diversity, it is important for the leader to be willing to listen to others' views and opinions, to be challenged, to take on board ideas that differ from their own and to be willing to adapt and change. Such an approach requires emotional intelligence: in particular, self-insight and self-regulation (Goleman, 1995) and an understanding of unconscious or cognitive biases.

Elevated sense making should incorporate time for reflection, coaching, mentoring and professional conversations. This allows for greater development and integration of the learning from heat experiences and understanding gained from colliding perspectives. Used effectively this develops a wider and more in-depth view of people, organisations and systems. This part of the process is all about the 'so what?' component of reflective practice; it requires the leader to make meaning and sense of their own role within the more complex system. Ideally this should lead to identification of learning needs including further heat experiences, knowledge and skills.

Source: Petrie (2015); Till et al. (2016).

How to co-create an integrated leadership approach

Peter Senge and colleagues (2015) argue for co-creation and have identified three core capabilities of system leaders: 1) they are profoundly committed to the health of the whole, which nurtures similar commitment in others; 2) they build relationships based on deep listening, so that networks of trust and collaboration begin to flourish; and 3) they are so convinced that something can be done that they don't wait for a fully developed plan, freeing others to step ahead and learn by doing.

Many students and clinicians seek work among underserved communities, but they can be unprepared to cope with the challenges. Relationships with mentors and peers have been shown to promote resilience and prevent burnout. To prepare students to work with vulnerable groups we need to foster leadership, advocacy and resiliency in our future workforce (Warde et al., 2014). Picking up the points made earlier, taking a 'constructionist' approach to leadership, rather than being viewed as subordinates, followers (or learners) are firmly established as active participants and hold equal importance to that of the leader (teacher) (Meindl, 1995). This emphasises the concept of leader–follower–manager relations being a dynamic set of activities and exchange of ideas. Here, teachers can help their learners to develop leadership skills through role modelling and facilitating the development of skills and insight to know when to take on leadership, followership and management roles and activities: the 'leadership triad' (Till & McKimm, 2016). People need to be supported and developed to appreciate, understand and accept this approach. An integrated, co created approach to leadership also requires power to be shared, even given away, and a flattening of hierarchies. This will help challenge the traditional autocratic leadership that tends to dominate education and healthcare, but it must be reinforced by positive organisational cultures, exemplified by the concept of collective leadership (West et al., 2014).

Leadership skills are not inherent, 'natural' skills of teachers and clinicians. Inclusive and person-centred leadership puts people at the heart of what we do, working positively with diverse people and ideas, recognising and addressing unconscious bias. Some key characteristics of leaders identified through the literature are resilience, grit, emotional intelligence, influencing skills, systems thinking, leadership self-efficacy, perspective-taking capacity, self-awareness and ambiguity tolerance. This is daunting but it is not a prescriptive checklist of personal qualities/skills that you must have to be a good leader, although there are some qualities and skills that can be learned and can help make you more effective.

McKimm (2017) suggests that the key personal qualities of effective, long-lasting leaders can be summed up from the literature as resilience, emotional intelligence and 'grit'. While 'grit' might sound quite 'masculine', it is actually a combination of resilience, passion, hard work, perseverance, determination and direction (Duckworth, 2016). 'To be gritty, you have to have a deep interest in what you're doing; take opportunities to practice skills and show self-discipline; cultivate a conviction and purpose about your work (it has to matter) and have hope and confidence that you can *do* leadership as well as *be* a leader' (McKimm, 2017, p 23). An awareness of these personal qualities will not make you a great leader but because taking on leadership roles (particularly senior positions) can be very challenging, knowing yourself (your strengths and limitations) can help shore you up when things get tough. To be an effective leader, you also need credibility. This can be developed through gaining a wide understanding of the context and 'industry' in which you work; having insight into the wider political, sociocultural and economic trends which might affect the organisation; becoming an expert in your area of work; and having a good understanding of your strengths and weaknesses, so you can build a team round you who can compensate for one another.

Learning coaches and clinical teachers can assist students to learn these skills, benefiting themselves and other workers in the health services, their families and ultimately their patients and the broader community (Grant et al., 2017). Furthermore, leadership is socially constructed and not simply a combination of personal qualities or attributes of an individual. Educators and healthcare leaders have an important role in the co-construction of the organisation in which they work.

Case study 23.1: Leading and establishing health professions education: collaboration and community engagement

Imagine that you had been asked to be part of a team to establish a new program to educate the next generation of doctors in an underserved community. This case study suggests a number of lessons for leadership and change in healthcare systems.

It began with an invitation to attend a community meeting in a small town. The town hall was 'packed to the rafters' with people who were keen to establish a medical education program. They invited a recent graduate and university leaders. They wanted to know what it would take to get the university to commit to sending medical students to their town. The local health services had been in decline and it was difficult to attract doctors to the town. While political commitment, community support and university policy supported the idea, infrastructure, policy formulation, planning and design processes are necessary, but they are not sufficient for ensuring implementation.

Strong community ownership and clinical leadership was vital to the change process. The team worked with the community to create a collective vision that attracted funding for some student accommodation and the council offered some space for a staff office and teaching area. The academics worked with the local clinic and hospital to arrange the clinical placements. They spent time explaining how the unique model of clinical supervision could be implemented. The model relied on the availability of a reasonable range of clinical conditions, continuity of supervision and continuity of patient care, and the students needed to be able to learn from visiting clinicians. Implementation was presented as a process of extending the program, building capacity and strengthening the local community and not as something totally new. This reassured key stakeholders that the program would be manageable and would be integrated into existing budgets and systems.

There were pre-existing nursing placements in the local hospital and this formed a good learning context for implementation. The implementation team included a combination of management experience and clinical education expertise. The manager was team leader and coordinated regular meetings, information sessions and negotiated the partnership agreement with the clinic and hospital.

The implementation process paid careful attention to establishing a manageable system through planning, information, training and selection of the students and staff. Communication and engagement with the community and local health service managers was also important. Local involvement in decision-making was a key feature of the project. These communications and a media campaign showed that there was high-level commitment to implementation, while simultaneously identifying and responding to challenges.

The implementation process followed the simple rules as discussed above and a broad project plan with just a few key milestones. While the project was strongly supported from the top, local people emerged as powerful players in the process. They were able to provide information about the delivery of healthcare and influenced how, when and where the students could see patients and what support would be provided. The team designed a simple evaluation framework as a mechanism for identifying and resolving problems and these were effective feedback loops.

After many years of declining health services the implementation of the new program reinvigorated the hospital and the clinic. However, it is difficult to implement clinical placements in small communities. Implementation required not only changes in practices but also the allocation of resources. Communication between local clinicians and managers appeared to be improved and there was a stronger culture of learning and sharing resources between the clinic and the hospital, which was governed by more hierarchy than consultation and collaboration. Some academic staff expressed reservations about the medical students' ability to achieve academically and to have enough clinical learning experiences. The evaluation found that there could have been more communication with the academics and administrators in the city. The value of nurses and other health professionals in accessing learning opportunities should not be underestimated as they have a crucial role of 'street level bureaucrats' in navigating the health system.

The establishment of health professional education in small communities is important in creating sustainable health services in underserved areas where it is difficult to attract doctors. This approach creates more capacity for clinical placements. Community engagement, communication and collaborative leadership are essential ingredients in facilitating these kinds of changes. The opportunity for students to learn in small communities is a solution to workforce shortages and can improve quality of care in communities.

Conclusion

An integrated, collaborative approach to leadership is based on complementary leadership theories such as transformative leadership, followership and complexity theory. These approaches challenge the traditional view that effective leadership is a constellation of individual traits, attributes and skills. There is an alternative view that leadership is a socially constructed process between multiple actors within education and healthcare systems. Educators can develop their leadership skills, knowledge, behaviours and values through formal education and training (horizontally) and engaging in vertical development, through sharing personal stories and gaining feedback on their performance from trusted colleagues. For students, alongside formal teaching, they can gain understanding through activities such as guided reflection or analysis of significant events, experiential clinical placements and service learning and professional conversations, which can be scaffolded throughout the curriculum.

Often learners are self-motivated to organise their own, and their peers', learning and development. Organising projects and collecting feedback can provide students with opportunities to develop expertise and practise leadership, management and quality improvement skills. Alternatively, extracurricular events can be delivered through a student society, allow for subjects to be discussed in more depth and complement an already crowded undergraduate curriculum. Leadership should be a core learning outcome for health professionals. Students find it interesting and appear to recognise the importance of leadership to their future careers (Matthews et al., 2017). Through IPE, educators can collaborate on effecting meaningful change and future students can co-create leadership learning and development that prepares them to practise in complex health systems.

References

Austin, J., Bentkover, J., & Chait, L. (2016). *Leading strategic change in an era of healthcare transformation.* Geneva: Springer.

Barrow, M., McKimm, J., & Gasquoine, S. (2011). The policy and the practice: early-career doctors and nurses as leaders and followers in the delivery of health care. *Advances in Health Sciences Education: Theory and Practice, 16*(1), 17–29. doi:10.1007/s10459-010-9239-2.

Bass, B. M., & Riggio, R. E. (2006). *Transformational leadership* (2nd ed.). Mahwah, NJ: Lawrence Erlbaum.

Bolden, R. (2011). Distributed leadership in organizations: a review of theory and research. *International Journal of Management Reviews, 13*(3), 251–269.

Cerra, F. B., & Brandt, B. F. (2015). The growing integration of health professions education. In S. Wartman (Ed.), *The transformation of academic health centers: meeting the challenges of healthcare's changing landscape.* London: Academic Press. www.sciencedirect.com/science/book/9780128007624.

Cilliers, P. (1998). *Complexity and postmodernism: understanding complex systems.* London: Routledge.

De Meuse, K. P., Dai, G., & Hallenbeck, G. S. (2010). Learning agility: a construct whose time has come. *Consulting Psychology Journal: Practice and Research, 62*(2), 119–130.

Dow, A. W., DiazGranados, D., Mazmanian, P. E., et al. (2013). Applying organizational science to health care: a framework for collaborative practice. *Academic Medicine, 88*(7), 952.

Duckworth, A. (2016). *Grit: the power of passion and perseverance.* US: Simon & Schuster.

Dzau, V. J., ElLaissi, W. F., & Udayakumar, K. (2015). Future directions. In S. Wartman (Ed.), *The transformation of academic health centers: meeting the challenges of healthcare's changing landscape.* London: Academic Press. www.sciencedirect.com/science/book/9780128007624.

Ford, R. (2009). Complex leadership competency in health care: towards framing a theory of practice. *Health Services Management Research, 22*(3), 101–114. doi:10.1258/hsmr.2008.008016.

George, B. (2017). *VUCA 2.0: A strategy for steady leadership in an unsteady world. Leadership, 17 February.* www.forbes.com/sites/hbsworkingknowledge/2017/02/17/vuca-2-0-a-strategy-for-steady-leadership-in-an-unsteady-world/#5fcdb4013d84.

Goleman, D. (1995). *Emotional intelligence: why it can matter more than IQ.* New York: Bantam Books.

Gordon, L., Rees, C., Ker, J., et al. (2017). Using video-reflexive ethnography to capture the complexity of leadership enactment in the healthcare workplace. *Advances in Health Science Education, 22*(5), 1101–1121. doi:10.1007/s10459-016-9744-z.

Gordon, L. J., Rees, C. E., Ker, J. S., et al. (2015). Dimensions, discourses and differences: trainees conceptualising health care leadership and followership. *Medical Education, 49*(12), 1248–1262. doi:10.1111/medu.12832.

Grant, A. M., Studholme, I., Verma, R., et al. (2017). The impact of leadership coaching in an Australian healthcare setting. *Journal of Health Organization and Management, 31*(2), 237–252. doi:10.1108/JHOM-09-2016-0187.

Heifetz, R. A. (2009). *The practice of adaptive leadership: tools and tactics for changing your organisational world.* Boston: Harvard Business Press.

Kean, S., Haycock-Stuart, E., Baggaley, S., et al. (2011). Followers and the co-construction of leadership. *Journal of Nursing Management, 19*(4), 507–516. doi:10.1111/j.1365-2834.2011.01227.x.

Magellan Horth, D. (2016a). *Navigating disruption. Centre for Creative Leadership, Insights and Research Blog, 10 March*. <insights.ccl.org/blog/navigating-disruption>.

Magellan Horth, D. (2016b). *Navigating disruption, part 2. Centre for Creative Leadership, Insights and Research Blog, 18 May*. <insights.ccl.org/blog/navigating-disruptio n-part-2>.

Matthews, J. H., Morley, G. L., Crossley, E., et al. (2017). Teaching leadership: the medical student society model. *The Clinical Teacher*, doi:10.1111/tct.12649. online.

McKimm, J., O'Sullivan, H., & Jones, P. (2017). A future vision for health leadership. In *E.A. Curtis & J Cullen, Leadership and change for the health professional* (pp. 254–269). London: Open University Press.

McKimm, J. (2017). Educational leadership. In J. McKimm, K. Forrest, & J. Thistlethwaite (Eds.), *Medical education at a glance*. Chichester: Wiley Blackwell.

McKimm, J., & Till, A. (2015). Clinical leadership effectiveness, change and complexity. *British Journal of Hospital Medicine*, 76(4), 166–170.

Meindl, J. R. (1995). The romance of leadership as a follower-centric theory: a social constructionist approach. *Leadership Quarterly*, 6(3), 329–341.

Meuser, J. D., Gardner, W. L., Dinh, J. E., et al. (2016). A network analysis of leadership theory. *Journal of Management*, 42(5), 1374–1403.

Petrie, N. (2015). *The how-to of vertical leadership development–part 2: 30 experts, 3 conditions, and 15 approaches. White Paper*. Greensboro, NC: Center for Creative Leadership.

Petrie, N. (2014). *Vertical leadership development–part 1: developing leaders for a complex world*. Greensboro, NC: Center for Creative Leadership. www.ccl.org/wp-content/uploads/2015/04/VerticalLeadersPart1.pdf.

Schneider, H., English, R., Tabana, H., et al. (2014). Whole-system change: case study of factors facilitating early implementation of a primary health care reform in a South African province. *BMC Health Services Research*, 14, 609. doi:10.1186/s12913-014-0609-y.

Senge, P. M., Hamilton, H., & Kania, J. (2015). *Co-creating the future: the dawn of system leadership*. Boston: Harvard Business Review.

Senge, P. M. (1990). *The fifth discipline: the art and practice of the learning organisation*. New York: Doubleday.

Stacey, R. D. (2007). *Strategic management and organisational dynamics: the challenge of complexity to ways of thinking about organisations*. Harlow, UK: Pearson.

Sturmberg, J. P., Martin, C. M., & Katerndahl, D. A. (2014). Systems and complexity thinking in the general practice literature: an integrative, historical narrative review. *The Annals of Family Medicine*, 12(1), 66–74.

Till, A., Dutta, N., & McKimm, J. (2016). Vertical leadership in highly complex and unpredictable health systems. *British Journal of Hospital Medicine*, 77(8), 471–475. doi:10.12968/hmed.2016.77.8.471.

Till, A., & McKimm, J. (2016). Doctors leading from the frontline. *BMJ Careers*.

Uhl-Bien, M., Riggio, R. E., Lowe, K. B., et al. (2014). Followership theory: a review and research agenda. *The Leadership Quarterly*, 25, 83–104.

Warde, C. M., Vermillion, M., & Uijtdehaage, S. (2014). A medical student leadership course led to teamwork, advocacy, and mindfulness. *Family Medicine*, 46(6), 459–462.

West, M. A., Armit, K., Loewenthal, L., et al. (2015). *Leadership and leadership development in healthcare: the evidence base*. London: Faculty of Medical Leadership and Management.

West, M., Eckert, R., Steward, K., et al. (2014). *Developing collective leadership for health care*. London: The King's Fund.

24

Disruptive innovation in health professions education
How might this model guide change?

Eric S. Holmboe

Introduction

Innovation is essential to scientific advancement and improvement in medicine and healthcare delivery. Health professions education should be no different. Simply defined, an *innovation* is a new idea or more effective device or process (*Merriam Webster Dictionary*, 2017). However, ample evidence exists that the health professions education enterprise is failing to keep pace with changes occurring in medical and healthcare delivery science. In some respects, innovative approaches are urgently needed to enable health professions education across the continuum to simply catch up. The question for educators across the health professions is how to effectively identify, choose and implement innovation moving forward.

In 1997, Clayton Christensen published a landmark management book, entitled *The innovator's dilemma*, which built on his previous work exploring the distinction between disruptive versus sustaining technologies (Christensen, 1997). As Christensen noted in 1997, *sustaining technologies* are 'new technologies that foster improved product performance'. Disruptive technologies bring to market a product with a 'very different value proposition'. *Disruptive technologies*, in the beginning, will often underperform relative to 'established products in the mainstream market' (Christensen, 1997, p xviii). Disruptive technologies are also characterised by often being cheaper, simpler and more convenient to use.

From a series of studies on several industries, Christensen moved beyond just technologies to an expanded concept of *disruptive innovation*. Disruptive innovations are innovations that create 'new markets or value networks' that, if successful, will ultimately displace and disrupt existing markets and networks. It is important to note that disruptive innovations are not 'breakthrough improvements'. Instead, the innovation is often not as good as the established product, but is more accessible to different groups of individuals. In fact, primary users of the established product may not be interested in the disruptive innovation at all. However, in the long run the result of this disruption may be the displacement of established market leaders and products. Disruptive innovations can also produce significant societal change, as witnessed by profound changes in computing over the past 40 years (Christensen, 1997).

Driven by pressure from the public and healthcare systems to improve quality and safety, the rise of outcomes-based medical education is certainly producing a number of changes from undergraduate medical education through continuous professional development. In medical education, outcomes-based education is more commonly referred to as competency-based medical education (CBME). In the United States, the triple-aim framework (see Box 24.1) now guides healthcare policy, and by extension the medical education enterprise (Berwick et al., 2008). Most medical education systems now use competency frameworks to enable the implementation of an outcomes-based approach to education (Holmboe et al., 2017). An outcomes-based approach, grounded in competency frameworks, has created an urgent need for innovation. It has become clear that older educational technologies and approaches, such as high-stakes examinations and short block rotations (e.g. four to six weeks in a specific specialty or location), can no longer sufficiently prepare future health professionals for twenty-first-century practice, and are ripe for disruptive change.

Box 24.1: The triple-aim framework for health policy

1. Health of the population
2. Costs of care
3. Aims of quality. Care that is:
   a. Safe
   b. Effective
   c. Efficient
   d. Patient-centred
   e. Timely
   f. Equitable

While disruption is a useful concept to explore innovation within health professions education, a deeper examination of innovation is needed to more fully understand some of the current areas of innovation pushing to be realised and recognised. In addition to disruption, two other critical innovation concepts explored in this chapter are diffusion and complexity. Both diffusion and complexity address core issues and attributes essential to effective implementation in health professions education. Without understanding diffusion and complexity, even the best disruptive innovations will not be realised.

This chapter will begin with a brief introduction to the concepts of diffusion of innovation, complexity, and de-innovation before turning attention to disruptive innovation and organisational change. Two case studies will be explored to highlight how these key concepts in innovation can be implemented, drawing specifically from current transformation efforts in medical education that are applicable across all health professions education. Case study 24.1 will explore the use of longitudinal integrated clerkships (LICs) as an attempt to move away from the block rotation model of health professions education. Case study 24.2 will describe innovation in workplace-based assessment methods to help realise the promise of outcomes-based education.

The second half of the chapter will bring in key educational theories that enable the innovations in the case studies, and describe how innovation and theory can be translated into pedagogical practice. The reader will hear from innovators in health professions education on how they use innovation and theory to bring about change in their own training programs. Finally, the chapter will provide some suggestions for future evaluation and research.

Diffusion of innovation

Everett Rogers, among others, explored how innovations get implemented and spread, or 'diffuse'. In his classic book, *The diffusion of innovations*, Rogers summarised the process of how innovations spread through a five-stage process, which is highlighted in Table 24.1 (Rogers, 1995).

TABLE 24.1: The five stages of the innovation adoption process

Stage of adoption	Description of stage
Knowledge	An individual or group is introduced to an innovation, but lacks key information and understanding about the innovation. Another important aspect of this stage is that the individual may not yet be inspired to learn more about the innovation.
Persuasion	The individual or group is now interested in the innovation, and will actively seek out more information.
Decision	An individual or group considers the advantages/disadvantages of using the innovation, and decides whether to adopt or reject the innovation. A number of factors will affect the decision to adopt or reject.
Implementation	An individual or group implements or tries the innovation to a varying degree, depending on the situation and context. During implementation, an individual or group will also determine the utility of the innovation. Depending on this initial experience, individuals or groups may seek additional information and evidence about the innovation.
Confirmation	The individual or group finalises their decision to continue or discontinue using the innovation. A key point about this stage is it is both intrapersonal *and* interpersonal. This helps the group to confirm it has made the right decision.

Source: Adapted from Rogers (1995) and Wikipedia (2017).

In addition to the stages of innovation, potential adopters also evaluate an innovation on five key attributes. The first is *relative advantage*. Is the innovation better than the current idea or approach in use? Stated another way, is the innovation *perceived* to be more effective and efficient compared to current tools or procedures? As Rogers has pointed out, it is the perception around the innovation that affects its rate of adoption (Rogers, 1995). The second attribute is compatibility. *Compatibility* refers to 'the degree to which an innovation is perceived as being consistent with the existing values, past experiences and needs of potential adopters'. Rogers also points out a critical lesson for medical education. Specifically, the adoption of an innovation perceived to be incompatible will usually require the adoption of a new value system *first*, and this is often a slow process, as anyone can attest when implementing major changes within an educational program.

The third attribute is *complexity*, which simply refers to the degree or magnitude of difficulty in understanding and/or using the innovation. *Trialability* is the fourth key attribute: the degree to which an innovation can be 'experimented' with before full adoption. In other words, can the potential end-user take the innovation for a test drive? The fifth attribute is observability. *Observability* relates to the degree others can view and understand the results. Rogers (1995, p 15) notes: 'the easier it is for individuals to see the results of an innovation, the more likely they are to adopt'.

While all five attributes are seen to affect success of adoption, relative advantage and compatibility appear to be especially important to the ultimate adoption of any innovation (Rogers, 1995).

Complexity and innovation

Healthcare and health professions education are both highly complex fields. Complexity has a different meaning in healthcare delivery than Rogers' definition of complexity in adopting an innovation. Most of the interventions we use to improve healthcare and medical education can be appropriately labelled as complex service interventions (CSIs) (see Table 24.2).

To help us understand the concept of a CSI, I will turn to a framework that Pawson and colleagues have used in the context of evaluating health care and policy interventions (Pawson et al., 2005). Complex interventions in the context of medical education operate on the hypothesis that if they are implemented (successfully) they will facilitate improved educational outcomes of learners and ultimately improve patient care outcomes.

TABLE 24.2: Milestones and the implications of complex service interventions (CSIs)

Characteristic	Implication for competencies and Milestones
1. CSIs operate on the hypothesis that if they are implemented effectively they will produce positive change	Competencies and Milestones are grounded in sound educational theory, but will require application of implementation theories to be most effective.
2. CSIs are active	Implementation requires the interdependent actions of multiple individuals. Implementation of any change requires a coalition with shared goals.
3. CSIs have a long journey	Transforming graduate medical education is a long, iterative process involving multiple stakeholders. This long journey requires a commitment on the part of all of the stakeholders to embrace change and engage in collaboration and co-production through civil discourse.
4. Implementation chains for CSIs are also non-linear	Implementation of competencies and Milestones will not be a simple, stepwise process. There will be 'ups and downs' along the journey. Some implementation strategies will be more impactful than others, and not always related to the magnitude of effort involved. It will be essential moving forward for the entire community to learn what triggers small and large intended and unintended effects.
5. CSIs are very fragile	Any change process, such as implementing Milestones, is fragile and can be easily disrupted by institutional changes, unanticipated events, frustration, inability to let go of ineffective approaches and cynicism. As a collective educational community, we must work together to work through and avoid such pitfalls.
6. CSIs are prone to mutate	Milestones will change and 'mutate' over time as they must. The current set of Milestones has always been labelled 'version 1.0'. There was a full realisation that they will need to change as programs learn, mutate and change Milestones during these early phases of implementation.
7. CSIs operate as 'open systems that will feed back on themselves'	There are multiple important feedback loops involving Milestones: feedback to and with residents and fellows; feedback within programs to help programs continually improve; feedback to help whole specialties evolve and improve through national reporting of Milestones data.

Source: Holmboe, ES. (2017b). The Journey to Competency-based Medical Education — Implementing Milestones. Marshall Journal of Medicine: 3:1; Article 2.

Secondly, CSIs are active, 'that is, they achieve their effects via the active input of [multiple] individuals (clinicians, educators, managers, patients [and learners])' (Pawson et al., 2005, p 22). Educational innovators must recognise that the knowledge, skills and actions of these interdependent actors will affect how and whether the innovation is adopted and implemented, and whether the innovation achieves its intended purposes within a program. Too often in health professions education we do not take sufficient time to reflect and try to understand the various roles and actions of individuals when implementing a change and building change coalitions.

Thirdly, CSIs have a long journey, especially if a new value system needs to be built and adopted. Implementation of any innovation or intervention must be accompanied by an evaluation plan to determine what works, for whom, in what circumstances, and why. Successful innovations will most often involve an iterative journey of learning and revision, embedded within complex adaptive systems (CAS) such as hospitals where medical education occurs. Complex adaptive systems are characterised by non-linear interdependence among people and activities that often operate on the edge of chaos (Plsek & Greenhalgh 2001). It is clear why implementation of CSIs would be challenging within healthcare institutions!

Fourthly, implementation chains for CSIs are non-linear. As noted above, non-linearity is a hallmark of all complex systems. Non-linearity can mean that 'large' interventions may have little to modest impact while, conversely, small interventions have large impact. Complex interventions in the early phases of implementation can actually cause regression (i.e. things get worse) as the actors in the system grapple with the changes necessary for effective implementation. It is important to monitor the relative influence and actions of all individuals involved in the implementation process in order to make iterative adjustments.

Fifthly, CSIs are very fragile, as they are embedded in multiple, dynamic social systems. In healthcare, many of these social systems are organised as microsystems. As defined by Nelson and colleagues (2007, p 7), a microsystem is simply a combination of a small group of people who work together on a regular basis to provide care and the subpopulation of patients who receive that care. It has clinical and business aims, linked processes, and a shared information environment, and it produces services and care that can be measured as performance outcomes. Many training microsystems are geographically located within hospitals, such as the emergency department, hospital ward, radiology suite, operating theatre, and so on. Our healthcare learners encounter multiple microsystems every day. These microsystems have profound influence on students' experiential learning and assessment, along with the social milieu (Bates & Ellaway, 2016; Ogrinc & Headrick, 2008).

Sixthly, CSIs will typically 'mutate', based on local context and needs, and not be implemented as entirely intended. Some refer to this as 'fidelity of implementation', but each program will confront its own contextual realities and make changes. This is not necessarily a bad thing, but rather represents the reality of potentially implementing innovations in more than one context. This observation calls out the need to embrace the likelihood of mutation as a learning opportunity that can guide the ongoing study and refinement of the innovation.

Finally, CSIs operate and function as 'open systems that will feed back on themselves'. The activities of implementation will themselves lead to further changes as learning occurs among those both performing and being affected by the innovation. This learning and ongoing change is part of the long journey, as well as the mutability and fragility of complex interventions (Pawson et al., 2005, p 23).

De-innovation

On the surface, innovation sounds fun and exciting, but using the lens of disruption, diffusion and complexity, innovation involves change. And change is, and always has been, hard! (Note: the concept of the difficulty of change is as old as dirt.) While it is beyond the scope of this chapter to cover all of the theories in change management, one does deserve a brief mention. Ubel and Asch introduced the concept of 'de-innovation' in healthcare delivery (Ubel & Asch, 2015). Essentially, de-innovation is an unlearning and letting-go process, so as to make space for innovation and change.

Otto Scharmer described this journey in his book *Theory U*, where the down-stroke, left-hand side of the U is letting go, so that something better can emerge on the upstroke, right-hand side of the U (Scharmer, 2016). For Scharmer, this journey starts with an open mind that moves to an open heart (emotion), to ultimately an open will to move forward with change. For example, the older clinical supervisor, based on their own training, may still believe in high-stakes testing as the predominant testing strategy, and more confrontational approaches to feedback, because these approaches have always worked for them. I often refer to this syndrome as *nostalgialitis imperfecta profunda* (i.e. profound and imperfect nostalgia about one's past training experiences). The letting-go stage starts with an open mind that new approaches to programmatic assessment approaches and feedback, based on new science and evidence, might be better and worth a try. The open-heart stage (emotion) depends on the supervisor's desire to make things better for their trainees and patients. Assuming these two stages are successfully engaged, the supervisor begins to build the will and motivation to try the change.

You can see this concept of de-innovation at work in Christensen's disruptive innovation model — individuals and organisations in the 'up-market' struggle with de-innovation — and Scharmer's open-mind stage (Christensen, 1997; Scharmer, 2016). In fact, Scharmer points out that many of us simply continue to download past patterns of beliefs and behaviours because, after all, they have worked for these individuals and organisations *until they don't*. And that is a critical message of disruptive innovation.

Disruptive innovation and organisational models

Let's briefly return to disruptive innovations in healthcare, with a particular focus on technology, as this will be useful later in exploring one of the medical education examples. Christensen and colleagues have explored why disruptive medical technologies have not yet substantially disrupted healthcare delivery, especially in North America (Christensen et al., 2009). After all, multiple innovative technologies already exist that could change healthcare delivery, such as artificial intelligence, wearable devices that can track multiple physiological parameters, and so forth. Their argument is that new technologies are almost always introduced as sustaining, not disruptive, technology. As Christensen and colleagues state, technology is almost always implemented 'primarily to help hospitals and doctors solve the most complex problems. There is nothing wrong with this, of course, but it does little to make health care more affordable and accessible.' (Christensen et al., 2009, p xxii).

One wonders whether a similar phenomenon is occurring in health professions education when new curricula are introduced to meet expanded expectations, simulation centres to supplement or even replace skills development previously done in the clinical work space, and so forth. Channeling Christensen, there is nothing inherently wrong with this, but does all of this produce a better healthcare professional who more effectively meets the needs of the public and with less cost (and by extension, in some countries, less student debt)?

As we think about 'disrupting' health professions education to improve outcomes, looking at the work of Norwegian economists Stabell and Fjeldstad can be instructive (Christensen et al., 2009; Stabell and Fjeldstad, 1998). They describe three essential business models: solution shops, value-added process businesses and facilitated user networks.

Solution shops are 'institutions built to diagnose and solve unstructured problems' (Christensen et al., 2009, pp 20–22). Academic medical centres are first and foremost solution shops. Patients with complex or undifferentiated problems often seek help from academic medical centres to find solutions. Many of our health professions students learn in solution shops. The good news is that they may see many interesting and unusual patients, patients with diseases and a combination of clinical problems they may never see again once in practice. On the surface this may seem like a useful educational experience, but it often comes at a cost. In my own experience training at a tertiary-care hospital, most of the patients I cared for as a resident were experiencing complications from their severe disease or were referred to the centre because they had an uncommon, and at times rare, medical problem. It was uncommon for me to evaluate and admit a patient to the hospital with one or more of the common diseases that cause the bulk of societal health problems. It was even rarer to spend time in an ambulatory setting, working with a panel of patients longitudinally. I truly trained in a solution shop.

Value-added process businesses 'transform inputs of resources, such as people, equipment, raw materials, energy, and capital, into outputs of greater value' (Christensen et al., 2009, pp 22–23). In essence, health professions schools are value-added type businesses. Schools often bristle at the thought of being a business, but they design educational processes that involve resources (e.g. library, information technology, etc.), people (i.e. faculty and others), equipment (e.g. simulators), raw materials (an entering student!), energy, and capital (tuition, endowments, etc.) to produce an output of greater value, namely a health professional (hopefully) prepared to meet societal needs. You can quickly see where tensions can arise when a learner, who has started their education in a value-adding health professions school (which is focused on building core competencies to meet common and pressing societal needs), is suddenly thrust into a solution-shop environment (which is more focused on rarer diseases and complications) to complete their training.

This framework also highlights another current philosophical problem plaguing health professions education — our learners as products. Instead, health professions education and healthcare should be grounded in a service, not product, logic (Holmboe & Batalden, 2015). The majority of training, after all, is experiential learning in the *service* of patients and families. Viewing healthcare and health professions education through a service logic lens is better aligned with person-centredness, and allows educators to move away from seeing students as simply widgets moving along a production line to graduation.

Finally, *facilitated user networks* are 'enterprises in which the same people buy and sell and deliver and receive things to and from each other' (Christensen et al., 2009, pp 24–25). For example, the Kaiser Permanente healthcare system in the United States is developing its own medical school, which will be added to its existing stable of graduate medical education (GME) programs. The system will put resources into its medical school and GME programs, with the goal of transitioning the most capable graduates into its own healthcare system (Kaiser Permanente School of Medicine, 2017). In other words, the Kaiser Permanente system will deliver and receive some health professionals from itself across the medical education continuum in a deliberate way. In other countries, such as the Netherlands, this also happens to a degree, as students move from medical school into graduate medical education programs within a country that has universal healthcare and allows medical students to graduate at variable times throughout the year.

Pulling it all together

We have now covered a number of important concepts around innovation. Before turning to our two medical education examples, let's briefly review and pull together these concepts.

Innovations simply represent new and hopefully better ideas, tools and approaches. The adoption of innovation depends on five key attributes: relative advantage, compatibility, complexity, trialability and observability (Rogers, 1995). However, since most innovations in health professions education can be classified as complex service interventions (CSIs), additional characteristics will come into play during adoption and implementation. CSIs are embedded in multiple social systems involving multiple agents, will mutate and reinvent themselves, are non-linear, will feedback on themselves and often have a long success journey (Pawson et al., 2005).

These attributes and characteristics of innovations can be disruptive in their own right. However, Christensen's concept of disruptive innovation may be viewed as a subtype or subset of innovation grounded in specific characteristics of innovations. Per Christensen, disruptive innovations are often cheaper, simpler and more convenient to use. Disruptive innovations are innovations that create 'new markets or value networks' that, if successful, will ultimately displace and disrupt existing markets and networks (Christensen 1997; Christensen et al., 2009).

As I will elaborate below, these characteristics do apply to parts of the two areas of innovation in medical education we will explore, but not necessarily all. In order to more fully understand innovation in health professions education, the challenge is to integrate and synthesise the lessons and research from disruptive innovation, the diffusion of innovation, and complex intervention science and economic theory — territory that we as health professions educators rarely tread.

Background to the case studies

Health professions education across the continuum is being buffeted and challenged by many factors across the globe. On the healthcare delivery side, quality, patient safety, healthcare costs, ageing populations, the growing burden of chronic disease, new infections and epidemics, and patient engagement are some of the factors forcing the health professions education community to critically examine its educational designs and processes. Frenk and colleagues in 2010 argued passionately that medical education programs globally must align with the health and healthcare needs of the populations served (Frenk et al., 2010).

These population and healthcare system challenges have helped to catalyse a push to move health professions education to a more outcomes-based model. Competency frameworks have been developed over the past 25 years as a mechanism to describe the abilities, or educational outcomes, needed by healthcare professionals for twenty-first-century clinical practice (Holmboe et al., 2017). Table 24.3 provides examples of several competency frameworks.

More recently, as covered in the chapters in the assessment section of this book, the newer concepts of milestones and entrustable professional activities (EPAs) have been introduced into several national medical education systems, as educational frameworks to assist in the implementation and operationalisation of the competencies and to help achieve the desired outcomes (Holmboe et al., 2017; ten Cate & Scheele, 2007).

If the goal is truly to move to an outcomes-based approach to improve health professions education and, more importantly, patient care, then how might disruptive innovations help? To help answer this question, let's explore two current case studies, one primarily targeting curricular change through longitudinal integrated clerkships (LICs), and another primarily targeting assessment, specifically new approaches to workplace-based assessment.

TABLE 24.3: The competencies of physicians as described by four organisations*

Canada	United Kingdom	United States
Medical expert	Good clinical care	Medical knowledge
Communicator	Maintaining good medical practice	Interpersonal and communication skills
Collaborator	Teaching and training appraising and assessing	Patient care
Leader	Relationships with patients	Professionalism Systems-based practice
Health advocate	Working with colleagues	Practice-based learning and improvement
Scholar	Probity	Systems-based practice
Professional	Health	—

*The organisations represented are: the Royal College of Physicians and Surgeons of Canada; the United Kingdom General Medical Council; the Accreditation Council for Graduate Medical Education; and the American Board of Medical Specialties.
Source: Adapted from E. S. Holmboe. (2017). The journey to competency-based medical education — implementing milestones. *Marshall Journal of Medicine, 3*, 1; article 2.

Case study 24.1: Longitudinal integrated clerkships

Longitudinal integrated clerkships (LICs) are receiving increasing interest globally as a potentially better educational model to prepare medical students for graduate medical education and twenty-first-century medical practice (Hirsh et al., 2012b; Poncelet & Hirsh, 2016). Unlike the traditional 'block rotation' model of medical school, where a student spends a prescribed amount of time (usually one to three months) in a specialty rotation (e.g. family medicine, surgery, internal medicine, and others), medical students in an LIC model are assigned a group of patients they follow longitudinally over the course of the year (Hirsh et al., 2007). The model affords students 'educational continuity' (Hirsh et al., 2007, p 858) as the students accompany the patients for medical appointments, hospitalisations, surgeries or other healthcare interactions as they occur. LIC students also have 'continuity of supervision' through year-long longitudinal supervisors and mentors they meet with regularly as part of their learning (Hirsh et al., 2007, p 859). Comparable to the block rotation model, students receive structured education in key topics through didactics and workshops.

In their recent textbook, Poncelet and Hirsh state that LICs are 'driven by a commitment to training the best physicians to meet the health care needs of individuals and communities' (Poncelet & Hirsh, 2016, p 1). This commitment is well aligned with the goals of outcomes-based medical education (Frenk et al., 2010; McGaghie et al., 1978). Evidence exists that students trained in LIC programs perform at least as well as their block rotation counterparts on national board exams and on high-stakes licensing examinations (Hirsh et al., 2012a; Poncelet & Hirsh 2016). Students also 'demonstrate significant public orientation in their ethos and many choose to contribute to the community in which they study' (Walters & Cosgrove, 2016, p 235).

LICs in their various configurations are all 'based upon five guiding principles: continuity relationships with patients over time, continuity relationships with faculty preceptors over time, a continuous learning community of peer learners, continuity of setting and system of practice, and a longitudinal developmental pedagogy' (Mazotti & Ogur, 2016, p 29). These principles of continuity as an organising principle align with contemporary educational learning theories that take into account the complex interplay between cognition and sociocultural factors in learning (Hirsh et al., 2007). The LIC is also grounded in several other educational theories, such as interleaved learning and meaningful deliberate practice (Ericsson, 2004; Rohrer & Pashler, 2010).

While LICs are certainly innovative and have disrupted the status quo at those institutions that have implemented them, they do not necessarily meet the pure definition of Christensen's disruptive innovation (Christensen, 1997). Whereas the cost of LICs is *not* demonstrated to be more expensive, LICs may not be necessarily cheaper (when considering initial start-up time), or simpler, or more convenient for the consumer (notions Christensen describes). Accordingly, Dr David Hirsh, a leader in the LIC movement, reflects that LICs are 'innovative and disruptive, but require consideration as to how they connect to Christensen's original definition of disruptive innovation' (Hirsh, personal communication, 2017). Hirsh notes that LICs are in some respects 'up-market' compared to traditional block clerkship rotations, because LICs call for:

> *educational considerations, deliberate design, and dynamic scheduling to maximize [sic] the student's experience. LICs are designed and managed in a co-production and collaborative model with faculty and students (and at times, patients) to continually refine and improve the LICs. Through co-planning and co-creation, students have real and meaningful input into their LIC experience. To sum up our LIC philosophy, LICs do not overly ascribe to hierarchy except when it is in the best interest of learning and caregiving; there is less an 'us and you' philosophy but rather an 'all of us in this together' approach to medical education and the care delivery that students engage. (Hirsh, personal communication, 2017)*

LICs require effort to implement and, as a dynamic program, to maintain over time. The quality of the experience may in fact be better, as highlighted above, potentially signifying that LICs may be a breakthrough change. They are certainly creating a 'new market', but one embedded within, not outside, the traditional medical school. LICs may also be attracting a particular subset of students interested in innovation and longitudinal relationships (Ogur & Hirsh, 2009). At this point, you may logically ask: How do we recognise and understand LICs as disruptive innovations?

The early LIC experience highlights an important paradox; that the current model of medical education using block rotations for the clinical years has been designed to be the most convenient and efficient model for faculty and training institutions. Rotations are more predictable, administratively more manageable, and can be standardised to some degree. In other words, students are treated as interchangeable widgets (a product mentality in a value-added network) plugged into an existing educational scaffold (Holmboe & Batalden, 2015). While this model possesses many convenient attributes, multiple studies over time have demonstrated that too many students are not sufficiently prepared to enter postgraduate medical training (Frischknecht et al., 2014; Lypson et al., 2004). Furthermore, costs for medical education overall have continued to increase, akin to an up-market mentality and consistent with the kind of markets that become disrupted, according to Christensen's framework (Christensen, 1997).

The situation is no better in many postgraduate (aka GME) training programs that use a rotational model. A number of recent studies also show that too many graduates of postgraduate programs (called 'residencies' in the United States) are not prepared to enter unsupervised practice after graduation (Crosson et al., 2011; Mattar et al., 2013). Perhaps most concerning is recent research that demonstrates that patient harm, including increased mortality, is associated with trainee transitions between one clinical rotation to another (Bernabeo et al., 2011; Denson et al., 2016; Holmboe et al., 2011).

LICs do not have such abrupt transitions for the learner, the faculty adviser and, perhaps most importantly, the patient. LICs may therefore be the canary in the coalmine, surfacing the substantial flaws in current structural models of medical education, especially at the undergraduate level. This clearly makes LICs both innovative and disruptive, if not necessarily a classic disruptive innovation in terms of cost and simplicity.

Interest is accelerating in exploring other innovative training models likely to be disruptive, such as early entry into postgraduate training programs from medical school for capable learners, earlier transition into subspecialty training, shortening undergraduate health professions education (e.g. nursing, medicine, etc.) using competency-based models and distance learning, and mid-career shifts using the site of practice as a learning setting with distance mentoring. All of these new curricular approaches have the potential to disrupt current medical education paradigms; whether they are cheaper and simpler to use is yet to be determined.

One reason for the hesitancy around all of these new models of training is the concern that less capable trainees could 'slip through', a situation not tolerable to the public. It is one thing to work with a less powerful personal computer compared to a mainframe computer than to see a less competent physician. Interestingly, LICs appear to do the opposite; LICs provide particular real-world practice challenges — self-organising, managing multiple competing commitments, and, perhaps most importantly, understanding patients, health and healthcare holistically — that may 'expose' learners in need (Hirsh et al., 2012b).

Case study 24.2: Workplace-based assessment in medical education

Outcomes-based medical education places greater pressure on assessment; medical education programs now must determine with a high degree of confidence that graduating trainees can actually do what the program says a graduate should be able to do in unsupervised clinical practice (Lockyer et al., 2017). No longer is it sufficient to simply complete a course of study without any missteps or problems and pass a high-stakes test as a proxy for overall competence to be a healthcare professional. For nearly a hundred years, however, education in medicine, like education across most health professionals programs, has relied heavily on proxy assessments, such as high-stakes licensing and certification examinations, as the primary measure of competence.

This is especially true in the United States, where medical trainees must pass four examinations (United States Medical Licensing Examinations) to obtain a licence, followed by another specialty examination for certification. These examinations can be expensive to develop (the development cost for a single question on a certification examination can cost several thousand dollars) and deliver. Candidates often incur additional expenses due to the travel necessary to complete an examination at a testing centre.

Despite these costs, there were, and are, several logical and rational reasons why testing became and remains the central component of assessment systems in many countries. First, knowledge remains an essential component of being a healthcare professional. However, the assessment of knowledge is overemphasised, based partly on the belief that if someone is really smart they must be equally proficient in the other competencies. This is the classic correlational rater error, more commonly called the *halo effect* (Pangaro et al., 2018). For the surgical discipline, this same error extends to procedural skills. How many times have you heard someone say a physician has lousy communication skills but 'they're really smart', or they 'are a great surgeon in the operating theatre but not a warm and fuzzy person', therefore justifying a diminution of other competencies such as communication, professionalism, quality and patient safety?

Secondly, the science of testing, psychometrics, clearly advanced during the twentieth century, enabling organisations to deliver high-stakes examinations with increasing quality and rigour (Downing, 2006). Psychometrics enabled the assessment of knowledge effectively and efficiently, at least in a controlled setting. Psychometrics also enabled tests to be evaluated for validity and fairness, critical elements in high-stakes assessment.

Thirdly, research has found a correlation between performance on high-stakes examinations and some aspects of patient care quality, an important component of validity. However, the amount of variance explained by test performance and clinical practice is modest at best (Holmboe et al., 2010; Lipner et al., 2013).

In essence, these high-stakes examinations are the 'up-market' in the Christensen model. Organisations that produce the tests continue to make important refinements and improvements, but the tests have gone up in price, not down. What a test can tell us about a health professional has likely 'peaked' — there is only so much a test can tell you about all of the abilities needed by healthcare professionals. The end-users of the test results, akin to Christensen's observations, also continue to drive, for the moment, the testing organisation's drive to maintain and refine this somewhat expensive system. For example, residency programs in the United States — those programs that prepare physicians for specialty practice — continue to rely heavily on the results of the first step of the licensing examination for the selection of students into postgraduate training (Prober et al., 2016). On the certification side, health systems and hospitals use certification in their initial selection and credentialling processes for new graduates entering practice. Finally, the public is rightly looking for assurance that physicians are properly trained and possess sufficient knowledge to care for them effectively.

As the twentieth century closed, however, signals emerged suggesting that this over-reliance on high-stakes multiple-choice tests for medical education was problematic. Health services and systems science began to mature, and developed new methods and approaches to measure the quality, safety and costs of care. The results globally were sobering, as many problems in the quality and safety of care were uncovered (Frenk et al., 2010, Mossialos et al., 2015).

In the United States, the Institute of Medicine's too seminal reports, *To err is human* and *Crossing the quality chasm*, laid out in stark detail the breadth and magnitude of patient safety and quality problems affecting the US healthcare system (Institute of Medicine 2000, 2001). These reports, among others, helped to catalyse the US outcomes-based medical education movement, culminating in the launch of the six general competencies in 2001 (see Table 24.3). Similar pubic pressure also catalysed the development of the CanMEDS roles in Canada in 1995 (see Table 24.3).

Subsequent research has continued to find pernicious problems throughout the healthcare system. In 2015, the National Patient Safety Foundation (NPSF) concluded that progress in improving safety had been agonisingly slow over the previous decade (National Patient Safety Foundation, 2016). The National Academy of Medicine released a report, *Improving diagnosis*, arguing that diagnostic error was a highly serious *patient safety* problem (National Academy of Medicine, 2015). They found that diagnostic errors remain deeply problematic, and noted that *every* American — a country of over 320 million people — will experience at least one diagnostic error in their lifetime. Finally, Makary and Daniel, in a provocative article argued that medical errors, the combination of both diagnostic and therapeutic errors, are now the third leading cause of death in the United States (Makary & Daniel, 2016).

On a personal note, these data hit close to home. Both of my parents experienced multiple life-threatening diagnostic errors in their lifetime. For my father, one of his would prove to be fatal. All of their physicians had passed the multiple licensing examinations and their initial specialty certification examinations. I honestly believe my parents' physicians wanted to provide high-quality care. However, a logical question is whether examinations at any stage of a career help keep physicians up to date and, perhaps more importantly, attend to other critical competencies necessary for twenty-first-century practice, including the complexities of clinical reasoning.

The point of all this may now be clear: relying solely on high-stakes testing is clearly insufficient to address the issues underlying these sobering statistics. Medicine has become highly complex, and must move beyond an over-reliance on episodic proxy assessments, such as high-stakes multiple-choice question examinations. New approaches to assessment are clearly needed to help all healthcare professionals continuously improve, and to assure the public that those of us in medicine are keeping up (Cook et al., 2015).

The realisation that high-stakes tests, even for practising physicians, are not meeting current healthcare needs helped to catalyse the creation of the competencies, and more recently the accelerated development of workplace-based assessments. Many of these new assessments are designed to capture the direct observations of faculty, patients, peers and interprofessional colleagues about a trainee's ability. Others are rethinking how to assess medical knowledge in the clinical workspace to address the serious problems in clinical reasoning and medical errors. And all, at the moment, share characteristics of disruptive innovations by being simpler to deliver, are being pushed by advocates outside the traditional regulatory system, and have also not yet achieved the psychometric bar pushed by regulators. In other words, workplace-based assessments are messy and less standardised, but may in the end be more meaningful and impactful.

Competencies such as history-taking, physical examination, counselling and shared decision-making and interprofessional teamwork, to name just a few, require a workplace-based, in-vivo approach. Workplace-based assessments targetting the other competencies usually consist of a rating scale and narrative comments. For years these assessments were mostly captured through paper-based forms. However, many are now being adapted and developed as applications for mobile devices, and we may now have truly disruptive innovations emerging in medical education. For purposes of illustration, I will highlight a major change in postgraduate medical training in the United States, and how technology is helping to implement this new approach to assessment. The first innovation currently being attempted in postgraduate education (aka GME) is the use of Milestones.

By definition, a 'milestone' is simply a significant point in development. For GME programs in the United States, the Milestones provide narrative descriptors of the competencies and subcompetencies along a developmental continuum with varying degrees of granularity (Holmboe et al., 2016). Simply stated, the Milestones describe the performance levels that trainees are expected to demonstrate for knowledge, skills, attitudes and especially behaviours in the six clinical competency domains. They lay out a framework of observable behaviours and other attributes associated with a resident's or fellow's development as a physician. The basic terminology used within the Milestones is included in Fig. 24.1.

Milestone description: template				
Level 1	**Level 2**	**Level 3**	**Level 4**	**Level 5**
What are the expectations for a beginning resident?	What are the milestones for a resident who has advanced over entry, but is performing at a lower level than expected at mid-residency?	What are the key developmental milestones mid-residency? What should they be able to do well in the realm of the specialty at this point?	What does a graduating resident look like? What additional knowledge, skills and attitudes have they obtained? Are they ready for certification?	Stretch goals — Exceeds expectation
☐ ☐ ☐ ☐ ☐ ☐ ☐ ☐ ☐				
Comments:				

Figure 24.1: General description of Milestone levels
Source: Milestone Guidebook for Residents and Fellows (2017). Accreditation Council for Graduate Medical Education, https://www.acgme.org/Portals/0/PDFs/Milestones/MilestonesGuidebookforResidentsFellows.pdf

The Milestones describe the learning trajectory within a subcompetency that takes the trainee from a beginner in the specialty or subspecialty, to a proficient trainee or early practitioner. Milestones are different from many other assessments, in that there is an opportunity for the learner to also demonstrate the attainment of aspirational levels of the subcompetency, and, just as importantly, allows for a shared understanding of the expectations for the learner and the members of the faculty. Milestones can provide a framework for all GME programs that allows for some assurance that graduating trainees across the United States have attained a high level of competency. At the current time, the Milestones are intended for formative purposes only, to help learners and the training programs improve their educational and assessment processes (Holmboe et al., 2016).

Programs use the Milestones rubric twice a year to judge a trainee's progress. This process is accomplished through programmatic assessment, where a group of educators, called a clinical competency committee (CCC), reviews data from a combination of workplace-based assessments to determine where a trainee is developmentally. Typical assessment methods used to inform the CCC discussion are faculty evaluations, direct observation, multi-source feedback and performance data using quality measures from the trainee's clinical practice. In other words, Milestones facilitate a synthetic, more holistic judgment across multiple workplace-based assessment methods and tools. When the assessment program works well, the trainee receives meaningful feedback that they use to create an individualised learning plan for the next six months. You may have quickly noticed that a high-stakes examination is not a part of this package. While many residents and fellows take a standardised knowledge examination called an in-training examination (ITE), it is given only once a year, meaning that the majority of the assessment of clinical reasoning will indeed occur via workplace-based assessment.

How is technology helping to operationalise the Milestones developmental approach to assessment? One example is called Mobile Medical Milestones (M3), which marries mobile technologies and workplace-based assessment (Page et al., 2017). The M3 mobile app allows faculty working with a trainee in any setting to simply dictate their observation and feedback into their smartphone. The M3 app uses natural language processing to convert the dictation to text. The faculty then simply 'tags' the narrative assessment to a specific Milestone, and the assessment encounter is then uploaded into a learning management system. The trainee also has instant access to the feedback text for their own learning. There are a growing number of these types of tools that can capture assessment in real time with increasing efficiency, and allow this information to be captured in a central repository to aid learner reflection on performance across time (Bohnen et al., 2016; Page et al., 2017).

Sounds pretty compelling, right? Will these types of assessments delivered by mobile technologies be the disruptive innovation that enables outcomes-based education to become a reality? Time will tell, but a quick review of the current limitations of workplace-based assessment is warranted, given we are using a disruptive innovation lens. From a traditional validity point of view, workplace-based assessment probably isn't yet as good as a high-stakes test (but it may be getting closer than educators and regulators think). For one, faculty assessments are prone to multiple rater cognitive problems, such as the halo effect, leniency error, contrast effects, and so forth (Gingerich et al., 2014; Kogan et al., 2017). Faculty also tend to use themselves as their primary assessment frame of reference to judge trainee performance. This is fine so long as the faculty possess expertise in the very competency they are judging; unfortunately, many of our faculty are struggling with the very competencies they are being asked to assess (Kogan et al., 2010). Faculty also tend to possess their own idiosyncrasies, which can be a bad or good thing, depending on whether the idiosyncrasy is a strength and up-to-date or a weakness and out-of-date (Gingerich et al., 2014).

However, all of these limitations describe the characteristics of a disruptive innovation in its early phases. Furthermore, all of the challenges just laid out are addressable. Reliability can be improved simply through increasing the amount of sampling longitudinally. The M3 app is a good example of using technology to simplify the assessment data collection process (Page et al., 2017), enabling learners to keep a record of multiple assessments over time. Faculty can also be trained to improve their own clinical skills, including in clinical reasoning, and also be trained to be better observers of clinical skills (Kogan et al., 2015; Kogan et al., 2017). Group process can maximise the quality of judgments (Andolsek et al., 2017; Hauer et al., 2016a; van der Vleuten 2016). Data analytics is increasingly being used to assist these group judgments by systematically and rigorously organising and interpreting different types of data into useful formats (Warm et al., 2016).

While much, much more research and evaluation needs to be done, as Milestones are still in early days, national validity studies on the specialty Milestones now exist for five specialties (Beeson et al., 2015; Conforti et al., 2017; Hauer et al., 2016b; Li et al., 2017; Peabody et al., 2017).

The innovation concepts of diffusion and complexity also apply to Milestones implementation. For example, early research shows that Milestone implementation has varied across programs on several of Rogers' key diffusion characteristics. As you might expect, the innovators and early adopters are finding more relative advantage and value in the Milestones (Warm et al., 2016). Compatibility appears to depend on the program's perceived need for change in graduate medical education, and on the users' ability to 'unlearn' (Holmboe, 2017). Table 24.3 views Milestones through the lens of a complex service intervention, expanding on the lessons of Rogers' diffusion model.

Implementing Milestones involves many individuals, is deeply embedded in social networks, and the process is fragile and long (Pawson et al., 2005). The rise of new workplace-based assessments are helping in this major change, and are beginning to disrupt prior approaches to assessment overall. What are the implications for high-stakes testing? While it is unlikely in the short term, workplace-based assessments will completely displace high-stakes testing because, as is often seen with disruptive innovations, it is becoming clear that there is a rebalancing afoot, especially in the United States.

Educational theory and innovation

To this point we have discussed how key theories and insights from disruptive innovations, diffusion of innovation, and complexity will influence the ultimate adoption of LICs (a complex service intervention itself), Milestones and point-of-care workplace-based assessment tools. However, all of these innovations are grounded in robust educational theories. Use of educational theory is important in the development of innovations. Theory should underlie the why and how of an innovation as it connects a hypothesis to a desired outcome. As Pawson and colleagues note, CSIs operate on the hypothesis that if the CSI is implemented effectively, a pre-defined better outcome will result (Pawson et. al., 2005).

For LICs, the hypothesis is that a longitudinal integrated educational experience will 'better' prepare medical students for postgraduate training and for practice beyond residency (Gaufberg et al., 2014; Hirsh et al., 2012b; Poncelet & Hirsh 2016). But what constitutes 'better'? The early LIC literature suggests that students in LICs may retain more compassion and build better relationships and communication skills (Gaufberg et al., 2014; Latessa et al., 2017; Walters and Cosgrove, 2016). The acquisition of knowledge, as measured by tests, appears to be equivalent with medical students in traditional clerkships (Walters & Cosgrove, 2016).

LICs operate on several key theories. One is *interleaved learning*, the weaving of different types of learning and topics longitudinally (Poncelet & Hirsh, 2016). So, instead of learning mostly psychiatry in a four-week rotation, psychiatry training is interleaved throughout the year with repeated opportunities to learn and apply key principles and communication skills in caring for patients who often have multiple conditions needing care.

The second theory highlighted by this example is *holism* (Givon & Simanton, 2016, p 81). Instead of seeing patients as parts related to the medical service where the students are training, students are assigned a panel of patients they follow throughout the year. They go to where the patient needs care. For example, if their patient with coronary heart disease and diabetes suddenly needs bowel surgery, they will participate in the admission and the surgical procedure.

Another key set of theories and principles revolve around *coaching and feedback*. Students are assigned a coach adviser, who works with the student throughout the year to engage in feedback and develop and refine the student's learning plans (Hirsh et al., 2007; Poncelet & Hirsh 2016). While I have covered only a few here, you can see how this innovative approach to medical school is grounded in a number of educational theories and principles.

Workplace-based assessment is no different. As highlighted in Chapters 18, 19 and 20, accurate assessment is a critical precursor to effective feedback and coaching. Without it, effective feedback and coaching are simply not possible. As many have pointed out, the development of expertise is extremely difficult, if not impossible, without practice under observation, feedback and coaching (Ericsson, 2004). Second, workplace-based assessments, especially direct observation, sit at the top of the Miller pyramid (i.e. what the trainee actually can do in the clinical setting) (Miller, 1990). Workplace-based assessments, unlike tests and other proxy assessments, can incorporate the critical element of context. Yes, dealing with variable and ever-changing contexts is messy, but in the end it is the reality our learners and patients experience. Workplace-based assessments incorporate key theories from validity and programmatic assessment (Schuwirth & van der Vleuten, 2011; van der Vleuten and Schuwirth, 2005).

Finally, workplace-based assessments are also tapping into the importance of activating learners to engage in assessment as co-producers (Holmboe & Batalden, 2015). For example, learners should be activated to seek out observation and feedback. Learners can audit their own clinical practice through the medical record. They can ask patients for feedback about their performance. All of these activities are what Sargeant and colleagues have called *informed self-assessment* (Sargeant et al., 2011). While this informed self-assessment process is both complex and complicated, it is essential for the ongoing development of expertise. Without active engagement, learners risk experiencing arrested development, or, put another way, the flattening of their developmental trajectory. Both LICs and workplace-based assessments facilitate co-production and informed self-assessment process.

Directions for evaluation and research

Longitudinal integrated clerkships

While there are multiple areas of research still needed for LICs, assessment is clearly a critical area (Poncelet & Hirsh, 2016). We can now bring the previous lessons of the chapter together to explore some potential directions for research around assessment and LICs. LICs rely predominantly on workplace-based type assessments, which should be combined and integrated as a program of assessment (Hirsh et al., 2014). As we noted above, programmatic assessment models emphasise multiple formative assessments (Schuwirth & van der Vleuten, 2011; van der Vleuten & Schuwirth, 2005). Programs of assessment are increasing the utilisation of narrative, and qualitative judgments from multiple sources, such as patients, peers and interprofessional faculty. The mobile app described for Milestones is an example of this shift (Page et al., 2017).

LICs are tailor-made for informed self-assessment approaches. However, the work of Sargeant and colleagues has demonstrated that many factors are in play in order for the promise of informed self-assessment to be fully realised (Sargeant et al., 2011). LICs present an opportunity to study these factors in a context where the power dynamic (medical student to faculty) can be wide. The LIC represents an interesting opportunity to marry research examining the impact of the LIC approach and programmatic assessment and informed self-assessment, all grounded in workplace-based assessments.

Workplace-based assessments

The most pressing research and evaluation need for workplace-based assessments is how to implement and use them more effectively. While continuing to improve the rating scales and assessment items is useful work, in the end any workplace-based assessment is only as good as the person using it. We have an abysmally small amount of research in this area. New concepts such as Milestones, using narrative, and developmental rubrics represent a major shift. Mobile technology is making it easier to capture assessment data, often de-emphasising the use of rating scales over narrative judgment. Research will be needed to explore how to most effectively use and combine qualitative and quantitative assessment. This research will require embracing new models, such as realist strategy, complex intervention models, systems science and health services models (Holmboe & Batalden, 2015; Pawson et al., 2005).

The disruptive innovations discussed in this chapter primarily focus on pedagogical design and assessment changes needed *now*; changes that are in fact long overdue based on available evidence. Other likely areas of disruption, diffusion and complexity in health professions education coming in the near future include: artificial intelligence (e.g. Watson computer); big data increasingly informing competency decisions among health professions students; the increasing use of simulation; more care delivered at a distance from the health care facility (e.g. telemedicine); major shifts in roles between healthcare professionals; and greater co-production of healthcare with patients, families and communities.

As one modest data example, the Milestones project discussed above generates over 3.4 million data points for over 130,000 residents in the United States every six months. These data, evaluating the six general competencies, is enabling more robust feedback to training programs using national benchmarks (Holmboe et al., 2016).

Co-production is beginning to change the way care is delivered with much greater involvement by patients and families, and will require educators to rethink the patient interaction and encounter (Batalden et al., 2016). Finally, evidence is beginning to accrue that simulation training can translate to real benefits for patients. It is highly likely in the near future that no trainee should perform a procedure, at a minimum, on a patient without first demonstrating mastery in a simulated setting (Barsuk et al., 2014).

To paraphrase the Greek philosopher Heraclitus, the only constant is change (Holmboe & Batalden, 2015). Educators should embrace innovation and change as necessary for the improvement and evolution of health professions education.

PRACTICAL TIPS

Here are some practical tips for clinical educators wanting to embrace disruptive innovations, diffusion of innovations, and complexity.

1. First and foremost, be open (i.e. open mind, open heart) to innovation. Become familiar with the key theories and implementation strategies discussed in this chapter. Health professions education is not, and should not be, a static enterprise. As changes and innovation in medical science and healthcare delivery accelerate, the need for health professions education to do the same will only grow in importance.
2. Innovations require a passionate champion who can bring energy and excitement. As Dr David Hirsh shared (personal communication, 2017): 'from energy and excitement flows resilience. When trying to make change, we will always face barriers. We hold the idea that meaningful change matters, so when things are not going well, those are the times that most call us.' Champions are those who spend more time listening, engage all stakeholders, possess a strong sense of volunteerism and mission, and are willing to let go and change things as innovations unfold.
3. Share ideas and innovations within and across health professions as much as you can. Too often in health professions education we keep ideas and innovation to ourselves, for fear of either embarrassment or someone else usurping or taking our ideas. Sharing almost always leads to improvement and further learning through group wisdom.

4. Utilise the principles and observations of the diffusion of innovations and complex service intervention models. These models will provide a roadmap to help plan, to indicate what to expect and what to measure, and to monitor during implementation.
5. Reflect and review often. Once you implement an innovation, by default you immediately change conditions on the ground. Build observation, reflection and evaluation into the implementation of innovations as part of a continuous quality-improvement process.
6. Finally, engage in 'abject humility'. Humility supports reflection, learning, curiosity and improvement in innovation. Turn to find wonder with each new experience. Practise 'bright-eyed observation' before and during the implementation of innovation (e.g. we should wonder 'Why did that happen?', or 'I wonder why that individual has reacted to this innovation in that way?', with the authentic belief that we can learn and improve by pausing to wonder) (Hirsh, personal communication, 2017).

Conclusion

With the intense interest worldwide in outcomes or competency-based medical education (CBME), improved patient and population outcomes represent the ultimate goal for all health professions training. One of the primary tenets of CBME is that a medical education program must start with the end in mind: the needs of patients and healthcare systems (Frenk et al., 2010; McGaghie et al., 1978). Policy-makers and public constituencies across the globe have increasingly expressed frustration and concern over the ability of undergraduate and graduate medical education programs to meet current and future societal needs. Multiple studies have highlighted deficiencies in key, 'newer' competencies, such as interprofessional teamwork, care coordination, stewardship of resources and cost-consciousness, health information technology, quality improvement, patient safety and informed decision-making (Institute of Medicine, 2000, 2001).

LICs provide a disruptive model to medical education that may address many of the limitations currently plaguing traditional block-rotation models. While LICs may not be necessarily cheaper, they are more firmly grounded in strong pedagogical and assessment theories and evidence. LICs are forcing a critical examination of medical education models on outcomes for both learners *and* patients.

Workplace-based assessments more closely align with Christensen's disruptive innovation model. They are messy, often cheaper, do not possess the same level of validity evidence, are increasingly easier to deliver through mobile technologies, and have begun to threaten up-market assessments, such as high-stakes multiple-choice question examinations (as evidenced by the US experience using high-stakes examinations for the maintenance of certification among practising specialists) (Cook et al., 2015). Programmatic assessment, built predominantly as a combination of workplace-based assessments, has the potential to be an excellent platform from which to build empirical models of trainee competence and robust assessment tools for inter- and intrapersonal competencies — both of which are lacking in the current assessment environment.

Health professions educators should embrace the principles, theories and lessons from disruptive innovations, diffusion of innovations, and complexity. This may be an uncomfortable space for many of us, not having much prior experience in these disciplines. However, the major challenge facing most health professions education programs is not lack of innovative curricular models or innovative workplace-based assessments, but rather how best to implement, refine and improve them. If done well, the current innovations available to all of us hold great promise to improve the lives of our patients, families, populations and, yes, learners.

References

Andolsek, K., Padmore, J., & Holmboe, E. S. (2017). *Clinical competency committees. A guidebook for programs.* Chicago: Accreditation Council for Graduate Medical Education. http://www.acgme.org/Portals/0/ACGMEClinicalCompetencyCommitteeGuidebook.pdf?ver=2015-11-06-115643-130. (Accessed 2 September 2017).

Barsuk, J. H., Cohen, E. R., Potts, S., et al. (2014). Dissemination of a simulation-based mastery learning intervention reduces central line-associated bloodstream infections. *BMJ Quality and Safety, 23*(9), 749–756. doi:10.1136/bmjqs-2013-002665.

Batalden, M., Batalden, P., Margolis, P., et al. (2016). Coproduction of healthcare service. *BMJ Quality and Safety, 25*(7), 509–517.

Bates, J., & Ellaway, R. H. (2016). Mapping the dark matter of context: A conceptual scoping review. *Medical Education*, 50(8), 807–816. doi:10.1111/medu.13034.

Beeson, M. S., Holmboe, E. S., Korte, R. C., et al. (2015). Initial validity of the emergency medicine milestones. *Academic Emergency Medicine*, 22(7), 838–844. doi:10.1111/acem.12697.

Bernabeo, E. C., Holtman, M. C., Ginsburg, S., et al. (2011). Lost in transition: The experience and impact of frequent changes in the inpatient learning environment. *Academic Medicine*, 86(5), 591–598.

Berwick, D. M., Nolan, T. W., & Whittington, J. (2008). The triple aim: Care, health, and cost. *Health Affairs (Millwood)*, 27(3), 759–769. doi:10.1377/hlthaff.27.3.759.

Bohnen, J. D., George, B. C., Williams, R. G., et al. (2016). The feasibility of real-time intraoperative performance assessment with SIMPL (System for Improving and Measuring Procedural Learning): Early experience from a multi-institutional trial. *Journal of Surgical Educucation*, 73(6), e118–e130. doi:10.1016/j.jsurg.2016.08.010.

Christensen, C. M. (1997). *The innovator's dilemma*. New York.: Harper Business.

Christensen, C. M., Grossman, J. H., & Hwang, J. (2009). *The innovator's prescription. A disruptive solution for health care*. New York.: McGraw-Hill.

Conforti, L. N., Yaghmour, N. A., Hamstra, S. J., et al. (2017). Effect and use of Milestones in the assessment of neurological surgery residents and residency programs. *Journal of Surgical Education*, S1931-7204(17)30278-7. doi:10.1016/j.jsurg.2017.06.001. [Epub ahead of print].

Cook, D. A., Holmboe, E. S., Sorensen, K. J., et al. (2015). Getting maintenance of certification to work: A grounded theory study of physicians' perceptions. *JAMA Internal Medicine*, 175(1), 35–42. doi:10.1001/jamainternmed.2014.5437.

Crosson, F. J., Leu, J., Roemer, B. M., et al. (2011). Gaps in residency training should be addressed to better prepare doctors for a twenty-first-century delivery system. *Health Affairs (Millwood)*, 30(11), 2142–2148.

Denson, J. L., Jensen, A., Saag, H. S., et al. (2016). Association between end-of-rotation resident transition in care and mortality among hospitalized patients. *JAMA: The Journal of the American Medical Association*, 316(21), 2204–2213. doi:10.1001/jama.2016.17424.

Downing, S. M. (Ed.), (2006). *Handbook of test development*. Mahwah, NJ: Lawrence Erlbaum Associates.

Ericsson, K. A. (2004). Deliberate practice and the acquisition and maintenance of expert performance in medicine and related domains. *Academic Medicine*, 79(10 Suppl.), S70–S81.

Frenk, J., Chen, L., Bhutta, Z. A., et al. (2010). Health professionals for a new century: Transforming education to strengthen health systems in an interdependent world. *The Lancet*, 376(9756), 1923–1958. doi:10.1016/S0140-6736(10)61854-5.

Frischknecht, A. C., Boehler, M. L., Schwind, C. J., et al. (2014). How prepared are your interns to take calls? Results of a multi-institutional study of simulated pages to prepare medical students for surgery internship. *American Journal of Surgery*, 208(2), 307–315.

Gaufberg, E., Hirsh, D., Krupat, E., et al. (2014). Into the future: Patient-centredness endures in longitudinal integrated clerkship graduates. *Medical Education*, 48(6), 572–582.

Gingerich, A., Kogan, J., Yeates, P., et al. (2014). Seeing the 'black box' differently: Assessor cognition from three research perspectives. *Medical Education*, 48(11), 1055–1068.

Givon, L., & Simanton, E. (2016). Clinical curriculum, developmental trajectory, and continuity with peers. In A. Poncelet & D. Hirsh (Eds.), *Longitudinal integrated clerkships. principles, outcomes, practical tools, and future directions* (pp. 81–90). North Syracuse, NY: Gegensatz Press.

Hauer, K. E., Cate, O. T., Boscardin, C. K., et al. (2016a). Ensuring resident competence: A narrative review of the literature on group decision making to inform the work of clinical competency committees. *Journal of Graduate Medical Educucation*, 8(2), 156–164. doi:10.4300/JGME-D-15-00144.1.

Hauer, K. E., Vandergrift, J., Hess, B., et al. (2016b). Correlations between ratings on the resident annual evaluation summary and the internal medicine milestones and association with ABIM certification examination scores among US internal medicine residents, 2013–2014. *JAMA: The Journal of the American Medical Association*, 316(21), 2253–2262. doi:10.1001/jama.2016.17357.

Hirsh, D., Gaufberg, G., Ogur, B., et al. (2012a). Educational outcomes of the Harvard Medical School-Cambridge integrated clerkship: A way forward for medical education. *Academic Medicine*, 87(5), 1–8.

Hirsh, D., Walters, L., & Poncelet, A. N. (2012b). Better learning, better doctors, better delivery system: Possibilities from a case study of longitudinal integrated clerkships. *Medical Teacher*, 34(7), 548–554.

Hirsh, D. A., Holmboe, E. S., & ten Cate, O. (2014). Time to trust: Longitudinal integrated clerkships and entrustable professional activities. *Academic Medicine*, 89(2), 201–204.

Hirsh, D. A., Ogur, B., Thibault, G. E., et al. (2007). Continuity' as an organizing principle for clinical education reform. *New England Journal of Medicine*, 356(8), 858–866.

Holmboe, E. S. (2017). The journey to competency-based medical education — implementing milestones. *Marshall Journal of Medicine*, 3, 1; article 2.

Holmboe, E. S., & Batalden, P. (2015). Achieving the desired transformation: Thoughts on *Next Steps for Outcomes-based Medical Education*. *Academic Medicine*, 90(9), 1215–1223.

Holmboe, E. S., Edgar, L., & Hamstra, S. (2016). *The Milestones guidebook*. Chicago: Accreditation Council for Graduate Medical Education. http://www.acgme.org/Portals/0/MilestonesGuidebook.pdf?ver=2016-05-31-113245-103. (Accessed 12 April 2018).

Holmboe, E. S., Ginburg, S., & Bernabeo, E. C. (2011). The rotational approach to medical education: Time to confront our assumptions? *Medical Education*, 45(1), 69–80.

Holmboe, E. S., ten Cate, O., Durning, S. J., et al. (2017). Assessment challenges in the era of outcomes-based education. In E. S. Holmboe, S. J. Durning, & R. E.

Hawkins (Eds.), *Practical guide to the evaluation of clinical competence* (2nd ed.). Philadelphia.: Elsevier.

Holmboe, E. S., Weng, W., Arnold, G., et al. (2010). The comprehensive care project: Measuring physician performance in ambulatory practice. *Health Services Research, 45*(6 Pt. 2), 1912–1933. doi:10.1111/j.1475-6773.2010.01160.x.

Institute of Medicine. (2000). *To err is human: Building a safer health system*. Washington, DC: National Academy Press.

Institute of Medicine. (2001). *Crossing the quality chasm*. Washington, DC: National Academy Press.

Kaiser Permanente School of Medicine. https://schoolofmedicine.kaiserpermanente.org/. (Accessed 4 July 2017).

Kogan, J. R., Conforti, L. N., Bernabeo, E., et al. (2015). How faculty members experience workplace-based assessment rater training: A qualitative study. *Medical Education, 49*(7), 692–708.

Kogan, J. R., Hatala, R., Hauer, K. E., et al. (2017). The do's, don'ts and don't know of direct observation. *Perspectives on Medical Education, 6*(5), 286–305. doi:10.1007/s40037-017-0376-7.

Kogan, J. R., Hess, B. J., Conforti, L. N., et al. (2010). What drives faculty ratings of residents' clinical skills? The impact of faculty's own clinical skills. *Academic Medicine, 85*(10 Suppl.), S25–S28. doi:10.1097/ACM.0b013e3181ed1aa3.

Latessa, R. A., Swendiman, R. A., Parlier, A. B., et al. (2017). Graduates' perceptions of learning affordances in longitudinal integrated clerkships: A dual-institution, mixed-methods study. *Academic Medicine, 92*(9), 1313–1319. doi:10.1097/ACM.0000000000001621.

Li, S. T., Tancredi, D. J., Schwartz, A., et al. (2017). Competent for unsupervised practice: Use of pediatric residency training milestones to assess readiness. *Academic Medicine, 92*(3), 385–393. doi:10.1097/ACM.0000000000001322.

Lipner, R. S., Hess, B. J., & Phillips, R. L., Jr. (2013). Specialty board certification in the United States: Issues and evidence. *Journal of Continuing Education in the Health Professsions, 33*(Suppl. 1), S20–S35. doi:10.1002/chp.21203.

Lockyer, J., Carraccio, C., Chan, M. K., et al. (2017). Core principles of assessment in competency-based medical education. *Medical Teacher, 39*(6), 609–616. doi: 10.1080/0142159X.2017.1315082.

Lypson, M. L., Frohna, J. G., Gruppen, L. D., et al. (2004). Assessing residents' competencies at baseline: Identifying the gaps. *Academic Medicine, 79*(6), 564–570.

McGaghie, W. C., Miller, G. E., Sajid, A. W., et al. (1978). *Competency-based curriculum development in medical education: An introduction*. Geneva: World Health Organization.

Makary, M. A., & Daniel, M. (2016). Medical error: The third leading cause of death in the United States. *BMJ (Clinical Research Ed.), 353*, i2139. doi:https://doi.org/10.1136/bmj.i2139.

Mattar, S. G., Alseidi, A. A., Jones, D. B., et al. (2013). General surgery residency inadequately prepares trainees for fellowship: Results of a survey of fellowship program directors. *Annals of Surgery, 258*(3), 440–449. doi:10.1097/SLA.0b013e3182a191ca.

Mazotti, L. A., & Ogur, B. (2016). LIC guiding principles and goals. In A. Poncelet & D. Hirsh (Eds.), *Longitudinal integrated clerkships: Principles, outcomes, practical tools, and future directions* (pp. 29–36). North Syracuse, NY: Gegensatz Press.

Merriam Webster Dictionary. https://www.merriam-webster.com/dictionary/innovation. (Accessed 4 July 2017).

Miller, G. E. (1990). The assessment of clinical skills/competence/performance. *Academic Medicine, 65*(9 Suppl.), S63–S67.

Mossialos, E., Wenzl, M., Osborn, R., et al. (2015). *International profiles of health care systems, 2014: Australia, Canada, Denmark, England, France, Germany, Italy, Japan, The Netherlands, New Zealand, Norway, Singapore, Sweden, Switzerland, and the United States*. New York: The Commonwealth Fund. http://www.commonwealthfund.org/publications/fund-reports/2015/jan/international-profiles-2014. (Accessed 4 July 2017).

National Academy of Medicine. (2015). *Improving diagnosis*. Washington DC.: National Academy Press.

National Patient Safety Foundation. (2016). *Free from harm: Accelerating patient safety improvement fifteen years after To err is human*. http://www.npsf.org/?page=freefromharm. (Accessed 28 May 2016).

Nelson, E. C., Batalden, P. B., & Godfrey, M. M. (2007). *Quality by design. A clinical microsystems approach*. San Francisco.: Jossey-Bass.

Ogrinc, G. S., & Headrick, L. A. (2008). Understanding and making changes in a system. In G. S. Ogrinc & L. A. Headrick (Eds.), *Fundamentals of health care improvement* (pp. 99–115). Oakbrook Terrace, IL: Joint Commission Resources.

Ogur, B., & Hirsh, D. (2009). Learning through longitudinal patient care: Narratives from the Harvard Medical School–Cambridge integrated clerkship. *Academic Medicine, 84*(7), 844–850.

Page, C., Reid, A., Coe, C. L., et al. (2017). Piloting the Mobile Medical Milestones Application (M3App©): A multi-institution evaluation. *Family Medicine, 49*(1), 35–41.

Pangaro, L. N., Durning, S. J., & Holmboe, E. S. (2018). Evaluation frameworks, forms and global rating scales. In E. S. Holmboe, S. J. Durning, & R. E. Hawkins (Eds.), *Practical Guide to the Evaluation of Clinical Competence* (2nd ed., pp. 37–60). Philadelphia: Elsevier.

Pawson, R., Greenhalgh, T., & Harvey, G. (2005). Realist review — a new method of systematic review designed for complex policy interventions. *Journal of Health Services Research and Policy, 10*(Suppl. 1), 21–34.

Peabody, M. R., O'Neill, T. R., & Peterson, L. E. (2017). Examining the functioning and reliability of the Family Medicine Milestones. *Journal of Graduate Medicine Education, 9*(1), 46–53.

Plsek, P. E., & Greenhalgh, T. (2001). The challenge of complexity in health care. *BMJ (Clinical Research Ed.), 323*(7313), 625–628. doi:https://doi.org/10.1136/bmj.323.7313.625.

Poncelet, A., & Hirsh, D. (2016). Background, definitions, history. In A. Poncelet & D. Hirsh (Eds.), *Longitudinal integrated clerkships; Principles, outcomes, practical tools, and future directions* (pp. 1–9). North Syracuse, NY: Gegensatz Press.

Prober, C. G., Kolars, J. C., First, L. R., et al. (2016). A plea to reassess the role of United States Medical Licensing Examination Step 1 scores in residency selection. *Academic Medicine*, *91*(1), 12–15.

Rogers, E. M. (1995). *Diffusion of innovations* (5th ed.). New York: Free Press.

Rohrer, D., & Pashler, H. (2010). Recent research on human learning challenges conventional instructional strategies. *Educational Researcher*, *39*(5), 406–412.

Sargeant, J., Eva, K. W., Armson, H., et al. (2011). Features of assessment learners use for informed self-assessments of clinical performance. *Medical Educcation*, *45*(6), 636–647. doi:10.1111/j.1365-2923.2010.03888.x.

Scharmer, C. O. (2016). *Theory U: Leading from the future as it emerges*. Oakland, CA: Berrett-Koehler.

Schuwirth, L. W. T., & van der Vleuten, C. P. (2011). Programmatic assessment: From assessment of learning to assessment for learning. *Medical Teacher*, *33*(6), 478–485. doi:10.3109/0142159X.2011.565828.

Stabell, C. B., & Fjeldstad, O. D. (1998). Configuring value for competitive advantage: On chains, shops and networks. *Strategic Management Journal*, *19*, 413–437.

ten Cate, O., & Scheele, F. (2007). Competency-based postgraduate training: Can we bridge the gap between theory and clinical practice? *Academic Medicine*, *82*(6), 542–547.

Ubel, P. A., & Asch, D. A. (2015). Creating value in health by understanding and overcoming resistance to de-innovation. *Health Affairs (Millwood)*, *34*(2), 239–244. doi:10.1377/hlthaff.2014.0983.

van der Vleuten, C. P. (2016). Revisiting 'Assessing professional competence: From methods to programmes. *Medical Education*, *50*(9), 885–888.

van der Vleuten, C. P., & Schuwirth, L. W. (2005). Assessing professional competence: From methods to programmes. *Medical Education*, *39*(3), 309–317.

Walters, L., & Cosgrove, E. M. (2016). LIC outcomes. In A. Poncelet & D. Hirsh (Eds.), *Longitudinal integrated clerkships: Principles, outcomes, practical tools, and future directions* (pp. 233–244). North Syracuse, NY: Gegensatz Press.

Warm, E. J., Held, J. D., Hellmann, M., et al. (2016). Entrusting observable practice activities and milestones over the 36 months of an internal medicine residency. *Academic Medicine*, *91*(10), 1398–1405.

Wikipedia. (2017). *Diffusion of innovation*. https://en.wikipedia.org/wiki/Diffusion_of_innovations. (Accessed 4 July 2017).

25

Translating educational research into educational practice

Rola Ajjawi, Jason M. Lodge and
Christopher Roberts

Introduction

Educational research has in recent decades added substantially to the body of knowledge on effective learning and teaching processes and practices. There is, however, an inherent difficulty in making meaning of this research (Thomas & Steinert, 2014); particularly in identifying and bridging the gap between educational theory and practice, and how research can contribute to informing decision-makers on their choices and priorities (Botwe et al., 2017; Molesworth & Lewitt, 2016; Tolsgaard et al., 2017). Little is known about how educational theories and research outcomes produced under optimal research conditions in highly controlled settings generalise to real-life educational contexts, including the clinical workplace (Tolsgaard et al., 2017). Much of this research is being conducted on aspects of learning that occur over short timespans, using specialised language, in highly controlled settings. Yet the clinical workplace is anything but highly controlled. Similarly, educational research conducted in the workplace requires expertise to unpack notions of quality, and to make the necessary translations to different contexts.

In the developed world, the education and healthcare landscapes are both rapidly changing. For example, technology has resulted in the use of multiple applications of social media, high-fidelity simulation, and exposure to breakthroughs in new scientific and clinical treatments, which in turn has led to increased complexity and sophistication of knowledge and practice. In addition, machine learning, artificial intelligence and associated automation of knowledge-based work are poised to create significant upheaval in society in the next decade (see, e.g., Hodges, 2018); therefore, this situation is likely to become even more complex. By contrast in the developing world, students are eschewing rural practice, and the health workforce is suffering under the strain of high levels of migration (Budhathoki et al., 2017). Such complex, changing and uncertain workplaces offer significant challenges to simple views of knowledge dissemination and transfer; instead, requiring greater sophistication of knowledge translation of educational research to practice.

In this chapter, we take a sociocultural perspective on knowledge translation, drawing parallels between design thinking and shared-decision making. We start by defining 'knowledge translation', and examining the challenges of research utilisation within health professions education that necessitate a shift from knowledge dissemination to knowledge translation. We then present an approach to faculty development activities, from higher education, that incorporates the tenets of design thinking in shaping plans to implement any educational intervention (Elliott & Lodge, 2017). A key aspect of design thinking for clinical educators is the process of interdisciplinary knowledge exchange between educationalists (e.g. specialist faculty members, education researchers or peers) and clinical educators, in order to design education in an evidence-informed way that prioritises what learners do, and is sensitive to context (Goodyear, 2015).

In this first example, collaborative decision-making forms a subset of the overall design process. In health, shared decision-making (SDM) is an approach to facilitating knowledge exchange between clinicians and their patients, where designed decision aids operate as an enabler of the overall SDM process. SDM entails a social and cultural approach to the tailoring of evidence to specific problems. By bringing design thinking and SDM together, we highlight the importance of interdisciplinary and collaborative design thinking, which helps to bring to the surface and negotiate the differing beliefs among educators about learning and curricular problems (Hawick et al., 2017), in order to create evidence-based, contextual solutions. We suggest that these two approaches dovetail well, and can be used strategically to advance the translation of educational research into educational practice within a broad range of educational contexts, taking into account the sociocultural factors that govern practice.

Defining knowledge translation

Knowledge translation describes a process to address the 'slow' and 'haphazard' under-utilisation of available scientific findings and evidence-based research (Graham et al., 2006). Its main aim is to bridge research and practice through interactive, non-linear and interdisciplinary processes spanning knowledge creation to application (Thomas & Steinert, 2014). Knowledge translation is defined by the Canadian Institutes of Health Research as a dynamic and iterative process that includes the synthesis, dissemination, exchange and ethically sound application of knowledge to improve health, provide more effective health services and products, and strengthen the healthcare system. This goes beyond simple dissemination of knowledge, to knowledge integration and exchange (Thomas & Steinert, 2014). It requires shifting from notions of knowledge transfer from one location to another, to translation as 'renovation and expansion of previous knowledge', requiring ongoing processes of change and boundary-crossing between research and practice (Hager & Hodgkinson, 2009). Those involved in the activities of knowledge translation aim to promote the uptake of evidence-based research in systems of care, thereby informing decision-making. Applied to clinical education, the aim of knowledge translation activities is to improve the uptake of evidence-based findings from educational research into educational practice.

Best evidence medical education

The claims for increasing research utilisation within health professions education are not new. In 1995, van der Vleuten (1995) highlighted the paradox of how health professions educators held different attitudes towards their clinical practice compared with their teaching practice. He commented that teachers tended to abandon their usual attitude of critical appraisal, which they adopted in relation to their field of clinical expertise, and instead relied on personal beliefs and opinions when it came to teaching and learning. Best evidence medical education (BEME) as a movement has grown since. BEME involves a professional judgment by the teacher about their teaching, taking into account evidence of the effectiveness of medical education interventions (Harden et al., 2000). Harden and colleagues (2000) drew parallels with the evidence-based movement in medicine, which involved that now well-known refrain that practice should involve 'the conscientious, explicit and judicious use of current best evidence in making decisions about the care of individual patients' (Sackett et al., 1996). BEME evolved from critiques of the 'lemming-like' approach to implementation of educational practice in the absence of evidence, alongside repeated pleas for evidence instead of intuition to inform educational practice, because traditions and intuitions can be misguided (Harden et al., 2000; van der Vleuten et al., 2000).

Traditions and intuitions rely on assumptions that can readily be proved wrong when subjected to scrutiny (Hart & Harden, 2000). This is increasingly the case as rigorous research calls into question some broadly accepted notions, such as the benefits of instruction aimed at catering for modality-based learning styles (Lodge et al., 2016; Norman, 2009). In a commentary typical of Norman's acerbic wit, he asked 'when will learning style go out of style?'; that is, when will this medical education myth be busted? Rightly, he argued that, although individual learners may have an affinity with a particular learning approach, there was a lack of empirical evidence supporting the concept of learning styles-based instruction. Instead, the primary deciding factor for the learning approach taken by a student is the design of the task (Lodge et al., 2016). Yet learning styles instruction continues to enjoy broad acceptance in practice (Cuevas, 2015).

Another example is the persistence of feedback as 'one-way' information transmission within clinical education (Molloy, 2009; Urquhart et al., 2018), even though there is considerable evidence that feedback is a more complex process involving dialogue, feedback loops and goal co-construction (Barton et al., 2016; Farrell et al., 2017; Telio et al., 2016). Therefore, it seems that even with the presence of educational research evidence, clinical educators' practice may be stubbornly resistant to change.

Similar critiques have been made in the fields of higher and classroom education, with the argument that there is little value in simply providing teachers with the results of systematic reviews, laboratory or neuroimaging studies and expecting them to make sense of these results for their context (Lodge, 2016). The distance from the laboratory to the classroom is simply too great for this approach to be viable. Indeed, it has often been described as a 'bridge too far' (Bruer, 1997). The risk in attempting to bridge this gap without careful consideration of the translation process is that neuromyths can be both created and perpetuated. These include such incorrect notions as the idea that students only use 10% of their brains, or that students can be 'left-brained' or 'right-brained' and have education tailored for their dominant hemisphere. Such 'neuromyths' have been found to be common among classroom educators, and may lead to detrimental approaches being adopted on the basis of these false assumptions about how the brain and mind learn (Howard-Jones, 2015). This problem can also be compounded when technology is added to the mix. The hype around brain training applications — despite an almost complete lack of evidence of effectiveness — demonstrates how alluring the combination of emerging technologies and neuroscience can be for educators and policy-makers (Lodge & Horvath, 2017).

Challenges to the uptake of evidence in clinical education

Although clinical educators value the role of educational evidence, they do not view it as their responsibility to translate this evidence (i.e. to find relevant articles and to critically evaluate this evidence and then apply it) (Delany & Bailocerkowski, 2011). BEME might seem a natural solution, as it seeks to review and synthesise the evidence for a particular topic from multiple studies and to draw specific recommendations for practice from this evidence. Putting aside arguments about what constitutes evidence and the problems with aggregating it that compromises reliability and validity of reviews (see, e.g., Dauphinee & Wood-Dauphinee, 2004), even once the evidence is synthesised there are many reasons for its lack of uptake by clinical educators. These reasons can be considered at the epistemicological, individual, interpersonal, and organisational levels.

At the epistemological level, working on real-world problems usually requires the combination of different kinds of specialised and context-dependent knowledge, as well as different ways of knowing. People who are flexible and adept with respect to different ways of knowing about the world can be said to possess epistemic fluency (Markauskaite & Goodyear, 2017). Medical education research is a contested interdisciplinary field where a broad range of disciplines, including education, psychology and the social sciences, feature (Albert, 2004). Clinicians would be more familiar with clinical research, which tends to be positivist in nature, and hence reading original research or BEME papers might be quite challenging given its interdisciplinary nature (Goodyear & Zenios, 2007). Therefore, in order to meaningfully engage in educational research, clinical educators require a level of epistemic fluency in a number of fields.

The professionalisation of medical education is resulting in recognition that being a good clinical educator requires more than specialised disciplinary knowledge, for example, in a particular body system, or communication skills. The clinical educator also needs to be expert in the knowledge, skills and behaviours of educators. Although Biesta (2015) has emphasised the teleological character of education — the fact that education always raises the question of its purpose — we found very little on the teleogical position of health professional educators. Some have argued that the purpose of health professional education research is to lead to improved patient healthcare outcomes through improved educational practice (Bligh & Parsell, 1999; McGaghie, 2010). However, health professional education research may also be theoretical and pure (serving the purpose of knowledge expansion) rather than being applied (Albert, 2004).

One of the most difficult aspects of the complexity faced by health professions educators is the growing body of knowledge across each of the domains of practice they are engaged in (Jorm & Roberts, 2018). If considered through the lens of the technological, pedagogical, content knowledge model (Mishra & Koehler, 2006), not only are there significant changes in the evidence and practice of medicine (i.e. the content knowledge), there are also similar advances in both the pedagogical and technical knowledge related to learning and teaching. The combination of advances across three disparate but related knowledge domains creates a difficult situation for educators in these contexts. It is difficult enough to keep up with advances in the content area, let alone also being on top of a rapidly changing landscape in adult education and educational technologies. For this reason, we recommend interdisciplinary and collaborative decision-making processes when it comes to knowledge translation.

At the individual level, clinical educators are juggling many roles and responsibilities, where typically their primary role is to deliver patient care. Time for education can be limited, and, when educators are time-pressured, education tends to be sacrificed to ensure that patient care is attended to (Sholl et al., 2017). Given that educating students and trainees is itself an additional burden on busy clinicians, it is not surprising that for some clinicians searching, reading and applying knowledge from BFME reviews to their practice can be a real struggle (Sethi et al., 2017). A claim that 75 minutes a day are needed for a clinician to keep themselves up-to-date with the medical education literature (Faux, 2000) is likely an underestimate now, in an age of increasing numbers of open-access journals. This hardly seems practical given workload demands in the healthcare sector.

At the interpersonal level, educational practice, and by extension research, is seen as the poor cousin to medicine (Sethi et al., 2017). While education and educational research is undervalued, clinical educators are less likely to prioritise spending time on it. This is despite the fact that it has been argued that the science and practice of education is the most difficult of all areas of research, given the complexity of human learning and how it occurs in complex formal and informal educational settings (Berliner, 2002). Supervisory support and mentorship are necessary mechanisms for the translation of continuing professional activities into the workplace (Sholl et al., 2017), yet can be lacking in the clinical workplace, particularly in relation to education.

At the organisational level, many clinical educators may not have a formal educational role as part of their work-plans, in effect teaching voluntarily. Hence, there are no minimal requirements to be a volunteer clinical educator, although this is changing at a policy level in some countries. For example, the General Medical Council in the United Kingdom recently mandated that all doctors who have a formal supervisory role must have achieved minimum educational requirements. In several countries, such as Australia and the United Kingdom, specialist postgraduate training colleges have implemented manadatory faculty development sessions that introduce clinicians to educational principles and strategies. Such workshops tend to be theory-light with no follow-up on application in the clinical environment, and no requirement for clinical educators to continue to examine educational evidence and to implement it in their practice. This is common to many faculty development programs oriented towards information transmission and exchange. These challenges to research utilisation collectively highlight the need to shift to more active and collaborative knowledge translation processes rather than passive dissemination.

Increasing uptake of educational evidence in practice

How can educational research be better tailored to, and used by, clinical educators who face so many barriers to evidence use? We can draw parallels with higher education and from health, where, in order to improve evidence-based practice, research translation into guidelines for health professionals to follow became common. Much like the use of clinical guidelines to inform practice, designs for learning operate in the same capacity as translations of educational evidence to inform teaching practice. Also much like the production of guidelines alone is not enough to ensure their adequate use in practice, we propose SDM in order to embed guidelines into practice. First, we highlight who might be involved in such activities, then present the parallel examples from higher education and health.

Knowledge brokering

One approach to addressing the challenges outlined above has been the development of health professional education units, which are seen as a response to increased public expectations about healthcare, the need for increased transparency in the demonstration of the competence of graduates, calls for social accountability, educational developments on how to educate clinicians, and the need to train more doctors. The functions of a dedicated education unit within the university sector (centrally or within schools of health) or even in healthcare settings, include research, teaching, service provision and career development of the staff (Davis et al., 2005). Staff working in these units may act as brokers in facilitating knowledge translation.

Dedicated faculty development through funded units can support clinical educators to take new approaches to knowledge translation and design-thinking-inspired decision aids. Ward, House and Hamer (2009) describe knowledge brokers as intermediaries between the worlds of researchers and decision-makers, who use a combination of active dissemination and translation activities. Depending on their expertise, clinical educators may act as knowledge brokers or they may work in collaboration with educational experts (e.g. faculty developers, educational researchers and/or peers) to effect knowledge brokering in practice, in order to change their educational practice.

Knowledge translation in higher education: design thinking

Within the discipline of higher and classroom education, several methods have been proposed to break down the distance between the laboratory and the classroom. One of the more established ways of helping educators to understand and implement evidence-based practice is to provide them with principles derived from the science of learning. This is an approach that has been widely adopted in the field of educational psychology. One of the most prominent examples are the multimedia learning principles developed by Mayer (2009). This research has been highly successful in informing educators about the processes students engage in while learning in multimedia environments, distilled into a set of principles with suggestions about how these principles might be applied. Despite the impact of this work, there is still much of the translation process that is left to educators. The principles do not inherently provide clear guidance to educators about how to implement the ideas into their own context, with their students. So, while the development of principles of learning has gone some way to bridging the gap between the laboratory and the classroom, there remains some distance between these principles and educational practice. This is perhaps why large-scale projects — such as those under the 'what works' agenda in the United States in the early 2000s (see Bransford et al., 2000) — did not have the impact that was hoped for.

More recently, a different approach is emerging for helping educators make sense of, and use, evidence from the science of learning. This approach still relies on principles to an extent, but is more focused on giving educators a means of systematically incorporating this evidence into practice. The approach involves assisting educators to develop their capacity for design thinking. Bennett, Agostinho and Lockyer (2017a) have found that teachers in higher education contexts already engage in a complex intuitive design process. By this, it is meant that these educators rely on tacit knowledge to make decisions about aspects of their teaching practice in a loosely systematic way. The purpose of developing their capacity for design thinking is largely to make this process more conscious (Elliott & Lodge, 2017). In doing so, this process of helping educators to be more mindful of the decisions they make has the potential to encourage them to consider each element of the educational situation more carefully; recasting their role as 'designers' of education.

While there is some conjecture as to whether design thinking is different from other forms of analysis or synthesis of information, design, as a means of reflecting and acting on teaching, has been receiving increased attention in education broadly (Laurillard, 2013). Cross (2011) contrasts the typical modes of thinking in the sciences and humanities with design thinking. The latter is about synthesising, forming patterns and creating the artificial world through iterative cycles of problem-solving, prototyping and creating solutions. This way of approaching education is dynamic, and assumes that the educational situation requires constant adaptation and modification in response to the complex forces within it (Mouasher & Lodge, 2016). This can be a different way of being for educators from diverse disciplinary backgrounds. The level of uncertainty inherent in design-based approaches to pedagogy can be some distance from the more structured scientific view of the universe, while the artificial nature of the designed products can be foreign to those from the humanities. The same is also true for health professions educators, who may similarly find design thinking to be somewhat different to the approaches to analysis and problem-solving they would engage in within the domain of the health professions.

Many examples of the impact of design thinking on education are emerging in the literature. One such example is reported in Venema, Drew and Lodge (2015). In this case, design thinking was used as part of a peer review of a lecture session. The problem with the lecture in this case was that handwritten elements formed a critical part of the session. It involved calculations and transformations on a set of numbers to make them useful in a digital environment. In order for students to understand the calculations, the lecturer worked through examples by hand. The problem is that material drawn on the whiteboard was not available for students to review. Additionally, the need to write on the whiteboard meant that the lecturer spent a large proportion of the class with his back to the students, which they found disengaging. This situation was analysed using Goodyear's (2005) design problem space framework as a basis, starting with expanding and reframing the understanding of the problem. Designing thinking was enabled through the structure provided by this framework, through analysing the assumptions made by the lecturer at a number of levels: the pedagogical philosophy, approaches, strategies and tactics employed in the session in relation to the evidence about student learning. The solution developed involved the use of a USB tablet that allowed for 'digital ink' to be collected and projected using the equipment in the lecture room. This solution meant that the lecturer could work through examples in a digital environment while maintaining eye contact with the class, and allowing the handwritten elements to be recorded and provided to students in video form for review. (For a description of the knowledge translation process and solution, see Venema and Lodge, [2013].)

This case study provides a concrete example of how design thinking was used to draw on evidence of quality student learning to solve a specific problem in an adult education context. The critical aspect of this example is that the peer review (i.e. knowledge exchange) process deliberately included a reviewer with expertise in the science of learning. The collaborative structure provided by the peer review process then allowed this foundational knowledge to be translated into practice through design-based discussions between the learning scientist and the educator. This form of interdisciplinary collaboration could prove valuable to clinical educators if appropriate knowledge brokers can be identified across the typically siloed practices of university settings.

Knowledge translation in health: shared decision-making

Shared decision-making (SDM) is a collaborative process that allows patients and their providers to make healthcare decisions together. It takes into account the best clinical evidence available, as well as the patient's values and preferences (Hoffmann et al., 2014). SDM is thought to appropriately balance the benefits of treatment with the possible harms (Barry & Edgman-Levitan, 2012; Hoffmann et al., 2014; Stiggelbout et al., 2012). Professional action which integrates an appreciation of the best evidence and the unique considerations of every patient is thought to lead to a more sustainable health system with the appropriate use of treatments and resources (Elshaug, 2015). A systematic review of studies on the practice of SDM identified the three most commonly reported barriers as: time constraints, lack of applicability due to patient characteristics, and lack of applicability due to the clinical situation (Gravel et al., 2006).

Patients are thought to want more involvement in health decisions; where there are preventive healthcare issues, situations with potential negative future consequences (e.g. chronic diseases), where the evidence is lacking, or where there are decisions involving potential side-effects (e.g. antihypertensive therapy) (Müller-Engelmann et al., 2013). One approach to involving patients in decision-making is through the use of decision aids, for which there is increasing evidence of their value (Austin et al., 2015; Légaré et al., 2008). Decision aids may include short videos or print material that digests the available evidence and offers flowcharts or decision trees to aid knowledge exchange or SDM of treatment preferences between clinicians and patients.

Haynes and colleagues have visualised the SDM process as a dynamic interplay between four differing ways of knowing: the research evidence; the patient's preferences; the context and circumstances in which the encounter is taking place; and the judgment of the clinician based on their findings (Haynes et al., 2002). We reconfigure these to suit the clinical education context, and the ways of knowing necessary to solve educational problems in the workplace, which takes into account: research evidence; student/educator and program preferences; the context and circumstances; and the educational judgments necessary for educational knowledge translation. We operationalise these in case study 25.1 below.

Shared decision-making and design thinking in health professions education

How, then, can SDM and design thinking be applied as a model to integrate a clinical educator's educational judgments and the evidence around educational theory and practice? Typically, clinical educators' practice will include numerous requests for problem-solving about education and training matters, or they may encounter multiple problems in their own practice. These may include problems or situations posed by academics (e.g. clinical liaison academics) and colleagues in clinical practice who have a teaching role. Problem-solving issues might include: 'What works in faculty development to enhance clinical educators' teaching skills?', 'When should I schedule feedback opportunities, and how can I make these most effective?'. In our model, we propose that collaborative decision-making occur between those with educational expertise and practitioners. For the sake of case study 25.1, we refer to the former as the health professional educator (HPE) and the practitioner requesting the advice as the client. We acknowledge that clinical educators may hold extensive educational expertise and may be the ones providing the advice (i.e. be the HPE). The process may also work with peers.

SDM enables a health professional educator and the client to participate jointly in making an appropriate educational decision based on existing evidence, having discussed the options, and the benefits and unintended consequences of any educational intervention, and having considered the client's values, preferences and circumstances. In health professions education, SDM should not be considered as a single consultation but rather an iterative process. The benefits of SDM include: enabling evidence and client's preferences to be incorporated into the consultation process; improving the knowledge of both the clinical educator and, in the case of education and training institutions, the committees and teachers involved. This can allow a greater appreciation of the risks of unintended consequences, or the likelihood of interventions that promote more effective ways of learning.

Various approaches can be used by the HPE to guide clinicians through the process. The following five simple questions can be used when approached about a potential educational intervention. These questions begin to unpack the problem, context, preferences and potential sources of evidence that could be sought, as highlighted in Fig. 25.1.

1. What is the fundamental problem we are trying to overcome?
2. How do we believe learners learn?
3. What are the benefits and the potential unintended consequences of each option?
4. Is there enough information to make a choice?
5. How will we judge whether we have made the optimal choice? What refinements to the design might be needed?

If the process of SDM is to become part of the HPE's skillset, it is important to consider what type of decision support tools might already exist or might need to be developed to support SDM. One approach in medical education has seen the journal *Academic Medicine* invite researchers to summarise their work (or others') into digestible infographics, which have been collated by the Association of American Medical Colleges (AAMC) for its members (see the 'Online resources' section at the end of this chapter).

In order to demonstrate how SDM using design thinking might guide an expert educator's academic judgment with a client, we bring a fictionalised case drawn from the authors' experience. Although in case study 25.1 we focus on the clinical educator seeking advice from a specialist educationalist at a university,

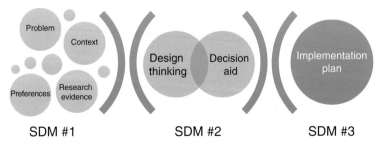

Figure 25.1: Iterative opportunities for educational shared decision-making (SDM) mediated through design thinking

clinical educators might choose to work in pairs/groups with other clinical educators to design education within their own contexts.

The collaborative approach, we feel, is important for the knowledge exchange and design process. The relationship formed during the SDM can help maintain motivation throughout the problem-solving and implementation stages. Potentially, the value of the discussions and questions raised may serve to build curiosity and accountability in clinical educators as co-producers and partners. Furthermore, helping clinical educators to exercise their educational judgments through design thinking for the local context is likely to be more satisfying than slavishly following guidelines or more guesswork through trial and error. The reciprocal benefit for HPE units and health professions academics/researchers whose expertise is not always capitalised on, often within the same universities they work in, is to apply their own research and expertise to inform curriculum development and clinical education processes.

Case study 25.1

A senior clinical educator, Rosa, who is based in general practice, approaches the health professional education unit at her local university for some advice about the re-design of their eight-week primary care placement. She wants to develop her students' clinical reasoning. She also isn't certain about the right mix of formal and immersive learning opportunities, especially as she feels that the students aren't adequately prepared for the placement but do not want to repeat what they have learned on campus. Rosa feels that she is providing more formal instruction, but that this is not necessarily effective for the students. She also believes that the formative assessment and feedback elements of the primary care placement could be strengthened. She struggles with balancing her service and educational roles while giving more to her learners.

A question of curriculum re-design

Using the model in Fig. 25.1, Fern, the university-based health professional educator, might refer first to the client's (Rosa's) context and circumstances. Rosa is part of the primary and community care teaching committee, as well as working as a clinician and being constrained for time; her committee is made up mainly of clinicians who are distributed around a wide area, and usually meet on campus once or twice a year, but most meetings use video-conferencing. Curriculum design and assessment in community and primary care is problematic. Health professional education and assessment have traditionally taken place in more controlled environments, such as hospitals with access to learning facilities. On community placements, students are geographically dispersed, the clinical experiences are highly varied, and there is an emphasis on self-directed learning.

In addressing the first question of SDM, as to what problem needs solving, Rosa reports that leading members of the committee are concerned around two major issues: the loss of facts related to the change in curriculum time allocated to knowledge about chronic disease management; and a lack of confidence that the integrative learning activities will do anything to promote clinical reasoning. Following discussion, Rosa rephrases the decision point as a question: How can students evidence clinical reasoning, and yet at the same time demonstrate appropriate knowledge in managing important chronic care conditions, during an immersive clinical experience in general practice? In terms of the second question, of how learners learn, Rosa has been doing some reading on clinical reasoning and the teaching of it in a case-based way in small groups (Kassirer, 2010; Norman, 2005), and specifically in primary care, which included the attraction of having virtual cases to work with (Adams et al., 2011). She has also read of methods that clinical educators can use in their practice (Atkinson et al., 2011; Wolpaw et al., 2012).

In considering the benefits and unintended consequences of these options (the third question of the SDM), it becomes apparent that it is beyond the resources of the committee to implement the faculty development issue of teaching all of the small-group tutors how to teach clinical reasoning, to prepare the students, and to get the IT support to develop computer-based cases. Fern then introduces the option of considering whether peer teaching might work; that is, the students present a case that they have seen. In considering the benefits, the cases they choose might be prepared by the students, and the significant content of the management of chronic conditions might be reduced. The unintended consequences might be that the students see this as a polished oral presentation rather than engaging in discussion, in which case the full benefit of peer learning for developing clinical reasoning will not be realised.

Further dialogue between Fern and Rosa focuses on whether the students could develop their clinical reasoning through peer learning, leaving the expert tutor to be a silent but expert facilitator. The first question is whether there is any evidence that peer learning activities have worked in similar contexts. Fern is able to offer a wealth of research evidence (Burgess et al., 2014; Tai et al., 2016). A second question is whether there is any evidence around the utility of assessing for clinical reasoning beyond the multiple-choice questions and long cases they are already using. Fern surmises that, other than Rosa, the committee by and large believes in a disciplinary approach to knowledge transfer, and might well be sceptical about the premises of the underlying problem or case-based learning, learning models which have driven curriculum reform for years.

Rosa and Fern have now jointly decided on a possible solution to the problem, which Rosa can take back to the committee (addressing the fourth question). In small groups, each student will develop one of several cases from a selection of chronic disease clinical problems, and present them to the group. Working together, Fern and Rosa design a pedagogical pattern for these sessions (SDM#2 in Fig. 25.1). They also co-create a rubric for the assessment of the clinical reasoning session run by the student, to be scored by the tutor. Rosa also recognises that the content the students research for their student presentations can be examined by using the existing multiple-choice questions in the basic and clinical sciences exams, and the long cases can be used formatively in the clinical setting with an emphasis on dialogic feedback.

Fern recognises that the committee could consider viewing their assessment from a programmatic perspective, and one which would better drive both the assessment of learning and the actual learning, (van der Vleuten et al., 2015) and take account of learning technologies (Bennett et al., 2017b). In thinking about question 5 — how Rosa will know whether the curriculum intervention is successful — Rosa recognises that her approach had been a traditional linear approach to developing curriculum, then the assessment, and then as time is almost done, the evaluation strategy. A more iterative approach in encouraging moving back and forth between the intended learning outcomes, the teaching and learning activities, the assessments, and evaluative goals is encouraged instead. Fern considers introducing the notion of non-linear approaches to health professional program evaluations (Jorm & Roberts, 2018) later on in the conversion. However, she is also highly pragmatic, and knows that the key to the success of her change to the program lies in a focused presentation that identifies the learning and teaching problem she is addressing, the compelling reason as to why it is important, and the benefits of the educational intervention she is proposing. She arranges a further meeting with Rosa after her presentation at the committee to discuss question 5 of the SDM in terms of evaluating the quality of educational judgments made in developing the implementation plan (SDM #3 in Fig. 25.1).

PRACTICAL TIPS

- Identify possible collaborators (educational researchers, educational experts, academics and/ or peers) who can scaffold the design thinking and contribute to shared decision-making (SDM).
- Recognise that sociocultural approaches to knowledge translation through design thinking and SDM are active processes that are iterative, collaborative, complex and emergent.
- Discuss pedagogical beliefs, approaches, strategies and tactics in relation to your specific context to help reframe the problem and create solutions.
- Reflect on the following five questions, and the forms of evidence that might inform the design.
  1. What is the fundamental problem we are trying to overcome?
  2. How do we believe learners learn?
  3. What are the benefits and the potential unintended consequences of each option?
  4. Is there enough information to make a choice?
  5. How will we judge whether we have made the optimal choice? What refinements to the design might be needed?

Conclusion

In this chapter, we have highlighted the challenges to research utilisation in the clinical context at the epistemological, individual, interpersonal and organisational levels. The aim of knowledge translation activities in clinical education is to overcome these challenges, and thus to improve the uptake of evidence-based findings into educational practice. We propose an interdisciplinary and collaborative framework for knowledge translation that utilises SDM and design thinking. Design thinking recasts the clinical educators' role to developing blueprints through making judgments in collaboration with educational experts about what is educationally desirable in particular situations, prioritising what the student does. The interdisciplinary and SDM perspective enables knowledge exchancement and the tailoring of evidence to the relevant context. This iterative approach takes into account the complexities of practice, helping to develop clinical educators' design thinking and to overcome the challenges to the uptake of educational research findings.

Online resources

Association of American Medical Colleges: https://www.aamc.org/download/355222/data/giaamlastpage.pdf.

References

Adams, E., Rodgers, C., Harrington, R., et al. (2011). How we created virtual patient cases for primary care-based learning. *Medical Teacher, 33*(4), 273–278.

Albert, M. (2004). Understanding the debate on medical education research: A sociological perspective. *Academic Medicine, 79*(10), 948–954.

Atkinson, K., Ajjawi, R., & Cooling, N. (2011). Promoting clinical reasoning in general practice trainees: Role of the clinical teacher. *The Clinical Teacher, 8*(3), 176–180. doi:10.1111/j.1743-498X.2011.00447.x.

Austin, C., Mohottige, D., Sudore, R. L., et al. (2015). Tools to promote shared decision making in serious illness: A systematic review. *JAMA Internal Medicine, 175*(7), 1213–1221. doi:10.1001/jamainternmed.2015.1679.

Barry, M., & Edgman-Levitan, S. (2012). Shared decision making — the pinnacle of patient-centred care. *New England Journal of Medicine, 366*(9), 780–781.

Barton, K. L., Schofield, S. J., McAleer, S., et al. (2016). Translating evidence-based guidelines to improve feedback practices: The interACT case study. *BMC Medical Education, 16*, 53–doi. https://doi.org/10.1186/s12909-016-0562-z.

Bennett, S., Agostinho, S., & Lockyer, L. (2017a). The process of designing for learning: understanding university teachers' design work. *Educational Technology Research and Development, 65*(1), 125–145. doi:10.1007/s11423-016-9469-y.

Bennett, S., Dawson, P., Bearman, M., et al. (2017b). How technology shapes assessment design: Findings from a study of university teachers. *British Journal of Educational Technology, 48*(2), 672–682. doi:10.1111/bjet.12439.

Berliner, D. C. (2002). Comment: Educational research: The hardest science of all. *Educational Researcher, 31*(8), 18–20.

Biesta, G. (2015). What is education for? On good education, teacher judgement, and educational professionalism. *European Journal of Education, 50*(1), 75–87. doi:10.1111/ejed.12109.

Bligh, J., & Parsell, G. (1999). Research in medical education: Finding its place. *Medical Education, 33*(3), 162–163.

Botwe, B. O., Arthur, L., Tenkorang, M. K. K., et al. (2017). Dichotomy between theory and practice in chest radiography and its impact on students. *Journal of Medical Radiation Sciences, 64*(2), 146–151. doi:10.1002/jmrs.179.

Bransford, J. D., Brown, A. L., & Cocking, R. R. (2000). *How people learn*. Washington, DC: National Academies Press.

Bruer, J. T. (1997). Education and the brain: A bridge too far. *Educational Researcher, 26*(8), 4–16.

Budhathoki, S. S., Zwanikken, P. A. C., Pokharel, P. K., et al. (2017). Factors influencing medical students' motivation to practise in rural areas in low-income and middle-income countries: A systematic review. *BMJ Open, 7*(2), 013501. doi:10.1136/bmjopen-2016-013501.

Burgess, A., McGregor, D., & Mellis, C. (2014). Medical students as peer tutors: A systematic review. *BMC Medical Education, 14*(1), 115.

Cross, N. (2011). *Design thinking: Understanding how designers think and work*. New York: Berg.

Cuevas, J. (2015). Is learning styles-based instruction effective? A comprehensive analysis of recent research on learning styles. *Theory and Research in Education, 13*(3), 308–333.

Dauphinee, W. D., & Wood-Dauphinee, S. (2004). The need for evidence in medical education: The development of best evidence medical education as an opportunity to inform, guide, and sustain medical education research. *Academic Medicine, 79*(10), 925–930.

Davis, M. H., Karunathilake, I., & Harden, R. M. (2005). The development and role of departments of medical education. AMEE Guide No. 28. *Medical Teacher, 27*(8), 665–675. doi:10.1080/01421590500398788.

Delany, C., & Bailocerkowski, A. (2011). Incorporating evidence in clinical education; barriers and opportunities in allied health. *Internet Journal of Allied Health Sciences and Practice, 9*(1), 7.

Elliott, K., & Lodge, J. M. (2017). Engaging staff in design thinking: Harnessing contemporary educational technologies. In R. James, S. French, & P. Kelly (Eds.), *Visions for the future of Australian tertiary education* (pp. 55–66). Melbourne: Melbourne Centre for the Study of Higher Education.

Elshaug, A. (2015). Choosing treatments wisely. *The Lamp: Magazine of the NSW Nurses and Midwives' Association*, 26–27.

Farrell, L., Bourgeois-Law, G., Ajjawi, R., et al. (2017). An autoethnographic exploration of the use of goal oriented feedback to enhance brief clinical teaching encounters. *Advances in Health Sciences Education, 22*(1), 91–104. doi:10.1007/s10459-016-9686-5.

Faux, D. (2000). Information overload. *Medical Teacher, 22*(1), 5–6. doi:10.1080/01421590078724.

Goodyear, P. (2005). Educational design and networked learning: Patterns, pattern languages and design practice. *Australasian Journal of Educational Technology, 21*(1), 82–101.

Goodyear, P. (2015). Teaching as design. *HERDSA Review of Higher Education, 2*, 27–50. www.herdsa.org.au/herdsa-review-higher-education-vol-2/27-50.

Goodyear, P., & Zenios, M. (2007). Discussion, collaborative knowledge work and epistemic fluency. *British Journal of Educational Studies, 55*(4), 351–368. doi:10.1111/j.1467-8527.2007.00383.x.

Graham, I. D., Logan, J., Harrison, M. B., et al. (2006). Lost in knowledge translation: Time for a map? *Journal of Continuing Education in the Health Professions, 26*(1), 13–24. doi:10.1002/chp.47.

Gravel, K., Légaré, F., & Graham, I. D. (2006). Barriers and facilitators to implementing shared decision-making in clinical practice: A systematic review of health professionals' perceptions. *Implementation Science, 1*(1), 16. doi:10.1186/1748-5908-1-16.

Hager, P., & Hodkinson, P. (2009). Moving beyond the metaphor of transfer of learning. *British Educational Research Journal, 35*(4), 619–638.

Harden, R. M., Grant, J., Buckley, G., et al. (2000). Best evidence medical education. *Advances in Health Sciences Education, 5*(1), 71–90. doi:10.1023/A:1009896431203.

Hart, I. R., & Harden, R. M. (2000). Best evidence medical education (BEME): A plan for action. *Medical Teacher, 22*(2), 131–135. doi:10.1080/01421590078535.

Hawick, L., Cleland, J., & Kitto, S. (2017). Getting off the carousel: Exploring the wicked problem of curriculum reform. *Perspectives on Medical Education, 6*(5), 337–343. doi:10.1007/s40037-017-0371-z.

Haynes, R. B., Devereaux, P. J., & Guyatt, G. H. (2002). Physicians' and patients' choices in evidence based practice. Evidence does not make decisions, people do. *BMJ (Clinical Research Ed.), 324*(7350), 1350. doi:10.1136/bmj.324.7350.1350.

Hodges, B. D. (2018). Learning from Dorothy Vaughan: Artificial intelligence and the health professions. *Medical Education, 52*(1), 11–13. doi:10.1111/medu.13350.

Hoffmann, T., Légaré, F., Simmons, M. B., et al. (2014). Shared decision making: What do clinicians need to know and why should they bother? *Medical Journal of Australia, 201*(1), 35–39.

Howard-Jones, P. A. (2015). Neuroscience and education: Myths and messages. *Nature Reviews. Neuroscience, 15*, 817–824. doi:10.1038/nrn3817.

Jorm, C., & Roberts, C. (2018). Using complexity theory to guide medical school evaluations. *Academic Medicine 93*(3), 399–405, doi:10.1097/acm.0000000000001828.

Kassirer, J. P. (2010). Teaching clinical reasoning: case-based and coached. *Academic Medicine, 85*(7), 1118–1124. doi:10.1097/ACM.0b013e3181d5dd0d.

Laurillard, D. (2013). *Teaching as a design science: Building pedagogical patterns for learning and technology*. New York: Routledge.

Légaré, F., Ratté, S., Gravel, K., et al. (2008). Barriers and facilitators to implementing shared decision-making in clinical practice: Update of a systematic review of health professionals' perceptions. *Patient Education and Counseling, 73*(3), 526–535, doi. http://dx.doi.org/10.1016/j.pec.2008.07.018.

Lodge, J. M. (2016). Do the learning sciences have a place in higher education research? *Higher Education Research and Development, 35*(3), 634–637, http://dx.doi.org/10.1080/07294360.2015.1094204.

Lodge, J. M., Hansen, L., & Cottrell, D. (2016). Modality preference and learning style theories: Rethinking the role of sensory modality in learning. *Learning: Research and Practice, 2*(1), 4–17.

Lodge, J. M., & Horvath, J. C. (2017). Science of learning and digital learning environments. In J. C. Horvath, J. M. Lodge, & J. A. C. Hattie (Eds.), *From the laboratory to the classroom: Translating learning sciences for teachers* (pp. 122–136). Abingdon: Routledge.

McGaghie, W. C. (2010). Medical education research as translational science. *Science Translational Medicine, 2*(19), 19 cm18. doi:10.1126/scitranslmed.3000679.

Markauskaite, L., & Goodyear, P. (2017). *Introduction. Epistemic fluency and professional education: Innovation, knowledgeable action and actionable knowledge* (pp. 1–18). Dordrecht: Springer Netherlands.

Mayer, R. E. (2009). *Multimedia learning*. New York, NY: Cambridge University Press.

Mishra, P., & Koehler, M. J. (2006). Technological pedagogical content knowledge: A framework for teacher knowledge. *Teachers College Record, 108*(6), 1017–1054.

Molesworth, M., & Lewitt, M. (2016). Preregistration nursing students' perspectives on the learning, teaching and application of bioscience knowledge within practice. *Journal of Clinical Nursing, 25*(5–6), 725–732. doi:10.1111/jocn.13020.

Molloy, E. K. (2009). Time to pause: Feedback in clinical education. In C. Delaney & E. K. Molloy (Eds.), *Clinical education in the health professions* (pp. 126–146). Sydney: Elsevier.

Mouasher, A., & Lodge, J. M. (2016). The search for pedagogical dynamism: Design patterns and the unselfconscious process. *Educational Technology & Society, 19*(2), 274–285. http://www.ifets.info/journals/19_2/20.pdf.

Müller-Engelmann, M., Donner-Banzhoff, N., Keller, H., et al. (2013). When decisions should be shared. *Medical Decision Making, 33*(1), 37–47. doi:10.1177/0272989X12458159.

Norman, G. (2005). Research in clinical reasoning: Past history and current trends. *Medical Education, 39*(4), 418–427. doi:10.1111/j.1365-2929.2005.02127.x.

Norman, G. (2009). When will learning style go out of style? *Advances in Health Sciences Education, 14*(1), 1–4. doi:10.1007/s10459-009-9155-5.

Sackett, D. L., Rosenberg, W. M. C., Gray, J. A. M., et al. (1996). Evidence based medicine: what it is and what it isn't. *BMJ (Clinical Research Ed.), 312*(7023), 71–72. doi:10.1136/bmj.312.7023.71.

Sethi, A., Ajjawi, R., McAleer, S., et al. (2017). Exploring the tensions of being and becoming a medical educator. *BMC Medical Education, 17*(1), 62. doi:10.1186/s12909-017-0894-3.

Sholl, S., Ajjawi, R., Allbutt, H., et al. (2017). Balancing health care education and patient care in the UK workplace: A realist synthesis. *Medical Education, 51*(8), 787–801. doi:10.1111/medu.13290.

Stiggelbout, A. M., van der Weijden, T., de Wit, M. P. T., et al. (2012). Shared decision making: Really putting patients at the centre of healthcare. *BMJ (Clinical Research Ed.), 344*, e256. doi:10.1136/bmj.e256.

Tai, J. H.-M., Canny, B. J., Haines, T. P., et al. (2016). The role of peer-assisted learning in building evaluative judgement: Opportunities in clinical medical education. *Advances in Health Sciences Education, 21*(3), 659–676. doi:10.1007/s10459-015-9659-0.

Telio, S., Regehr, G., & Ajjawi, R. (2016). Feedback and the educational alliance: Examining credibility judgements and their consequences. *Medical Education, 50*(9), 933–942. doi:10.1111/medu.13063.

Thomas, A., & Steinert, Y. (2014). Knowledge translation and faculty development: From theory to practice. In Y. Steinert (Ed.), *Faculty development in the health professions: A focus on research and practice* (pp. 399–418). Dordrecht: Springer Netherlands.

Tolsgaard, M. G., Kulasegaram, K. M., & Ringsted, C. (2017). Practical trials in medical education: Linking theory, practice and decision making. *Medical Education, 51*(1), 22–30. doi:10.1111/medu.13135.

Urquhart, L. M., Ker, J. S., & Rees, C. E. (2017). Exploring the influence of context on feedback at medical school: A video-ethnography study. *Advances in Health Sciences Education, 23*(1), 159–186. doi:10.1007/s10459-017-9781-2.

van der Vleuten, C. P. M. (1995). Evidence-based education? *Advances in Physiology Education, 269*(6), S3.

van der Vleuten, C. P. M., Dolmans, D. H. J. M., & Scherpbier, A. J. J. A. (2000). The need for evidence in education. *Medical Teacher, 22*(3), 246–250. doi:10.1080/01421590050006205.

van der Vleuten, C. P. M., Schuwirth, L. W. T., Driessen, E. W., et al. (2015). Twelve tips for programmatic assessment. *Medical Teacher, 37*(7), 641–646. doi:10.3109/0142159X.2014.973388.

Venema, S., Drew, S., & Lodge, J. M. (2015). Peer observation as a collaborative vehicle for innovation in incorporating educational technology into teaching: A case study. In C. Klopper & S. Drew (Eds.), *Teaching for learning and learning for teaching: Cases in context of peer review of teaching in Higher Education* (pp. 209–226). Rotterdam: Sense Publishers.

Venema, S., & Lodge, J. M. (2013). Capturing dynamic presentation: Using technology to enhance the chalk and the talk. *Australasian Journal of Educational Technology, 29*(1), 20–31. http://dx.doi.org/10.14742/ajet 62

Ward, V., House, A., & Hamer, S. (2009). Knowledge brokering: The missing link in the evidence to action chain? *Evidence and Policy: A Journal of Research, Debate and Practice, 5*(3), 267–279. doi:10.1332/174426409X463811.

Wolpaw, T., Côté, L., Papp, K. K., et al. (2012). Student uncertainties drive teaching during case presentations: More so with SNAPPS. *Academic Medicine, 87*(9), 1210–1217.

26

Improving clinical education
Attending to the processes of designing and becoming

Elizabeth Molloy and Clare Delany

Introduction

In this final chapter, we discuss how this book challenges traditional approaches to clinical education based on apprenticeship. Throughout the book, the contributors have demonstrated how theoretical framings can be used to underpin educational strategies and have provided illustrative examples in the form of case studies to help bring to life the propositions for doing things better. It is this blend of the practical, theoretical and illustrative that sets this book apart from other texts on clinical education. We propose that the use of theory and the privileging of context through illustrative case studies may serve as a productive formula for professional development of clinical educators.

In editing this book, two key concepts became apparent to us, and we have framed them as questions. The first is: 'What is the role of design in facilitating learning in unpredictable work settings?' This theme relates to the merits of educators using design principles in their approach to teaching, and provides an alternative to the often-reactive way that clinical educators operate because of the complex, demanding and unpredictable nature of healthcare practice.

We argue that clinical educators need to become better designers of experiences in the workplace so that learners can make the most of the educational value within these opportunities. We further elaborate on what it means to 'design', drawing on principles from the industrial design community and 'design thinking' in higher education, to help provoke insights into the thoughtful crafting of activities with consideration of context. We also attempt to address anticipated scepticism that it is impossible to design, a priori, experiences in the workplace when there is little assurance on 'who walks in, or is wheeled in, the door', let alone the regulatory, environmental, cultural and individual variables that intersect to produce the complex process of learning through work.

The second prominent concept is the importance of focusing on clinical educator identity development: 'How can we better understand and facilitate the process of "becoming" a clinical educator?' The contributors, in exploring different aspects of clinical education, have charted the complex and often idiosyncratic pathway of 'becoming' both for students aspiring to be clinicians and for clinicians aspiring to be better educators. Many of the chapters highlight that clinical educator development should draw from the same educational principles that frame student learning and professional growth. The identity shifts involved for both learners and educators in their ongoing trajectory towards 'becoming' require an openness to new experiences, insight and reflection to learn from mistakes and a willingness to co-construct knowledge with others (whether it be patients, peers or supervisors).

Clinical educators may feel an added layer of discomfort in their transition when they are moving from high levels of expertise in the clinical domain, and yet at times exhibit novice educational capacities (despite the not insignificant crossover in skill sets). What people think it means to be an educator shifts with increasing experience. Reading the illustrative case studies throughout the book, there is a strong sense that 'becoming an educator' involves less instructing and more designing of conditions and activities that support the learner's trajectory towards clinical expertise. This means that we need faculty-development (or capacity-building) activities that support clinical educators in developing broader-based educational capabilities to: establish safe learning environments; set up connected tasks that adequately stretch the learner; and provide cues for learners to self-evaluate and regulate.

Throughout this chapter, we highlight design considerations for clinical educators who have responsibilities for facilitating students' learning in work-based settings, along with considerations for leaders who develop professional development programs for health professional educators.

The role of design in clinical education

Education as design work is not a simple undertaking. There are certain features in clinical education that make it difficult to translate educational principles into practice. For example, the tension between attending to learning and attending to patient care is a hallmark of workplace learning and is well described by contributors to this book, along with the wider literature (Frenk et al., 2010; Watling et al., 2016; Damodaran, 2017). Most leaders in the health professions education community acknowledge that this tension is not one that is likely to be resolved anytime soon. The contributors to this book, however, through reference to their own empirical studies and critiques of the literature, are optimistic that learners, particularly with adequate priming and feedback, can squeeze more educational value from work-based experiences. Despite the need to privilege service demands over student learning priorities, the embedded nature of learning through work holds many advantages over classroom-based learning. Through their orientation to the patient, and therefore orientation to feeling fundamentally useful, learners can also leverage off intrinsic motivation and can watch for the impact. This ability to see firsthand the impact of 'performance' on others, and on a system, is a unique characteristic of learning through work.

However, a premise of this book is that clinical educators have a rather formidable task in facilitating learners' professional trajectories, tapping into learners' intrinsic motivation to become professionals, while also managing their own professional learning. The contributors describe the experience of both learners and educators in attempting new tasks in high-stakes environments and making leaps from student to clinician, and from clinician to clinical educator, respectively. These transitions in identities occurring within complex and dynamic environments resonate with a disorienting world described by German industrial designer, Dieter Rams (Kemp & Ueki-Polet, 2010). Concerned by the state of the world around him, 'an impenetrable confusion of forms, colours and noises' (http://en.wikipedia.org/wiki/Dieter_Rams), Dieter Rams developed 10 fundamental design principles to cut through this confusion. His central idea was that form should follow function (Rodgers & Bremner, 2011). The need for careful and purposeful design of educational experiences with consideration of the complexity of the environment and goals of learning is a central tenet in nearly all the case studies in the book, picked up most explicitly by Ajjawi, Lodge and Roberts in Chapter 25 with their discussion on design thinking, and by Reedy and Jones in Chapter 22 with their discussion of how clinicians/teachers can reframe their professional role from 'custodians of knowledge' to 'facilitators of learning'.

The illustrative case studies vividly portray the confusion of noises and tasks for the clinical educator, including: balancing their own roles as lifelong learner, educator and clinician; managing expectations of patients, students, colleagues, regulators and administrators; developing and assessing learner competencies;

> **Box 26.1:** Design principles tailored to the clinical education setting
>
> Good educational design should strive to be:
>
> 1. **innovative** — educational design *develops in tandem* with innovative technology and is therefore not an end in and of itself (e.g. simulation is an example of using technology to achieve specific educational goals)
> 2. **useful** — *not only functional*, but also meeting the emotional needs of the learner as a developing professional capable of meeting the needs of patients
> 3. **aesthetic** — where the *quality* or *tenor* of the educational experience is elegant, considered and temporal (including set, middle and closure)
> 4. **understandable** — so that learners can see the *relevance and utility* of their tasks or experiences in the clinical setting
> 5. **unobtrusive** — that is, both neutral and restrained, to leave room for *learners' self-expression and autonomy*
> 6. **honest** — and not attempt to make a product or an activity seem more innovative, powerful or valuable than it really is; it should strive *not to manipulate* the learner with promises that cannot be kept (e.g. certain technology may help you to manage patient data in the hospital, but won't do the thinking for you)
> 7. **long-lasting** — *avoid being fashionable* or part of a teaching fad where the new ideas seem so seductive that they are not challenged or tested
> 8. **thorough down to the last detail** — reduce the elements that are *arbitrary or left to chance* as care in the design process shows respect towards patients, students and clinicians
> 9. **environmentally friendly** — learners and clinical educators make a *positive contribution* to the healthcare system
> 10. **as little design as possible** — where it is not so much 'less is more' as 'less, but better' because of a focus on the *essentials of the learning encounters*. 'Over design' can create too many inputs and can constrain learner volition and engagement.

Source: Adapted from the 10 principles of design by Dieter Rams (Kemp & Ueki-Polet, 2010).

and recognising and being ready to exploit learning moments within clinical practice. Each contributor examines the confusion head-on using three threads of 1) educational theory, 2) practical teaching strategies and 3) illustrative cases.

The use of educational theory can provide clinical educators with a platform from which they can more flexibly respond to the specific needs of learners and the particular affordances of a given context. It frees them to become designers of education. A fundamental principle of design thinking is that the *form* of an object (teaching encounter) should be led by its particular intended functional outcome (student learning). Applied to education practice, this design principle highlights the need to think about the learning needs of the student and work backwards to shape aspects of the teaching encounter. Such design thinking may help address the warning from Bearman, Castanelli and Denniston in Chapter 17, that 'if you notice yourself saying or doing the same thing over and over again, it might be time to think differently'. In Box 26.1 we take Deiter Rams' industrial design principles and apply them to the clinical education setting as examples of the thinking required to optimise student learning.

These 10 principles may act as useful reflective prompts when considering educational design in clinical education. Sharing some of these properties articulated by Rams, 'design thinking' is increasingly being studied within the context of higher education (Elliott & Lodge, 2017; Laurillard, 2013). Many contributors in this book engage both implicitly and explicitly with this design focus. An example of the latter is Chapter 25, where Ajjawi, Lodge and Roberts mount an argument for how this way of thinking encourages educators to redistribute their energies and invest in a problem-solving process, where they consider and dismantle elements such as context, values and purpose, and reconfigure these to form a learning and teaching solution. Principle 1 promotes innovation as a process that is led by the needs of the user/consumer, rather than motivated by a perceived need to innovate per se. Holmboe expands on this eloquently in Chapter 24, describing the hallmarks of diffusion and complexity along with disruptive innovation. He outlines how these principles can be applied to longitudinal clerkships and to workplace-based assessment with an outcomes-led agenda.

Thoughtful educational design performs a double duty. Not only does it promote learner engagement in the task itself, but it can also build, as stated by principle 5, self-regulatory and critical thinking capacities in the learner, needed for future work. For example, a learner who sets their own topic for a research project or quality improvement initiative in the workplace, and commits to regular feedback cycles during the completion of this project, is more likely to produce better work in the short term, as well as develop capabilities in making judgments about what constitutes a quality research project. In Chapter 19 Ajjawi and Boud provide good illustrative examples of how sustainable assessment performs this double duty. Similarly, in Chapter 11 Delany and Beckett suggest that educators need to find a balance between 'throwing the learner in the deep end', relying completely on survival as a form of learning, and a 'shallow end' approach where each progression in learning is sequential and supported. They argue for less focus on the role of the educator in providing information about professional ideals, and instead suggest that the educator's role is one of fostering, in students, sensitivity to the worldview of others and a commitment to establishing shared or common understandings about the meaning of health. In Chapter 12, Tai, Sevenhuysen and Dawson reinforce that a capable clinical educator, through activating peer learning opportunities, will be able to design themselves out of the picture (metaphor only) for the benefit of the learner.

These discussions point strongly to the role of the educator as a designer and creator of conditions that function to encourage students to learn through work. Based on these ideas, a 'design' approach to clinical education should focus on outcomes of helping learners to be aware of their own needs and responses to others, and to recognise the value of their patients and peers as sources of knowledge and insight. The key goal is to produce practitioners who can work interdependently, not independently. Therefore, educational goals focus on helping to develop a practitioner who is self-regulating through seeking internal cues and external cues from the environment, to form judgments about the quality of their work.

Design thinking can also be applied to temporal phases in workplace learning. A recurring theme within this book is the richness of the *before*, *during* and *after* in the workplace, reflective of principle 8. This temporally oriented lens broadens our attention to spaces either side of the task itself. Billett (2016) describes this useful framework of before, during and after in his research on workplace learning in the healthcare setting. In Chapter 15 Billett, Noble and Sweet discuss how learners can be oriented to the 'invitational qualities' of handovers, ward rounds and team meetings, and how debriefing after these events can also enhance knowledge development. The simulation community is well versed in the merits of before, during and after, and has purposefully manipulated, or designed, these qualities into simulation-based programs as described in Chapter 13 by Nestel and Gough. In Chapter 21, Molloy and van de Ridder describe the model of Feedback Mark 2, where learners ask supervisors not only to observe them in practice, but also to watch for certain aspects of performance they are concerned about. For example, 'Can you focus on my anastomosis? This is what I struggled with most last time' or 'Can you listen for how I respond to the patient's concerns while I'm conducting the interview? I'm concerned that I'm too brash when I move onto the next topic.' Designing in a priming phase for both learners and teachers, before task engagement, helps to generate feedback conversations that are meaningful for the learner, and more likely to be acted on (Boud & Molloy, 2013).

Helping educators and learners to better capitalise on the role of priming and debriefing in workplace learning (the work either side of the work) may be an important focus for curriculum designers. Chapters in the first section of this book particularly pay tribute to these preparatory initiatives to develop 'workplace learning ready' students as distinct from 'work ready' students.

Designing approaches to research in workplace learning and teaching

Scholarship in health professions education continues to grow, and increasingly journals are requiring researchers to explicate the theoretical tradition in which their work is situated, and how theory is used in their work (Nestel & Bearman, 2015). Clinical educators have reported that theory can be difficult to access, and we see this is partly because it takes time to immerse yourself in different grand, middle and micro theories, and partly because health professions education researchers have not paid enough attention to explaining how theory has been used to sensitise their understanding, or illuminate certain qualities in their data. Principle 7 provides some guidance in this area. It highlights the importance of good design being 'long-lasting' (for education, grounded in established and relevant theory) rather than being 'fashionable' or part of a 'teaching fad'. Researchers and faculty developers may need to be more transparent about how theory can be used to ground and contribute to the sustainability of their research and practice.

Many of the chapter contributors chose to declare their allegiance to constructivism or social constructionism, and in particular, we see many examples of how sociocultural learning theories help researchers to better understand and design socially embedded processes of learning and teaching in the workplace. Nearly all of the contributors call for more longitudinal study designs so that we can attend to the effects of educational approaches on learners over time (longitudinal audio-diaries being one such approach to monitor processes of becoming). They also argue for more observation-based studies to complement stakeholder self-report on particular educational activities or phenomena.

In summary, design thinking is conscious, solution-oriented, accounts for context and, necessarily so in the clinical environment, accounts for changing variables and relationships between these variables. There is an emphasis on looking for effects (does the product achieve the job it was set out to do?) and a refinement in design until the consumers and designers are happy with the process and outputs. Principle 10 is 'less, but better'. This sentiment is reinforced in many chapters, with practical strategies calling for clinical educators to work smarter, not harder. Discussions within Section 3 about assessment and feedback literacy also focus on the role of educators to assist students to prepare to learn in the workplace, but not as an isolated activity slotted into the academic calendar. Instead both assessment and feedback need to be integrated or 'designed' into curricula, with tasks that progressively extend students and expand their understanding and awareness of their own professional identity as they gain more knowledge and skills relating to what it means to be a learner and a clinician.

Identity: a focus on 'becoming'

Intersecting with the concept of educators as designers of learning experiences, a key message throughout the book is that developing expertise as a clinical educator requires time on the job as well as wrestling with underpinning educational theory. Expertise applied to all types of professional practice is not a state or status that is passively achieved but is a dynamic and ongoing process of professional development (Jensen & Delany, 2016; Billett, 2015; Billett, 2016). It requires commitment and motivation to continue learning, improving and creating.

In other professional domains, experts have been shown to build extensive and well-organised practical knowledge through the use of self-monitoring or meta-cognitive skills (Ericsson et al., 2006). In health professional clinical practice, such reflective skills manifest in skills of careful listening and observation so as to integrate the lived experience of the patient with foundational and more formal professional knowledge (Benner, 2000; Edwards et al., 2004; Hager & Hodkinson, 2013; Jensen & Delany, 2016). We suggest that a similar integration of educational theory and teaching experience on the ground is required in the process of becoming a clinical educator. Having a static repertoire of teaching strategies may not be enough to develop as a teacher in the face of challenges and change in clinical work places. In Chapter 17 Bearman, Castanelli and Denniston highlight the need for constant preparation and the feeling of vulnerability for clinical educators (and students) if insufficient attention is given to a 'Plan B'. Each student and each clinical situation will generate different learning opportunities, and guiding educational principles may enable clinical educators to be nimble in their approaches.

Throughout this book, and particularly in Chapters 7 (workplace context), 8 (professional identities and professionalism), 9 (scaffolding for independence) and 22 (faculty development), contributors attend to the development of professional identities through work, that is 'who one is and who one wants to become' (Monrouxe, 2016). We read about the learner becoming a clinician and the clinician becoming a clinical educator and the rewards and strains this 'becoming' brings. Competence in any professional area is mediated through sociocultural influences. It is something that evolves and is embodied within a practice community, rather than a set of knowledge, skills and attitudes owned by the individual. This view of expertise as a dynamic, context-dependent construct means that, in essence, there is no end point to 'becoming'.

Another consideration when viewing expertise from this sociocultural frame is that learners, through their participation in workplaces, help to change the set of practices that make up the workplace. This is one of the reasons why academic medical centres or university-based hospitals are valued commodities (Frenk et al., 2010).

Many contributors mount arguments consistent with the discourse in the wider literature about becoming a clinical educator or healthcare professional, and this discourse is a direct counter to a culture of 'arrival'. There are of course formal transition points recognised within health professions education. Finishing medical school, starting postgraduate training, achieving specialisation or being awarded a PhD are all milestones that afford capital and capacity to perform different tasks compared with earlier career stages. Learners who are striving towards formal gates (such as graduation) have typically invested enormously in time, money and self (identities). The quest for proving oneself and 'making the cut' can render learners vulnerable. For those learners who are underperforming, it can be a steep ask to expect them to take risks in choosing tasks that will stretch them, to hunt down supervisors and request direct observation and feedback, to self-evaluate and expose their deficits to their supervisor (among a sea of already exposed deficits). So, while research can illustrate the benefits of learners articulating their own evaluative judgments (Bearman & Molloy, 2017; Tai et al., 2015), throughout this book the contributors acknowledge that this intellectual risk-taking is often easier for those who are already accepted as experts, secure in their identities. As argued by Bates, Ellaway and Watling (Chapter 7), Bearman, Castanelli and Denniston (Chapter 17), and Molloy and van de Ridder (Chapter 21), reciprocal vulnerability between educator and learner is one way to establish richer environments for learning in the workplace.

In Chapter 8, Shaw, Crampton, Rees and Monrouxe describe the process of becoming a clinician and outline how the theories of professionalism, embodiment and identity can shed light on the shifting identities of the learner. Generating safe environments for storytelling, reflective practice and expression of vulnerability/struggles is also described by Delany, McDougall, Gillam and Johnston in Chapter 5 (ethics education), with accompanying examples of ways to cultivate a culture for learning and becoming.

These same notions and practical strategies could also be applied to the clinical educator in their move towards expertise within a new practice community (that of health professions education). As many clinicians report, the tea room serves as an important informal space for this type of work. Skilled facilitation of discussion within education-based coursework and the use of simulation-based education with debriefing can also create rich learning opportunities for clinical educators who are becoming more serious about education (Steinert et al., 2016). As we stated in Chapter 1, the majority of clinicians do not set out to be a clinical educator. For many, the role is set upon them as part of clinical work (Dory et al., 2015). Some take on teaching roles with reticence (e.g. 'I was the last to duck') and discover that they want to be career clinician educators. Others continue to take on a small educational role, and improve through experience and trial and error. The nature of the pathway, including the speed of trajectory, in the development of educational expertise is largely influenced by clinicians' own interests and strengths or by the opportunities or constraints within their own workplace. This includes the richness of the 'educational culture' in the department or wider health service (Frenk et al. 2010).

In designing and becoming, context is everything

Learning cannot be separated from context (Bates & Ellaway, 2016). Many of the chapters describe the changing landscape of healthcare and the subsequent impact on educating practitioners equipped to meet the changing needs of the community. For example, changes such as increasing chronic disease, team-based care, trends towards development of specialised care centres (e.g. focused centres devoted to multidisciplinary cancer treatment), increasingly empowered patients/consumers with higher health literacy on account of the accessibility of knowledge, and the shift from hospital-based to community-based care, all influence the type of clinician we would like to shape.

The chapter contributors also describe the changing expectations of higher education with increasing student numbers, a preference for online learning, and fragmentation of educational experiences with content experts recruited to teach one-off sessions. There are also regulatory changes in universities that can afford and constrain educational activities. The results of these initiatives designed to improve educational practice are not always favourable. For example, for some institutions, rules around turnaround time for marking and maximum number of assignments per unit, designed to help the learner, have produced unintended negative consequences. Educators have become pushed into 'timely feedback' but are failing to set up connected tasks that allow learners to translate the feedback information into the next task (Boud & Molloy, 2013). It could be that, in some instances, these system-level changes designed to improve feedback may have resulted in poorer learning outcomes.

The contributors in this book argue that assessment practices have a large bearing on learning in the workplace. We are seeing more examples of assessment oriented to learner and peer self-assessment (Tai et al., 2015), a larger emphasis on learner goal-setting (rather than prescription of learning outcomes) and programmatic assessment approaches where the learner has more responsibility for gathering 'data' to build a picture of their learning and performance over time (Boud & Molloy, 2013). The contributors in Section 3 (workplace assessment) argue for careful assessment design that accounts for multiple 'functions' of assessment, including for certification and for learning. One of the outcomes of assessment should be helping learners to develop as independent practitioners with capacities to recognise good work (standards) and to understand how their own work relates to such benchmarks. The properties of the local assessment system (context), along with the assessment literacy of learners and clinical educators, will influence the type of activities learners engage in, and the results of this engagement.

Supporting 'becoming' through clinical educator capacity-building

Given the framing of learning as a situated practice, and the increased focus on the need for learner investment in their own goal-setting in the literature, why do faculty development workshops for clinical educators often continue to focus on how educators can 'teach or tell'? There needs to be more emphasis on thinking about what learning means, the processes of problem-solving through design, and how to set expectations for dialogic exchanges about performance (Bearman et al., 2018).

As Reedy and Jones state in Chapter 22: 'What faculty development does, when done well, is it problematises education. Rather than teaching being a "commonsense" activity that can be done by anyone who knows their own discipline, faculty development encourages us to think critically about education and to question the decisions (tacit as well as overt) that are made. And it encourages us to find a thoughtful, well-grounded rationale for the decisions that we make.'

There are considerable problems with quick tricks, or 'three-step models' that frequently feature in professional development initiatives for clinical educators. On the one hand, clinicians may argue that some frameworks are better than none. But in fact, the frameworks, if they are not built on theoretically sound foundations, may cause more damage to educational practice than clinicians relying on their gut instinct (Molloy & Boud, 2013). For this reason, in thinking about the 'design' of this book, we wanted to ensure that practical strategies or tips were well grounded in educational principles or theory.

The contributors in this book suggest that faculty development for the clinical educator should help to expose the unique properties of learning in the healthcare system. There is a strong argument throughout the book for more consideration of the patient's voice in clinical education. The high-stakes nature of healthcare practice is recognised, and contributors pay tribute to the potentially dire consequences of making errors for novice and experienced practitioners alike. The context of caring for others renders both learners and expert practitioners vulnerable. For learners, this set of stressors can be further amplified given the competitive nature of postgraduate training/specialisation where excellence is demanded, and discussions of failure or fallibility are hidden (or not valued) within the practice culture. Part of the agenda in faculty development might be to remind clinical educators of the elements of the training culture they are embedded within (and therefore may not see).

Part of the 'role burden' described by clinical educators may be tied with the expectation that they are responsible for 'providing' the answers, 'crafting' the feedback and 'picking' the right tasks that will challenge the learner, based on the learner's current demonstrated capacity. We have summarised contributors' suggestions for faculty development for the clinical educator in Box 26.2. In keeping with the practical strategies identified throughout this book, Box 26.2 describes methods that incorporate the design thinking necessary to build the identities and expertise of clinical educators. We suggest that this shift in focus may not only improve learning outcomes in the workplace, but may also reduce some of the pressure described by educators 'to carry the learners over the line' (Bearman et al., 2012).

In this book, we wanted to acknowledge the importance of context and provide examples of how educational strategies might be incorporated into the 'swampy lowlands' of clinical practice. We gave little instruction to contributors to prompt the writing of the case studies, other than a request to provide an illustrative example of how the topic or issue of focus might play out in practice. When we read all the case studies prior to publication, we were struck by the richness in detail, the authentic setting of the scenes and the nuance rather than 'hit you over the head', 'caricature-style problems' in clinical education. Despite lack of formal prompting, most contributors seem to describe a situation, complication, question

---

Box 26.2: Practical considerations for building clinical educator capacity

More emphasis on

- Educational design, including the role of priming and feedback to make the most of the 'doing' in clinical practice
- Task selection in the clinical environment (how to pick the right task to adequately and safely extend the learner)
- Task connection (overlapping competencies) so that learners can put into practice the new strategies
- Direct observation — nothing can replace the power of direct observation (videoing being the one exception)
- Connecting educational theory with practical strategies *and* illustrative case studies
- Problematising context in clinical education, including how the discipline domain, local culture, regulatory requirements and individual and relational factors might promote or constrain learning
- Talk — giving space for clinical educators to discuss their triumphs, struggles, uncertainties and shifting identities between learner, clinician, coach, supervisor, assessor, expert and novice

Less emphasis on

- Three-step models to improve teaching

---

and outcome, described as four pillars in storytelling by Minto (2008). While we recognise we have aspiring and published novelists within our group of contributors, most are not trained in this storytelling and yet do it very well. These four pillar prompts may be helpful for clinical educators or faculty developers new to case writing, and we hope the level of detail showcased may also assist with this development of local cases. Alternatively, faculty developers may draw directly on the cases to trigger discussion in their sessions. The cases may enable educators to more fully appreciate the how and why of their teaching approaches and we anticipate that the interprofessional focus will help orient educators to different and rewarding educational practices.

Conclusion

In this book, the contributors provide a challenge to think differently about learning through work, with the help of theory and evidence. Clinical educators are encouraged to try things on for size and, most importantly, as they do in their clinical practice, to reflect on the effect of the approaches they employ in terms of student learning and patient outcomes. The evaluative judgment capacities they are trying to cultivate in learners aspiring to be clinicians are exactly the capacities that clinical educators need to exercise in an ongoing commitment to quality education in the workplace. The two pathways of 'becoming' have more similarities than differences.

Historically, clinical education has resided in the realm of the reactive. Both learners and clinical educators have been asked to respond nimbly to challenges or stimuli that arise in the busy workplace. The contributors in this book privilege the role of design in workplace education. Clinical educators are asked to be proactive, anticipatory and design-focused in the way they help to build conditions that support and challenge the learner to move towards expertise. Building learner self-regulatory capacity does not lessen the workload of educators. The illustrative case examples and associated empirical evidence suggest that clinical educators still need to work hard to support learners' trajectories, but need to work differently. Preparation of learners for how to look for opportunities and engage in opportunities for developing clinical skills in the workplace is paramount. The more 'workplace learning literate' students are when they arrive in the clinical setting, the more they are likely to gain from the affordances that present.

Professional development of clinical educators has characteristically focused on tips and tricks, with award-bearing courses such as graduate certificate and masters' programs bearing responsibility for providing underpinning educational theory to support educator strategies. This book has demonstrated that articulating theoretical frameworks as a way to sensitise 'the learner' (in this case, the reader) to new ideas or practices, along with providing clear, authentic case examples about how principles can be enacted at the coalface, can be achieved. The compelling argument for strong theoretical foundations in clinical education is that if particular strategies do not work for learners (or teachers), other strategies that align with the same underpinning educational notion can be devised. This gives the clinical educator both security and flexibility — states that are not often described in the discourse of becoming a clinical educator.

Dieter Rams asked himself the question 'Is my design good design?' This simple question sparked a revolution in product design. If clinical educators and educational researchers invest in this sense of curiosity, and commit to looking for the effects of educational approaches beyond the immediate task, we might just see a substantial shift in workplace learning in healthcare.

References

Bates, J., & Ellaway, R. (2016). Mapping the dark matter of context: A conceptual scoping review. *Medical Education*, 50, 807–816.

Bearman, M., & Molloy, E. (2017). Intellectual streaking: The value of teachers exposing minds (and hearts). *Medical Teacher*, 39(12), 1284–1285. doi:10.1080/0142159X.2017.1308475.

Bearman, M., Molloy, E., Ajjawi, R., et al. (2012). 'Is there a plan B?' Clinical educators supporting underperforming students in practice settings. *Teaching in Higher Education*, 1–14. doi:10.1080/13562517.2012.752732.

Bearman, M., Tai, J., Kent, F., et al. (2018). What should we teach the teachers? Identifying the learning priorities of clinical supervisors. *Advances in Health Sciences Education: Theory and Practice*, 23(1), 29–41. doi:10.1007/s10459-017-9772-3.

Benner, P. (2000). Learning through experience and expression: skilful ethical comportment in nursing practice. In D. Thomasma & J. Kissell (Eds.), *The health care professional as friend and healer* (pp. 49–64). Washington, DC: Georgetown University Press.

Billett, S. (2015). Readiness and learning in health care education. *The Clinical Teacher*, 12, 1–6. doi:10.1111/tct.12477.

Billett, S. (2016). Learning through health care work: Premises, contributions and practices. *Medical Education*, 50(1), 124–131.

Boud, D., & Molloy, E. (2013). Rethinking models of feedback for learning: The challenge of design. *Assessment & Evaluation in Higher Education*, 38(6), 698–712.

Damodaran, A. (2017). Time to say goodbye to learner-centredness? *Medical Education*, 52(1), 7–9.

Dory, V., Audetat, M., & Rees, C. (2015). Beliefs, identities and educational practice: A Q methodology study of general practice supervisors. *Education for Primary Care: An Official Publication of the Association of Course Organisers, National Association of GP Tutors, World Organisation of Family Doctors*, 26, 66–78.

Edwards, I., Jones, M., Carr, J., et al. (2004). Clinical reasoning strategies in physical therapy. *Physical Therapy*, 84(4), 312–335.

Elliott, K., & Lodge, J. M. (2017). Engaging staff in design thinking: harnessing contemporary educational technologies. In R. James, S. French, & P. Kelly (Eds.), *Visions for the future of Australian tertiary education* (pp. 55–66). Melbourne: MCSHE.

Ericsson, K. A., Charness, N., Feltovich, P., et al. (Eds.), (2006). *The Cambridge handbook of expertise and expert performance*. New York: Cambridge University Press.

Frenk, J., et al. (2010). Health professionals for a new century: Transforming education to strengthen health systems in an interdependent world. *Lancet (London, England)*, 376(9756), 1923–1958.

Hager, P., & Hodkinson, P. (2013). Becoming as an appropriate metaphor for understanding professional learning. In L. Scanlon (Ed.), *'Becoming' a professional: an interdisciplinary analysis of professional learning* (pp. 33–56). Dordrecht, Netherlands: Springer.

Jensen, G., & Delany, C. (2016). Ethics and expert practice. In J. Higgs & F. Trede (Eds.), *Professional practice discourse marginalia* (pp. 73–82). Amsterdam: Sense.

Kemp, K., & Ueki-Polet, K. (2010). *Less and more: the design ethos of Dieter Rams*. Berlin: Die Gestalten Verlag.

Laurillard, D. (2013). *Teaching as a design science: building pedagogical patterns for learning and technology*. London: Routledge.

Minto, B. (2008). *The pyramid principle* (3rd ed.). London: Prentice Hall.

Molloy, E., & Boud, D. (2013). Changing conceptions of feedback. In D. Boud & E. Molloy (Eds.), *Feedback in higher and professional education* (pp. 11–33). London: Routledge.

Monrouxe, L. V. (2016). Theoretical insights into the nature and nurture of professional identity. In R. L. Cruess, S. R. Cruess, & Y. Steinert (Eds.), *Teaching medical professionalism* (Vol. 2, pp. 37–53). Cambridge: Cambridge University Press.

Nestel, D., & Bearman, M. (2015). Theory and simulation-based education: Definitions, worldviews and applications. *Clinical Simulation in Nursing*, 11, 349–354.

Rodgers, P., & Bremner, C. (2011). Alterplinarity: 'Alternative disciplinarity' in future art and design research pursuits. *Studies in Material Thinking*, 6, 1–16.

Steinert, Y., Mann, K., Anderson, B., et al. (2016). A systematic review of faculty development initiatives designed to enhance teaching effectiveness: A 10-year update—BEME Guide No. 40. *Medical Teacher*, 38, 769–786. doi:10.1080/0142159X.2016.1181851.

Tai, J., Canny, B., Haines, T., et al. (2015). Building evaluative judgement through peer-assisted learning: Opportunities in clinical medical education. *Advances in Health Sciences Education: Theory and Practice*, 21, 659–676.

Watling, C., LaDonna, K., Lingard, L., et al. (2016). 'Sometimes the work just needs to be done': Socio-cultural influences on direct observation in medical training. *Medical Education*, 50, 1054–1064. doi:10.1111/medu.13062.

Index

Page numbers followed by 'f' indicate figures, 't' indicate tables, and 'b' indicate boxes.